NECK PAIN

Medical Diagnosis
and
Comprehensive Management

NECK PAIN

Medical Diagnosis
and
Comprehensive Management

DAVID G. BORENSTEIN, M.D.
Professor of Medicine
Medical Director
The Spine Center
Associate Director for Education and Research
Division of Rheumatology
The George Washington University Medical Center
Washington, D.C.

SAM W. WIESEL, M.D.
Professor and Chairman
Department of Orthopaedic Surgery
Georgetown University School of Medicine
Washington, D.C.

SCOTT D. BODEN, M.D.
Associate Professor of Orthopaedics
Director, The Emory Spine Center
Emory University School of Medicine
Atlanta, Georgia

W.B. SAUNDERS COMPANY
A Division of Harcourt Brace & Company
Philadelphia   London   Toronto   Montreal   Sydney   Tokyo

W.B. SAUNDERS COMPANY
A Division of Harcourt Brace & Company

The Curtis Center
Independence Square West
Philadelphia, Pennsylvania 19106

Library of Congress Cataloging-in-Publication Data

Borenstein, David G.

Neck pain : medical diagnosis and comprehensive management /
David G. Borenstein, Sam W. Wiesel, Scott D. Boden.—1st ed.

p.   cm.

Includes index.

ISBN 0–7216–5412–6

1. Neck ache.   I. Wiesel, Sam W.   II. Boden, Scott D.
   III. Title.   [DNLM: 1. Neck.   2. Pain—diagnosis.
   3. Pain—therapy.   4. Cervical Vertebrae—physiopathology.
   WE 708 B731n 1996]

RC936.B586 1996   617.5′3—dc20

DNLM/DLC   95–50015

NECK PAIN: Medical Diagnosis and Comprehensive Management   ISBN 0–7216–5412–6

Copyright © 1996 by W.B. Saunders Company.

All rights reserved. No part of this publication may be reproduced or transmitted in any form or by any means, electronic or mechanical, including photocopy, recording, or any information storage and retrieval system, without permission in writing from the publisher.

Printed in the United States of America.

Last digit is the print number: 9   8   7   6   5   4   3   2   1

For my teachers who inspired me to become a rheumatologist. This book is dedicated to Lawrence Shulman, M.D., and in memory of Mary Betty Stevens, M.D.

DAVID G. BORENSTEIN, M.D.

It is with special thanks and appreciation for her outstanding work that I dedicate this book to Sandy Dudley.

SAM W. WIESEL, M.D.

This book is dedicated to the five women in my life, Mary, Stephanie, Allison, Lauren, and Suzanne, for allowing me the time away to contribute to this project.

SCOTT D. BODEN, M.D.

PREFACE

Since the publication of *Low Back Pain: Medical Diagnosis and Comprehensive Management,* readers have asked the authors questions regarding the diagnosis and therapy of cervical spine disorders. After reviewing the available texts, we believed that a companion volume to *Low Back Pain* would be a useful addition to the literature discussing neck pain.

Neck Pain: Medical Diagnosis and Comprehensive Management has a dual purpose. The book is a practical guide to the diagnosis and management of patients with neck pain. The text is also a reference book for the disorders associated with the symptoms of neck pain.

Many disorders affect the entire axial skeleton, including the cervical and lumbar spine. Components of therapy are effective for disorders of the entire axial skeleton. Therefore, this book contains passages, tables, and illustrations that are similar to those in *Low Back Pain.* However, extensive portions of this book cover topics that are not discussed in the other book, including a new algorithm for the diagnosis and management of neck pain.

Clinicians should use *Neck Pain: Medical Diagnosis and Comprehensive Management* as an independent, complete treatise on neck pain. We hope that this volume will be as helpful for neck pain as the other volume is for low back pain.

DAVID G. BORENSTEIN, M.D.
SAM W. WIESEL, M.D.
SCOTT D. BODEN, M.D.

ACKNOWLEDGMENTS

The authors would like to recognize those individuals who supplied support, encouragement, constructive criticism, and expertise.

Members of the George Washington University and Georgetown University medical communities have been essential for the development and completion of this book. They have included the professional and support staff of the Division of Rheumatology; William M. Steinberg, M.D., Professor of Medicine; Joseph M. Giordano, M.D., Professor of Surgery; Werner Barth, M.D., Professor of Medicine; Laligam N. Sekhar, M.D., Professor and Chairman of Neurological Surgery; Robert Irving, Photographer; and Judith Guenther, Medical Illustrationist, all of the George Washington University Medical Center; and Thomas Welsh, Chief Physical Therapist, Georgetown University Hospital.

Individuals at other institutions have also been willing to share their expertise, patient histories, and radiographs when requested, and their kindness is greatly appreciated: Anne Brower, M.D., Professor and Chairperson of Radiology, Eastern Virginia Medical School (Author of *Arthritis in Black and White*); and Alan Borenstein, M.D., Private Neurologist, Florida Medical Center, Ft. Lauderdale, Florida.

We wish to acknowledge the constructive criticism of the editorial and production staff of W.B. Saunders Company.

DAVID G. BORENSTEIN, M.D.
SAM W. WIESEL, M.D.
SCOTT D. BODEN, M.D.

CONTENTS

Section I

ANATOMY AND PHYSIOLOGY OF NECK PAIN

Anatomy and Biomechanics of the Cervical Spine

The structure of the cervical spine is complex. To diagnose and treat this area effectively, one must have a clear knowledge of the normal anatomy. The purpose of this chapter is to present a working description of the anatomy and biomechanics of the cervical spine. This information will provide a keystone from which to build as the various pathologic entities affecting the cervical spine are discussed.

CERVICAL VERTEBRAE

The osseous anatomy of the cervical spine includes seven cervical vertebrae and the occiput (base of the skull). The first two cervical vertebrae, which compose the upper cervical segment, have a unique structure in comparison with other components of the spine. The lower cervical vertebrae (C3–C7) are similar and compose the lower cervical segment. Between each vertebral body below the second vertebra is an intervertebral disc. From cephalad to caudad the size of each subsequent vertebra increases progressively.

The atlas, or first cervical vertebra, possesses no vertebral body (Fig. 1–1). The bone that comprises the body of the atlas is joined to that of the second cervical vertebra, the axis, to form the odontoid process, or dens. The atlas consists of an anterior and posterior arch, joining to form the heavy lateral masses that bear the superior and inferior articular surfaces. The superior facets articulate with the occiput, and the inferior facets with the axis.[1] The axial articular masses are broader and deeper than other masses because they bear

the weight of the skull without any assistance from the odontoid process. Spanning the lateral masses anteriorly is the slender anterior arch, which lies in front of the dens. It has on its internal surface a facet for articulation with the dens, and in the front it has an anterior tubercle for muscular attachments. The posterior arch is longer and bears a small posterior tubercle in place of a spinous process. Each transverse process has a transverse foramen for the vertebral artery. The transverse processes of the atlas are wider than those of other vertebrae. This increased width provides greater leverage and mechanical advantage to the muscles inserted into the transverse process.[2] This transverse process is the only one in the cervical spine that is not grooved to allow exit of a nerve root.[3]

The second cervical vertebra, or axis, is identified by the projection of the odontoid process, or dens, that develops from the embryologic body of the first vertebra (Fig. 1–2). The dens is continuous with the body of the second vertebra. The dens acts as an eccentric point about which the atlas pivots. The posterior surface of the dens has a facet that accommodates the synovial bursa that separates it from the transverse band of the cruciate ligament. The spinous process of the dens is elongated and bifid. The superior articular surfaces are large and face upward, posteriorly, and laterally. They are placed on heavy masses arising from the body and pedicles. The axis does not form a neural foramen for spinal roots.

The third, fourth, fifth, and sixth vertebrae exhibit identical anatomic features (Fig. 1–3). The body of a typical cervical vertebra is elongated transversely so that its width is approxi-

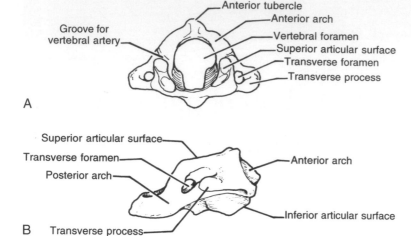

A

Figure 1–1. First cervical vertebra (atlas): *A*, cranial view; *B*, lateral view.

B

mately 50% greater than its anteroposterior dimension. The upper surface is concave from side to side, and this concavity is deepened by an uncinate process, which is a bony protuberance projecting upward from the posterior lateral aspect of the rim of the body. These vertebral projections act as a barrier to the extrusion of disc material posterolaterally, preventing compression of the nerve roots. The upper surface is also concave in the anteroposterior direction. A prominent inferior overhanging lip is noted on the anteroinferior surface of the vertebral body. The inferior and slightly posterolateral aspects of the vertebral body are

beveled and lie in apposition to the uncinate process of the body below, forming the bony components of the joints of Luschka, otherwise known as the uncovertebral joints. Bland has reported data from dissection of 191 cervical spines, stating that the joints of Luschka are not true synovial articulations.[2] This fact proves to be important in the consideration of areas of the cervical spine that may be at risk of being damaged by disorders that cause systemic synovitis, such as rheumatoid arthritis.

The seventh cervical vertebra is the vertebra prominens as its spinous process is usually larger than the process associated with the

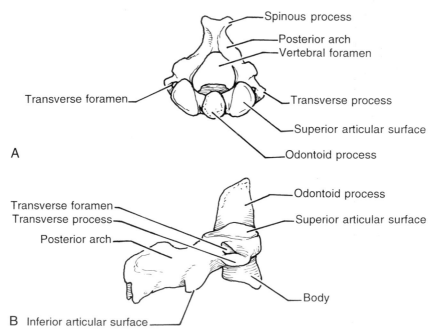

A

B

Figure 1–2. Second cervical vertebra (axis): *A*, cranial view; *B*, lateral view.

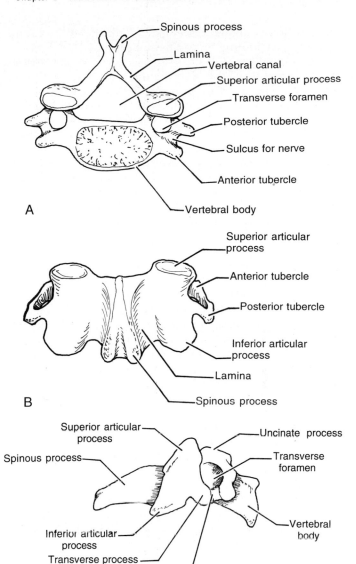

Figure 1–3. Fifth cervical vertebra: A, cranial view; B, dorsal view; C, lateral view.

first thoracic vertebra. The C7 vertebra is the transitional vertebra of the cervicothoracic region. The C7 vertebra has anatomic characteristics that are similar to those of T1. The dimensions of the vertebrae increase with size, whereas the dimensions of the spinal canal decrease at C6 and C7, representing a transition from the cervical to the thoracic spine. The spinous process is large and single. The transverse process of the seventh vertebra does not contain a foramen for the vertebral artery and its accompanying veins and sympathetic nerves.

The pedicles of the lower cervical segment vertebrae are short and bear superior and inferior articular processes that form the zygapophyseal joints. The pedicles have a height of about 7 mm and a width of 6 mm.[4] In the

cervical spine, the facet joints start at the C2–C3 level and range to the C7–T1 level. The articular processes of the superior facets face upward and posteriorly, whereas those of the inferior articular facets face downward and anteriorly at a 45° angle. Their surface area is about two thirds that of the intervertebral disc joints. The facet joints are enclosed in a fibrous capsule that is lax to allow movement in different planes. Synovial tissue lines the joint capsules. The joints contain a fibrofatty, fibrocartilaginous meniscus that separates the hyaline cartilage that covers the articular bone. The curvature of the facets allows for complex movements of these joints on lateral flexion and rotation of the neck, but the joints do not have the architectural stability of the joints of the thoracic or lumbar spine. A total of 37 separate joints allows movement of the head and neck, including 14 zygapophyseal and 12 joints of Luschka.[5]

On either side of the body are the transverse processes. The anterior portion of the transverse process is developmentally a rib, whereas the posterior portion is a true transverse process. These portions fuse, but between them persists the transverse foramen, which allows for passage of the vertebral artery. One exception is the transverse foramen of the seventh vertebra, which does not generally contain the vertebral artery. The transverse processes contain a gutter that runs obliquely from back to front for the spinal nerves. Posteriorly the laminae terminate in a short, slender spinous process that is bifid; however, the large spinous process of the seventh vertebra is not bifid and is called the vertebra prominens.

At each cervical segment nerve roots exit from the spinal canal through the intervertebral foramina. Each foramen is bordered by the pedicles inferiorly and superiorly. The dorsal wall of the neural foramen consists of the facet joint and its capsule. Ventrally, it is defined by the posterolateral corner of the disc, the posterior portion of the uncovertebral joint, and the vertebral artery. The foramina are essentially small canals approximately 4 mm in length, and they exit obliquely in an anterior and inferior direction. They are ovoid in shape, and they have a vertical diameter of approximately 10 mm in height; the anteroposterior diameter is approximately half this. The foramina are largest at the C2–C3 level. They decrease in size progressively to the C6–C7 level. The roots and floors of the foramina fill the grooves in the bases of the adjacent vertebral arches (Fig. 1–4).

All of the cervical spinal nerves, except the first and second, are contained within the intervertebral foramina. In contrast to the nerves in the thoracic and lumbar spine, the nerves in the cervical spine take the name of the pedicle above which they exit. For example, the C5 nerve root exits between the fourth and fifth cervical vertebrae. The exception is the eighth cervical root, which exits between the seventh cervical and first thoracic vertebrae. The nerve roots and mixed spinal nerve completely fill the anteroposterior diameter of the intervertebral foramen. The nerve roots of the cervical spine pass almost directly laterally at each level to exit from the spinal canal at the same foraminal level as their origin from the spinal cord. The horizontal position contrasts with the more vertical orientation of the lumbar nerve roots. The upper quarter of the foramen is filled with areolar tissue and small veins. In addition to these structures, small arteries arising from the vertebral arteries and the sinuvertebral nerves traverse the canals. Any space-occupying lesion that encroaches on the anteroposterior diameter of the intervertebral foramen can be expected to cause compression of the nervous tissue elements traversing this limited space. The close proximity of the contents of the intervertebral foramen to the uncovertebral joints anteromedially and to the apophyseal (facet) joints posterolaterally should be noted because these are potential sites of hyperplastic processes that can constrict the canal. Flexion of the cervical spine increases the vertical diameter of the neural foramen, whereas extension decreases it.

The vertebral canal is triangular with rounded angles. The posterior aspect of the vertebral body is the base of the triangle. The pedicles and the transverse foramina comprise part of the sides of the triangle, along with the zygapophyseal joints, the laminae, and the ligamenta flava. The canal has a funnel shape in the sagittal orientation. The canal is widest at the atlantoaxial level and narrowest at the lamina of C6. The lateral width of the canal is significantly greater than the anteroposterior depth at all levels. Normal sagittal diameters of the cervical spine are 17 to 18 mm at C3 through C6, and 15 mm at C7.[4] The cervical canal is capacious from the level of the atlas to C3. The cervical spinal cord enlargement extends from C3 to T2. The enlargement corresponds to the increase in nerves supplying the limbs. The cervical cord fills a greater portion of the canal in the area of the cervical enlargement. The relationship of the size of the canal and spinal cord differs significantly among individuals. The vertebral canal is narrower in women than in men.[2]

SPINAL CORD

The spinal cord is surrounded by the dura mater, which is firmly attached to the rim of the foramen magnum.[6] The dura merges with the periosteum of the skull inside the foramen magnum, but it is separated from the walls of the spinal canal by fat, forming the epidural space (Fig. 1–5). The dura is lined by the arachnoid. A capillary subdural space separates the dura from the arachnoid. The subarachnoid space is filled with cerebrospinal fluid. The pia mater covers the spinal cord and forms a linear fold that extends longitudi-

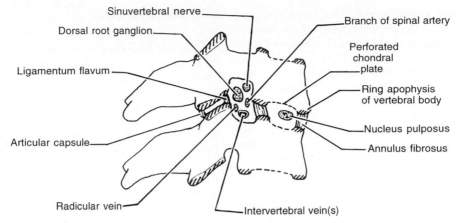

Figure 1–4. Schematic of a sagittal section of the cervical spine showing contents of an intervertebral foramen in relation to an intervertebral disc. The two vertebral bodies and disc along with the supporting structures constitute a motor unit, which includes all components of a somite in an embryo.

nally the length of the spinal medulla. This fold is the source of 20 dentate ligaments that line both sides of the cord. The dentate ligaments extend between the ventral and dorsal nerve roots to attach to the dura and suspend the spinal medulla in the spinal fluid. This organization of ligaments limits the motion of the spinal cord while allowing movement of the dura.

The ventral motor roots exit the cervical spinal cord through the ventral lateral sulcus, and the dorsal sensory roots enter the cord through the lateral longitudinal sulcus. The dorsal root is three times thicker than the ventral root, except at C1 and C2, because of the greater amount of sensory input mirrored by the greater number of sensory fibers. The six to eight rootlets at each level join together to be surrounded by the dura. Anastomoses may exist between contiguous levels of sensory nerve rootlets as they enter the spinal cord.[7] The presence of intrathecal anastomoses may explain some of the deviation from classic dermatome patterns found in patients with cervical spine pathology. The two nerve roots enter independently an outpouching of the dura

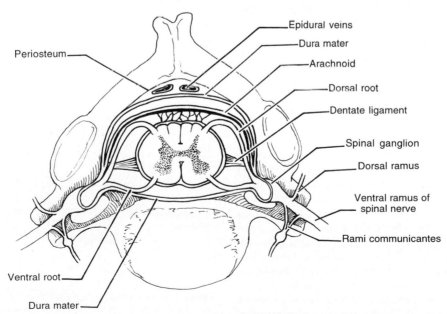

Figure 1–5. Cross-sectional view of the cervical spine demonstrating the position of the spinal cord, nerve roots, dorsal root ganglion, and spinal nerve. The dentate ligaments secure the spinal cord within the vertebral canal. The spinal cord is covered by the pia mater and suspended in the cerebrospinal fluid contained by the arachnoid membrane.

and exit the spinal canal. The dural sleeves are attached to the bony margin of the intervertebral foramen.[2] Within the confines of the intervertebral foramen, the dorsal spinal root is enlarged by the spinal ganglion cells. The ventral nerve root is in apposition to the uncinate process of the vertebral body; the dorsal root is in apposition to the zygapophyseal joint; and the vertebral artery is anterior to the nerve root. The spinal root, containing motor and sensory fibers, loses its dural covering and splits into dorsal and ventral branches. The gray rami from the sympathetic cervical ganglia join the ventral primary divisions of the spinal roots lateral to the intervertebral foramen. No white rami communicantes are located in the cervical spine. The three sympathetic ganglia that supply nerve fibers to the gray rami in the cervical cord are in the connective tissue ventral to the transverse process of the cervical vertebra, are between the longus colli and the longus capitis, and are embedded in the dorsal aspect of the carotid sheath. The three ganglia are the superior cervical ganglion, the middle cervical ganglion, and the inferior ganglion. When the inferior and first thoracic ganglia are fused, the structure is referred to as the stellate ganglion. These ganglia are highly variable in their anatomic position. The cervical sympathetic system consists of preganglionic and postganglionic autonomic fibers. The preganglionic fibers originate in the interomediolateral gray column of the T1–T5 spinal cord segments. White rami communicantes leave the corresponding thoracic ventral roots and ascend in the sympathetic trunk. The largest ganglion is the superior ganglion, located at the C2–C3 level. The middle ganglion, the smallest, is located at C6. The inferior ganglion lies between the transverse process of C7 and the first rib.

Sympathetic nerves from the first four cervical nerves supply components of nerves innervating the pharynx. The fifth cervical spinal nerve root provides sympathetic innervation to the arteries of the head and neck. The sixth root has fibers to the subclavian artery and brachial plexus. The seventh root has components supplying the cardioaortic plexus, the subclavian and axillary arteries, and phrenic nerves.[2] Sympathetic nerve fibers surrounding the internal carotid artery provide branches to the posterior orbit, orbital muscles, dilator muscles of the pupils, and smooth muscles of the upper eyelid. Those nerves surrounding the vertebral arteries reach the vestibular portion of the ear.[2]

INTERVERTEBRAL DISCS

The intervertebral discs form approximately 25% of the length of the vertebral column above the sacrum. In the cervical region the discs contribute 22% of the length of the column. The discs are the major structural link between adjacent vertebrae. They serve to allow greater motion between the vertebral bodies than would occur if the vertebrae were in direct apposition. More important, the discs distribute weight over a large surface of the vertebral body during bending motions—weight that would otherwise be concentrated eccentrically on the edge toward which the spine was bent.

Each intervertebral disc is composed of a gelatinous nucleus pulposus surrounded by a laminated, fibrous annulus fibrosus (Fig. 1–6). Each disc is situated between the cartilaginous end plates of two vertebrae. The discs are contained more closely in the cervical spine than at other levels owing to the deeply concave structure of the superior surface of the caudal vertebra and the more convex inferior surface of the rostral vertebra.

The annulus fibrosus forms the outer boundary of each disc. It is composed of fibrocartilaginous tissue and fibrous protein, which are arranged in concentric layers, or lamellae, and run obliquely from one vertebra to another. Successive layers of these fibers slant in alternate directions so that they cross each other at different angles depending on

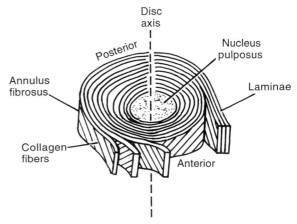

Figure 1–6. The intervertebral disc. The outer portion, the annulus fibrosus, is composed of 90 sheets of laminated collagen fibers that are oriented vertically in the peripheral layers and more obliquely in the central layers. Successive laminae run at angles to each other.

the intradiscal pressure of the nucleus pulposus. Thus, the annulus fibrosus can absorb stress by expanding and contracting like a Japanese fingertrap. Its peripheral fibers pass over the edge of the cartilaginous end plate to unite with the bone of each vertebral body. The most superficial fibers blend with the anterior and posterior longitudinal ligaments. With age, these fibers deteriorate, become fissured, and lose their capacity to restrain the nucleus pulposus. If there is sufficient internal stress, the nucleus pulposus material can penetrate through the annulus, and the resulting injury is termed a herniated disc. Aging may also alter the integrity of the nucleus. After 50 years of age, the nucleus pulposus becomes a fibrocartilaginous mass that is similar to the characteristics of the inner zone of the annulus fibrosus. The nucleus may no longer be distinguishable from the annulus in later life.[8]

The nucleus pulposus is situated posteriorly and centrally within the disc and consists of collagen fibrils enmeshed in a mucoprotein gel. The nucleus pulposus occupies about 40% of the disc's cross-sectional area. At birth, it has a high water content (88%), which mechanically allows it to absorb a significant amount of stress; however, with age, the percentage of water decreases, reflecting both an absolute decrease in available proteoglycans and a change in the ratio of the different proteoglycans present. This desiccation (loss of water) reduces the functional ability of the nucleus pulposus to withstand stress.

In the cervical spine, the discs are thicker anteriorly than posteriorly and are entirely responsible for the normal cervical lordosis. They do not conform completely to the surfaces of the vertebral bodies with which they are connected, being slightly smaller in width than the vertebral bodies. The discs bulge anteriorly beyond the adjacent vertebrae. The nucleus pulposus in the cervical spine is located more anteriorly than in other portions of the spine.

LIGAMENTS OF THE CERVICAL VERTEBRAL COLUMN

The vertebral bodies are bordered front and back by two major ligaments. The anterior longitudinal ligament is a broad, strong ligament on the anterior and anterolateral aspects of the vertebral bodies from the atlas to the sacrum (Fig. 1–7). Superiorly, the ligament attaches to the anterior arch of the atlas and the anterior atlanto-occipital membrane. Its deepest fibers blend with the intervertebral disc and extend from the body of one vertebra, to the disc, and to the body of the adjacent vertebra. These deep fibers bind the disc and the margins of the vertebra. Most of the superficial fibers extend over several vertebrae, occasionally spanning as many as five. This ligament is most firmly attached to the vertebral bodies at their periphery. The edges of the ligament are thinner than the centermost portion.

The posterior longitudinal ligament lies on the posterior surface of the bodies of the vertebrae from the axis to the sacrum. The ligament is continuous with the tectorial membrane as it passes onto the occiput. The ligament is attached most firmly to the ends of the vertebrae and most deeply to the in-

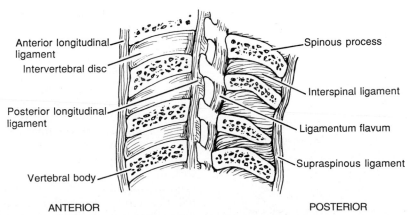

Figure 1–7. Lateral view of the cervical spine demonstrating the ligaments that support the anterior (anterior longitudinal, posterior longitudinal) and the posterior (supraspinous, interspinous) elements of the vertebral column. Note the position of the ligamentum flavum forming a smooth posterior wall of the neural foramen.

Anterior longitudinal ligament
Intervertebral disc
Posterior longitudinal ligament
Vertebral body

Spinous process
Interspinal ligament
Ligamentum flavum
Supraspinous ligament

ANTERIOR   POSTERIOR

tervening discs. The midportion of the body is only loosely attached to this ligament. Unlike the anterior longitudinal ligament, which is ribbonlike, the posterior longitudinal ligament is waisted over the vertebral bodies and fans out over the intervertebral discs. The posterior longitudinal ligament is wider in the upper cervical spine than in the lower cervical spine.[6] The lateral expansions over the discs are rather weak and represent a more vulnerable area for disc herniation compared to the strong central band (Fig. 1–8).

The articulations between the vertebral arches are maintained by the supraspinous ligaments, which become the ligamentum nuchae in the cervical spine; the interspinous ligaments; the ligamentum flavum; and the synovial facet joints and capsules.

Supraspinous and interspinous ligaments are found between adjacent spinous processes. The supraspinous ligament is thin, is composed of a high percentage of elastic tissue, and runs over the tips of the spinous processes. In some quadruped animals, the ligamentum nuchae is an essential structure for maintaining the head in an extended position. In humans, this structure extends from the vertebra prominens to the external occipital protuberance, and although considered rudimentary compared to its configuration in quadrupeds, it is probably a major stabilizer of the head and neck. Its deeper fibers attach to the spinous process of each of the cervical vertebrae and reinforce the interspinous ligaments, which in the neck appear less developed than in other regions of the spine. The interspinous ligaments attach in an oblique orientation from the posterosuperior aspect of the anteroinferior aspect of the spinous process below.

The highly elastic ligamentum flavum, or yellow ligament, is found posteriorly between adjacent laminae. There are two of these ligaments at each level, a right and a left, and they are separated by a small cleft. The ligamenta flava merge with the interspinous ligaments posteriorly and with the fibrous capsule of the synovial facet joints anteriorly. They extend from the bases of the articular processes on one side to those on the opposite. They extend laterally into the intervertebral foramen, forming a portion of the roof of the foramen. They are attached to the inferior aspect of the lamina above on the anterior surface and to the superior aspect of the lamina below on the dorsal surface. This unique attachment, combined with anterior tilting of the lamina, has the effect of creating an extremely smooth posteroinferior wall of the spinal canal, which remains smooth in the various postural positions and serves to protect the spinal cord.

The facet joints in the lower cervical spine are diarthrodial joints with typical synovial membranes and fibrous capsules. The joints are distinctive in that the facets are oriented more obliquely than in the thoracic or lumbar spine. In addition, the joint capsules are more lax than in other regions of the spine to permit a gliding motion. They contain menisci that protect articular surfaces from damage during cervical motion. These menisci may become entrapped in the joint and cause cervical dysfunction.[9, 10]

The articulation of the occiput, atlas, and axis differs considerably from that of the lower cervical spine and must be considered separately. The occiput and the atlas articulate through two joints. Each of these joints is formed by the deeply concave, oval, superior articular surface of the lateral mass of the atlas and the corresponding convex condyle of the occiput. These joints are condyloid in configuration, and the articular surfaces are reciprocally curved. In spite of the massive size of the atlanto-occipital joint, strong accessory ligaments are necessary to provide stability.

The anterior atlanto-occipital membrane is a strong, dense band composed of thick fibers that stretch across the anterior margin of the foramen magnum above to the upper border of the anterior arch of the atlas below. In the midline there is a round, tough band of fibers connecting the anterior tubercle of the atlas with the occiput. This structure may be considered a continuation of the anterior longitudinal ligament. The posterior atlanto-occipital membrane is thinner than its anterior counterpart and connects the posterior margin of the foramen magnum with the upper border of

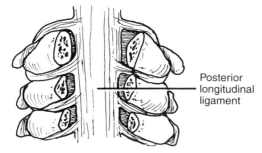

Posterior longitudinal ligament

Figure 1–8. Posterior view of the cervical spine with the spinous processes removed. The posterior longitudinal ligament covers the posterior portion of the cervical vertebrae with lateral expansions to cover the intervertebral discs.

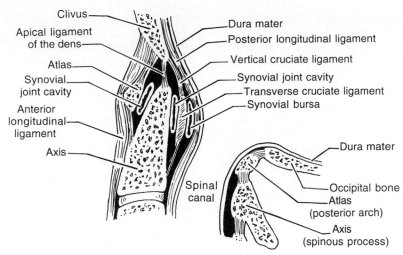

Figure 1–9. Sagittal view of the skull and upper cervical spine shows the atlantoaxial joint and surrounding synovial structures.

the posterior arch of the atlas. Inferiorly and laterally, there is an arched defect that permits the passage of the vertebral artery and the first cervical nerve. The articular capsules of the atlanto-occipital joints are loose, thin structures connecting the condyles of the occiput with the superior articular processes of the axis (Fig. 1–9).

In addition to the stability provided by the ligaments between the occiput and the atlas, stability of the head on the vertebral column is further enhanced by a group of ligaments between the occiput and the axis. The alar ligaments are short, strong bundles of fibrous tissue directed obliquely upward and laterally from either side of the upper part of the odon-

toid process to the medial aspect of the condyles of the occiput. Because these ligaments restrict motion of the head on the atlas, they are often referred to as check ligaments. The apical odontoid ligament is a tough fibrous cord arising from the apex of the odontoid process between the alar ligaments. It inserts into the anterior margin of the foramen magnum (Fig. 1–10).

The tectorial membrane, or occipitoaxial ligament, is a broad strong band in the vertebral column that lies immediately behind the body of the axis and its ligaments. Inferiorly, it is anchored to the posterior surface of the body of the axis and superiorly to the basilar groove of the occiput. The structure is essen-

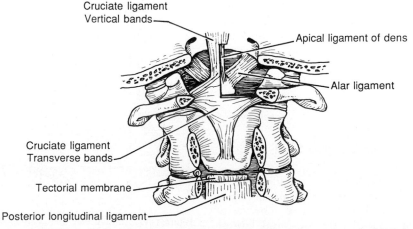

Figure 1–10. Coronal view of the skull and upper cervical spine shows the transverse-cruciate ligaments, the primary stabilizers of the odontoid process. Secondary stabilizers of the odontoid are the alar ligament, which arises from the sides of the dens to the condyles of the occipital bone, and the apical ligament, which arises from the apex of the dens to the foramen magnum as a remnant of the notochord.

tially a continuation upward of the posterior longitudinal ligament.

There are three true synovial articulations between the atlas and the axis—the two lateral atlantoaxial joints and the median atlantoaxial joint. The lateral joints are formed by the inferior articular surfaces of the atlas and the superior articular surfaces of the axis. They are a large mass of arthrodial, or gliding, joints. Their broad surfaces are directed slightly downward and laterally. The median atlantoaxial joint is essentially a pivot joint with two synovial cavities, one anteriorly between the odontoid and the posterior surface of the anterior arch of the atlas, and the other between the posterior aspect of the odontoid and the front of the transverse ligament of the atlas.

The transverse ligament of the atlas is undoubtedly the most important component of the ligamentous system in this region. It is a broad, strong, triangular ligament arching across the ring of the atlas and firmly anchored on each side to a tubercle in the medial surface of the lateral masses of the atlas. It divides the ring of the atlas into a small anterior and a large posterior compartment. In the anterior compartment lies the odontoid process, which is held firmly against the anterior arch of the atlas by the transverse ligament. There are two synovial cavities, one between the arch of the atlas and the odontoid anteriorly, and the other between the transverse ligament and the odontoid posteriorly (Fig. 1–9). A bursa lined with synovium is interposed between the transverse ligament of the atlas and the posterior longitudinal ligament. The posterior compartment is occupied by the spinal cord and its membranes; this compartment is equally divided between free space and the spinal cord. The transverse ligament gives off two strong fasciculi. The superior fascicle is elongated upward to the basal part of the occiput. The inferior fascicle is attached to the posterior surface of the body of the axis. This gives the transverse ligament a cruciate configuration.

BLOOD SUPPLY OF THE CERVICAL SPINE

The vertebral artery is the major source of blood supply for the cervical spine and the cervical portion of the spinal cord. The vertebral arteries are usually the first and largest branch of the subclavian artery on each side. The vertebral arteries enter the foramen transversarium of C6 and ascend to the atlas, where

they wind posteriorly around the lateral masses of the atlas and pass over the posterior arch of C1 just behind the lateral mass of that vertebra (Fig. 1–11). The left artery is larger in diameter than the right artery. The position of the vertebral artery in the transverse process is anterior to the exiting spinal nerve root just distal to the cervical ganglion. The vertebral arteries give off branches that supply the bone, joints, muscles, as well as the neural elements. As a consequence of its relationship at the superior edge of the atlas, the vertebral artery is particularly vulnerable to injury during posterior surgery in the atlanto-occipital area (Fig. 1–12). Rotation of the cervical spine may compress the vertebral artery if it is atheromatous at this same location.[2]

The vertebral arteries join together after passing through the foramen magnum to form the basilar artery. Just before joining, one or both of the vertebral arteries give off a branch that joins with the branch from the other side and descends in the ventral medial fissure on the anterior aspect of the spinal cord as the anterior spinal artery. The posterior cord is supplied by the two posterior spinal arteries that descend from the vertebral arteries and give rise to a plexus of vessels on the dorsal aspect of the cord. The vertebral arteries also give off medullary feeders to the anterior and

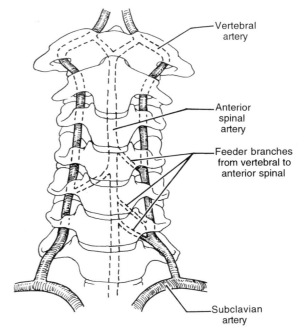

Figure 1–11. Anterior view of the cervical spine shows the course of the vertebral arteries from C6 to C1 through the transverse foramen. The course of the arteries is tortuous at the C1 and C2 levels, corresponding to a potential location for stenosis.

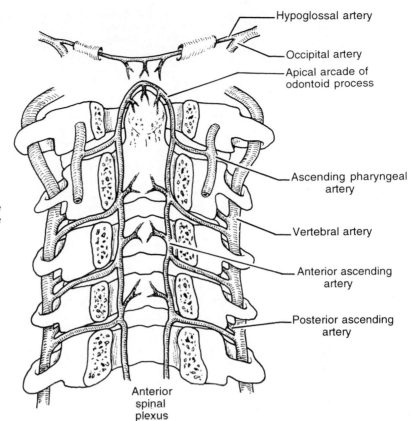

Hypoglossal artery

Occipital artery

Apical arcade of odontoid process

Ascending pharyngeal artery

Vertebral artery

Anterior ascending artery

Posterior ascending artery

Anterior spinal plexus

Figure 1–12. Posterior view of the upper cervical spine shows the vertebral arterial blood supply.

posterior spinal arteries. The medullary feeders are inconsistent branches of the segmental arteries that are evident at each level of the spine. The segmental vessels enter the intervertebral foramen at each level and supply the vertebrae and surrounding soft tissues (Fig. 1–13). In neck flexion, an intervertebral disc herniation may cause compression of the spinal cord, with loss of pulsation and obliteration of venous channels. Neck extension allows for return of blood flow.

Venous blood returns from the spinal cord through a system analogous to the anterior and posterior arterial channels. The venous drainage of the vertebrae is divided into an external and an internal system. The external system is arranged in the same distribution as the anterior, central, and posterior laminar arteries. The system inside the spinal canal consists of a series of valveless sinuses in the epidural space clustered anteriorly and just medial to the pedicles over the midportion of the vertebral bodies. The anterior portion of the external venous plexus drains into the venae comitantes of the vertebral arteries, and the posterior portion of the plexus drains into the deep cervical veins bilaterally. These ve-

nous systems drain into the brachiocephalic veins. The valveless complex of veins in the spine forms a continuous connection between the pelvis and the cerebral sinuses and connects with the caval and azygos systems. The absence of valves allows the reversal of blood from the pelvis to the cervical spine[11] (Fig. 1–14).

MUSCLES AND FASCIA OF THE CERVICAL SPINE

The muscles of the neck can be defined by anatomic limits, innervation, or function. Because the cervical spine is the most mobile section of the spine, it contains the most elaborate and specialized muscle system of the spine.

The posterior muscles of the neck are divided into superficial, intermediate, and deep groups. The trapezius muscle is the most superficial muscle of the posterior group and is innervated by the spinal accessory nerve—the eleventh cranial nerve. This muscle originates from the spinous processes of C2 through T12 and occipital protuberance to insert on the

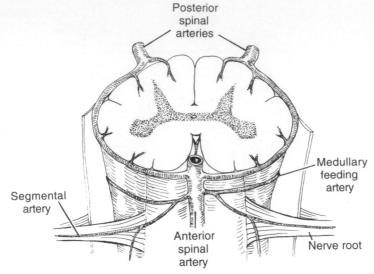

Figure 1–13. The anterior and posterior spinal artery blood supply to the spinal cord. A medullary feeding artery, originating from the segmental artery, also contributes to the vascularity of the spinal cord.

scapula, acromion, and clavicle (Fig. 1–15). It functions to stabilize and elevate the scapula and extend the head. The trapezius muscle is a frequent source of pain in individuals with muscular strain of the cervical spine. Another muscle, the levator scapulae, elevates the medial scapula and rotates it medially. It is inner-

vated by the nerve to the levator scapulae and runs from the transverse process of the upper cervical spine to the superior medial scapula.

The intermediate muscles surrounding the spine function primarily as spinal extensors. The muscles include the splenius capitis and the splenius cervicis. The muscles originate

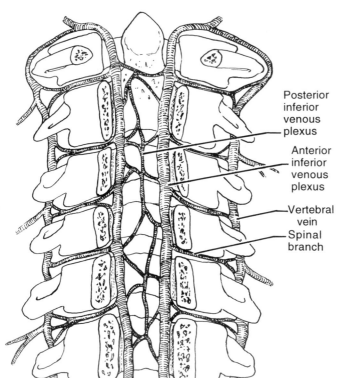

Figure 1–14. Posterior view of the cervical spine shows the internal and external system of venous channels that drain into the brachiocephalic veins.

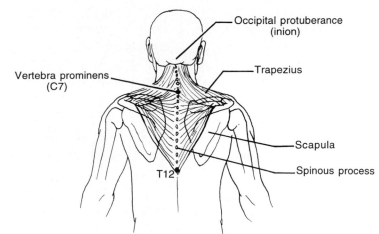

Figure 1–15. Posterior view of the cervical spine demonstrating the trapezius muscle, a primary extensor of the cervical spine.

from the spinous processes of the lower cervical and upper thoracic spine and insert on the transverse processes of the upper cervical spine and the mastoid process (Fig. 1–16). Biomechanical studies have documented the importance of the splenius capitis and cervicis as prime muscles for extension of the head and neck.[12]

In the deep layer, the erector spinae muscles from the thoracolumbar spine continue to the cervical region, including the iliocostalis cervicis laterally; longissimus cervicis and longissimus capitis centrally; and spinalis cervicis, semispinalis capitis, and semispinalis cervicis medially (Fig. 1–17). The iliocostalis extends

from the angles of the upper six ribs to the posterior tubercles of the transverse processes of the lower cervical vertebrae. The longissimus group extends from the transverse processes of the upper thoracic vertebrae to the posterior tubercles of the transverse processes of the lower cervical vertebrae and to the mastoid process as part of the longissimus capitis. The semispinalis group arises on the posterior tubercles of the transverse processes of the upper thoracic and lower cervical vertebrae and inserts into the area between the superior and inferior nuchal line of the occiput. Beneath the semispinalis muscle lie the multifidus from C4 to C7 and rotatores muscles that

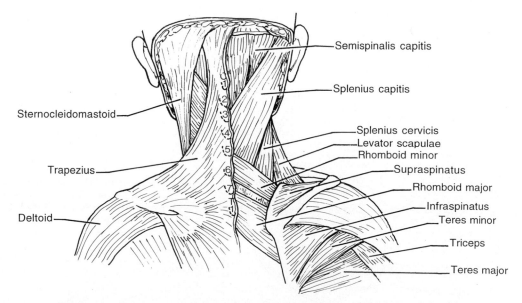

Figure 1–16. Posterior view of the superficial muscles of the cervical spine and shoulders.

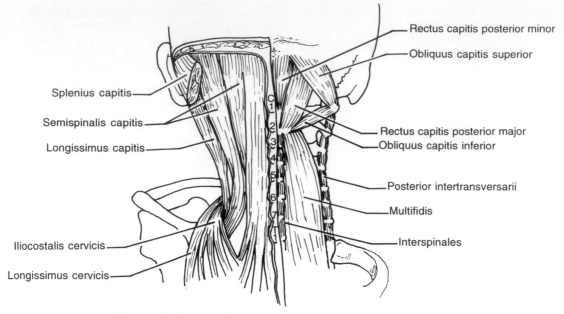

Rectus capitis posterior minor

Obliquus capitis superior

Splenius capitis

Semispinalis capitis

Longissimus capitis

Rectus capitis posterior major

Obliquus capitis inferior

Posterior intertransversarii

Multifidis

Interspinales

Iliocostalis cervicis

Longissimus cervicis

Figure 1–17. Posterior view of the deeper muscles of the cervical spine.

cross one segment of the spine and extend from the transverse process to the spinous process. In the upper cervical spine, suboccipital muscles (rectus capitis posterior major and minor and the obliquus capitis inferior and superior) attach from the occiput to the C2 vertebra. Most posterior muscles are involved in producing extension of the neck and head; some muscles, particularly the deeper muscles, produce rotation and lateral flexion (Table 1–1). Posterior deep muscles are innervated segmentally by the branches of primary dorsal rami of one or more cervical nerves. This arrangement is related to the embryonic development and is termed segmental innervation (Fig. 1–18).

The anterolateral cervical muscles function to flex and rotate the head and neck. These muscles include the platysma, sternocleidomastoid, and hyoid muscles; strap muscles of the larynx; and scalenes, longus colli, and longus capitis (Fig. 1–19). The platysma is a thin muscle below the subcutaneous tissue that spans the deltoid to the pectoral fascia and

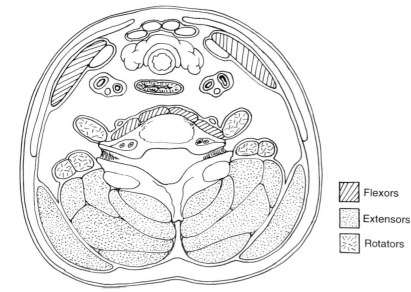

Figure 1–18. Cross section of body musculature through the sixth cervical vertebrae. Flexors are anterior to the spine and extensors are posterior. The muscles that cause lateral bending and rotation are contiguous to the vertebral bodies in a lateral position.

Flexors

Extensors

Rotators

TABLE 1-1. MUSCLES OF THE CERVICAL SPINE

FLEXION

Sternocleidomastoid
Longus colli
Longus capitis
Rectus capitis anterior

EXTENSION

Splenius capitis
Splenius cervicis
Semispinalis capitis
Semispinalis cervicis
Longissimus capitis
Longissimus cervicis
Trapezius
Interspinalis
Rectus capitis posterior major
Rectus capitis posterior minor
Obliquus capitis superior
Sternocleidomastoid

ROTATION AND LATERAL BENDING

Sternocleidomastoid
Scalene group
Splenius capitis
Splenius cervicis
Longissimus capitis
Levator scapulae
Longus colli
Iliocostalis cervicis
Multifidi
Intertransversarii
Obliquus capitis inferior
Obliquus capitis superior
Rectus capitis lateralis

the clavicle, and it inserts on the mandible, muscles of the lip, and lower face skin. The platysma depresses the lower jaw and lip and tightens the skin of the anterior neck. The other anterolateral muscles are divided into two large triangles by the sternocleidomastoid muscle. The sternocleidomastoid is innervated by the spinal accessory nerve. The muscle arises from two heads: sternal and clavicular. When the sternocleidomastoid muscles contract simultaneously, the head is flexed or the thorax raised if the head is held in a fixed position. Medial and deep to the sternocleidomastoid muscle is the carotid sheath containing the internal carotid artery, vagus nerve, and internal jugular vein. The "strap muscles" attach to the hyoid, thyroid cartilage, and sternum and are medial to the sternocleidomastoid except for the posterior aspect of the omohyoid muscle (Fig. 1–20). These muscles are innervated by segmental branches of the cervical anterior primary rami. The muscles above the hyoid are innervated by the hypoglossal nerve and are rarely encountered in anterior cervical spine surgery. The hyoid mus-

cles do not control motion of the cervical spine, but they are important in controlling movement of the hyoid bone and larynx. Deep and medial to the carotid sheath are the anterior cervical spine vertebral bodies covered by a prevertebral fascia. The prevertebral muscles of the neck are the longus colli and longus capitis. These muscles are paired with one on each side of the spine. The longus colli muscles extend from C1 to T3, spanning the lateral portions of the vertebral bodies and having lateral attachment to the anterior tubercles of the lateral masses of C3–C6. The longus capitis muscles arise on the anterior tubercles of C3–C6 and extend cephalad to the basiocciput where they are supplemented by the rectus capitis anterior and the rectus capitis lateralis. These muscles are flexors of the cervical spine.

The sternocleidomastoid is the dividing boundary for the anterior and posterior triangles of the neck (Fig. 1–21). The posterior triangle is formed by the sternocleidomastoid, trapezius, and clavicle, with a floor consisting of the semispinalis capitis, levator scapulae, splenius capitis, scalenus medius, and scalenus anterior. The omohyoid muscle runs obliquely across the inferior portion of the posterior triangle to form the omoclavicular triangle. The anterior triangle is bounded by the midline of the neck, the lower border of the mandible, and the sternocleidomastoid. The anterior triangle is further divided into the submental, submandibular, muscular, and carotid triangles. The carotid triangle is bounded by the anterior border of the sternocleidomastoid, posterior belly of the digastric muscle, and the superior belly of the omohyoid muscle and contains the carotid sheath.

As in other parts of the body, muscles, blood vessels, nerves, and viscera of the neck are contained within fascial coverings of connective tissue. These fasciae form planes and compartments in which deeper structures of the neck are organized (Fig. 1–22). The three fascial layers of the cervical spine are superficial, intermediate, and deep.[13] The superficial fascia surrounds subcutaneous fat, the platysma muscle, the external jugular vein, and cutaneous sensory nerves. The superficial layer surrounds all the deeper structures of the neck. The superficial fascia exists as a single sheet over the anterior and posterior cervical triangles. Immediately anterior to the cervical spine are the esophagus, trachea, and thyroid gland. These structures are covered by an intermediate fascial layer separate from the prevertebral fascia. The alar fascia spreads behind the esophagus and surrounds the carotid sheath.

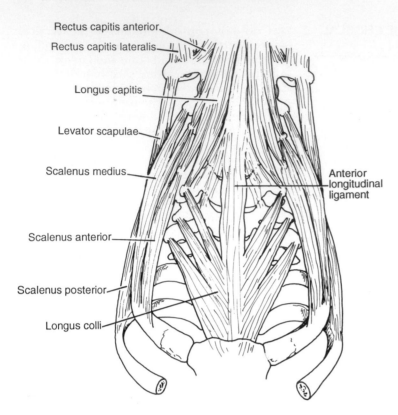

Rectus capitis anterior
Rectus capitis lateralis
Longus capitis
Levator scapulae
Scalenus medius
Scalenus anterior
Scalenus posterior
Longus colli
Anterior longitudinal ligament

Figure 1–19. Anterior view of the superficial muscles of the cervical spine.

The carotid sheath encloses the carotid artery, internal jugular vein, and the vagus nerve. The outer layer of the deep fascia extends from the trapezius muscle over the posterior triangle and then splits to enclose the sternocleidomastoid muscle. The middle layer of the deep cervical fascia encloses the strap muscles and extends laterally to the scapula. The deepest layer of the deep fascia is the prevertebral fascia, which covers the scalenus muscles, longus colli muscles, and the anterior longitudinal ligament.

A number of important structures are located between these fascial layers. In the relatively avascular space between the anterior vertebral body and the carotid sheath pass several important nerves, arteries, and veins. The superior laryngeal nerve travels at the C3–C4 level with the superior thyroid artery. The inferior thyroid artery and vein pass caudally at

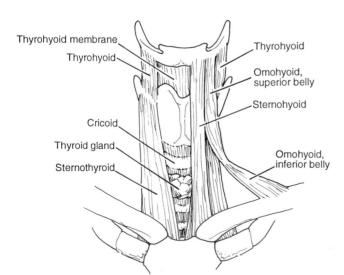

Thyrohyoid membrane
Thyrohyoid
Cricoid
Thyroid gland
Sternothyroid
Thyrohyoid
Omohyoid, superior belly
Sternohyoid
Omohyoid, inferior belly

Figure 1–20. Anterior view of the deeper anterior muscles of the cervical spine.

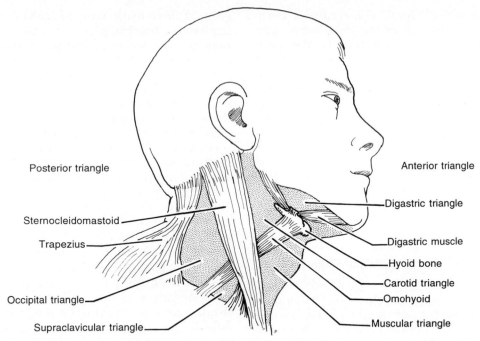

Figure 1–21. Triangle organization of the neck. The posterior triangle is formed by the trapezius, clavicle, and sternocleido-mastoid, with the omohyoid muscle dividing this triangle into the occipital and supraclavicular areas. The anterior triangle is bounded by the midline of the neck, the lower border of the mandible, and the sternocleidomastoid. The anterior triangle is subdivided by the digastric and omohyoid muscles.

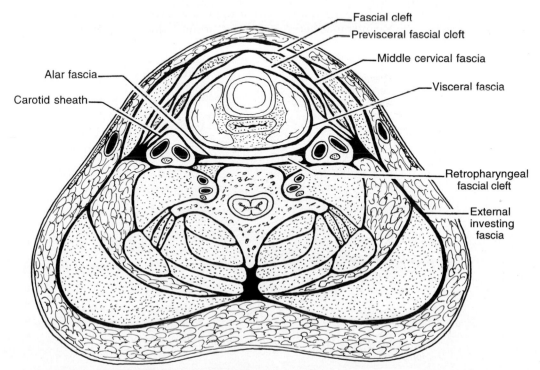

Figure 1–22. Sagittal view of the cervical spine demonstrating the division of neck structures into fascial planes.

about the C6–C7 level. The recurrent laryngeal nerve, a branch of the vagus nerve, provides an essential innervation to the vocal cord. The recurrent laryngeal nerve crosses this plane at different levels on the left and right sides. On the right side, the nerve loops around the subclavian artery before it enters the visceral fascia between the esophagus and the trachea. Its course is somewhat variable. On the left side, the nerve loops around the arch of the aorta before entering the visceral fascia as on the right. Its course is more predictable and lower in the interval between the vertebrae and the carotid sheath.

NERVE SUPPLY OF THE CERVICAL SPINE

The nerve supply to the spinal column is derived from the spinal nerve root once it passes out the neural foramina. There are eight cervical nerve roots, and the first cervical nerve exists between the atlas and the occiput. Subsequently, the cervical nerve roots C2 to C8 exit from the neural foramina so that the lower cervical nerve root exits after crossing the intervertebral disc numbered one higher (for example, C5 crosses the C4–C5 disc).

The mixed spinal nerve contains motor fibers, sensory axons of the dorsal root ganglia, as well as preganglionic fibers from the autonomic nervous system. The main spinal nerve gives off three major branches before continuing into the brachial plexus: primary posterior rami; primary anterior rami; and the sinuvertebral nerve of Luschka. The primary anterior and the posterior rami supply the muscles about the spine and chest wall. The sinuvertebral nerve contains only sensory and sympathetic fibers, and each nerve branches to two adjacent levels within the spinal canal. The cervical sinuvertebral nerves supply the level of entry and the disc above. Branches of the vertebral nerve supply the lateral aspects of the cervical discs. The nerve provides sensory endings for the posterior longitudinal ligament, annulus fibrosus, and ventral dura mater. Nerve fibers are present within the outer third of the annulus fibrosus.[14] The ventral nerve plexus, consisting of interconnections between the gray rami, the perivascular vertebral artery plexus, and the sympathetic trunk, innervates the anterior longitudinal ligament, the outer annulus fibrosus, and the anterior vertebral body[15] (Fig. 1–23). Structures that are not highly innervated include the nucleus pulposus and the ligamentum flavum. The sinuvertebral nerve is very sensitive to stretch and possibly ischemia. The facet joints are innervated by a branch of the primary dorsal rami and descend to at least one vertebral level below.

From the preceding discussion it is obvious that there are several possible sources of pain in and around the spinal column. The phe-

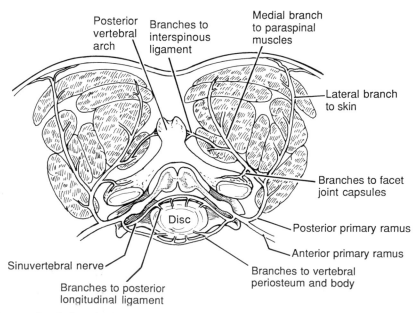

Figure 1–23. Cross-sectional view depicting nerve supply to the anterior (sinuvertebral) and posterior (posterior ramus) portions of the cervical spine.

nomenon of referred pain, or pain distant from the source, follows the anatomic course of the given nerve. This helps demonstrate why cervical spine disease is often referred to the scapular area, the shoulder, or the chest wall. The concept of referred versus radicular pain is discussed in more detail in Chapter 3.

NEIGHBORING STRUCTURES IN THE CERVICAL SPINE

A working knowledge of the overall anatomy of the neck is helpful in understanding the possible sources of pain in this part of the human body. Structures other than the spine itself may cause neck or arm pain. Examples of the structures include the temporomandibular joints, the pharynx, cervical lymph nodes, esophagus, thyroid, and apex of the lungs. The clavicle and its articulations with the sternum and acromion process of the scapula may also be a source of cervical pain.

Correlating surface anatomy and structures in the neck and cervical spine is helpful in localizing important landmarks. The angle of the mandible is at the first cervical vertebra. The transverse process of the second cervical vertebra is between the angle of the mandible and the mastoid process. The hyoid bone is anterior to the third cervical vertebra. The thyroid cartilage is anterior to the fourth cervical vertebra. The sixth vertebra is at the level of the cricoid cartilage (Fig. 1–24).

BIOMECHANICS OF THE CERVICAL SPINE

Familiarity with the anatomy of the cervical spine helps identify those structures that are at risk of developing pain, but such familiarity is not adequate to explain all the mechanisms by which neck pain develops. The normal function of the cervical spine requires both flexibility to move the head and endurance of the musculature. The neck normally moves more than 600 times each hour, whether a person is awake or asleep.[5] Recognition of deviations from normal biomechanical function, such as a hypermobile segment and excessive cervical kyphosis, may help explain the source of pain in some individuals who do not have specific anatomic abnormalities. A basic understanding of the clinically relevant biomechanics of the cervical spine is necessary for making a complete assessment of the neck of patients who have cervical problems.

Much of what is known about the normal biomechanics and pathomechanics of the cervical spine has been learned from static mechanical testing of cadaveric specimens in the laboratory. There is a wealth of information available about the dynamic mechanics of all aspects of the spine. It is well established that forces and stresses can be applied to the spine in any combination of flexion, extension, rotation, and shear. These stresses affect the entire motion segment, including the intervertebral disc, zygapophyseal joints and capsules, anterior and posterior longitudinal ligaments, uncovertebral joints, and the other ligamentous structures. The muscles and the fascial attachments interact with the cervical spine to accommodate load, alter forces, and direct motion. Whereas the lumbar spine is well suited to accommodate heavy loads and provide stability, the cervical spine is better suited for mobility and is not required to transmit heavy loads. The head weighs only 5 to 7 pounds. However, all vital nerve centers are in the skull and allow coordination of vision, vestibular balance, and auditory direction. Precise control of head position and movement is essential for normal functioning of these senses.[16]

The architecture of the axial skeleton is designed to maintain the center of gravity in a functional position. The two lordotic curves, cervical and lumbar, and the two kyphotic curves, thoracic and sacral, balance each other. The center of gravity passes the external meatus of the ear and transects the odontoid process and the bodies of T1 and T12. The line then passes through the sacral promontory, courses slightly posterior to the center of the hip joint, and passes anteriorly to the center of the knee joint, through the calcaneocuboid joint of the foot, and ends slightly anterior to the lateral malleoli. In the coronal plane, the center of gravity descends from the foramen magnum and passes along the superior spinous processes of each vertebra, the tip of the sacrococcyx, to a point midway between the two navicular bones of the feet.[16] Alterations in the degree of curvature in one area of the spine results in reciprocal alterations in curvature in other areas of the spinal column in order to preserve the orientation of the body over the center of gravity. For example, an increase in lumbar lordosis will result in increased cervical lordosis.

The cervical spine is composed of functional units. Each functional unit consists of two contiguous vertebrae that may be divided into an

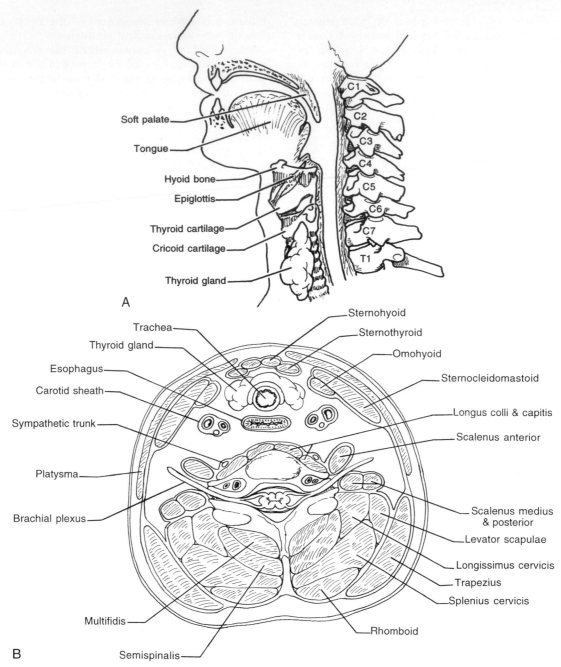

Figure 1–24. Diagrammatic views (*A* and *B*) of the anatomic relationships of the visceral organs in the anterior portion of the neck and the cervical spine.

anterior column, composed of the vertebral body, longitudinal ligaments, and intervertebral disc, and a posterior column, composed of the osseous canal, the zygapophyseal joints, and the erector spinae muscles. The anterior portion is a weight-bearing, shock-absorbing, flexible structure (Fig. 1–25). The posterior portion protects the neural elements, acts as a fulcrum, and guides movement for the functional unit (Fig. 1–26).

The biomechanical studies involving the cervical spine have concentrated on two major areas: clinical stability and kinematics. Stability as it applies to the spine may be defined as the ability of the spine under physiologic loads to limit patterns of displacement so as not to damage or irritate the spinal cord and nerve roots and, in addition, to prevent incapacitating deformity or pain due to structural changes.[17] While the issue of clinical instability

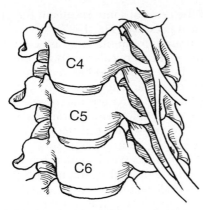

Figure 1–25. Anterior view of the cervical spine showing the anterior segments of C4 through C6 vertebral bodies. The structure of the anterior segment allows for the exit of spinal nerves and flexibility of the intervertebral discs for maximum motion.

is particularly germane to traumatic injuries of the cervical spine, the subject also applies to inflammatory disorders such as rheumatoid arthritis and degenerative spondylolisthesis. Range of motion in the subaxial cervical spine can be helpful in making decisions about instability. The maximum anteroposterior translation on a lateral radiograph under physiologic loads has been measured. Direct measure-

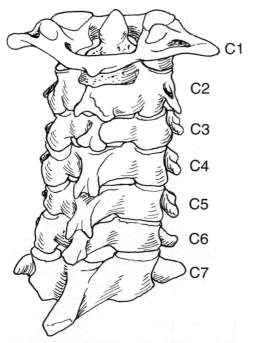

Figure 1–26. Posterior view of the entire cervical spine shows the posterior segments that offer maximum protection to the spinal cord and organized movement of the neck.

ments from cadavers suggest that the upper limit of normal is 2.7 mm. On a radiograph, with magnification due to tube distance, the guide for the upper limit of normal has been 3.5 mm.[18] An intervertebral disc space separation increase with traction of more than 1.7 mm is also abnormal.[19] A difference in angulation greater than 11° between two cervical segments on a lateral radiograph also suggests abnormal motion.[18]

Kinematics is the examination of the motion of bodies without consideration of the influencing forces. The two factors that determine the kinematics of vertebral motion are the geometry of the articulating surfaces and the mechanical properties of the connecting structures. At each level of the spine, the planes and extent of motion of each unit are dictated by the orientation of the articular surfaces as well as the surrounding ligaments and integrity of the intervertebral disc. The motion in the cervical spine between the atlas and the axis, for example, is influenced by the specific geometry of the articular surfaces and the elastic properties of the ligaments.

The function of the cervical spine may be divided into two sections, that of the upper segment above C3 and that of the lower segment from C3 to C7. The upper cervical segment includes five articulations, consisting of two between the occiput and atlas, two between the atlas and axis, and one between the dens and atlas. The occipitoatlantoaxial complex is the most complicated series of articulations in the body. The occipitocervical angle is sharp so that the head is in a horizontal plane. The occipitoatlantal joint has about 13° of flexion and extension and the atlantoaxial joint has about 10°.[20] Thus, there are about 23° of flexion/extension at the occipitoatlantoaxial complex. The orientation of the condyles prevents any lateral flexion or rotation.

Most of the axial rotation in the upper cervical spine occurs at the atlantoaxial joint.[21] The articular surfaces are convex with a horizontal orientation, allowing for maximum mobility. Atlantoaxial rotation averages 47°, which represents about 50% of the axial rotation in the neck, with the lower cervical spine contributing the other 50% of rotation. There are also about 4° of axial rotation at the occipitocervical junction.[22] The rotation of C2 on C3 is physically limited by the anatomic locking of the anterior tip of the articular process of C3 on the lateral process of the axis. A summary of the normal range of motion of the various cervical segments is shown in Table 1–2.

TABLE 1–2. MEAN RANGE OF CERVICAL SPINE MOTION (DEGREES)

LEVEL	FLEXION/ EXTENSION	LATERAL BENDING	ROTATION
0–C1	13	8	0
C1–C2	10	0	47
C2–C3	8	10	9
C3–C4	13	11	11
C4–C5	12	11	12
C5–C6	17	8	10
C6–C7	16	7	9
C7–T1	9	4	8

The lower cervical segment includes C3 through C7 with foraminal openings for the spinal nerve roots that supply the upper extremities. Motion in the lower cervical spine includes flexion, extension, lateral flexion, and rotation. No motion occurs in a single plane. Cervical lateral flexion also requires rotation. Motion also requires deformation of the intervertebral disc. In forward flexion, the anterior disc space undergoes compression with widening posteriorly. Simultaneous separation and shear of the posterior elements occur. An anterior shearing force is placed on the disc with elongation of annular fibers. Forward gliding of the superior vertebra occurs on the inferior vertebra with widening of the facet joint. In extension of the cervical spine, the posterior aspect of the disc compresses, and the anterior portion elongates. The facet joint glides posteriorly. Positions of the cervical spine affect intradiscal pressure: pressure is least in the supine position; exten-

sion of the cervical spine results in the greatest intradiscal pressure (Fig. 1–27).

The neural foramina are affected by the position of the cervical vertebrae. In cervical flexion, the vertebral bodies separate, thereby opening the neural foramina. In cervical extension, the foramina are narrowed. In lateral bending or rotation, the foramina close on the side toward which the neck moves, while opening on the contralateral side.

Flexion of the cervical spine is limited by the posterior longitudinal ligament, the posterior intervertebral ligaments that attach to the transverse processes, the posterior superior spine, and the limited elasticity of the fascia of the extensor musculature. Excessive extension of the cervical spine is limited by the direct contact of the vertebral laminae, the zygapophyseal joints, and the posterosuperior spinous process.[16]

Movement of the cervical spine affects the dura and the spinal cord. As the neck flexes, the spinal canal lengthens, with the posterior wall elongating to a greater degree than the anterior wall. Conversely, when the neck extends, the canal shortens, with the anterior wall lengthening in comparison with the posterior wall. The structures within the canal must follow a similar pattern. The spinal cord ascends and descends in the spinal canal as the neck is flexed and extended, respectively. In flexion, the plastic character of the cord allows elongation. The dura unfolds its plications within flexion. In extension, the spinal cord shortens and descends in the canal. The dura shortens and becomes pleated. The nerves connected to the spinal cord are affected in a

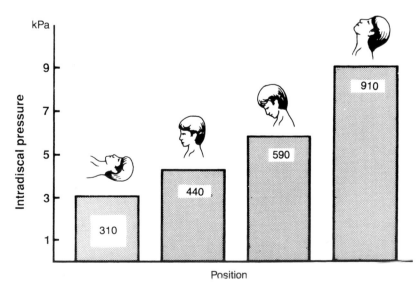

Figure 1–27. Normal intradiscal pressure in various positions of the cervical spine. (Adapted from Hattori S, Oda H, Kawai S: Cervical intradiscal pressure in movements and traction of the cervical spine. J Orthop 119:568, 1981.)

manner similar to the cord. The nerve roots are elongated, assuming a more acute angle with the boundaries of the foramen. Compression of the nerve root is minimized because the flexion of the neck not only angulates the nerve but also widens the neural foramen, allowing greater room for the neural elements.

The combination of all these biomechanical factors results in a static and dynamic posture of the cervical spine. An individual has good posture if it can be maintained for extended periods in an effortless, nonfatiguing fashion. In the cervical spine, the antigravity action of the extensor muscles plays a predominant role as the source of support. Because the cervical curve is the uppermost curve in the axial skeleton, proprioceptive impulses from the lower extremities and the lower parts of the spine play a crucial role in determining the position of the neck and head by maintaining appropriate muscular tone. Posture is a neuromuscular reaction to proprioceptive impulses from the periphery, and the feeling that posture is appropriate is a learned process.[16] Eventually, the position that is assumed during the years the musculoskeletal system develops results in the person's posture. This posture will be considered "normal" by the nervous system even if it places the musculoskeletal system at a mechanical disadvantage. In later life, these positions may result in fatigue and neck pain. In addition, emotional states may have an effect on the physical position of the neck. Depression, anxiety, anger, or happiness are only a few of the psychological states that may result in the head being bent forward or upright. Consideration of these anatomic, biomechanical, and physiological factors by the clinician may help in understanding the source of an individual's neck pain.

References

1. Ellis JH, Martell W, Lillie JH, Aisen AM: Magnetic resonance imaging of the normal craniovertebral junction. Spine 16:105, 1991.
2. Bland JH: Disorders of the Cervical Spine: Diagnosis and Medical Management, 2nd ed. Philadelphia: WB Saunders Co, 1994.
3. Jeffreys E: Disorders of the Cervical Spine, 2nd ed. Oxford: Butterworth-Heinemann Ltd, 1993, p 164.
4. Panjabi MM, Duranceau J, Goel V, et al: Cervical human vertebra: Quantitative three-dimensional anatomy of the middle and lower regions. Spine 16:861, 1993.
5. Nakano KK: Neck Pain. In: Kelley W, Harris E, Ruddy S, Sledge C (eds): Textbook of Rheumatology, 4th ed. Philadelphia: WB Saunders Co, 1994, p 397.
6. Parke WW, Sherk HH: Normal Adult Anatomy. In: Sherk HH, Dunn EJ, Eismont FJ, et al. (eds): The Cervical Spine, 2nd ed. Philadelphia: JB Lippincott, 1988, pp 11–32.
7. Schwartz HG: Anastomoses between cervical nerve roots. J Neurosurg 13:190, 1956.
8. Bland JH, Boushey DR: Anatomy and physiology of the cervical spine. Semin Arthritis Rheum 20:1, 1990.
9. Mercer S, Bogduk N: Intra-articular inclusions of the cervical synovial joints. Br J Rheumatol 32:705, 1993.
10. Yu S, Sether L, Haughton VM: Facet joint menisci of the cervical spine: Correlative MR imaging and cryomicrotomy study. Radiology 164:79, 1987.
11. Batson OV: The vertebral vein system. Am J Roentgenol 78:195, 1957.
12. Nolan JP, Sherk HH: Biomechanical evaluation of the extensor musculature of the cervical spine. Spine 13:9, 1988.
13. An HS: Anatomy of the Cervical Spine. In: An HS, Simpson JM (eds): Surgery of the Cervical Spine. Baltimore: Williams & Wilkins, 1994, pp 1–39.
14. Bogduk N, Windsor M, Inglis A: The innervation of the cervical intervertebral discs. Spine: 13:2, 1988.
15. Bogduk N: The clinical anatomy of the cervical dorsal rami. Spine 7:319, 1982.
16. Cailliet R: Neck and Arm Pain, 3rd ed. Philadelphia: FA Davis Co, 1991.
17. White AA, Panjabi MM: The basic kinematics of the human spine. Spine 3:12, 1978.
18. White AA, Johnson RM, Panjabi MM, Southwick WO: Biomechanical analysis of clinical stability in the cervical spine. Clin Orthop 109:85, 1975.
19. White AA, Panjabi MM: Clinical Biomechanics of the Spine. Philadelphia: JB Lippincott, 1978.
20. Werne S: Studies in spontaneous atlas dislocation. Acta Orthop Scand Suppl 23:1, 1957.
21. Penning L: Normal movements of the cervical spine. Am J Roentgenol 130:317, 1979.
22. Dvorak J, Panjabi MM, Gerber M, Wichmann W: CT-functional diagnostics of the rotatory instability of the upper cervical spine. Part 1. An experimental study on cadavers. Spine 12:197, 1987.

2

Epidemiology of Neck Pain

Epidemiology, the study of the incidence, prevalence, and control of disease in a population, can provide important insights to the physician caring for patients with neck problems. Through epidemiology, linkages between pain and individual or external factors can be determined, which allows risk elements to be identified and minimized. More important, epidemiology provides an understanding of the natural history of a condition, which is relevant to counseling patients about prognosis, and it provides a standard by which the efficacy of various treatments may be verified.

DEFINITIONS

No discussion of epidemiology can begin without reviewing the two most basic definitions. Incidence is the rate at which healthy people develop a symptom or disease over a specified period. Incidence is solely the rate at which the disease occurs. Prevalence is the number of people in a population who have the symptom or disease at a particular time. The 1-year prevalence of neck pain, for example, is a measure of all those with neck pain during a 1-year period, regardless whether the problem began during or before the survey period. Therefore, prevalence depends on both incidence and duration.

Although information on the prevalence and incidence of neck pain is available from multiple sources, including insurance and hospital data, interviews and questionnaires, and clinical studies, it is somewhat limited because it is grouped with shoulder or back problems. The quality of the databases is variable, especially when their primary purpose is financial

accounting rather than scientific. Another problem that alters the prevalence measured is a lack of a uniform definition of the problem. For example, a study that defines neck pain as an episode lasting 1 week would report a much higher prevalence than a survey defining neck pain as an episode lasting more than 2 weeks. Further, the information that is available is often confusing because of the variety of terms used to describe post-traumatic neck injuries. Terms such as whiplash, acute neck sprain, acute cervical strain, cervical syndrome, hyperextension-hyperflexion neck injury, acceleration-deceleration neck injury, tension neck syndrome, and others are frequently used to describe what appear to be similar conditions. These cervical injury syndromes have not been clearly defined, making meaningful analysis of the recorded neck injuries difficult.

PREVALENCE OF NECK PAIN

Neck pain is a far less frequent cause of work absenteeism than low back pain, but in certain occupations it results in a substantial amount of lost productivity. The 1-year prevalence of neck pain is approximately 20% in most industrialized countries. Scandinavian studies have reported a 1-year prevalence rate of 16% in men and 18% to 20% in women.[1, 2] In a study of 2,684 male employees, Anderson reported cervical problems occurred one-half to one-quarter as often as lumbar spine abnormalities.[3]

If the definition of neck pain is an episode lasting 2 weeks, as it was in the National Health and Nutrition Examination Survey II, the prevalence of neck pain in men and women was 8.2% among persons 25 through 74 years of age (Table 2–1).[4] The highest prevalence (10.1%) was among persons 45 through 64 years of age. Rates were higher for white (8.6%) than either black (5.6%) or other racial groups (7.2%).

Bovim and colleagues[5] reported on the results of a questionnaire inquiring about neck pain within the last year sent to randomly selected 10,000 Norwegian adults. A total of 34.4% of the respondents had experienced back pain within that year. A total of 13.8% reported neck pain that continued for more than 6 months.

PREVALENCE OF CERVICAL DISC HERNIATIONS AND ARM PAIN

The first step in establishing the prevalence of a disease is to define the clinical syndrome. Varied definitions of herniated disc are used in epidemiologic surveys. In general, brachialgia is considered to be pain radiating along the course of one of the cervical nerve roots to the shoulder or arm. A herniated nucleus pulposus is one but not the only cause of brachialgia. Arm symptoms are present in a minority of patients with neck problems.

The incidence of cervical disc herniations is difficult to estimate. A study in Rochester, Minnesota, showed an annual incidence of 5.5 per 100,000.[6] The most frequently affected disc level was C5–C6, followed by C4–C5 and C6–C7. Studies in New Haven and Hartford, Connecticut, surveyed people who had cervical disc herniation (confirmed by radiograph) and radicular pain.[7–9] These studies calculated odds ratios, showing an increased risk of herniation in men, frequent lifters, cigarette smokers, and springboard divers.

PREVALENCE OF OCCUPATIONAL NECK PAIN

The relationship between occupational factors and neck pain is difficult to study because exposure to those factors is usually difficult or impossible to quantify. Workers may be exposed to multiple risk factors in the same job; workers in the same occupation may have substantially different exposure; and workers with neck pain may shift to less strenuous jobs, leaving healthy workers on the heavy tasks, thereby shifting the apparent prevalence of neck pain. In addition, workers' memory of occupational exposure is notoriously poor and is often influenced by financial manipulation of the insurance system.

Occupational neck pain represents less than 2% of all workplace injuries. The majority of work-related neck injuries are diagnosed as a sprain or strain. Certain occupations appear to have a predisposition to neck symptoms. For example, the lifetime prevalence of neck and shoulder symptoms is 81% for machine operators, 73% for carpenters, and 57% for office workers.[10] Manual workers have more symptoms than office workers, and the type of manual labor also seems to affect the risk. A history of twisting and bending during work

TABLE 2–1. PREVALENCE OF JOINT PAIN BY SITE OF JOINT AND SELECTED DEMOGRAPHIC CHARACTERISTICS

		(RATE PER 100 PERSONS)			
		Back, Neck, or Other Joint Pain	Back Pain[1]	Neck Pain[2]	Other Joint Pain[3]
Total ages	25–74 years	21.0	16.0	8.2	19.0
Male		19.6	16.0	7.0	16.6
Female		22.4	16.0	9.4	21.3
Age	25–44 years	15.8	12.3	6.6	12.3
	45–64 years	38.4	20.3	10.1	25.1
	65–74 years	40.1	18.2	9.3	28.1
Race	White	21.9	16.5	8.6	19.4
	Black	15.5	13.2	5.6	16.8
	Other	13.7	11.3	7.2	12.5

[1]Have you ever had pain in your back on most days for at least 2 weeks?
[2]Have you ever had pain in your neck on most days for at least 2 weeks?
[3]Have you had pain or aching in any joint other than the back or neck on most days for at least 6 weeks?
From Praemer A, Furner S, Rice DP: Musculoskeletal conditions in the United States. Illinois: American Academy of Orthopaedic Surgeons 1992, pp 23–33. Source: National Center for Health Statistics, NHANESII, 1976–1980.

and the age of the employee are strong risk indicators. Others have suggested that non-physical factors, such as job satisfaction and general dissatisfaction, play an important role in neck pain syndrome.[11] Hult studied the experience of 1,137 working men, aged from 25 through 54 years, who were evenly distributed between light- and heavy-duty jobs.[12] Neck pain occurred in 27% who were younger than 30 years of age, and 50% who were older than 45 years of age. Arm pain occurred in only 8% of those younger than 30 years but in over 38% of those older than 45 years. Heavy-duty laborers were not at a significantly increased risk of developing arm pain secondary to neck symptoms.

Other studies have shown an increased incidence of neck pain in dentists in comparison with office workers and farmers. Meat carriers, miners, and "heavy workers" have significantly higher rates of cervical degenerative changes in comparison with reference groups.[13] Keyboard operators have been shown to have an increase in tension neck syndrome.[14]

The increased presence on radiographs of neck symptoms and cervical degenerative changes in various occupational groups is of great interest but limited practical value. Neck symptoms and cervical degenerative changes are quite prevalent in the general population, and it is often difficult to implicate a job-related accident as the root of the problem.

PREVALENCE OF WHIPLASH INJURIES

Whiplash injuries have been known since the First World War, when airplane pilots were often injured during catapult-assisted takeoffs because of inadequate fixation of the cockpit seat. Following the early recognition and description of this condition, which then involved a limited number of people in a specialized occupational area, the prevalence of this type of injury has continued to increase. It is a frequently described injury almost universally associated with automobile accidents.

Whiplash is the most commonly used term to describe this type of post-traumatic, hyper-extension-hyperflexion neck injury. Whiplash is a nonmedical term, first used by Crowe in 1928,[15] to describe a hyperextension injury to the neck resulting from an indirect force, usually a rear-end automobile collision. This syndrome was later redefined in 1953 by Gaye and Abbott,[16] and the term has been used extensively since then to describe this type of injury. Therefore, the authors use the term, in spite of its lack of scientific specificity, because of its common public use and its frequent use in the medical literature. This term has also been accepted as a neck injury code for hospital discharges and for insurance reimbursement.

The National Safety Council has stated that 20% of all automobile accidents are rear-end impacts. It has been estimated that 85% of all neck injuries seen clinically result from automobile accidents. Of the automobile accidents that result in neck injuries, 85% are rear-end impacts. The remaining 15% of neck injuries result from some other type of impact.[17–19] McNab[20] estimated that one fifth of exposed occupants sustains neck injuries.

The National Accident Sampling System (NASS) estimated that in 1979 there were 530,000 cases of minor whiplash injury.[21] These 530,000 people represented 2.8% of all victims in police-reported automobile accidents. The number of whiplash injuries to people in automobiles that did not require towing from the scene of the accident was significantly higher than the number of injuries to people in automobiles that did require towing. The NASS also found no correlation between the severity of damage to the automobile and the severity of an individual's complaints of neck pain.

When considering such statistics, one must also keep in mind the development of late whiplash syndrome.[22] This syndrome has been defined as a collection of symptoms and disabilities that occur more than 6 months after a neck injury resulting from an automobile accident. The physical and emotional implications of this syndrome are discussed at the end of the section on Neck Injuries and Litigation. Balla[22, 23] found a striking difference in the development of this syndrome when he compared individuals with acute neck injuries in Australia and Singapore. When he compared groups of similar patients 2 years after the initial diagnosis, none of the Singapore patients had symptoms of late whiplash syndrome; however, it was a common finding among the Australian patients. The significance and possible causes of this finding are likely to be related to the rate of litigation in the local area. From this and similar studies, one certainly must conclude that the number of people suffering from late whiplash syndrome will vary significantly in different cultural environments.

Factors Influencing Neck Injuries. Because the majority of acute neck injuries are the result of rear-end automobile accidents, it is appropriate to review certain factors concerning automobile accidents and automobile passengers that might influence the development of such injuries. These factors include the use of seat belts, shoulder straps, and head restraints; the sitting location of the injured individual; and the age, sex, and size of the occupants.

There is general agreement that acute neck injuries are more frequent among front seat passengers than among rear seat passengers.[19, 24] The person most frequently injured is the front seat passenger. The number of injuries to drivers and rear seat passengers is essentially the same.

The influence of seat belts on acute neck injuries depends on other factors, the most important of which is the presence or absence of head restraints (head rests). If head restraints are present, the use of seat belts alone results in fewer injuries. Without head restraints, the use of seat belts alone appears to cause a slight increase in injuries.[19] Using seat belts with a shoulder strap reduces the incidence of injuries, even without head restraints. The combined use of seat belts, shoulder strap, and head restraint significantly reduces the number of injuries.

Various studies have evaluated the effectiveness of head restraints. Data from different sources show a reduction in neck injuries by 10% and more with the use of head restraints. In one study[25] adjustable head restraints reduced injuries by approximately 10%, and head restraints that were an integral part of the seat reduced injuries by 17%. This study noted that 72% of the cars sold during 1960–1981 had adjustable restraints, and 25% had head restraints that were an integral part of the seat. As a result of this mix of adjustable and integral head restraints, the study estimated that head restraints prevented more than 64,000 injuries per year. Other studies have estimated a significantly higher rate of protection with head restraints. Although an exact percentage cannot be given, the best estimate is that use of head restraints has reduced the incidence of acute neck injuries in rear-end automobile accidents by about 20%.

Studies have also shown that 75% of head restraints that are adjustable are kept in the lowest possible position,[25] not an appropriate position for most automobile occupants. A visual survey of drivers in 4,983 moving domestic automobiles with adjustable head restraints in the Los Angeles and Washington, D.C., metropolitan areas indicated that, in the former, 74% of the male drivers and 57% of the female drivers had their head restraints positioned improperly; in the latter, the respective figures were 93% of the males and 80% of the females.[26] Although this is a relatively small sample, it is evident that a significant majority of the head restraints now in use in automobiles in the United States are not in the appropriate position to protect the automobile occupants. Proper positioning would undoubtedly increase their protective value significantly.

The studies that have concentrated on the position of the head restraint have found that the restraint protects women more than men. This probably results from the restraints being in the lowest position and thereby providing more protection for women, whose height is less on average than that of men.

The possible use of head restraints in the rear seats of automobiles has also been considered. Many studies have shown, however, that their use in rear seats is not justified because they would not significantly reduce the number of acute neck injuries.

A relatively new safety feature in many cars is the driver- and/or passenger-side air bag. The air bag used together with a seat belt, shoulder strap, and head restraint will more than likely further reduce the incidence of cervical spine injuries from rear-impact accidents and may also play an important role in head-on collisions.

There are conflicting data concerning the incidence of neck injuries in men and women. A majority of studies show a higher incidence of whiplash injuries in women; some studies show the frequency of neck injury among women to be twice as high as among men.[24] Kahane found that significant injuries of the cervical spine were more common in men (in the ratio of 3:2) but that whiplash injuries occurred more often in women (70%).[25] This observation, which is apparently contradictory, has been confirmed by a number of other authors.[20, 27–28] The reason for this may be that women travel more often as passengers and the injury occurs while they are in a state of muscular relaxation. The driver, more often a man, may anticipate the impact and be able to neutralize whiplash partially by keeping his head flexed and by gripping the steering wheel.

Age does not seem to be an important factor in acute neck injuries. The assumption that with increasing age and the development of osteoarthritic changes in the cervical spine there would be an increased incidence of acute neck injuries in older people has not been documented. The usual age distribution for whiplash injuries is between the ages of 30 and 50 years. Another explanation may lie in the decreased frequency of automobile accidents among older people, who spend less time driving.

Lightweight people appear to be more susceptible to acute neck injury than heavier people. There is also a positive correlation between increased height and neck injuries.[19]

Neck Injuries and Litigation. Effective litigation in acute neck injuries has received much attention.[18, 27, 29, 30] Many articles have been written, with such titles as ''The Whiplash: Tiny Impact, Tremendous Injury''[28] and ''Whiplash Injury of the Neck—Fact or Fancy.''[31] Television programs have shown characters in a minor automobile accident hiring a lawyer to sue for whiplash injury. Anecdotal incidents are prevalent, such as the city bus filled with passengers that is rear-ended by a small car with no damage to the car or bus and the only injury sustained being that of the bus driver, who suffers an acute whiplash injury. This has led to speculation that litigation and compensation are the most important factors in the incidence and severity of whiplash.

A unique factor is present in the type of accident that commonly leads to whiplash. The striking vehicle is almost invariably at fault and, therefore, this removes the burden of proof of liability for the accident. In addition, because the person with the injured neck rarely presents an objective, demonstrable abnormality, one is left with a blameless victim incapacitated by subjective symptoms, the existence of which are difficult to prove or disprove. This combination of accident events and subjective symptoms makes the accident victim a candidate for legal intervention and disability remuneration.

How frequently do people with whiplash injuries seek remuneration? This is difficult to determine because of the lack of follow-up in reporting of minor injuries and the current trend to settle out of court. However, in a few controlled studies, more than 50% of the accident victims eventually received some type of settlement.[26]

A number of studies have been undertaken to determine if the awarding of a monetary settlement has resulted in significant improvement of the symptoms of injured people.

Among people with only subjective complaints, more than 50% improved significantly after litigation claims were settled. In patients with objective findings, such as reduced range of neck movement or evidence of neurologic loss, the percentage that improved after litigation is lower than 25% after settlement.[26]

Emotional factors that might contribute to a person's symptoms and disability cannot be overlooked. These might be classified as conscious malingering, conscious exaggeration of underlying complaints, or subconscious exaggeration or modification of an underlying acute neck injury. In studies of low back injuries, the conscious malingerer is relatively infrequent. The more frequent circumstance appears to be the conscious exaggeration of an underlying complaint.

Although it is sometimes difficult to separate the conscious from the subconscious exaggeration, under many circumstances this differentiation can be made fairly accurately by a careful examiner performing a detailed history and physical examination. The typical conscious manipulator is the person who arrives at the physician's office with extensive documentation of the accident or injury, demonstrates a persistently defensive attitude, is often overly hostile, withholds information, involves an attorney to the extent that simple questions are not answered without consulting the attorney, and shows variable and inconsistent hysterical symptoms.

The person with a subconscious emotional overlay often demonstrates a significantly different pattern. This person often shows a lack of concern for documentation and also starts with a defensive attitude. This attitude may alternate with transient episodes of anger, and the patient does not knowingly withhold information. If hysterical symptoms are present, they are usually constant. This person usually has an attorney but has a much more passive involvement.

Although these are general descriptions that do not apply in all cases, this type of differentiation has served the authors well in managing the course of treatment and particularly in the early use of independent medical examiners for employees suffering from acute neck injuries.

LONG-TERM OUTCOME OF NECK PAIN

Neck pain in the majority of patients resolves with time. Gore and colleagues reported on the evaluation of patients with neck pain 10 years after the initial episode.[32] Seventy-nine percent had decreased pain, 43% were free of pain, and 32% had moderate or severe pain. Patients who had an injury and severe pain in the initial episode were the individuals at greatest risk of developing persistent pain. A radiograph of the cervical spine did not predict the degree of pain an individual experienced. A prediction of final outcome based on initial symptoms or radiographic findings was not possible.

SUMMARY

The epidemiology of neck pain and brachialgia is both critical and confusing. All epidemiologic information on this topic must be carefully analyzed relative to the source from which it is taken as well as to the potential motivation for gain on the part of the patients or physicians who provide the information. Knowledge of the incidence, prevalence, and natural history of degenerative neck problems is much more extensive than knowledge of the frequency of true acute neck injuries. In addition, acute neck injuries have resulted in a great deal of discussion but very little verifiable medical information. Although it is apparent that the most common initiating factor is a rear-end automobile impact, it also appears clear that the number of resulting injuries could be significantly reduced by the proper use of the safety equipment in the automobiles. Patients with neck strain or whiplash injury should be treated according to the same protocols that are presented in the following chapters. The physician should recognize that those with a whiplash injury may have a protracted recovery of 12 to 18 months, compared to those with more acute exacerbations of degenerative problems, which tend to be more often an acute strain unrelated to litigation and generally resolve within several weeks. Understanding and knowledge of the physical and psychosocial risk factors that have been confirmed can help prevent and minimize the severity of recurrences.

References

1. Takala J, Sievers K, Klaukka T: Rheumatic symptoms in the middle-age population in southwestern Finland. Scand J Rheumatol Suppl 47:15, 1982.
2. Westerling D, Jonsson BG: Pain from the neck-shoulder region and sick leave. Scand J Soc Med 8:131, 1980.
3. Anderson JAD: Rheumatism in industry: A review. Br J Ind Med 28:103, 1971.
4. Praemer A, Furner S, Rice DP: Musculoskeletal Conditions in the United States. Illinois: American Academy of Orthopaedic Surgeons, 1992, pp 23–33.
5. Bovim G, Schrader H, Sand T: Neck pain in the general population. Spine 19:1307, 1994.
6. Kondo K, Molgaard CA, Kurland LT, Onofric BM: Protruded intervertebral cervical disc. Minn Med 64:751, 1981.
7. Kelsey JL, Githens PB, O'Connor T, et al.: Acute prolapsed lumbar intervertebral disc: An epidemiologic study with special reference to driving automobiles and cigarette smoking. Spine 9:608, 1984.
8. Kelsey JL, Githens PB, Walter SD, et al.: An epidemiological study of acute prolapsed cervical intervertebral disc. J Bone Joint Surg Am 66:907, 1984.
9. Kelsey JL, Githens PB, White AA, et al.: An epidemiologic study of lifting and twisting on the job and risk for acute prolapsed lumbar intervertebral disc. J Orthop Res 2:61, 1984.
10. Tola S, Riihimaki H, Videman T, et al.: Neck and shoulder symptoms among men in machine operating, dynamic physical work and sedentary work. Scand J Work Environ Health 14:299, 1988.
11. Kiesler S, Finholt T: The mystery of RSI. Am Psychol 43:1004, 1988.
12. Hult L: Cervical, dorsal, and lumbar spinal syndromes. Acta Orthop Scand Suppl 17:1, 1954.
13. Hagberg M, Wegman DH: Prevalence rates and odds ratios of shoulder-neck diseases in different occupational groups. Br J Ind Med 44:602, 1987.
14. Hagberg M, Sundelin G: Discomfort and load on the upper trapezius muscle when operating a wordprocessor. Ergonomics 29:1637, 1986.
15. Crowe HE: Injuries to the cervical spine. Paper presented at the meeting of the Western Orthopaedic Association, San Francisco, 1928.
16. Gay JR, Abbott KH: Common whiplash injuries of the neck. JAMA 152:1698, 1953.
17. Jackson R: The positive findings in alleged neck injuries. Am J Orthop 6:178, 1964.
18. Jackson R: Crashes cause most neck pain. Am Med News, Dec. 5, 1966.
19. States JD, Korn MW, Masengill JB: The enigma of whiplash injury. NY State J Med 70:2971, 1970.
20. McNab I: Acceleration injuries of the cervical spine. J Bone Joint Surg Am 46:1797, 1964.
21. Partyka S: Whiplash and other inertial force neck injuries in traffic accidents. Paper presented at the meeting of the Mathematical Analysis Division, National Center for Statistics and Analysis, 1981.
22. Balla JI: The late whiplash syndrome. Aust N Z J Surg 50:610, 1980.
23. Balla JI: The late whiplash syndrome: A study of an illness in Australia and Singapore. Cult Med Psychiatry 6:191, 1982.
24. Kihlberg JK: Flexion-torsion neck injury in rear-end impacts. Proceedings of 13th Annual Conference of American Association for Automotive Medicine, 1969.
25. Kahane CJ: An evaluation of head restraints. Federal Motor Vehicle Safety Standard 22. Technical Report 2982:308, 1982.
26. O'Neill B, Haddon W, Kelley AB, Sorenson W: Automobile head restraint—Frequency of neck injury claims in relation to the presence of head restraints. Am J Publ Health 62:399, 1972.

27. Cammark KV: Whiplash injuries to the neck. Am J Surg 93:663, 1957.
28. Guy JE: The whiplash: Tiny impact, tremendous injury. Industr Med Surg 37:688, 1968.
29. Gotten N: Survey of one hundred cases of whiplash injury after settlement of litigation. JAMA 162:856, 1956.
30. Hohl M: Soft-tissue injuries of the neck in automobile accidents: Factors influencing prognosis. J Bone Joint Surg Am 56:1675, 1974.
31. Braaf MM, Rosner S: Whiplash injury of neck—Fact or fancy? Int Surg 46:176, 1966.
32. Gore DR, Sepic SB, Gardner GM, Murray MP: Neck pain: A long-term follow-up of 205 patients. Spine 12:1, 1987.

Sources of Neck Pain

3

The patient with neck pain presents a challenge to the family practitioner, internist, rheumatologist, orthopedist, neurosurgeon, psychiatrist, osteopathic physician, and physical therapist. The patient's complaint is a symptom, not a diagnosis. The number of anatomic parts of the cervical spine that have the potential to cause pain is substantial. In addition, the spectrum of disease processes that may affect neck structures is broad. Compounding the problem are the patients who have neck pain that is associated with a work-related or motor vehicle injury. The extent and intensity of symptoms may be exaggerated by nonphysiologic factors. The physician's task in treating patients with neck pain is to identify the likely source of pain and the pathologic process causing it. Only then may the physician feel reasonably confident in implementing appropriate therapy.

Unfortunately, in many circumstances, a physician may not fully examine a patient with neck pain. There are many reasons for an incomplete examination, including the number of patients with the symptom of neck pain, the natural history of the neck pain, the effect of nonphysiologic factors on the severity and duration of symptoms, and the physician's degree of knowledge of the functional anatomy of that part of the body.

Although neck pain is less common than back pain, physicians see many patients with cervical spine symptoms. The natural history of neck pain is one of rapid improvement, similar to that of low back pain. Eighty percent to 90% of patients with neck pain are better within 2 months, with or without intervention of a physician. The need for making a specific diagnosis at the initial visit is not important from a practical standpoint. Most patients will improve, and most patients have a mechanical,

noninflammatory, cause for their neck pain (muscle strain, annular tear of an intervertebral disc), not an underlying serious, systemic illness. Identifying the source of a patient's pain to be ligamentous, muscular, or articular in origin in this acute circumstance does not significantly alter therapy or hasten recovery. Furthermore, some physicians may have developed a skepticism about the severity of patients' symptoms of neck pain. Physicians are taught to believe that patients will be honest about the severity of their symptoms because it is in their self-interest. When that honesty seems questionable, the physician believes there is a breach of trust. This skepticism occurs among physicians whose patients are involved in motor vehicle accidents or work-related injuries. Some physicians see so many of these patients that they have stopped "evaluating" them. A patient may have a motive for continuing to have pain—to increase a monetary reward or to get a light-duty job at work. This distrust is destructive to the physician-patient relationship and results in patients who might be helped being denied appropriate care. The manipulation of workers' compensation or insurance systems by a few individuals should not influence the way a physician treats patients with neck pain.

It is not uncommon for a physician to be more familiar with the functional anatomy of organs of the chest and abdomen than with those of the cervical spine. It is left to the orthopedists and neurosurgeons to be concerned with anatomic relationships and sensory innervation of the structures of the neck. Unfortunately, this is a shortsighted view of a complicated problem. Only with familiarity with anatomic sources of pain in the cervical spine and the mechanism of pain transmission and inhibition can a physician adequately evaluate patients with neck pain. With greater knowledge of functional anatomy and patho-physiologic effects of disease processes on the structures of the cervical spine, a physician is better able to differentiate those individuals with a potentially more ominous cause of neck pain from those with mechanical abnormalities. The physician may also be better able to differentiate the various causes of mechanical neck pain. The significant differences between acute and chronic pain take on greater importance in regard to goals for therapy. Not only does understanding of the sources of pain help in the differential diagnosis of diseases of the cervical spine, it also provides a rationale for a variety of therapeutic modalities used for patients with neck pain. These therapies treat the mechanisms that cause continued pain in areas of healed, structural injury. The purpose of this chapter is to review pain physiology and to discuss the sources and character of pain associated with abnormalities involving the anatomic structures of the cervical spine.

PAIN PRODUCTION AND TRANSMISSION

Pain is defined by pain specialists (algologists) as an unpleasant sensory and emotional experience associated with actual or potential tissue damage, or an experience described in terms of such damage. Pain is a subjective, individual perception related to mechanical and chemical alterations of body tissues. This means that pain is perceived in the cortical portions of the central nervous system; it is not dependent on the precise nature or absolute amount of tissue destruction peripherally. This potential separation of tissue destruction from the perception of pain emphasizes the fact that pain messages can be modified at many levels of the nervous system.

The peripheral nervous system contains a wide range of nerve fibers. Myelinated somatic nerves are called A fibers and are subdivided into four groups according to decreasing size: alpha, beta, gamma, and delta. The largest are the alpha fibers, which conduct impulses that serve motor function, proprioception, and reflex activity. Beta fibers also innervate muscle and convey touch and pressure sensations. For example, in the skin, A-beta fibers respond to light touch and the bending of hairs. Gamma fibers control muscle spindle tone. Delta fibers subserve pain and temperature functions. The thinly myelinated B fibers are preganglionic autonomic axons that innervate smooth muscle. The unmyelinated C fibers transmit nociceptive impulses (Table 3–1).

Bare nerve endings and specialized corpuscular receptors are the two kinds of receptor organs serving body sensory function.[1] They differ in their capacity to transform mechanical, thermal, and chemical energy into electrical impulses. The corpuscular receptors (mechanoreceptors) are most sensitive to mechanical vibratory energy. They are larger myelinated fibers (A-alpha and A-beta) that rapidly transmit information about innocuous mechanical stimuli to the cerebral cortex.

Another set of fibers responds only to stimuli associated with actual tissue damage. These fibers are called nociceptors. Mechanoreceptors and polymodal nociceptors are two primary forms of these nerve fibers. Mechanoreceptors transmit information about mechanical forces that cause tissue injury. Bare nerve

TABLE 3–1. PERIPHERAL NERVE FIBER CHARACTERISTICS

	MYELINATION	RECEPTOR TYPE	TRANSMISSION (m/sec)	THRESHOLD	DISTRIBUTION	MODALITY
A-alpha	+	Mechanoreceptor	Rapid (70–120)	Low	Local	Vibration (proprioception) Pain (prick)
A-beta	+	Mechanoreceptor	Rapid (40–70)	Low	Local	Vibration (proprioception) Reflex withdrawal
A-gamma	+	Mechanoreceptor	Rapid (20–40)	Low	Local	Muscle spindle
A-delta	+	Mechanonociceptor	Slow (5–15)	High	Local	Damaging pressure
A-delta	+	Thermal mechano-nociceptor	Slow (5–15)	High	Local	Noxious Temperature (sharp)
B	+	Autonomic	Slow (10–15)	High	Diffuse	Preganglionic fibers
C	−	Mechanonociceptor	Slow (0.2–1.5)	High	Diffuse	Noxious
C	−	Polymodal nociceptor	Slow (0.2–1.5)	High	Diffuse	Pressure (sharp) Any noxious stimulus (dull)

endings, in contrast, are sensitive to all physical modalities (such as heat and chemical injury) but differ in their individual sensitivity and threshold to different stimuli.

Nociceptors have two mechanisms to differentiate innocuous from noxious stimuli. These mechanisms are the association of intensity of tissue damage with frequency of nerve impulses and a high threshold for stimulation. The highest neural firing rates occur when nociceptors respond to stimuli in the noxious range.

Nociceptive impulses are carried by two sizes of nerve endings. The largest of the two types of pain fiber is the A-delta fiber, 6 to 8 μm in diameter, which is thinly myelinated and conducts impulses relatively quickly (12 μm/sec). Some A-delta fibers respond mainly to mechanical energy and accurately locate a site of injury. Others respond to chemical or thermal stimulation in proportion to the degree of injury. More frequent nerve firings are associated with greater tissue damage.[2] Some A-delta fibers may be polymodal responders, which fire after a high threshold has been reached and tissue damage has occurred. These fibers lower their active thresholds once they have been exposed to other noxious stimuli.[3] In the sensitized state, innocuous mechanical stimuli that previously evoked no response produce nociceptive impulses that continue following cessation of the stimulus. Sensitization plays a role in the prolongation of acute pain and the development of chronic pain. Complete destruction of a receptor does not block the sensitized transmission of impulses from undamaged receptors of the same axon.[4] Focal areas of demyelination caused by chronic irritation may give rise to spontaneous action potentials that travel in an anterograde or retrograde direction. In these injured nerves, normal stimulation may evoke sustained after-discharges.

The smaller, unmyelinated C fibers, 0.3 to 1.0 μm in diameter, conduct impulses slowly (0.4 to 1.0 m/sec), are polymodal responders (mechanical, chemical, heat), and are activated only by tissue destruction. These receptors show continued or delayed firing after the physical stimulus has been discontinued. After repeated or prolonged stimulation, their threshold for activation can diminish to levels of intensity that are usually innocuous.[5] Humoral mediators and chemical substances released during acute inflammation and tissue destruction may play a role temporally in C fiber transmission. Peptides, such as bradyki-

nin, are released after a latency of 15 to 30 seconds and reach a peak 15 seconds after the latency period, which may contribute to the delayed and continued firing of high-threshold receptors. Other factors that may play similar roles in nociceptive potentiation are potassium, histamine, substance P, serotonin, and prostaglandins.[6, 7] In combination, these nociceptive A-delta and C fibers detect noxious stimuli that damage body structures. For example, muscle pain is mediated by both A-delta and C fibers. The A-delta fibers are activated by release of histamine, serotonin, and bradykinin during intense exercise. The C fibers respond to rapid contractions of muscle but not to by-products of muscle metabolism.

The interaction of the chemical mediators of inflammation, peripheral inflammatory cells, and neuropeptides that mediate nociceptive stimulation is complex.[8] The products of inflammation released during tissue destruction sensitize and stimulate peripheral nociceptors. The nociceptors produce neurotransmitters that stimulate the C fiber (Table 3–2). The excitation of the primary afferent also produces an axon reflex that results in the peripheral release of neuropeptides such as substance P, neurokinin A, and calcitonin gene-related peptide. Other identified sensitizing factors include interleukin-1, neutrophil-chemotactic peptides, and nerve growth factor-derived octapeptide.[9] A combination of chemical mediators and peripheral white blood cells affects the transmission of nociceptive impulses (Fig. 3–1). Some of these neuropeptides are the same mediators that stimulate second-order neurons in the spinal cord. The tissue damage caused by the direct stimulation of peripheral nociceptive fibers is called neurogenic inflammation.[10]

The two groups of pain fibers are associated with two dissociable types of sensory input. The pinprick type of sensation, which is quick in onset and well localized, is carried in the larger, myelinated A fibers. These fibers be-

TABLE 3–2. MEDIATORS OF PERIPHERAL NOCICEPTIVE TRANSMISSION

CHEMICAL MEDIATORS	NEUROTRANSMITTERS
Bradykinin	Substance P
Prostaglandins	Norepinephrine
Leukotrienes	Neurokinin A
Histamine	Calcitonin gene-related peptide
Serotonin	

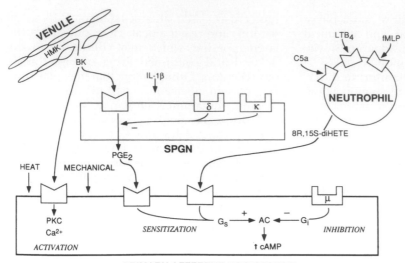

Figure 3–1. Sites of peptide action in peripheral pathways of pain and hyperalgesia. The inflammatory peptide bradykinin (BK), cleaved from high-molecular-weight kininogen (HMK) circulating in the venules, can activate the primary afferent nociceptor (PAN) in a protein kinase C (PKC)- and Ca^{2+}-dependent mechanism or sensitize the PAN through the production of PGE_2 in sympathetic postganglionic neurons (SPGN). Opioid ligands can do so at the level of the PAN via the inhibitory G protein. Interleukin-1β is IL-1β; leukotriene B_4 is LTB_4; prostaglandin E_2 is PGE_2. (From Levine JD, Fields HL, Basbaum AI: Peptides and the primary afferent nociceptor. J Neurosci 13:2275, 1993.)

long to a phylogenetically newer sensory system that ascends to the sensory cortex with few interposed relays. This type of pain results in rapid movement, quick protection, and reflex withdrawal from a potentially damaging stimulus. The later, dull, aching, less localized sensation is carried by the unmyelinated C fibers. These smaller fibers belong to a phylogenetically older sensory system with multiple relays in the medulla and thalamus.[11] The pain associated with C fiber stimulation produces tonic contraction, which functions to guard and protect the injured part.

The Dorsal Horn

Dorsal horn neurons are classified according to their response to primary afferent input. Low-threshold neurons respond only to non-noxious stimuli such as hair movement or touch. High-threshold neurons are nociceptive specific, responding to excessive joint movement. Dorsal horn neurons stimulated by noxious and non-noxious stimuli are classified as wide dynamic range neurons. These neurons have graded responses that increase with increasing intensities of stimulation. Wide-dynamic-range neurons respond to hair movement, pressure, pinch, or pinprick.

The nociceptive A-delta and C fibers with nerve endings in the periphery and their cell bodies in the dorsal root ganglion have destination points in the dorsal horn of the spinal cord.[12] Of the six specialized layers (laminae) of nerve endings that are laminated in the dorsal horn, layers I, II, and V receive nociceptive fibers (Fig. 3–2). Laminae III and IV receive primary afferent input from large-fiber, low-threshold neurons involved with spinal cord processing of proprioception. Lamina VI has low-threshold and wide-dynamic-range neurons that may share some function with lamina V in transmission of nociceptive information to supraspinal sites. This organization of the dorsal horn has physiologic importance. Small-caliber myelinated fibers ascend or descend in Lissauer's tract for one or two segments before entering the dorsal gray matter. They terminate in lamina I and the bottom of lamina II. Lamina I receives A-delta mechanoreceptors and some polymodal C afferents. The sensory input is from the skin and muscle nociceptors that have a small peripheral receptive field. These neurons are important in signaling the presence of pain, but they are unlikely to transmit information concerning the intensity or nature of the painful stimulus.[13] In contrast, cells in lamina V receive more specific information because of the convergent input of rapidly conducting A-beta fibers and of the more slowly conducting A-delta and C nociceptive fibers (wide dynamic range neurons). These fibers respond to mechanical or thermal stimuli, steadily increasing their discharge frequency with the intensity of the noxious stimulus. Lamina V conveys the information concerning the location, intensity, and form of harmful stimuli. These axons contain substance P, a neurotransmitter that is most highly concentrated in the superficial layers of the dorsal horn.[14] Substance P plays an important role in dorsal horn transmission of nociception. Dorsal horn nociceptors are substantially stimulated by substance P. Capsaicin, the active ingredient in hot peppers, has

PAIN RELATED FIBERS IN THE DORSAL HORN OF THE SPINAL CORD

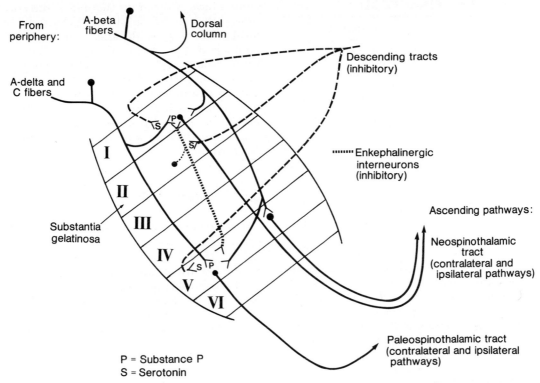

P = Substance P
S = Serotonin

Figure 3–2. The dorsal horn: this graphic demonstrates the organization of the pain-related fibers in the dorsal horn. Nociceptive A-delta and C fibers carry pain messages from the periphery to laminae I and V. These nerves release substance P. These neurons synapse with second-order relay neurons, which ascend in the rapid pathway (neospinothalamic tract) and/or the slow pathway (paleospinothalamic tract). The nociceptive messages of these neurons are modified presynaptically by collateral branches of the large low-threshold cutaneous mechanoreceptors (A-beta fibers) whose main branches ascend in the ipsilateral dorsal columns. The nociceptive fibers are also inhibited by enkephalinergic interneurons whose cell bodies are situated in lamina II. The enkephalinergic cells are driven by the large peripheral A afferents or the serotoninergic fibers descending in the dorsolateral white funiculus of the spinal cord. Descending tracts also attach presynaptically to nociceptors in laminae I and V to inhibit pain transmission.

a significant effect on the transmission of nociceptive impulses.[15] Initially, capsaicin activates nociceptors selectively. A later effect of capsaicin on nerve fibers is the depletion of substance P. Depletion of substance P in the spinal cord with capsaicin is associated with decreased transmission of nociceptive impulses.[16]

Substance P is an undecapeptide that is present in 20% of dorsal root ganglion neurons. Substance P is a member of a group of peptides, the tachykinins or neurokinins. Although substance P is present in nociceptors, this neurotransmitter is not solely associated with pain transmission because it is also found in non-nociceptive fibers.[17] Dorsal root ganglion nerves contain a variety of neurotransmitters. Afferents innervating different organs differ consistently in their peptide content. The peptide content of primary afferents is determined by specific factors in the tissues they innervate. In addition, peptide content changes dramatically in response to certain prolonged stimuli or nerve damage. However, control of substance P levels does not totally eliminate the production of pain transmission in the nociceptor.

Substance P, along with other chemical mediators, may contribute to the severity of injury associated with joint inflammation.[18] Depletion of substance P concentrations in animal models of arthritis is associated with less severe joint damage.[19] Substance P is only one of an ever-increasing number of neuropeptides associated with modulation of sensory input in the spinal cord[8] (Table 3–3). Many fibers produce more than one neuropeptide. For example, substance P and calcitonin gene-re-

TABLE 3–3. NEUROPEPTIDES MODULATING NOCICEPTIVE INPUT IN THE SPINAL CORD

STIMULATORY	INHIBITORY
Substance P	Serotonin
Neurokinin A	Somatostatin
Glutamate	Cholecystokinin
Aspartate	Norepinephrine
Vasoactive intestinal polypeptide	Gamma-aminobutyric acid
Calcitonin gene-related peptide	Glycine
	Endogenous opioid peptides
	β-endorphin
	Enkephalin
	Dynorphin

lated peptide are released simultaneously by neurons in the spinal cord.[20] Excitatory amino acids, such as aspartate and glutamate, are also neurotransmitters in the spinal cord. One hypothesis has suggested that excitatory amino acids are the mediators of fast nociceptive transmission, and the neuropeptides are the mediators of slow transmission.[16] The repertoire of neuropeptides and excitatory amino acids associated with a specific noxious stimulus has not been determined. These neuropeptides have effects not only at the level of their nerve source but may also diffuse to act at a distance from their site of release (Fig. 3–3).

The unmyelinated fibers from lamina V supply not only the skin and muscles but also other somatic structures such as joints and ligaments. In addition, visceral afferents converge on the wide-dynamic-range neurons in lamina V that supply sensory innervation for somatic structures, including skin. It is important to remember that on entering the spinal cord the visceral fibers travel caudally or cranially for several segments in the posterior horn of gray matter before synapsing with neurons in the dorsal horn. The "referred pain" associated with visceral disease processes occurs secondarily to "cross-talk" between visceral sensory afferents and the wide-dynamic-range neurons that supply sensation to cutaneous structures. This convergence of afferent nerves allows for the summation of nociceptive input on a spatial and temporal basis. Stimulation of the visceral afferents results in a wide field of cutaneous nerve stimulation, which activates secondary neurons ascending to the midbrain. This diffuse stimulation results in the perception that the skin has been stimulated when in fact the actual source of the sensory input is the visceral afferents.[21]

Lamina II (substantia gelatenosa) receives the majority of the slow, unmyelinated C afferents. Although a small number of cells in this lamina have projections that reach the cortex, most cells in the substantia gelatinosa have local connections with other neurons in other laminae at the same segmental level and with the substantia gelatinosa on the opposite side of the spinal cord. This connection is accomplished through commissural fibers that cross the spinal cord. These nerves have inhibitory effects on pain transmission. Most of the C fibers interconnect with descending inhibitory neurons.[22]

Spinothalamic Tract

The majority of the second-order neurons connect with incoming afferent neurons in laminae I and V of the dorsal horn and cross to the contralateral side at the same spinal cord level to ascend rostrally in the anterolateral spinothalamic tract (neospinothalamic tract) (Fig. 3–4). Phylogenetically, the neospinothalamic tract is the newer pain sensory tract in the human nervous system. The neo-

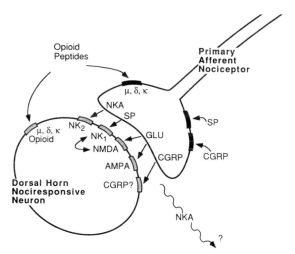

Figure 3–3. Primary afferents and peptide actions in the CNS. The PAN releases a variety of co-occurring neuropeptides (NKA, SP, CGRP) and excitatory amino acids (e.g., glutamate [GLU]). These act at several postsynaptic receptors: the NK_1 and NK_2 tachykinin receptors, the CGRP receptor, and the NMDA and AMPA excitatory amino receptors. NKA may diffuse to act at a distance from its site of release. There is evidence that SP and CGRP also act at autoreceptors at neuropeptide-containing primary afferent terminals. In addition, opioid peptides act upon both pre- and postsynaptic μ-, δ-, and κ-opioid receptors to modulate transmitter release and the firing of second-order nociresponsive neurons. (From Levine JD, Fields HL, Basbaum AI: Peptides and the primary afferent nociceptor. J Neurosci 13:2279, 1993.)

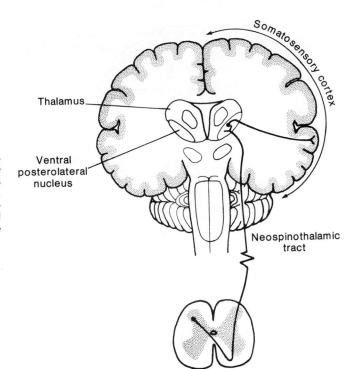

Figure 3–4. The neospinothalamic tract consists of a rapid three-neuron relay system from the dorsal horn to the ventral posterolateral nucleus of the thalamus to the somatosensory cortex. This rapid system, with its somatotopic organization, allows for analysis of the site, intensity, and nature of pain but provides no means to activate evasive motor action.

spinothalamic tract courses upward in the spinal cord with new fibers, at each spinal level, joining medially pushing axons from more caudal segments laterally. This organization preserves the somatotopic organization of the tract in the spinal cord. These fibers terminate in the posterior nuclear group of the thalamus, particularly the ventral posterolateral nucleus. Third-order neurons carry impulses from the thalamus to the posterior central gyrus of the parietal cortex. This rapid system, with its somatotopic organization, allows for analysis of the site, intensity, and nature of pain (pricking, pressing, throbbing, stabbing, or burning). However, this rapid transit system provides no means to mediate reflexes to activate the motor system for evasive action or to alter cortical function to increase alertness. The neospinothalamic tract also has a polysynaptic portion with fibers branching with collaterals that enter the reticular system of the brainstem. Some of these collaterals synapse on cells that provide nociceptive information to the descending inhibitory system.[23]

The phylogenetically older anterior division, the paleospinothalamic tract, supplies the connections for the cortical response to pain (Fig. 3–5). These include suffering, which is a negative affective response to pain; fear; and depression. The second-order neurons of this tract send multiple connections to the reticular formation of the brain stem while traveling to the midline and intralaminar nuclei of the thalamus. The higher-order neurons that emerge from the reticular formation and thalamic nuclei connect with other thalamic nuclei, the hypothalamus, the basal ganglia, and the midbrain central gray area. From these structures, a multitude of higher-order neurons synapse with a number of cortical areas, including the frontal lobe (pain perception), temporal lobe (recent and long-term memory), and hypothalamus (autonomic sympathetic and parasympathetic reflexes).[24] These cortical functions work independently of each other; the intensity of nociceptive input does not necessarily result in a specific emotional response or autonomic reflexes such as increased heart rate and blood pressure or increased gastrointestinal secretion and motility.

The connections of the nociceptors with a number of different areas of the cerebral cortex underscore the definition of pain as a subjective response that is a summation of total sensory input. Pain has sensory-discriminative, motivational-affective, and cognitive-evaluative dimensions.[25] The neospinothalamic tract contributes to the sensory-discriminative dimension. The cortical projection of this system transmits information that characterizes the spatial, temporal, and magnitude properties of a noxious stimulus. The brainstem retic-

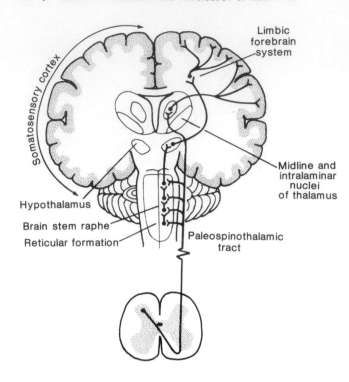

Figure 3–5. The paleospinothalamic tract consists of a slow multineuron relay system from the dorsal horn to the brain stem, hypothalamus, thalamus, and limbic forebrain system. This tract mediates reflexes and integrated responses (fear, memory, suffering) related to nociceptive impulses.

ular formation and the limbic system play a significant role in the motivational-affective dimension. The paleospinothalamic tract supplies the nerves with multiple synapses in the reticular system. These nerves do not carry spatial or temporal information because target cells in the brain stem and cortex have wide receptive fields covering half or more of the body surface. Effects of sight and sound on pain perception occur through connections in the reticular system. Escape and protective behaviors are mediated through the reticular-limbic system. This system acts as an intensity monitor and contributes to the quality of unpleasantness, mobilizes internal defenses, and elicits behavior geared to avoiding or stopping the distress.

Cognitive functions—memory, cultural values, and anxiety—also play a significant role in the perception of pain. A new pain with little associated damage may be perceived as severe because of the fear of the unknown, whereas a pain associated with greater tissue damage may not elicit the same degree of discomfort because its cause is familiar. This central cognitive system evaluates and analyzes input in terms of past experience, probability of outcome, and symbolic importance. This system facilitates or inhibits activities in the sensory and motivational systems by modulating activity of inhibitory neurons in the substantia gelatinosa.

Another important connection between nerves at the level of the dorsal horn is the synapse between dorsal horn sensory fibers and anterior horn motor fibers. Through direct synapse with internuncial nerves, input from sensory nerves stimulates motor neurons at the same or neighboring segmental levels. This stimulation may result in reflex action that causes an instantaneous contraction of a muscle or a more tonic contraction (spasm) with repeated stimulation of nociceptive fibers.

Descending Analgesic Pathways

In addition to the two distinct sensory pathways that transmit nociceptive signals to brainstem and cortical structures, the cortex and midbrain have descending pathways that modulate pain input at the level of the dorsal horn[26] (Fig. 3–6). Neurons surrounding the cerebral aqueduct of the midbrain and the brain stem raphe in medullopontine reticular formation terminate on interneurons present in lamina II (substantia gelatinosa).[27] The entire descending network extends from the frontal cortex and hypothalamus, through the periaqueductal gray zone to the rostral ventromedial medulla, and then via the dorsolateral funiculus to the dorsal horn of the spinal cord. The dorsolateral pontomesencephalic tegmen-

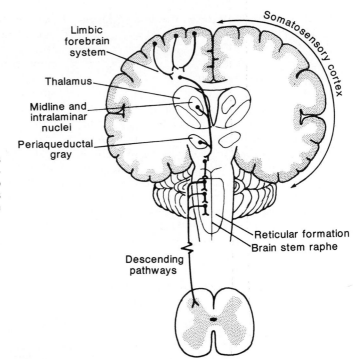

Figure 3–6. Descending pathways carry signals from higher brain centers through the periaqueductal gray and the brain stem raphe back to the dorsal horn, whereas its associated neurons release serotonin and inhibit pain transmission through nociceptive fibers.

tum is a parallel system projecting to the rostral ventromedial medulla that also modulates pain signals generated in the spinal cord.[28] The neurotransmitter for this descending pathway is serotonin (5-hydroxytryptamine). Serotoninergic cells activate enkephalinergic interneurons that exert presynaptic inhibition of the small unmyelinated nociceptors that produce substance P.

Enkephalins are pentapeptides that are secreted by neurons where there are opiate receptors.[29] Substance P is produced by unmyelinated nociceptive fibers.[30] The release of enkephalin inhibits substance P–sensitive nociceptors, decreasing the ascending signals. This inhibitory process relies on opiate receptors for its action. Naloxone, an opiate antagonist, temporarily reverses the analgesic effects of activation of the periaqueductal gray and raphe neurons. Two other descending analgesic fiber systems include neurons from the locus ceruleus (neurotransmitter—norepinephrine) and Edinger-Westphal nucleus (neurotransmitter—cholecystokinin). The exact location for the interaction of these systems and neurons in the dorsal horn is unknown.

In addition to the descending analgesic pathways, segmental input from myelinated mechanoreceptors that synapse with small-diameter nociceptive afferents inhibits pain transmission. The modulation of nociceptive input by massage, compression, or vibration of tissues is the cornerstone of the "gate theory of pain."[31] A limited amount of sensory information can activate ascending fibers terminating in the brain stem and cortical portions of the nervous system. A gate at the level of the spinal cord can swing open to allow nociceptive impulses or proprioceptive impulses to pass through. Stimulation of myelinated A-beta (mechanoreceptor) fibers inhibits (closes the gate to) transmission of A-delta and C nociceptive fibers. The substantia gelatinosa (lamina II) is the location for this interaction. This inhibition is not related to opioid receptors because this effect is independent of naloxone (narcotic antagonist).[32] The enkephalinergic interneurons and the descending inhibitory neurons also serve to close the gate to pain transmission.

The clinical correlation of pain moderation by proprioceptive stimulation is the practice of rubbing the area after it has been injured. This maneuver activates large low-threshold fibers, reducing the effects of small fiber input to a level at which pain is less severe. The procedure of transcutaneous electrical nerve stimulation in diminishing pain is based on this principle. On the other hand, disease processes that diminish large fiber input may magnify painful stimuli. Herpes zoster viral infection, which preferentially damages large-fiber vibratory, dorsal ganglion cells, may result in hyperesthesia in the sensory field of the affected nerve secondary to the loss of large-fiber, proprioceptive input.

Visceral Sensory System

The sensory nerves for the thoracic, abdominal, and pelvic viscera have cell bodies in the dorsal root ganglia but do not use the spinal nerves to reach the target organ. Instead these nerves pass through the pathways of the sympathetic and parasympathetic nervous systems. The sympathetic trunks are longitudinal strands of nerve fibers and sympathetic ganglia that lie anterolateral to the vertebral column from the level of the first cervical vertebra to the front of the coccyx. The sympathetic trunk in the neck does not receive white rami communicantes, but it contains three cervical sympathetic ganglia (interior, middle, and superior) that receive their preganglionic fibers from the upper thoracic spinal nerves via white rami communicantes whose fibers leave the spinal cord on the ventral roots of thoracic spinal nerves. From the sympathetic trunk in the neck, fibers pass to the structures as postganglionic fibers in cervical spinal nerves or leave as direct visceral branches (e.g., to the thyroid gland). Branches to the head run with arteries, especially the internal and external carotid arteries (Fig. 3–7).

The inferior cervical ganglion lies at the level of the neck of the first rib, where it is wrapped around the posterior aspect of the vertebral artery. It is usually fused with the first thoracic ganglion (and sometimes the second) to form a large ganglion known as the cervicothoracic ganglion (stellate ganglion). It lies

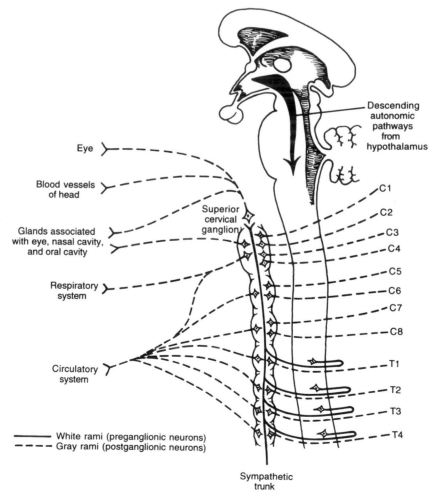

Figure 3–7. The autonomic nervous system. The sympathetic (thoracolumbar) division of the autonomic nervous system. Preganglionic fibers extend from the intermediolateral nucleus of the spinal cord to the peripheral autonomic ganglia, and postganglionic fibers extend from the peripheral ganglia to the effector organs as shown. Sympathetic outflow from the spinal cord. The preganglionic fibers are shown in heavy lines, and the postganglionic fibers are in dashed lines.

anterior to the transverse process of C7, just above the neck of the first rib on each side, posterior to the origin of the vertebral artery. Some postganglionic fibers from this ganglion pass into the seventh and eighth cervical nerves and to the heart and the vertebral plexus around the vertebral artery.

The middle cervical ganglion is small and lies on the anterior aspect of the middle thyroid artery at about the level of the cricoid cartilage and the transverse process of C6, just anterior to the vertebral artery. Postganglionic branches pass from it to the fifth and sixth cervical nerves and to the heart and the thyroid gland.

The superior cervical ganglion is large. It is located at the level of the atlas and axis. Postganglionic branches from it pass along the internal carotid artery and enter the head. It also sends branches to the external carotid artery and into the upper four cervical nerves.

It is important to remember that the segmental innervation of a visceral organ is not dependent on its location in the fully mature human but rather on its embryologic segment of origin because sensory nerves grow into the viscera early in their development before they migrate to their final anatomic destination. An example is subdiaphragmatic irritation, which presents as referred pain to the shoulder. In addition, the organization of visceral afferents in the dorsal horn also plays an important role in the distribution of visceral pain. Visceral afferents synapse in lamina V with wide dynamic range neurons. These visceral neurons have a wide field of innervation. A single visceral fiber may synapse with a number of cutaneous afferents. Stimulation of the visceral afferent activates a wide field of cutaneous nociceptors whose activity is perceived as referred pain (Fig. 3–7). The visceral afferents are also closely associated with activation of sympathetic and parasympathetic nerves. Stimulation of visceral afferents, in the appropriate circumstances, activates autonomic nerve fibers, resulting in, for example, vasoconstriction, vasodilation, flushing, or tachycardia. The field of activated nociceptors may be transmitted to several segmental levels, whereas somatic pain is transmitted to a single level.

Segmental Innervation

A brief review of the embryologic origin of the axial skeleton and the peripheral nervous system provides the anatomic background for understanding the clinical symptoms associated with disorders of the cervical spine. By the end of the second week, the notochord forms on the dorsum of the embryonic disc between the endoderm and ectoderm. The notochord is the central framework of the spine and is eventually absorbed into the vertebral column where its remnants form the nucleus pulposus of the intervertebral disc. By the third week, mesodermal cells that parallel the notochord start to segment into individual somites. The somites subsequently differentiate into three primary parts: skin (dermatome); muscle, tendon, and ligaments (myotome); and bone (sclerotome). Simultaneously, the corresponding spinal nerve for each somite develops from the neural tube, supplying innervation for three components of the somite. As the skin, muscle, and bone develop and migrate to their final location in the body, each segment takes along its corresponding nerve supply in its cells. Structures from one somite, which includes parts of the neck, shoulder, arm, and cervical spine, may all become painful if one component is damaged.

The embryologic organization of segmental structures is evident in the innervation of skin, muscle, and bones of the cervical spine and upper extremities. The sensory nervous system is organized segmentally. Each dorsal root ganglion supplies a particular segment. Topographically, on the surface of the body, the segments are ordered into cutaneous dermatomes. The same dermatomes cover areas both in the cervical spine as well as the upper extremity. Although this organization may seem confusing when viewing the body in an upright position, the organization becomes clearer when the body is placed in a quadruped orientation (Fig. 3–8). Dermatomes stretch from areas in the cervical spine to contiguous areas in the upper extremity. The C6, C7, and C8 segments have no cutaneous branches in the cervical spine. They supply cutaneous structures in the arm situated between the C5 and T1 segments.

It is important to remember that the distribution of these dermatomes is not absolute and may vary from individual to individual. The dermatomes overlap each other and extend slightly past the midline (Figs. 3–9 and 3–10). For deeper somatic structures (muscles, joint capsule, tendons), the sensory fibers correspond with the same spinal cord segment that supplies motor nerves to those muscles. On the other hand, as previously mentioned, the segmental innervation of the viscera that

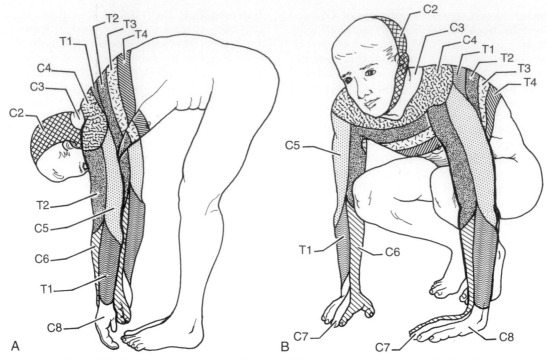

Figure 3–8. *A* and *B*, Organization of the cervical dermatomes in the quadruped orientation.

are supplied with visceral afferents corresponds with the level of embryologic origin rather than with the actual anatomic location. Figures 3–11 through 3–19 list the dermatome, myotome, and sclerotome for the cervical and first thoracic nerves. Review of these figures reveals the extent of the innervation of structures from individual spinal cord levels and marked overlap among the levels. The complexity of innervation of the cervical spine and surrounding organs occurs because of structural duplication and individual variation. It is important for physicians evaluating patients with neck, shoulder, or arm pain to keep the overlap and variation of innervation from individual to individual in mind when evaluating referred pain.

CLINICAL INTERPRETATION OF NECK PAIN

The challenge for the clinician is to translate the patient's description of pain into anatomic and physiologic correlates that will identify the structure that has been "injured" and the pathologic process that has resulted in pain. Anatomically, structures of the cervical spine receive specific types of sensory innervation that are associated with distinct qualities of pain (i.e., sharp, dull, aching, throbbing,

burning). An understanding of the quality of pain associated with pathologic processes in specific structures helps identify the source of the pain. In addition to quality, pain may be categorized by its intensity, location, onset and duration, aggravating and alleviating factors, and behavioral response (Table 3–4).[33, 34] The sources of neck pain are superficial somatic, deep somatic (spondylogenic), radicular, neurogenic, viscerogenic referred, and psychogenic.

Superficial Somatic Pain

The skin and subcutaneous fibers of the neck are innervated by nociceptive nerve fibers that cover small areas. Pathologic processes in the skin result in localized lesions whose intensity correlates with the extent of tissue distention and damage. The involvement of superficial tissues of the neck with trauma (laceration, burning, compression), ulceration, superficial neoplasms, or infections (cellulitis) is usually recognized rapidly because of location and is not of great diagnostic difficulty. The exception may be patients who present with the burning pain of herpes zoster infection prior to the appearance of vesicles. The acute onset and distribution in a dermato-

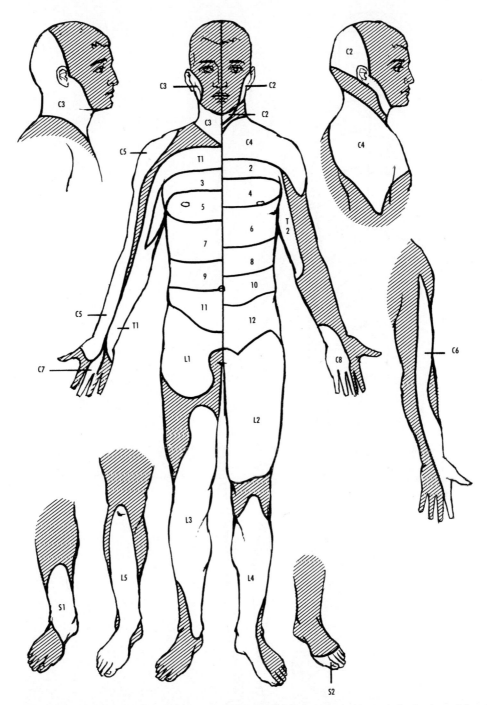

Figure 3–9. Dermatomal distribution (frontal view). The right and left halves show the total distribution of the alternating dermatomes, illustrating the overlap that may involve two or more dermatomes. The insets demonstrate the broad distribution of certain dermatomes. (Adapted from Gardner E, Gray DJ, O'Rahilly R: Anatomy, 4th ed. Philadelphia: WB Saunders Co, 1975.)

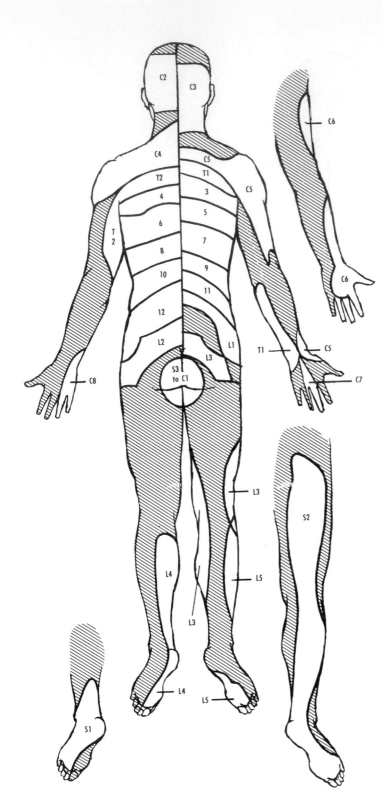

Figure 3–10. Dermatomal distribution (posterior view). (Adapted from Gardner E, Gray DJ, O'Rahilly R: Anatomy, 4th ed. Philadelphia: WB Saunders Co, 1975.)

C1

DERMATOME
- Posterior scalp
- Retro-orbital area
- Forehead

MYOTOME
Muscles
- Head flexors
- Head extensors
- Head rotators

SCLEROTOME
Bones
- Atlas
- Occiput

Ligaments
- Atlanto-occipital
- Medial atlanto-occipital
- Alar
- Apical dental
- Cruciform
- Accessory atlantoaxial
- Articular capsule
- Nuchal
- Atlanto-occipital (anterior, posterior)

(Pain perceived: forehead, retro-orbital area, and temple)

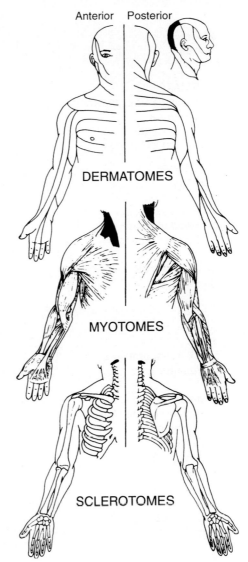

Anterior   Posterior

DERMATOMES

MYOTOMES

SCLEROTOMES

Figure 3–11. Dermatome, myotome, and sclerotome distribution for C1.

mal pattern should alert the clinician to this possibility.

Deep Somatic (Spondylogenic) Pain

The parts of the cervical spine that are the sources of deep somatic pain are the structures of the vertebral column, the surrounding muscles, and the attaching tendons, ligaments, and fascia. Processes that mechanically disrupt these structures result in neck pain. In addition, inflammatory processes that destroy tissue or increase tissue tension cause pain. Increased vascular pressure that results in distended vessels may also cause pain.

In general, with the exception of inflamma-

tory and neoplastic processes, spondylogenic pain is characterized by a deep, dull ache that is maximum over the involved site. The pain is exacerbated by specific motions and is relieved by recumbency. The most common cause of spondylogenic pain is the production of high tensions in the muscles of the neck, which leads to avulsion of tendinous attachments of muscles to bony structures or rupture of muscle fibers or tearing of muscles sheaths (sudden recruitment of muscle bundles when muscles are flexed and relaxed).[35] Pain associated with tendinous lesions is more severe than that associated with muscle injury proper. Either injury is associated with a sharp stab of pain at the moment of injury, followed by a dull ache that may persist for weeks along with

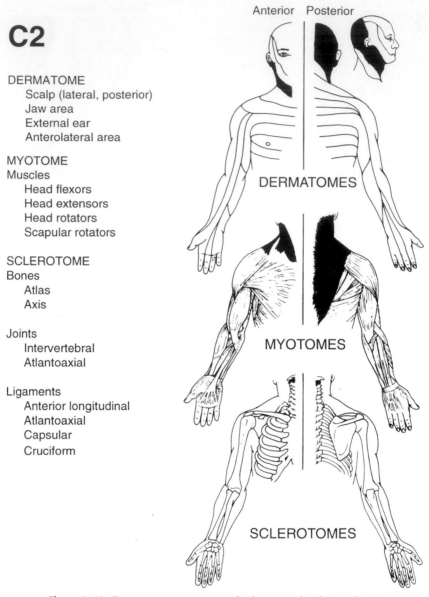

C2

DERMATOME
  Scalp (lateral, posterior)
  Jaw area
  External ear
  Anterolateral area

MYOTOME
Muscles
  Head flexors
  Head extensors
  Head rotators
  Scapular rotators

SCLEROTOME
Bones
  Atlas
  Axis

Joints
  Intervertebral
  Atlantoaxial

Ligaments
  Anterior longitudinal
  Atlantoaxial
  Capsular
  Cruciform

Figure 3–12. Dermatome, myotome, and sclerotome distribution for C2.

tenderness on palpation and reflex muscle spasm. The initial pain originates in the unmyelinated nerve fibers that are stimulated by the mechanical disruption of the tendons, fascial sheaths of muscles, or the surrounding intramuscular blood vessels. The prolonged aching pain is a result of the same nerve endings being stimulated by chemical mediators associated with the healing inflammatory response.[24]

Muscle pain may occur in the absence of true muscle injury. Persistent use of muscle groups results in muscle pain and, potentially, tonic contraction (spasm). The chronic use of a muscle, which occurs more commonly in untrained than in trained muscles, results in

increased metabolic activity and the production of chemical by-products that may stimulate unmyelinated nerve fibers. These by-products may include lactic acid and potassium. Physical factors (ambient temperature) and muscle training (sedentary versus athletic) may explain the reason for spondylogenic pain in the person whose abnormal posture results in persistent contraction of posterior cervical muscles, as often occurs with poorly designed data entry environments for typists. With increasing fatigue, primary muscles are unable to complete physical tasks, necessitating the recruitment of secondary muscle groups, at a greater risk for injury. The endurance of mus-

C3

DERMATOME
    Posterior, anterolateral neck
    Posterior scalp
    Clavicle

MYOTOME
Muscles
    Head flexors
    Head extensors
    Head rotators
    Lateral flexors

SCLEROTOME
Bones
    Vertebrae axis-C3

Joints
    Discs
    Luschka
    Sternoclavicular
    Zygapophyseal

Ligaments
    Anterior, posterior longitudinal
    Capsular
    Nuchal
    Ligamenta flava
    Interspinous

(Pain perceived: upper neck, jaw area,
 and anterior upper neck)

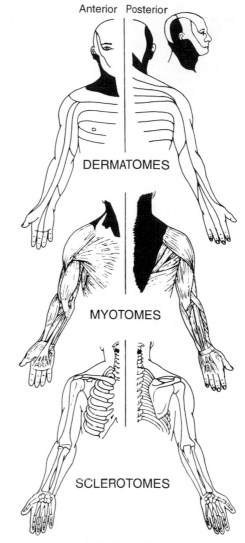

Anterior Posterior

DERMATOMES

MYOTOMES

SCLEROTOMES

Figure 3–13. Dermatome, myotome, and sclerotome distribution for C3.

cles may be more important as a predictor of pain than absolute strength of muscles.

Muscle hyperactivity may also develop secondary to nociceptive input from nonmuscular sources. Pathologic processes resulting in inflammatory or degenerative processes in facet joints, periosteum, skeleton, or visceral organs may cause muscle pain. It is difficult to differentiate reflex spasm secondary to mechanical, structural abnormalities from inflammatory lesions of the cervical spine or viscera. Taking a careful history and physical examination may help in suggesting the primary source of tissue injury. Of great importance in separating traumatic muscle spasm from reflex spasm is a history of partial injury. However, an episode of trauma is not always remembered by patients. In other circumstances, patients ascribe their symptoms of muscle pain to an insignificant episode of trauma when in fact their symptoms are secondary to a more serious illness (metastasis).

Other sources of spondylogenic nociceptive input are the anatomic components of the vertebral column, including joints, ligaments, bone, vessels, and the dural and epidural structures. Mechanical injury and resultant inflammation of the apophyseal joint capsule and ligamentous structure of the cervical spine may cause pain. Nerves that supply joints with sensory innervation frequently also supply surrounding muscle, bones and skin. There is usually an overlap of nerve innervation, with several nerves supplying a single joint. Terminal branches of unmyelinated and myelinated fibers are distributed through the synovium

C4

DERMATOME
    Summit of shoulder
    Region of clavicle
    Anterolateral neck

MYOTOME
Muscles
    Head and neck flexors
    Head and neck extensors
    Lateral flexors

SCLEROTOME
Bones
    Clavicle
    Vertebrae C3-C4

Joints
    Discs
    Luschka
    Zygapophyseal
    Sternoclavicular

Ligaments
    Anterior, posterior longitudinal
    Capsular
    Nuchal
    Ligamenta flava
    Interspinous

(Pain perceived: posterior neck,
scapular area, high thoracic spine)

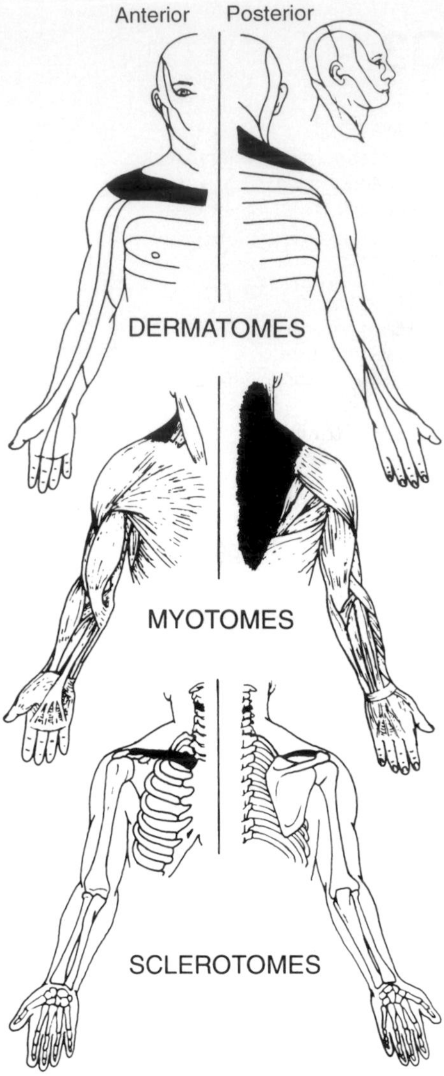

Figure 3–14. Dermatome, myotome, and sclerotome distribution for C4.

and periosteum. The joint capsule is richly supplied with sensory innervation. Sensory innervation to the joints includes mechanoreceptors in the joint capsule and nociceptors surrounding blood vessels and near the surface of synovial cells. The most painful stimuli to a joint are twisting, tearing, and stretching of the joint capsule or surrounding ligaments. The unmyelinated C nerve fibers of the posterior primary rami of multiple segments supply these structures. Therefore, patients have difficulty identifying the exact location for sources of their pain. Usually patients point to the midline or the occipitocervical joint area. Percussion tenderness does not cause as much discomfort in the joints as percussion over muscles in spasm. However, because of the distribution of the sensory and motor nerves, patients with articular and ligamentous disease may develop reflex spasm on both sides of the cervical spine and cutaneous hyperesthesia over the same areas.

Mechanical or inflammatory processes may cause joint pain. Mechanical stresses that stimulate nociceptors in the joint capsule may occur secondary to prolonged sitting or standing in inappropriate postures, atrophy of neck muscles, excess joint motion secondary to decreased disc or vertebral body height, or malformations. Inflammatory diseases of the axial skeleton joints may cause the production of joint swelling along with release of inflammatory mediators that are irritating to nociceptors in the fibrous capsule. Structural changes affecting articular cartilage and synovium may not be associated with pain because these tis-

C5

DERMATOME
  Anterior shoulder, arm, and forearm to wrist
  Lateral and ventral axial line
  Small area of back of neck

MYOTOME
Muscles
  Shoulder flexors
  Shoulder adductors
  Shoulder abductors
  Medial and lateral rotators
  Scapular elevators

SCLEROTOME
Bones
  Parts of humerus, scapula, proximal ulna
  Vertebrae C5-C6

Joints
  Acromioclavicular
  Glenohumeral
  Discs
  Luschka
  Elbow
  Zygapophyseal
  Sternoclavicular

Ligaments
  Anterior, posterior longitudinal
  Capsular
  Nuchal
  Ligamenta flava
  Interspinous

(Pain perceived: shoulder and arm,
 wider area than dermatome)

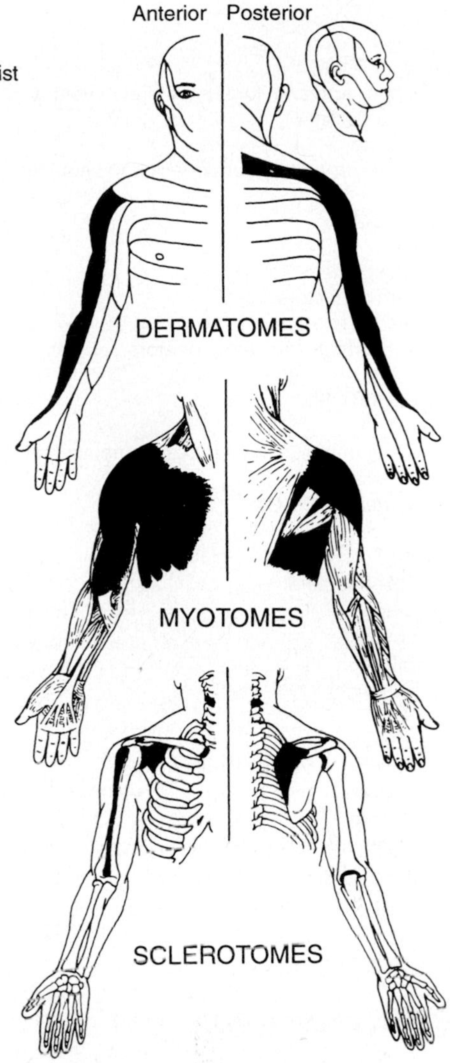

Figure 3–15. Dermatome, myotome, and sclerotome distribution for C5.

sues contain no free nerve endings. The clinical correlate of this fact is the lack of relationship between the extent of structural joint changes on radiographic evaluation of the neck and the severity of pain.[36]

Another source of spondylogenic pain are ligaments surrounding the vertebral column and fascia that attach muscles to each other and bone. Although noncontractile tissue, the ligaments of the cervical spine play an essential role in the static postural support of the neck in the upright, sitting, and flexed positions. When the neck is in its normal configuration (normal lordosis), the ligaments stretch to a natural length that supports the neck without muscular contraction other than what is generated by autonomic muscle tone. Pain is gener-

ated by nociceptors in the ligaments if they are placed under mechanical stress by poor posture, chronic contraction, excessive force, or a loss of elasticity due to aging. The same inflammatory disease that affects joints may also engulf ligamentous structures, resulting in pain that may spread beyond the margins of articular structures. The exact segmental distribution of pain arising from ligamentous structures is hard to define. Experiments injecting hypertonic saline into ligamentous structures have described locations of pain, but it is unclear whether the tension caused by the injection or the chemical irritation was the source of pain.[37] Whether pain generated in this fashion is the same as pain generated by a mechanical injury is conjecture because

C6

DERMATOME
    Upper arm and forearm lateral to ventral
       axial line
    Thumb
    Small area of posterior neck and shoulder

MYOTOME
Muscles
    Wrist extensors
    Arm adductors
    Medial rotators
    Forearm flexors and pronators

SCLEROTOME
Bones
    Parts of radius, humerus, first metacarpal,
       scapula
    Vertebrae C6-C7

Joints
    Glenohumeral
    Discs
    Luschka
    Elbow
    Zygapophyseal

Ligaments
    Anterior, posterior longitudinal
    Capsular
    Nuchal
    Ligamenta flava
    Interspinous

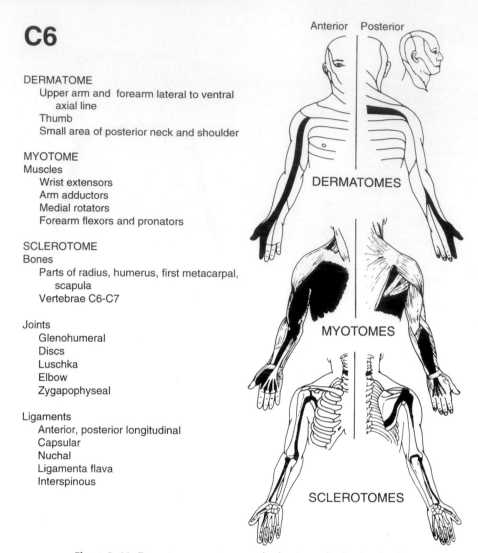

Figure 3–16. Dermatome, myotome, and sclerotome distribution for C6.

pain is related not only to the location of injury but also to the form of the noxious stimulus.

Bone pain is particularly intense when the periosteum is disrupted. Mechanical trauma, crush fractures, neoplasms, or infections may be causes of pain. Pain from a vertebral body may be insignificant despite destruction and replacement of trabecular bone if the process is slowly progressive and does not cause fractures or irritation of the periosteum. Once bone has been replaced to a significant degree, minor trauma may result in a pathologic fracture and intense pain.

Another potential cause of somatic neck pain is the distention of veins of the vertebral plexus.[24] Nociceptive fibers supply the venous plexus. When sufficiently stretched by prolonged coughing, vomiting, parturition, or ob-structed micturition, these fibers produce a dull, deep pain that may be associated with headache. In patients with herniated nucleus pulposus or intraspinal tumor, a moderate degree of increased pressure may provoke or exacerbate existing pain. These are patients who describe increased neck pain secondary to coughing or straining with a bowel movement.

The nociceptive innervation of the dura explains the association of pain with pathologic processes affecting the anterior dural membrane. The posterior dura has no nociceptive innervation. The anterior dura and the dural sleeves, which extend into the neural foramina, are densely innervated. Pain associated with dural lesions are of a deep, aching quality, located near the midline.

The annulus fibrosus receives nociceptive

C7

DERMATOME
　　Dorsum of hand and forearm
　　Dorsal and palmar 2nd and 3rd digits

MYOTOME
Muscles
　　Arm adductors
　　Forearm extensors
　　Wrist flexors
　　Finger extensors

SCLEROTOME
Bones
　　Radius, ulna, humerus, scapula

Joints
　　Discs
　　Luschka
　　Elbow
　　Zygapophyseal

Ligaments
　　Anterior, posterior longitudinal
　　Nuchal
　　Ligamenta flava
　　Interspinous

(Pain perceived: below elbow in area
overlapping and much larger than dermatome)

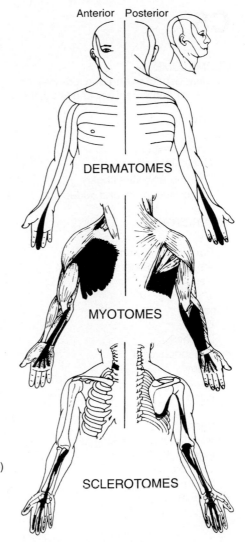

Figure 3–17. Dermatome, myotome, and sclerotome distribution for C7.

innervation, which is limited to the outer fibers of the annulus. Tears of the annulus fibrosus produce somatic pain that is predominantly located in the central neck. Abnormalities of the nucleus pulposus unassociated with disruption of annular fibers are devoid of pain. The nucleus pulposus does not receive any sensory innervation.

Kuslich and colleagues reported their observations, made during lumbar disc procedures performed under progressive local anesthesia,[38] on the pain sensitivity of various structures in the lumbar spine. Compressed and inflamed nerve roots were painful. The ventral dura mater, posterior longitudinal ligament, and annulus fibrosus were frequently pain-sensitive. Lesions on the left side of the annulus caused left-side back pain, and right-side lesions caused right-side back pain. The facet capsule, articular cartilage, and bone were less often pain-sensitive. These patterns of pain lend evidence in support of sclerodermal sensory innervation.

Radicular Pain

The source of radicular pain is not the peripheral sensory nerves but the proximal spinal nerves that form from the ventral and dorsal roots. Processes that decrease blood flow to the spinal nerve (ischemia) cause radicular pain. The large mechanoreceptor fibers, because of their large diameters, have greater

C8

DERMATOME
Ulnar aspect of arm and forearm
Palmar and dorsal 4th and 5th digits

MYOTOME
Muscles
Finger flexors
Metacarpal abductors
(thumb and little finger)
Finger abductors and adductors

SCLEROTOME
Bones
Parts of ulna, humerus
4th and 5th fingers (all bones)
Vertebrae C7-T1

Joints
Discs
Luschka
Zygapophyseal
Elbow
Wrist
Hand

Ligaments
Anterior, posterior longitudinal
Ligamenta flava
Interspinous
Supraspinous
Nuchal

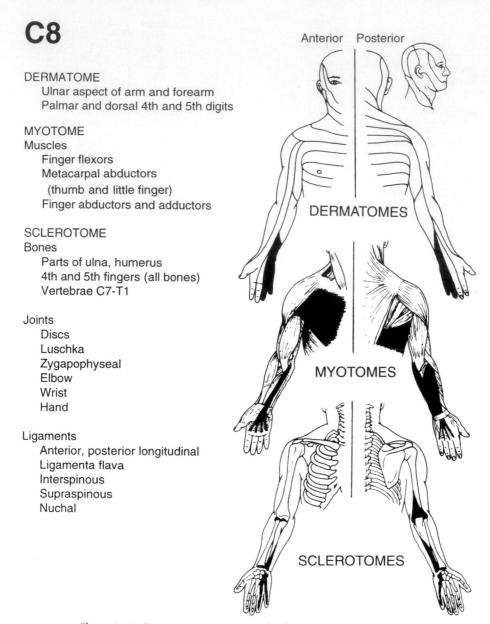

Anterior   Posterior

DERMATOMES

MYOTOMES

SCLEROTOMES

Figure 3–18. Dermatome, myotome, and sclerotome distribution for C8.

metabolic activity and are more sensitive to disturbances of blood flow. This results in the loss of inhibitory pain impulses, allowing for preferential nociceptive input into the dorsal horn. Another mechanism of pain production is inflammatory chemical irritation. Traction on a normal, noninflamed nerve root does not produce pain. However, slight tension on an inflamed root is associated with production of radicular pain.

Radicular pain has a lancinating, shooting, burning, sharp, tender quality that may radiate from the neck to the arm and hand in the distribution of the compromised spinal nerve.

This pain that radiates from the neck to the arm is commonly called brachialgia. In addition to arm pain, achiness and spasm may be experienced in neck and shoulder muscles. The pain is exacerbated by any motion that increases tension on the involved nerve root; immobilization and decreased axial loading relieve pain.

A frequent cause of compressive lesions, which result in radicular pain, are lesions of the cervical vertebral discs (most commonly the C5–C6 disc). Factors that cause disruption of normal disc architecture facilitate degeneration of discs and increase the potential of rup-

T1

DERMATOME
    Anterior thorax below clavicle
    Anterior medial arm and forearm to wrist
    Small area of back

MYOTOME
Muscles
    Little finger abductor
    Thumb adductor
    Finger abductors and adductors

SCLEROTOME
Bones
    Parts of ulna, humerus
    4th and 5th fingers (all bones)
    Vertebrae C7-T1

Joints
    Discs
    Luschka
    Zygapophyseal
    Elbow
    Wrist
    Hand

Ligaments
    Anterior, posterior longitudinal
    Ligamenta flava
    Interspinous
    Supraspinous
    Nuchal

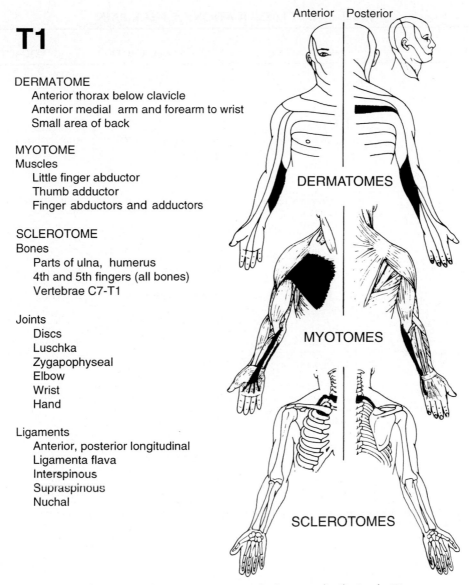

Figure 3–19. Dermatome, myotome, and sclerotome distribution for T1.

ture and the production of radicular pain. The majority of research in this area has involved the lumbar spine, and much of the work has been focused on the behavior of healthy and degenerated discs. The research effort has been multidisciplinary, focusing on biomechanical, biochemical, nutritional, immunologic, and nociceptive factors. A review of these factors helps in recognizing individuals who are at risk of developing this problem.

DISC BIOMECHANICAL FACTORS

Most of what is known about the pathomechanics of neck disorders has been gleaned by studying the mechanical behavior of cadaveric spinal motor segments. A motor segment is composed of two adjacent vertebral bodies, the interposed disc, and surrounding structures. It seems clear that under flexion, extension, rotation, and shear stress, the load distribution in the motor segment is not confined to the intervertebral disc alone but is shared between the strong anterior and posterior longitudinal ligaments, the facet joints and their capsules, and the other ligamentous structures, such as the ligamentum flavum and the interspinous and supraspinous ligaments. In vivo, these same structures, as well as the muscle and fascial attachments intrinsic and extrinsic to the vertebral column, interact to ac-

TABLE 3–4. CLASSIFICATION OF NECK PAIN

CATEGORY	SENSORY NERVES	PATHOLOGIC ENTITY	QUALITY
Superficial somatic (skin with subcutaneous tissue)	Cutaneous A fibers, small field	Cellulitis	Sharp
		Herpes zoster	Burning
Deep somatic (spondylogenic) (muscles, fascia, periosteum, ligaments, joints, vessels, dura)	Sinuvertebral	Muscular strain	Sharp (acute)
	Posterior primary ramus unmyelinated	Arthritis	Dull ache (chronic)
		Fracture Increased venous pressure	Boring
Radicular (spinal nerves)	—	Herniated vertebral disc	Segmental
		Foraminal stenosis	Radiating
			Shooting
Neurogenic	Mixed motor sensory nerves	Herpes zoster Brachial plexopathy	Burning
Viscerogenic referred (cardiac and carotid structures)	Autonomic sensory, unmyelinated C fibers, large field	Myocardial infarction	Deep, heaviness
		Carotidynia	Boring
		Esophageal spasm	Colicky
Psychogenic	—	Depression Conversion reaction Malingering	Variable

Modified from Engel GL: Pain. In: Blacklow R (ed): Signs and Symptoms: Applied Pathologic Physiology and Clinical Interpretation. Philadelphia: JB Lippincott Co, 1983, pp 41–60; and Macnab I: Backache. Baltimore: Williams & Wilkins, 1983, pp 16–18.

commodate the load-bearing requirements of the cervical spine.

When pure compressive loads are progressively applied to an intervertebral disc, the vertebral end plate gives way before the nucleus pulposus herniates. The disc itself behaves like a viscoelastic structure and protrudes circumferentially. It should be appreciated that there is no difference in the failure pattern between normal and degenerated intervertebral discs.

It has been suggested that abnormal torsional stresses, applied particularly to the lordotic motion segments, may be the mechanism by which radial and circumferential fissures are produced within the annulus fibrosus. Furthermore, these fissures tend to occur in the posterolateral segments of the annulus because of the eccentric geometry of the inter-

vertebral disc. The effects of this torsional stress concentration are also intensified in the presence of asymmetry of the facet joints as well as when there is advanced degeneration of the disc. In these situations the disc tends to fail after a few degrees of torsion.

Under tension, the disc is strongest in the anterior and posterior regions and weakest in the center. It is somewhat paradoxical to note that the tensile strength of the annulus has been found to be greatest in its posterolateral segment, which is usually the location where the nucleus pulposus herniates. This is the location where the posterior longitudinal ligament is weakest.

Most of the biomechanical knowledge of the cervical spine deals with the normal and abnormal function of the intervertebral disc. The bony elements have only recently been evalu-

TABLE 3–4. CLASSIFICATION OF NECK PAIN *Continued*

LOCATION	INTENSITY	ONSET AND DURATION	AGGRAVATING AND ALLEVIATING FACTORS	BEHAVIOR
Well localized	Correlates with intensity of nerve stimulation (mild to moderate)	Acute	Intensified by direct contact	Mild concern
		Correlates with status of lesions	Diminished by light touch in adjacent areas	Able to see lesion
Diffuse	Correlates with intensity of nerve stimulation (mild to severe)	Acute or chronic	Intensified with movement	Avoidance of movement
Multiple segments affected			Diminished with rest	Abnormal posture secondary to protective spasm
Neck pain	Mild to severe	Acute	Intensified with standing	Avoidance of movement
Afferent distribution of affected nerve root (superficial and deep)	Correlates with intensity of nerve impingement		Diminished with bedrest	
Peripheral nerve	Severe	Chronic Persistent	Intensified with palpation	Apprehension
Segmental with radiation inside body	Mild to severe	Acute or chronic	Related to factors affecting each organ system	Movement to find comfortable position
	Correlates with intensity of nerve stimulation			
Nondermatomal	Variable	Persistent	No consistent correlation	Emphasis on suffering

ated. It appears that the anterior elements provide the major support for the spinal column and absorb various impacts. The posterior structures share some of the loads, but they mainly influence the potential patterns of motion.

The facet joints resist most of the intervertebral shear force and in lordotic postures share in resisting intervertebral compression. The facet joints also serve to prevent excessive motion from damaging the discs. In particular, the posterior annulus is protected in torsion by the facet surfaces and in flexion by the capsular ligaments of the facet joints.

DISC BIOCHEMICAL FACTORS

On a microscopic level, the intervertebral disc consists of two adjacent hyaline cartilage end plates, an annulus fibrosus composed of collagen fibers obliquely aligned in layered sheets at angles varying between 40° and 80°, and a nucleus pulposus consisting of a loosely arranged network of collagen fibers and cells in an extracellular matrix. The annular fibers are attached to the end plates and, for a short distance, into the vertebral bodies. The annulus is thicker anteriorly than posteriorly and gradually thins out as it approaches the nucleus pulposus internally.

To function efficiently, the disc depends largely on the physical properties of the nucleus pulposus, which in turn are closely related to its water binding capacity. The higher the hydration content, the more effectively the disc functions. Unfortunately, the hydration of the disc drops progressively from early life, when the water content is 88%, to a level of 69% in the eighth decade of life.[39] Ultrastructurally, 99% of the tissue mass of the disc is formed by its matrix, which contains glycoproteins, proteoglycans, collagen, and other proteins. It is presently believed that structural insufficiency of the disc is accompanied by an alteration in this biochemical composition.

The bulk of the connective tissue matrix in an intervertebral disc is collagen. There are seven major subtypes of collagen identified in the intervertebral discs. The annulus fibrosus contains types I, II, III, V, VI, IX, and XI and the nucleus pulposus types II, VI, IX, and XI.[40] Type I, found predominantly in tendons, skin, bones, and ligaments, accounts for about 90% of the collagen in the body. Type II is absent from these tissues but is found in high concentrations in hyaline cartilage. In the human, the collagen in the annulus fibrosus is predominantly type I, with the remainder being type II. More than 80% of the collagen in the nucleus pulposus is type II. The significance is that type I collagen has a restricted water content and is thus better able to handle tensile stress; conversely, type II, with its hydrophilic physical properties, is ideally suited to absorb compressive forces. Types II, V, and XI are fibril-forming collagens. Type III is found in both the nucleus and the inner annulus fibrosus. Type V is distributed in noncartilaginous tissues in combination with type I collagen. Type V collagen forms a scaffold for type I, and these are copolymerized within the same fibril network in the annulus. Type XI copolymerizes with type II to control fibril diameter and may also serve as the site of binding of cartilage proteoglycans, heparin, and chondroitin sulfate. Type VI collagen is located in the nucleus pulposus and encircles interstitial collagen fibers, forming an independent network for organization of extracellular components, including proteoglycans. Type IX is found primarily in the nucleus pulposus and cross-links type II to bridge collagen fibrils covalently. In addition, collagens VI, IX, and XI form a porous capsule around chondrocytes that provides a compliant but inelastic barrier during compression. The interactions of the component collagens result in a three-dimensional meshwork of fibrils that influence the biologic properties of the disc.[40]

After collagen, the proteoglycans make up the major component of the extracellular matrix of the disc. These molecules consist of noncollagenous protein cores along with the attached sulfated glucose aminoglycans of chondroitin 4-sulfate, chondroitin 6-sulfate, and keratan sulfate. The proteoglycans are, in turn, attached to long chains of hyaluronic acid by small glycoprotein links. These molecules are found in great abundance within the nucleus pulposus but form only a small proportion of the dry weight of the annulus fibrosus. They are hydrophilic and therefore regulate the fluid content of the nucleus.

Proteoglycans are synthesized in chondrocytes. After the protein core is manufactured, up to 100 chondroitin sulfate and 50 keratan sulfate chains are added during post-translational processing in the chondrocyte.[40] The proteoglycan monomers aggregate as they encounter hyaluronate. The process of aggregation immobilizes the proteoglycans within the extracellular matrix. A link protein cements the proteoglycan to hyaluronate. Approximately 100 to 200 proteoglycan monomers are bound to a single hyaluronate chain.

Many age-related changes have been noted in disc proteoglycans. With time, these molecules lose their ability to associate with collagen, have a lower molecular weight, have a reduced aggregation potential, and develop an increased keratan sulfate content. These changes adversely affect the ability of the disc to imbibe water, which in turn decreases its capacity to dissipate energy when loaded. The changes in disc composition may also be related to topographic variations in the synthesis of disc proteoglycans.[41] Proteoglycan synthesis rates for annulus fibrosus in fetal discs are five times greater than for similar locations in adult discs. Synthesis rates are highest in the inner annulus for fetal discs and the midannulus for adult discs. The clinical correlate is that certain portions of an intervertebral disc are at risk of persistent injury secondary to inadequate production of proteoglycan. Injuries to the annulus fibrosus are unable to heal.[42] A greater understanding of the mechanisms by which chondrocytes synthesize and degrade extracellular matrix and collagen may help in differentiating between normal aging and pathologic degeneration of intervertebral discs.

DISC NUTRITIONAL FACTORS

The intervertebral disc is a relatively avascular structure and beyond 15 through 20 years of age has no direct blood vessels. Diffusion is the main transport mechanism for disc nutrition in the adult. Small uncharged solutes, such as glucose and oxygen, mainly gain access to the metabolizing cells through the vertebral end plates. The diffusion of negatively charged solutes such as sulfates, which are important for proteoglycan production, occurs mainly through the annulus fibrosus. Because the area available for diffusion of these negatively charged solutes is smaller in the posterior region of the annulus, turnover of both collagen and proteoglycan is slower in this critical zone. It is believed that this nutritional inadequacy in conjunction with the concentration of mechanical stress in the posterolateral annulus accounts for the high incidence of intervertebral disc ruptures in this area. Also, it is most likely that when fissures and cracks do occur in this area, even prior to the stage of rupture, the propensity for healing is liable to be low or inadequate at best.

Decreased oxygen concentrations throughout intervertebral discs result in increased lactate concentrations. The increased lactate levels result in decreased pH. The acid milieu causes decreased matrix synthesis and increased degradative enzyme activity. The eventual consequence of inadequate nutrients is degeneration and poor healing of disc constituents.[43]

DISC IMMUNOLOGIC FACTORS

In its normal state, the intervertebral disc, owing to its avascular structure, seems to be an immunologically privileged site. However, as the disc degenerates, its chemical constituent parts are exposed to the host's normal immune defense mechanism, causing an autoimmune reaction to some extent. The phenomenon was first demonstrated in rabbits when it was found that their nucleus pulposus can induce the production of autoantibodies. This autoimmune reaction has been confirmed in the human, and there is particularly strong evidence that this sequestration within the spinal canal elicits a strong cell-mediated immune response to the autogenous disc material.

These findings can help explain, in part, the etiology of the acute radicular pain associated with disc ruptures. It seems clear that the mechanical compression on the nerve root that is being irritated by the herniated disc material is an important factor in the production of pain. As for the inflammation that occurs around the nerve root, no one is certain whether it is related to an autoimmune phenomenon, ischemic neuropathy from alteration in blood flow patterns, or defects in the neuronal transport mechanism of the nerve root itself. Regardless, it has been shown that inflammation is a necessary ingredient in the production of root pain from disc herniations. This was demonstrated by the use of thin silk threads that were passed around lumbar nerve root sheaths at times of surgery for the removal of herniated discs. The threads were brought out through the skin during wound closure. Postoperatively, when pressure was applied to the roots that had not been compressed by the disc herniation, the patient experienced only paresthesias in the dermatomal distribution of the nerve. There was no pain. When tension was applied to the inflamed root that had previously been compressed by the disc herniation, radicular pain was perceived. This perhaps explains the reason why many patients with radicular symptoms can be treated effectively with anti-inflammatory medications.[44]

Radicular pain may occur in the absence of nerve root compression secondary to nucleus pulposus extrusion. The nucleus pulposus may have properties that inflame nerve roots without direct compression. Olmarker and colleagues developed a porcine model of nucleus pulposus herniation without mechanical compression.[45] The epidural application of nuclear material to a nerve root causes a pronounced reduction in nerve conduction velocity compared with application of retroperitoneal fat. Histologic evaluation of affected nerve roots could not explain the nerve conduction delay because of breakdown of axons and myelin sheaths in a minority of myelinated nerve fibers. This suggests that spinal nerve root dysfunction with disc herniation may be mediated by a number of factors, including autoimmune reactions, microvascular changes, and inflammatory phenomena independent of mechanical compression. The implication of this study is that nerve root dysfunction may occur without compression, suggesting that therapy of nerve root dysfunction may not always be improved by elimination of compression alone and should include anti-inflammatory drugs.

DISC NOCICEPTIVE FACTORS

In the cervical region, free nerve endings supplied by the sinuvertebral nerve and posterior primary ramus provide sensory innervation to the anterior and posterior longitudinal ligaments, the facet joint capsules, the superficial lamellae of the annulus fibrosus, the dural envelope, the periosteum of the vertebrae, and the blood vessels. A review of the anatomy of the neural foramina elucidates the structures at risk from compression by a herniated disc.

As the nerve roots descend from the C4

level, they cross the disc immediately at the level of the foramen they exit. They enter the foramen below the pedicle and leave the foramen in a downward and forward fashion. In the lower cervical spine, the roots exit at a more horizontal angle and the T1 root exits in a slightly cephalad direction. By virtue of this configuration, the nerve is located in the superior portion of the foramen. The nerve carries the arachnoid along with it until the confluence of the ventral and dorsal roots, and the dura, which invaginates in the foramen. The dura continues along the distal nerve and forms the outer sheath, the perineurium. There is some question whether the dural sleeves are firmly or loosely attached to the walls of the foramen.[24]

Flexion of the spine allows motion of these elements in the foramina. When tension is placed on the structures, the nerve will elongate, and the dura increases in tension. In the foramen, about 50% of the space is occupied by the nerve and its sheath. Connective tissue, adipose tissue, vessels, lymphatics, and the sinuvertebral nerve fill the remainder. The sinuvertebral nerve winds back into the foramen, supplying the posterior longitudinal ligament, fibrous tissue near the annulus, and the anterior but not the posterior dural sheath. The posterior dura has no nociceptive innervation.

In the initial stage of protrusion, the sinuvertebral nerve on the posterior longitudinal ligament is irritated, which gives rise to pain in the lower neck without brachialgia. As the impingement increases, the dural sleeves and nerve root are involved. As a result, neck pain becomes more severe and widely distributed. With greater pressure, pain in a radicular distribution is elicited along with paresthesias and numbness, and the motor fibers in the inferior portion of the spinal nerve are compressed, resulting in reflex muscle spasm. With greater duration and extent of nerve pressure, numbness replaces pain as a symptom and muscle weakness replaces spasm. Additional clinical features of herniated vertebral discs are discussed in Chapter 10.

It is known that not all radicular-like pain is related to disc herniation. Distention of degenerated lumbar intervertebral discs or facet joints with injections of saline or contrast material can produce pain in the low back that radiates down the leg.[46, 47] This is not true radicular pain. It is referred pain that appears in mesenchymal structures of the same embryonic sclerotome in the injured tissue. When this type of pain is referred into the neck and

arms, it has a dull, aching quality unlike the sharp, lancinating pain of true brachialgia.

Herniated vertebral discs are not the only cause of radicular pain. Overgrowth of bone from the facet joints intrudes into the spinal canal, decreasing the room for the neural elements. This is called spinal stenosis. A patient may experience neck and radicular pain in positions that decrease room in the spinal canal (positions of extension). In a severe case of central stenosis, spinal cord compression and clinical myelopathy may result. Alternatively, foraminal stenosis may be confined to an exiting nerve root.

Nerve root compression is also seen with fracture-dislocation of the spine, infections, and neoplasms. Neoplasms that cause radicular pain are usually extradural (metastatic) or intradural (neurofibroma). Intramedullary tumors are associated with neurogenic symptoms.

Neurogenic Pain

Neurogenic pain arises from abnormalities of the peripheral or central nervous system. The structures associated with neurogenic pain include the peripheral nerves, dorsal root ganglia, spinal cord, thalamus, and sensory area of the cerebral cortex. Damage to the sensory portion of the nervous system may result in pain produced spontaneously or produced by painless sensory stimulation (light touch). The pain follows a distribution that corresponds to the damaged neural structure. The response to simple light touch can be excruciating pain similar to that experienced in a case of causalgia or reflex sympathetic dystrophy.[48] The pain may be delayed or occur in paroxysms. The pain may be sustained for some time after cessation of the stimulus (hyperpathia). Particularly in injuries of the central nervous system, pain may begin abruptly without evident peripheral stimulation. Neurogenic pain is described as burning, tingling, crushing, gnawing, or skin-crawling (formication). In many circumstances, it is a unique pain that the patient has not experienced previously.[49] As opposed to what occurs in radicular pain, increases in intraspinal pressure produced by coughing or sneezing rarely exacerbate nerve pain. Instead, pain is intensified by sensory stimulation of the damaged nerve. Therefore, patients actively protect the limb from contact and develop behavior that protects the limb from the environment.

The abnormality causing neurogenic pain is

the loss of the pain inhibitory system in the peripheral nerves and/or central nervous system. Those processes that diminish the large, myelinated fiber input to the dorsal horn allow for increased transmission of nociceptive information. Also, nociceptive transmission is increased by diminished input from the nerves originating in the periaqueductal gray area of the midbrain.

An example of neurogenic pain is diabetic mononeuropathy of the femoral or sciatic nerve. The neuropathy presents with sudden onset of burning pain in the peripheral distribution of the nerve associated with loss of sensory and motor function. Herpes zoster preferentially affects dorsal root ganglion cells of mechanoreceptors and causes neurogenic pain distributed in a dermatomal pattern.

Viscerogenic Referred Pain

Viscerogenic referred neck or shoulder pain arises from abnormalities in organs that share segmental innervation with structures in the cervical spine. These organs include the thyroid, heart, esophagus, gallbladder, stomach, lungs, pancreas, and diaphragm. Visceral afferents that supply these organs transmit impulses to the dorsal horn, where somatic and visceral pain fibers share second-order neurons.[50] Impulses from visceral nerve endings arrive at the same reception point among the posterior horn cells as do impulses of somatic origin. Visceral pain is noted in the same somatic segment with which it shares neurons in lamina V of the dorsal horn.

The precise localization of somatic pain differs from the wider distribution of visceral pain because the latter is transmitted to multiple segments (Fig. 3–20). In addition to superficial cutaneous pain, reflex muscle spasm and vasomotor changes may also occur. The neck pain may have a gripping, cramping, aching, squeezing, crushing, tearing, stabbing, or burning quality, depending on the affected

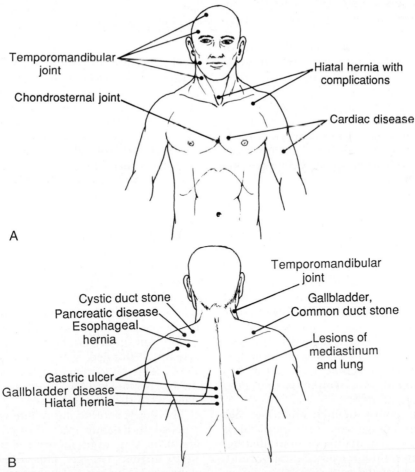

Figure 3–20. *A,* Anterior referral sites in the cervical spine arising from distant visceral or somatic structures. *B,* Posterior referral sites. (*A* and *B* modified from Nakano KK: Neck pain. In: Kelley WN, Harris ED Jr, Ruddy S, et al. [eds]: Textbook of Rheumatology, 4th ed. Philadelphia: WB Saunders Co, 1993.)

organ. The degree of tissue injury correlates with the intensity of the pain and is associated with recruitment of additional segmental levels above and below as well as those neighboring segments that have transmitted past or concurrent nociceptive impulses. A clinical correlate of this recruitment of segments is the radiating quality of visceral pain.

The duration and sequence of viscerogenic referred neck pain are helpful in identifying its organ of origin. For example, neck pain caused by referred impulses follows the periodicity associated with the diseased organ. Rhythmic peristaltic waves of a hollow viscus attempting to expel its contents against resistance produce pain that rises quickly to its greatest intensity in 20 to 30 seconds, lasts 1 to 2 minutes, and quickly subsides, only to recur again in minutes. Lesions in the esophagus are associated with this pattern of pain. Vascular lesions are associated with throbbing pain. Lesions that result in inflammation and the release of chemical mediators that facilitate pain are associated with pain that increases in intensity and lasts extended periods.[6]

Neck pain is rarely the sole symptom of visceral disease. Changes in gastrointestinal function may be clues to the potential source of pain. Viscerogenic pain may be differentiated from deep somatic pain by the response to activity and rest. Somatic pain is frequently exacerbated by activity and improved by rest. Patients with viscerogenic pain get no relief from bedrest. In fact, they may feel more comfortable by moving about, trying to achieve a comfortable position.

Psychogenic Pain

Psychogenic pain arises not from structures located in the cervical spine but at levels of the cerebral cortex. Patients with psychogenic pain experience discomfort, but the pain is not due to tissue damage. Patients with psychogenic pain may suffer from depression, hysteria, or conversion reaction. They respond to their environment with symptoms that help control their situation.[51]

The pain is poorly defined and does not follow dermatomal patterns. It is superficial or deep, sharp or dull, radiating or nonradiating, constant or intermittent, excruciating or mild. Pain may be associated with specific social activities, such as work and sexual intercourse, whereas activities that require similar kinds of physical effort elicit little pain.

The duration of pain defies physiologic time sequences. Pain may last for seconds or for years. Pain may be unrelenting and unmoved by therapy during an extended time. The language used to describe the pain may reflect a patient's thoughts of suffering or punishment. The patient may speak of pain as a "knife sticking you," "being hit," "burned with a red hot poker," or "having your skin peeled off."[52]

Psychogenic pain resists most conventional therapies that are effective in somatic causes of neck pain. Therapy must be directed not at the pain but at the reasons causing an agitated depression, conversion reaction, or reluctance to return to work. Patients with psychogenic pain experience pain that is just as incapacitating as that caused by muscle strain. These patients do not improve unless the source of their pain is recognized.

Duration of Pain

The function of pain as it affects the whole body is closely related to its duration. Acute pain frequently has an understandable cause (trauma), normally has a characteristic time course, and resolves once healing has occurred. The purpose of acute pain is to inform the host that tissue damage has occurred and to prevent further injury. The rapidly conducting systems (such as the neospinothalamic tract and dorsal column tract) are suited to the speedy relay of both nociceptive and light touch sensations necessary to determine the initial phase of tissue injury. The overlap between systems allows one to be responsive to proprioceptive stimuli and another to be primed to receive nociceptive stimulation. The organization of multiple ascending systems allows the individual to be constantly primed for nociceptive impulses, which are important to prevent injury while the central nervous system is flooded with non-nociceptive inputs.[53] This rapid system activates appropriate motor responses that attempt to minimize damage to the affected part.

The slowly conducting system, including the paleospinothalamic tract, carries information about the state of the injury and its susceptibility to further damage. This tonic stimulation determines the general behavioral state of the individual to prevent further damage and foster rest and care of the damaged area to promote healing. Tonic pain also resolves with healing of the injury. The functions of the rapidly and slowly conducting systems may be controlled by different neurochemical mechanisms. This may have therapeutic implications because the phasic and tonic components of pain may respond to different drugs.[53]

Chronic pain may persist long after the injury has healed. Chronic pain, which is continuous over several months, results from habituation of the sensory system to nociceptive stimuli. Constant stimulation activates the cerebral cortex function of memory. The central nervous system becomes habituated to sensory input to such an extent that pain is perceived in the absence of a detectable lesion. As the duration of pain continues, the area affected may spread to adjacent or distal body areas. Chronic pain also results in autonomic responses that are depressive (vegetative) in quality: poor sleep, decreased appetite, irritability, withdrawal of interests, strained interpersonal relationships, and increased somatic preoccupation.[54] Therefore, chronic pain is associated with significant depression.[55] In addition, resolution or reduction of pain reverses the reactive depression caused by the pain.[56] The marked psychological effects, including depression and anxiety associated with chronic pain, do not serve a useful purpose.

The changes associated with chronic pain that occur in the central nervous system are related to alterations in molecular control of neuropeptide synthesis and neuroreceptor production.[57] Immediate early genes (IEGs) are oncogenes that are activated by a variety of stimuli to nerve cells. IEGs, such as c-*fos* and c-*jun,* act as transcription messengers that control the transcription mechanisms of a cell. Repetitive noxious stimulation is a potent promoter of IEG activation.[58] Noxious stimulation of C fibers results in alterations in postsynaptic receptors for excitatory amino acids, such as N-methyl-D-aspartate (NMDA). The ensuing increase in sensory nerve cell excitability is related to the emergence of NMDA receptors at the afferent synapses of dorsal horn neurons.[59] Increased excitability may persist for weeks following a transient peripheral injury. The development of chronic pain modifies transmission of stimuli in the nervous system. The persistence of chronic pain may become independent of ongoing nociceptive stimulation if neural cells have been modified to have a lower threshold for stimulation. The nervous system is malleable. It changes according to environmental stimuli. In the future, therapy for chronic pain may be directed at control of cellular gene products that normalize receptor distribution on cell membranes or neurotransmitter production.

SUMMARY

Pain is a complex, subjective experience that is mediated through multiple components of the peripheral and central nervous systems. Factors at all levels of the neuraxis modulate pain perception. The sum of these inputs results in a perception that can be described in terms of its intensity, location, onset and duration, aggravating and alleviating factors, and elicited emotional responses. In acute circumstances, pain marks the onset and location of damage. It serves the purpose of protection. With chronic pain, the pain itself becomes the disease because the injury that initiated the nociceptive response has healed. The goals for therapy for patients who experience neck pain must take into account these anatomic, physiologic, and psychological factors. The choice of specific forms of therapy for neck pain patients should be made in light of these factors. The potential is great for individual patients to respond to a wide variety of therapeutic interventions, given the multitude of factors that result in pain.

References

1. Iggo A: Activation of cutaneous nociceptors and their actions on dorsal horn neurons. In: Bonica JJ (ed): International Symposium on Pain. Adv Neurol 4:1, 1974.
2. Collins WF, Nulsen FE, Randt CT: Relation of peripheral fiber size and sensation in man. Arch Neurol 3:381, 1960.
3. Fitzgerald M, Lynn B: The sensitization of high threshold mechanoreceptors with myelinated axons by repeated heating. J Physiol (Lond) 65:549, 1977.
4. Thalhammer JG, LaMotte RH: Spatial properties of nociceptor sensitization. Brain Res 231:257, 1982.
5. Bessou P, Perl ER: Response of cutaneous sensory units with unmyelinated fibers to noxious stimuli. J Neurophysiol 32:1025, 1969.
6. Keele CA: Chemical causes of pain and itch. Annu Rev Med 21:67, 1970.
7. Ferreira SH: Prostaglandins, aspirin-like drugs and analgesia. Nature 240:200, 1972.
8. Aimone LD: Neurochemistry and modulation of pain. In: Sinatra RS, Hord AH, Ginsberg B, Preble LM (eds): Acute Pain: Mechanisms and Management. St Louis: Mosby-Year Book, 1992, pp 29–43.

9. Levine JD, Fields HL, Basbaum AI: Peptides and the primary afferent nociceptor. J Neurosci 13:2273, 1993.

10. Lynn B: Neurogenic inflammation. Skin Pharmacol 1:217, 1988.

11. Bishop GH: The relation between nerve fiber size and sensory modality: phylogenetic implications of the afferent innervation of the cortex. J Nerv Ment Dis 128:89, 1959.

12. Maciewicz R, Landrew BB: Physiology of pain. In: Aronoff GM (ed): Evaluation and Treatment of Chronic Pain. Baltimore: Urban and Schwarzenberg, 1985, pp 17–38.

13. Christensen BN, Perl ER: Spinal neurons specifically excited by noxious or thermal stimuli: marginal zones of the dorsal form. J Neurophysiol 33:293, 1970.

14. LaMotte CC, de Lanerolle N: Substance P, enkephalin and serotonin: Ultrastructural basis of pain transmission in primate spinal cord. In: Bonica JJ, Lindblom V, Iggo A (eds): Advances in Pain Research and Therapy, vol 5. New York: Raven Press, 1983, pp 247–256.

15. Simone DA, Baumann TK, La Motte RH: Dose-dependent pain and mechanical hyperalgesia in humans after intradermal injection of capsaicin. Pain 380:99–107, 1989.

16. Yaksh TL, Farb D, Leeman S, Jessell T: Intrathecal capsaicin depletes substance P in the rat spinal cord and produces prolonged thermal analgesia. Science 206:481, 1979.

17. Plenderleith MB, Haller CJ, Snow PJ: Peptide coexistence in axon terminals within the superficial dorsal horn of the rat spinal cord. Synapse 6:344–350, 1990.

18. Meyer RA, Campbell JN, Raja SN: Peripheral neural mechanisms of nociception. In: Wall PD, Melzack R (eds): Textbook of Pain, 3rd ed. Edinburgh, Churchill Livingstone, 1994, pp 13–44.

19. Basbaum AI, Levine JD: The contribution of the nervous system to inflammation and inflammatory disease. Can J Physiol Pharmacol 69:647–651, 1991.

20. Morton CR, Hutchison WD: Release of sensory neuropeptides in the spinal cord: studies with calcitonin gene-related peptide and galanin. Neuroscience 31:807, 1989.

21. Procacci P, Zopp M: Pathophysiology and clinical aspects of visceral and referred pain. In: Bonica JJ, Lindblom V, Iggo A (eds): Advances in Pain Research and Therapy, vol 5. New York: Raven Press, 1983, pp 643–660.

22. Cervero F, Iggo A: The substantia gelatinosa of the spinal cord: a critical review. Brain 103:717, 1980.

23. Willis WD, Maunz RA, Foreman RD, Coulter JD: Static and dynamic responses of spinothalamic tract neurons to mechanical stimuli. J Neurophysiol 38:587, 1975.

24. Wyke B: Neurological aspects of low back pain. In: Jayson MIV (ed): The Lumbar Spine and Back Pain. New York: Grune & Stratton, 1976, pp 189–256.

25. Melzack R: Neurophysiological foundation of pain. In: Sternbach RA (ed): The Psychology of Pain. New York: Raven Press, 1986, pp 1–24.

26. Reynolds DV: Surgery in the rat during electrical analgesia induced by focal brain stimulation. Science 164:444, 1969.

27. Fields HL, Basbaum AI: Brainstem control of spinal pain-transmission neurons. Annu Rev Physiol 40:217, 1978.

28. Fields HL, Basbaum AI: Central nervous system mechanisms of pain modulation. In: Wall PD, Melzack R (eds): Textbook of Pain, 3rd ed. Edinburgh, Churchill Livingstone, 1994, pp 243–257.

29. Aronin N, DiFiglia M, Liotta AS, Martin JB: Ultrastructural localization and biochemical features of immunoreactive LEU-enkephalin in monkey dorsal horn. J Neurosci 1:561, 1981.

30. Hökfelt T, Kellerth JO, Nillsson G, Pernow B: Substance P: localization in the central nervous system and in some primary sensory neurons. Science 190:889, 1975.

31. Melzack R, Wall PD: Pain mechanisms: a new theory. Science 150:971, 1965.

32. Sjolund BH, Eriksson MBE: The influence of naloxone on analgesia produced by peripheral conditioning stimulation. Brain Res 173:295, 1979.

33. Engel GL: Pain. In: Blacklow R (ed): Signs and Symptoms: Applied Pathologic Physiology and Clinical Interpretation. Philadelphia: JB Lippincott Co, 1983, pp 41–60.

34. Macnab I: Backache. Baltimore: Williams & Wilkins, 1983, pp 16–18.

35. Floyd WF, Silver PHS: Function of erectores spinae and flexion of the trunk. Lancet 1:133, 1951.

36. Lawrence JS, Bremner JM, Bier F: Osteoarthrosis: prevalence in the population and relationship between symptoms and x-ray changes. Ann Rheum Dis 25:1, 1966.

37. Kellgren JH: On the distribution of pain arising from deep somatic structures with charts of segmental pain areas. Clin Sci 41:46, 1939.

38. Kuslich SD, Ulstrom CL, Michael CJ: The tissue origin of low back pain and sciatica: a report of pain response to tissue stimulation during operations on the lumbar spine using local anesthesia. Orthop Clin North Am 22:181, 1991.

39. Eyre DE: Biochemistry of the intervertebral disc. Connect Tissue Res 8:227, 1979.

40. Bayliss MT, Johnstone B: Biochemistry of the intervertebral disc. In: Jayson MIV (ed): The Lumbar Spine and Back Pain. Edinburgh: Churchill Livingstone, 1992, pp 111–131.

41. Bayliss MT, Johnstone B, O'Brien JP: Proteoglycan synthesis in the human intervertebral disc: variation with age, region, and pathology. Spine 13:972, 1988.

42. Hampton D, Laros G, McCarron R, Franks D: Healing potential of the annulus fibrosus. Spine 14:398, 1989.

43. Eyre D, Benya P, Buckwalter J, et al.: The intervertebral disc: Basic science perspectives. In: Frymoyer JW, Gordon SL (eds): New Perspectives on Low Back Pain. Park Ridge, Illinois: American Academy of Orthopaedic Surgeons, 1988, pp 147–207.

44. Smyth MJ, Wright V: Sciatica and the intervertebral disc: an experimental study. J Bone Joint Surg 40:1401, 1958.

45. Olmarker K, Rydevik B, Nordborg C: Autologous nucleus pulposus induces neurophysiologic and histologic changes in porcine cauda equina nerve roots. Spine 18:1425, 1993.

46. Hirsch C, Inglemark BE, Miller M: The anatomical basis for low back pain: studies on the presence of sensory nerve endings in ligamentous, capsular, and intervertebral disc structures in the human lumbar spine. Acta Orthop Scand 33:1, 1963.

47. Mooney V, Robertson J: The facet syndrome. Clin Orthop 115:149, 1976.

48. Melzack R, Loeser JD: Phantom body pain in paraplegics: evidence for a central "pattern generating mechanism" for pain. Pain 4:195, 1978.

49. Denny-Brown D: The release of deep pain by nerve injury. Brain 88:725, 1965.

50. Selzer M, Spencer WA: Convergence of visceral and cutaneous afferent pathways in the lumbar spinal cord. Brain Res 14:331, 1969.

51. Devine R, Merskey H: The description of pain in psychiatric and general medical patients. J Psychosom Res 9:311, 1965.
52. Klein RF, Brown W: Pain descriptions in medical settings. J Psychosom Res 10:367, 1967.
53. Dennis SG, Melzack R: Pain-signaling systems in the dorsal and ventral spinal cord. Pain 4:97, 1977.
54. Sternbach RA. Clinical aspects of pain. In: Sternbach RA (ed): The Psychology of Pain. New York: Raven Press, 1986, pp 223–239.
55. Krishnan KR, France RD, Pelton S, et al.: Chronic pain and depression. I. Classification of depression in chronic low back pain patients. Pain 22:279, 1985.
56. Sternbach RA, Timmermans G: Personality changes associated with reduction of pain. Pain 1:177, 1975.
57. Zimmermann M: Basic neurophysiological mechanisms of pain and pain therapy. In: Jayson MIV (ed): The Lumbar Spine and Back Pain. Edinburgh: Churchill Livingstone, 1992, pp 43–59.
58. Sheng M, Greenberg E: The regulation and function of c-*fos* and other immediate early genes in the nervous system. Neuron 4:477, 1990.
59. Davies SN, Lodge D: Evidence for involvement of *n*-methylaspartate receptors in ''wind-up'' of class 2 neurones in the dorsal horn of the rat. Brain Res 424:402, 1987.

Section II

CLINICAL EVALUATION OF NECK PAIN

4

History

TAKING THE HISTORY

Taking the history is the essential initial step in evaluating the patient with the symptom of neck pain. The history should include the patient's chief complaint, family history, past history, social history, review of systems, and present illness. Some physicians may concentrate only on the present illness, leaving out parts of the review of systems or social history. Others use reproduced forms that list a succession of questions that are complete for evaluating the patient's pain but do not integrate the neck symptoms with other medical, social, or psychological problems. In circumstances involving patients with acute spinal cord compression (from tumor, infection, or trauma), the necessity to do a complete history is reduced in the face of the need to evaluate the patient for emergency surgical decompression. In other patients with chronic neck pain, a thorough review of all the components of the patient's history is essential to understanding the patient's difficulties. Historical evaluation and physical examination are the major means of gathering data in diagnosing cervical disorders, and they are done superficially in many circumstances.[1]

Common sense is an essential component of this process. The astute clinician allows patients to tell their story in their own words and also steers them in directions that elicit the essential information needed for the diagnostic process. The clinician knows when the history must be abbreviated to administer essential therapy or prolonged to gather all the facts that may pertain to the patient's problem.

The expenditure of time in obtaining a complete history reaps the clinician great dividends in understanding the patient's disease. If not all the information is obtained during the initial evaluation, it is worthwhile to review the history on subsequent visits. The patient may have forgotten an essential piece of history. Repeated questions about the neck pain may jar the patient's memory. It also allows the patient to monitor response to therapy.

CHIEF COMPLAINT

The recording of the chief complaint describes the patient's age, sex, and duration of neck pain. It is at this point that the possibility of a life-threatening cause of neck pain needs to be considered. A tumor, infection, or traumatic disruption of the cervical spine is one of the few catastrophic causes of neck pain that may require emergency intervention. In addition to neck pain, progressive motor weakness, incontinence, progressive gait abnormalities, and lower extremity pain should be recognizable by the emergency room physician or general practitioner. In such instances only essential history needs to be obtained. Physical examination helps establish the potential causes of the paraplegia and spinal cord compression. Neurologic dysfunction, although not life-threatening, results from a spinal cord insult and requires immediate evaluation. If the level of insult to the spinal cord is high up in the cervical spine, it may present respiratory difficulties and thus become a life-threatening emergency. After the life-threatening causes of neck pain have been eliminated as potential diagnoses, a complete history should be obtained.

Age

Figure 4–1 lists the various causes of neck pain arranged by the age range at which they

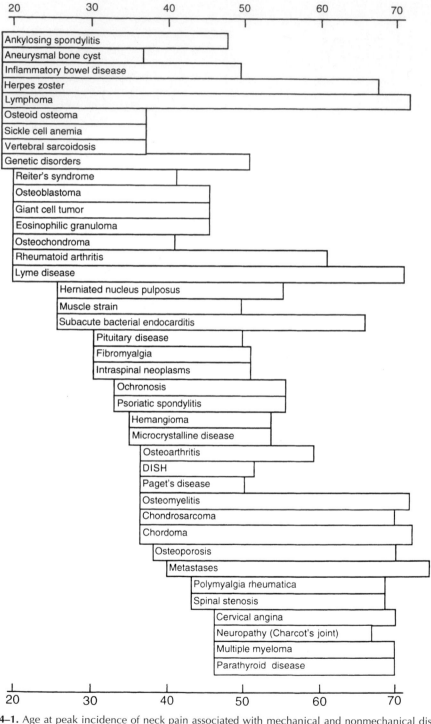

Figure 4–1. Age at peak incidence of neck pain associated with mechanical and nonmechanical disorders.

most frequently occur. Spondyloarthropathies, including ankylosing spondylitis, Reiter's syndrome, spondylitis associated with inflammatory bowel disease, and benign tumors of the spine (aneurysmal bone cyst, osteoid osteoma, osteoblastoma, and giant cell tumor) occur between the third and fourth decades. Trauma and spasmodic torticollis occur more commonly in younger individuals. A different set of diseases occurs more commonly during and following the sixth decade. These diseases include malignant disease (metastases), metabolic disease (chondrocalcinosis), and degenerative diseases. Diseases of middle age include diffuse idiopathic skeletal hyperostosis, gout, Paget's disease, and osteomyelitis.

Gender

Neck pain is common in men and women. Some studies indicate that the frequency of neck injuries may actually be higher in women. Occupational exposure for women who work at a desk and frequently type at computers may explain some of the increased prevalence of this symptom. Many medical illnesses, including the spondyloarthropathies, infections, and malignant and benign tumors, occur more commonly in men. Endocrinologic disorders, including parathyroid disorders and muscle disease (polymyalgia rheumatica and fibromyalgia), are more likely to occur in women. Psoriatic spondylitis, spondylitis associated with inflammatory bowel disease, hemangioma, herpes zoster, and skeletal metastases occur with equal frequency in men and women. A listing of illnesses associated with neck pain according to sexual predominance is presented in Table 4–1.

FAMILY HISTORY

Familial predisposition does occur in certain medical illnesses that are associated with neck pain. A prime example of a group of illnesses with such a predisposition is the spondyloarthropathies. In the presence of a particular histocompatibility locus antigen (HLA-B27), members of a family are at risk of developing ankylosing spondylitis, Reiter's syndrome, psoriatic spondylitis, and spondylitis associated with inflammatory bowel disease. Other spondyloarthropathies, such as those occurring in familial Mediterranean fever and Whipple's disease, occur more commonly in family mem-

TABLE 4–1. GENDER PREVALENCE FOR ILLNESSES ASSOCIATED WITH NECK PAIN

MALE PREDOMINANT

Ankylosing spondylitis	Multiple myeloma
Reiter's syndrome	Chordoma
Diffuse idiopathic skeletal hyperostosis	Lymphoma
	Gout
Osteomyelitis	Paget's disease
Eosinophilic granuloma	Osteoid osteoma
Osteoblastoma	

FEMALE PREDOMINANT

Rheumatoid arthritis	Osteoporosis
Polymyalgia rheumatica	Calcium pyrophosphate deposition disease
Fibromyalgia	
Giant cell tumor	Aneurysmal bone cyst

EQUAL FREQUENCY

Psoriatic spondylitis	Mechanical disorders
Enteropathic arthritis	Muscle strain (whiplash)
Hemangioma	Herniated disc
Herpes zoster	Osteoarthritis/spinal stenosis
Skeletal metastases	

bers without any specifically associated genetic factor. The ethnic background of the family may predispose members to specific illnesses. White women of northern European extraction are at greater risk of developing osteoporosis. Ashkenazic Jews may develop Gaucher's disease. Many of the other illnesses that cause neck pain have no specific familial predilection. However, it is always prudent for the examining physician to inquire about other family members with similar symptoms and the diagnoses that have been associated with their complaints. This information can help direct the clinician in formulating the diagnostic evaluation of the patient.

OCCUPATIONAL/SOCIAL HISTORY

The occupational history is essential for evaluating the risk of the patient for developing mechanical neck pain. Workers who have been required to do repetitive tasks with their upper extremity as well as prolonged sitting with their head in a flexed position, such as during typing, are at risk of developing mechanical neck pain. In addition, occupations that involve vibration or exposure to an environment filled with smoke may also predispose workers to this problem. However, neck pain is common and does not require occupational exposure to occur. The association of work and the onset of pain is important in evaluating the patient in regard to compensation. Whether or not the symptom of neck pain is related to the patient's work, it is important to discuss the association of the two from the patient's viewpoint.

Ankylosing spondylitis is not caused by any work-related actions. Patients may have difficulty accepting that the work they have been doing has no correlation with the onset of their illness. A positive therapeutic outcome has a better chance of occurring when patients realize the source of their difficulties and do not have false expectations about compensation for their symptoms. It is also appropriate to inquire about any pending litigation in regard to the patient's neck pain. It is incumbent on the physician not to assume that, because workers' compensation is involved or litigation is pending, the patient's symptoms are fictitious or exaggerated. Physicians should give the patient the benefit of the doubt. Patients who are hurt on the job or have an accident develop neck pain secondary to mechanical or medical causes. An incidental trauma may be assumed to be the source of pain while the actual cause of pain, such as a pathologic fracture secondary to a tumor, goes unrecognized. Only a thorough examination by the patient's physician can discover the true cause of the patient's neck pain.

Pressures to return to work may be different for the salaried employee versus the self-employed person. A self-employed individual may push the physician into cutting corners of evaluation and therapy to obtain the "quick fix" needed to allow a return to normal activities. On the other hand, the salaried employee may delay return because of the fear of reinjury. The treating physician must keep these concerns of patients in mind when developing an appropriate diagnostic and therapeutic program.

Social history also includes quantification of consumption of alcohol, coffee, cigarettes, and recreational drugs. Increased consumption of alcohol, coffee, or cigarettes is associated with osteoporosis, and illicit drug use results in immunosuppression and predisposition to infection.

Review of leisure time activities is another important way to measure level of function before the onset of neck pain. Are recreational activities limited to the same degree as work-related tasks? Response to therapy can often be measured by the patient's resumption of recreational activities. Inquiries about the new use of bifocals may also be significant. Repeated flexion and extension of the cervical spine may result in neck pain, occipital pain, or retro-orbital discomfort.[2]

PAST MEDICAL HISTORY

Past medical history should list in chronologic order all operations, hospitalizations, and previous severe injuries that affected the neck. Neck injuries remembered from childhood are usually significant in the amount of damage sustained by anatomic structures. A history of slipping on ice and hitting the head, resulting in bedrest for a few days, may be the initial episode that results in the development of disc disease in adulthood. Individuals may remember a swimming accident in which the neck was severely bent during bodysurfing or diving. Similarly, a car accident or any high-speed trauma with a whiplash injury may, in some instances, predispose to later degeneration, although this association has not been linked. All general medical problems should be reviewed. Certain diseases, including diabetes, other endocrinopathies, malignancies, and metabolic bone disease, may have a direct effect on structures in the cervical spine. Other disorders may not have a direct effect on the neck pain per se, but they may be associated with physical disorders (congestive heart failure and angina) or require specific medications (anticoagulants) that limit the therapeutic options for the treating physician. In addition, allergies to medications are listed on the history.

REVIEW OF SYSTEMS

Although frequently thought to be redundant or superfluous, review of systems is an essential part of neck pain history. A complete negative review is added evidence for the regional or mechanical nature of the pain. Positive responses help organize symptoms into patterns associated with systemic illness that cause neck pain. The presence of constitutional symptoms is a worrisome finding and requires a more thorough evaluation. Fever in the setting of new-onset neck pain may be associated with influenza, pyogenic discitis, or osteomyelitis.

Review of the integument system may reveal a history of scaling patches over the elbows that respond to topical agents (psoriasis) or nail opacification that never responded to antifungal therapy (Reiter's syndrome). History of conjunctivitis, iritis, or oral ulcers should raise the possibility of a spondyloarthropathy as the cause of neck pain. Temporomandibular joint dysfunction may be associated with a painful bite or limited jaw opening resulting in neck pain. Decreased cardiopulmonary function may be a manifestation of the spondyloarthropathy or endocrinopathy. Lesions of segments C3, C4, and C5 may affect the diaphragm and thus breathing. Patients may complain of dyspnea when the nerve supply to respiratory muscles is affected. Visceral causes of neck pain should be considered in the patient with a positive history for gastroesophageal reflux or diffuse esophageal spasm or malignancy. Dysphagia may be caused by disorders affecting the cervical spine. Pain with swallowing may be related to anterior disc protrusion, vertebral osteophyte, or vertebral subluxation into the esophagus. Difficulty forming a bolus of food may be related to muscular weakness secondary to a primary muscle disorder (polymyositis) or a neurologic disorder (myasthenia gravis). A history of anemia may be related to a systemic illness, gastrointestinal blood loss of an iatrogenic nature (drugs), or a primary hematologic disorder (sickle cell disease). A history of peptic ulcer disease may alter the ability to tolerate anti-inflammatory medications. Nausea and vomiting may accompany spinal cord compression.

A cardiovascular system history is relevant. Cervical angina consists of cardiac ischemic symptoms referred to regions innervated by the C5–T1 nerve roots, thereby mimicking an acute cervical radiculopathy.[3] Pain may radiate to the left shoulder or arm and be accompanied by upper extremity numbness. These symptoms are usually exacerbated by exertion, relieved by nitrates, and unaffected by neck movement. In older individuals, the coexistence of true angina and pseudoangina must be considered. Irritation of the C4 nerve root, which supplies the diaphragm and pericardium, may result in palpitations or tachycardia. Episodes of syncope may be indicative of insufficiency of vertebral circulation secondary to cervical spine disease.

Neuropsychiatric history should not be skipped. Headache is common in cervical syndromes. The occipital region is affected and is dull and aching in character. The headache pain may spread to the eye region on one or both sides. This pain may be related to occipital neuralgia. The pain is aggravated by straining, sneezing, and coughing, as well as by movements of the head and neck. Headache

may result from nerve root or sympathetic nerve compression, vertebral artery pressure, autonomic dysfunction, muscle spasm, or osteoarthritis of the apophyseal joints affecting the upper three cervical vertebrae.[4] In its most severe form, headache may awaken individuals from sleep. A number of factors should alert the clinician to potential, dangerous forms of headache that are unassociated with abnormalities in the cervical spine[5] (Table 4–2). Eye symptoms, such as blurred vision, increased tearing, eye pain, or retro-orbital pain, may be associated with cervical disorders. Irritation of the cervical sympathetic nerves that supply eye structures that are innervated by plexuses surrounding the vertebral and internal carotid arteries may cause neck symptoms. Abnormalities in equilibrium may also result from disorders of the sympathetic plexus surrounding the vertebral arteries. These abnormalities of gait may also be associated with decreased auditory acuity or tinnitus. These symptoms of autonomic disorders may persist during pain-free intervals.[6]

Descriptions of local versus generalized sensory and motor abnormalities help categorize neck symptoms as a component of a systemic neurologic disease or as a regional disturbance associated with local nerve dysfunction. Review

TABLE 4–2. DANGEROUS SIGNS INVOLVING HEADACHES

1. Headache is a new symptom or has markedly changed in character over the past 3 months.
2. Presence of sensory or motor deficits accompanying headache other than the typical visual prodromata of migraine with aura.
3. Headache solely on one side of the head.
4. Headache associated with unconsciousness after a trauma.
5. Headache is constant and unremitting.
6. Patient with tension-like headache has pain intensity steadily increasing over a period of weeks to months with little relief, is worse in the morning and less severe during the day, and is accompanied by vomiting.
7. Headache occurs in a patient with a history of cancer.
8. Headache is associated with change in personality, behavior, or intellectual function.
9. Headache is a new complaint in an individual who is older than 60 years of age.
10. Headache pain is sudden in onset and occurs during conditions of exertion.
11. Headache occurs in an individual with a family history of cerebral aneurysm, other vascular anomalies, or polycystic kidneys.

Modified from Andrasik F: Assessment of patients with headaches. In: Turk DC, Melzack R: Handbook of Pain Assessment. New York: The Guilford Press, 1992, p 345.

of any psychiatric disturbance is also essential. During this part of the examination it is helpful to have the patient describe his or her personality. Is the patient obsessive, compulsive, or driven? Is the patient passive? Is the patient depressed about the physical condition? Is the patient overly anxious or unconcerned about the potential cause of the neck pain (anxiety neurosis or hysteria)? Answers to these questions alert the physician to the individual who may have psychogenic neck pain.

PRESENT ILLNESS

The majority of the history taken about the present illness is directed toward the elaboration of the chronologic development of neck pain and its character, review of the results of previously obtained diagnostic tests, and response to therapy taken during the episode of neck pain.

Onset

Mechanical causes of neck pain (muscle strain and herniated nucleus pulposus) usually have an acute, sudden onset. The onset of pain is frequently associated with a specific task done in a mechanically disadvantaged position. Muscle bundles may be torn, fasciae stretched, and facet joints or uncovertebral joints irritated. Pain starts instantaneously or may come on gradually within a few hours.

Medical causes of neck pain tend to have a more gradual onset of pain. Tumor pain, for example, starts insidiously, except for episodes of acute pain associated with pathologic fractures of skeletal structures. Pain from inflammatory spondyloarthropathy may develop over months or years.

Duration and Frequency

Mechanical neck pain generally has a duration of a few days to a few months. Most muscle strains are relieved within 2 weeks. Disc herniations may require 8 weeks for resolution. Disc degeneration may cause a low-grade chronic discomfort that is exacerbated during acute attacks that last for 2 to 4 weeks. Most mechanical neck pain is intermittent. The frequency of episodes depends to a certain extent on exposure of the individual to mechanical stresses that worsen the condition.

Medical conditions, in contrast, cause chronic pain that is persistent rather than episodic. Patients with spondyloarthropathies develop chronic aching neck pain that has a long duration measured in months. In addition they may have associated thoracic or lumbar spinal pain. Tumors of the spine cause pain that is persistent, building in intensity over months. In addition a history of night pain is also frequent.

Psychogenic pains are constant and unrelenting. Histories of years of constant, excruciating pain are not uncommon.

Location and Radiation

Most mechanical and medical causes of neck pain are localized to the cervical spine. Damage to the musculoskeletal structures (discs and posterior apophyseal joints) may cause referred pain in surrounding areas of the neck and shoulders. These structures include adjacent paraspinous, anterior, and posterior cervical muscles. Abnormalities in facet joints, annular disc fibers, and supporting ligaments may also result in neck pain. Pain can be localized to a specific midline structure, such as a spinous process, or may be more lateral in the paraspinal tissues. The identification of the point of maximum tenderness in the midline often helps differentiate bone lesions from soft tissue lesions with paraspinal pain.

Pain that radiates into the arm from the cervical spine or that is exclusively in the arm is more suggestive of nerve root irritation. Lesions from C5 and below may cause arm symptoms. Discs that disrupt annular fibers cause pain in the arm. As the disc impinges the nerve root, pain is referred down the arm. Once the disc is extruded and the pressure on the annulus from disc protrusion is relieved, arm pain continues while neck pain may resolve. Spinal stenosis also causes radiation of pain into the arm. Disc herniation causes radiating pain that is present at rest, whereas radiating pain with spinal stenosis occurs in positions that extend the spine or decrease room in the spinal canal for the neural elements.

Radiation of pain to the upper extremity is not limited to mechanical abnormalities exclusively. Compression of the brachial plexus may occur from thoracic outlet syndrome, a cervical rib, or hypertrophy of the scalene muscles. Pathologic conditions in and around the shoulder may also result in nerve compression as well as compression of any point distally in the extremity itself. Common causes are compression of the ulnar nerve in the cubital tunnel and the median nerve in the carpal tunnel syndrome. In general it is easy to distinguish these problems from a herniated cervical disc, if their diagnosis is thought of and checked for. It is important to elicit a history of shoulder and arm pain that is related to position or movement of the arm. It is also important to remember that a subdiaphragmatic process such as an abscess can cause referred pain in the shoulder.

Psychogenic pain is not well localized. Large nondermatomal areas are affected. Radiation of pain follows no consistent anatomic pattern.

Aggravating and Alleviating Factors

Characteristically, mechanical lesions of the cervical spine improve with recumbency and worsen with increased activity. Increased activity includes long sitting or standing with the neck unsupported, particularly when looking down at a keyboard or reading. Patients with muscle strain improve with bedrest or controlled immobilization of the neck with a soft cervical collar. Not all cervical spine movements necessarily exacerbate muscle strain pain. Careful history defines those motions that are painless and put no stress on damaged muscles and those that irritate the injured muscle and result in reflex spasm.

Increases in cerebrospinal fluid pressure increase nerve root irritation caused by disc herniation. Coughing, sneezing, and Valsalva's maneuver increase pressure and may exacerbate radicular pain. Sudden, reflex motions associated with coughing or sneezing may increase muscle strain as well. However, pain caused by muscle strain remains localized and does not radiate into the upper extremities.

Some patients with mechanical neck pain feel worse with bedrest. Patients with spondyloarthropathy have exacerbated pain after they have been in bed for a few hours. Not infrequently they wake up during the night because of pain associated with rolling over in bed. Early morning is the worst time of day for the patient with spondyloarthropathy.

Pain from tumors involving bone, muscle, or the spinal cord is often increased with recumbency. Patients with such tumors seek relief by sleeping in a chair or pacing the floor.

Other patients do find relief of pain with recumbency. These individuals find relief only with absolute immobility. This is a sign of acute infection, compression fracture–related metabolic bone disease, or pathologic fracture secondary to a tumor or infiltrative disease.

Patients with viscerogenic referred pain rarely describe any association of the discomfort with position. Patients with psychogenic pain have difficulty describing factors that relieve or worsen their pain. The pain is present all the time. There is no position that is comfortable. Activities that involve little physical effort have an exaggerated effect on their pain.

Time of Day

Mechanical disorders (muscle strain, degenerative disc disease, spinal stenosis, and osteoarthritis) cause pain that increases with activity. The end of the day, after the patient has been up and around, is associated with the most pain. Medical disorders are problematic in the morning or after the patient has gone to sleep. Classically, inflammatory arthropathies cause morning stiffness. Patients have great difficulty getting out of bed in the morning because of stiffness and pain. As the patient ambulates, the stiffness and pain lessen.

Tumors of the spine and spinal cord cause pain that increases with recumbency. Therefore, most individuals with cervical spine tumors complain of pain that is maximal during the night. This characteristic of tumors is not solely reserved to malignant processes. Benign tumors, a prime example being an osteoid osteoma, cause severe nocturnal pain. Patients with spinal tumors may get up and ambulate at night to diminish their discomfort.

Sleeping position of the patient may have a significant effect on the extent of neck pain. Individuals with large pillows may be in a flexed posture for extended periods. An arm hyperabducted under the pillow may be associated with shoulder pain.

Quality and Intensity

Description of the quality of the pain can be helpful in identifying its source. The adjectives used to describe neck pain are numerous. Initially patients should describe the quality of pain themselves without suggestions from the examining physician. A list of words from the physician may alter the patient's responses to a category of terms that cannot really describe the discomfort. However, some patients are

McGill Pain Questionnaire

Patient's Name _____ Date _____ Time_____am/pm

PRI: S_____ A _____ E _____ M _____ PRI(T)_____ PPI ___
    (1–10)   (11–15)   (16)   (17–20)   (1–20)

1 FLICKERING
  QUIVERING
  PULSING
  THROBBING
  BEATING
  POUNDING

2 JUMPING
  FLASHING
  SHOOTING

3 PRICKING
  BORING
  DRILLING
  STABBING
  LANCINATING

4 SHARP
  CUTTING
  LACERATING

5 PINCHING
  PRESSING
  GNAWING
  CRAMPING
  CRUSHING

6 TUGGING
  PULLING
  WRENCHING

7 HOT
  BURNING
  SCALDING
  SEARING

8 TINGLING
  ITCHY
  SMARTING
  STINGING

9 DULL
  SORE
  HURTING
  ACHING
  HEAVY

10 TENDER
  TAUT
  RASPING
  SPLITTING

11 TIRING
  EXHAUSTING

12 SICKENING
  SUFFOCATING

13 FEARFUL
  FRIGHTFUL
  TERRIFYING

14 PUNISHING
  GRUELLING
  CRUEL
  VICIOUS
  KILLING

15 WRETCHED
  BLINDING

16 ANNOYING
  TROUBLESOME
  MISERABLE
  INTENSE
  UNBEARABLE

17 SPREADING
  RADIATING
  PENETRATING
  PIERCING

18 TIGHT
  NUMB
  DRAWING
  SQUEEZING
  TEARING

19 COOL
  COLD
  FREEZING

20 NAGGING
  NAUSEATING
  AGONIZING
  DREADFUL
  TORTURING

PPI
0 NO PAIN
1 MILD
2 DISCOMFORTING
3 DISTRESSING
4 HORRIBLE
5 EXCRUCIATING

BRIEF __   RHYTHMIC __   CONTINUOUS __
MOMENTARY __   PERIODIC __   STEADY __
TRANSIENT __   INTERMITTENT __   CONSTANT __

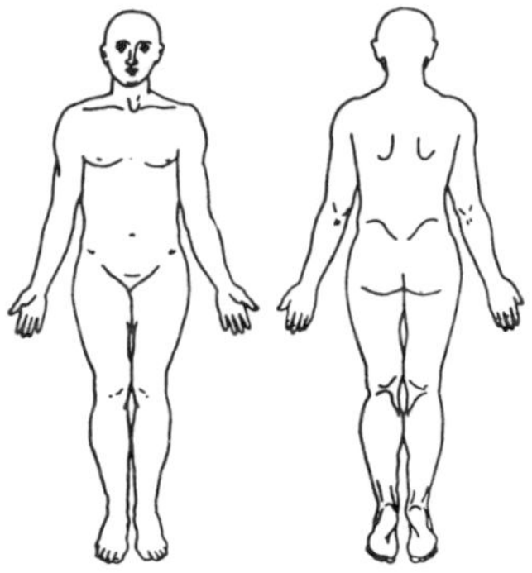

E = EXTERNAL

I = INTERNAL

COMMENTS:

Figure 4–2. The McGill Pain Questionnaire. (From Melzack R [ed]: Pain Measurement and Assessment. New York: Raven Press, 1983.)

unable to describe their pain in their own words. At this point it would be helpful to supply them with a list of choices. One example of such a list of pain descriptions is the McGill Pain Questionnaire[7] (Fig. 4–2). The questionnaire divides words into three major groups: those that describe the sensory quality of pain in terms of temporal, spacial, pressure, thermal, and other properties; those that describe the affective qualities of pain in terms of tension, fear, and autonomic properties; and those that describe the subjective, overall intensity of pain. In each category the words are listed according to increasing intensity. In addition a line drawing of the body is included, demarcating the location of pain. A pain rating index (PRI) is determined by adding together the rank values of origin in each subclass. The number of words chosen is quantified. The scale can be administered on successive visits to help quantify response to therapy. If the McGill Pain Questionnaire is not used, the examining physician should include a line drawing of the body in the patient's history. The pictorial representation of the patient's pain helps delineate its extent. The patient's response to therapy may also be monitored by review of the extent of painful areas on serial line drawings.

The intensity of pain may also be measured by visual means. The visual analogue scale (Fig. 4–3) is a visual way to quantify pain.[8] A visual analogue scale is a line, 10 cm in length, in which one end represents no pain and the other severe, incapacitating pain. Patients mark a point on the line corresponding to the severity of their pain. The distance from this point to the end of the line represents pain severity. The visual analogue scale has greater sensitivity quantifying pain than verbal descriptors. It is a continuum whereas verbal descriptors correspond to points along a line. There are not enough words to describe all the possible points along a line.

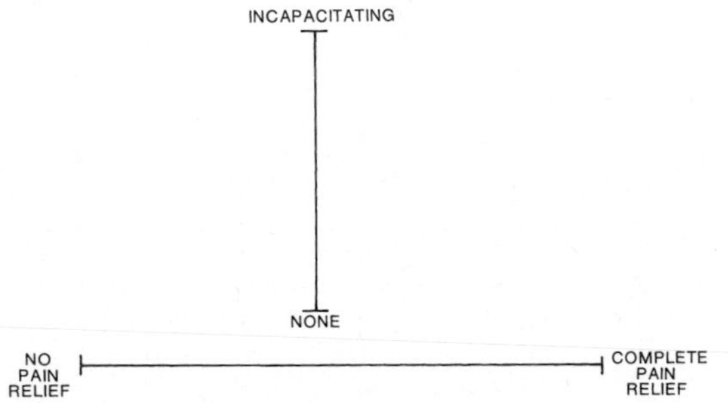

Leak and colleagues at Northwick Park Hospital in London, England, developed a validated questionnaire to measure neck pain and disability[9] (Fig. 4–4). Questions on duration and intensity of pain were good indicators of patients' global assessment of their condition. Improvement of symptoms over time was associated with a decrease in the severity of pain as measured by the questionnaire. This questionnaire is a useful tool to objectify the degree of neck pain experienced by patients with cervical spine disease.

Superficial somatic, deep somatic, neurogenic, viscerogenic referred, and psychogenic pain have qualities that differentiate them. Those qualities have been described in Chapter 3. Refer to this chapter for the characteristics of the various pain categories. Cramping, dull, aching pain is associated with muscle damage. Sharp, shooting pain is linked to nerve root disorders. Burning, stinging, pressure sensations are caused by disorders affecting sympathetic nerves. Deep, nagging, dull pain symptoms are associated with bone disorders, and severe, sharp pain is caused by fractures. Diffuse, throbbing pain is associated with vascular lesions.

Patients should list the physicians who have been consulted about their neck pain. Sometimes the length of this list is instructive in making the diagnosis of a malingerer. In addition, information about the diagnostic tests used for evaluation of the patient's neck pain and efficacy of previous therapies should be obtained from the patient. Finally, the history is not complete unless the physician has a clear understanding of why the patient "really" came to see the physician and what are the patient's true expectations from the encounter.

Figure 4–3. Visual analogue scales for pain (top) and pain relief (bottom). The physical orientation of the scales may be vertical or horizontal.

SUMMARY

The history is the foundation on which the rest of the diagnostic process is built. By listening carefully to the patient's description of the chief complaint, the clinician should be able to generate a list of potential diagnoses that could be causing the difficulties. The next step in the process is a complete and appropriate physical examination. With the myriad of tests that can be done during the physical

NECK PAIN QUESTIONNAIRE

Label

Surname: OTHER NAMES:	DATE OF BIRTH:
HOSPITAL NO:	CONSULTANT:
	DATE COMPLETED:

Please read:

This questionnaire has been designed to give us information as to how your NECK PAIN has affected your ability to manage in everyday life.

Please answer every section and mark in each section ONLY THE ONE BOX which applies to you. We realise you may consider that two of the statements in any one section relate to you, but PLEASE JUST MARK THE BOX WHICH MOST CLOSELY DESCRIBES YOUR PROBLEM.

Remember, just mark ONE box in each section.

1. NECK PAIN INTENSITY

☐ I have no pain at the moment
☐ The pain is mild at the moment
☐ The pain is moderate at the moment
☐ The pain is severe at the moment
☐ The pain is the worst imaginable at the moment

2. NECK PAIN AND SLEEPING

☐ My sleep is never disturbed by pain
☐ My sleep is occasionally disturbed by pain
☐ My sleep is regularly disturbed by pain
☐ Because of pain I have less than 5 hours sleep in total
☐ Because of pain I have less than 2 hours sleep in total

3. PINS & NEEDLES OR NUMBNESS IN THE ARMS AT NIGHT

☐ I have no pins & needles or numbness at night
☐ I have occasional pins & needles or numbness at night
☐ My sleep is regularly disturbed by pins & needles or numbness
☐ Because of pins & needles I have less than 5 hours sleep in total
☐ Because of pins & needles or numbness I have less than 2 hours sleep in total

4. DURATION OF SYMPTOMS

☐ My neck and arms feel normal all day
☐ I have symptoms in my neck or arms on waking, which last less than 1 hour
☐ Symptoms are present on and off for a total period of 1–4 hours
☐ Symptoms are present on and off for a total of more than 4 hours
☐ Symptoms are present continuously all day

5. CARRYING

☐ I can carry heavy objects without extra pain
☐ I can carry heavy objects, but they give me extra pain
☐ Pain prevents me from carrying heavy objects, but I can manage medium weight objects
☐ I can only lift light weight objects
☐ I cannot lift anything at all

6. READING & WATCHING T.V.

☐ I can do this as long as I wish with no problems
☐ I can do this as long as I wish, if I'm in a suitable position
☐ I can do this as long as I wish, but it causes extra pain
☐ Pain causes me to stop doing this sooner than I would like
☐ Pain prevents me from doing this at all

7. WORKING/HOUSEWORK ETC

☐ I can do my usual work without extra pain
☐ I can do my usual work, but it gives me extra pain
☐ Pain prevents me from doing my usual work for more than half the usual time
☐ Pain prevents me from doing my usual work for more than a quarter the usual time
☐ Pain prevents me from working at all

8. SOCIAL ACTIVITIES

☐ My social life is normal and causes me no extra pain
☐ My social life is normal, but increases the degree of pain
☐ Pain has restricted my social life, but I am still able to go out
☐ Pain has restricted my social life to the home
☐ I have no social life because of pain

9. DRIVING (Omit 9 if you never drive a car when in good health)

☐ I can drive whenever necessary without discomfort
☐ I can drive whenever necessary, but with discomfort
☐ Neck pain or stiffness limits my driving occasionally
☐ Neck pain or stiffness limits my driving frequently
☐ I cannot drive at all due to neck symptoms

10. Compared with the last time you answered this Questionnaire, is your neck pain:

☐ Much better
☐ Slightly better
☐ The same
☐ Slightly worse
☐ Much worse

Thank you very much for your help.

DATE: . . . .

TIME: . . . .

SIGNED . . . .

Figure 4–4. Neck Pain Questionnaire. (From Leak AM, Cooper J, Dyer S, et al.: The Northwick Park neck pain questionnaire devised to measure neck pain and disability. Br J Rheumatol 33:474, 1994. By permission of Oxford University Press.)

and laboratory evaluations, the history allows the clinician to select those parts of the examination that will help the clinician most efficiently make the correct diagnosis from the possibilities included in the differential diagnosis list.

References

1. Brain WR: Some unsolved problems in cervical spondylosis. Br Med J 1:771, 1963.
2. Bland JH: Clinical methods. In: Bland JH (ed): Disorders of the Cervical Spine: Diagnosis and Medical Management, 2nd ed. Philadelphia: WB Saunders Co, 1994, pp 113–146.
3. Mitchell LC, Schafermeyer RW: Herniated cervical disk presenting as ischemic chest pain. Am J Emerg Med 9:343, 1991.
4. Emeads J: The cervical spine and headache. Neurology 38:1874, 1988.
5. Andrasik F: Assessment of patients with headaches. In: Turk DC, Melzack R: Handbook of Pain Assessment. New York: The Guilford Press, 1992, pp 345–361.
6. Appenzeller O: The autonomic nervous system in cervical spine disorders. In: Bland JH (ed): Disorders of the Cervical Spine: Diagnosis and Medical Management, 2nd ed. Philadelphia: WB Saunders Co, 1994, pp 313–327.
7. Melzack R: The McGill Pain Questionnaire. In: Melzack R (ed): Pain Measurement and Assessment. New York: Raven Press, 1983, pp 41–47.
8. Huskisson EC: Visual Analogue Scales. In: Melzack R (ed): Pain Measurement and Assessment. New York: Raven Press, 1983, pp 33–40.
9. Leak AM, Cooper J, Dyer S, et al.: The Northwick Park neck pain questionnaire devised to measure neck pain and disability. Br J Rheumatol 33:469, 1994.

5

Physical Examination

After completion of the medical history, the physical examination is the next step in the diagnostic process. The history has alerted the physician to those individuals who have medical emergencies and require therapy to begin after only an abbreviated examination. These include patients with a lesion causing acute progressive cord compression (herniated intervertebral disc) or infection (meningitis). Patients with cervical spine cord compression may present with acute paraplegia, lower extremity weakness or awkwardness of gait, and urinary incontinence. These patients are evaluated expeditiously so that therapy may be instituted to minimize permanent damage to the spinal cord. Fortunately, the number of patients who present in this manner is extremely small.

GENERAL MEDICAL EXAMINATION

Examination of the cervical spine is done after completion of the general physical examination. This is a useful sequence of events for a number of reasons. Examining the part of the body that is painful is best left for the last portion of the evaluation. Putting the patient through various maneuvers needed to evaluate cervical spine function may leave the patient in a condition that limits cooperation with completing portions of a general medical examination. It also allows the physician an opportunity to observe the patient's motions and posture at a time when the cervical spine is not being examined. The patient may be unaware of the fact that observation is the initial portion of the physical examination. In fact, unbeknownst to the patient, the chief complaint is being evaluated starting with the physician's introduction to the patient.

Clues to the systemic character of neck pain are discovered during the general physical examination. Vital signs can document the presence of fever associated with an infection or neoplasm. Tachycardia may be the sympathetic nervous system's response to the patient's pain. Normotension in a patient with hypertension suggests acute blood loss. Discrepancies in blood pressure between the arms occurs in neck pain patients who have compression of vascular structures in the cervical spine. A reduction of blood pressure in one arm and bruit heard in one or both subclavian arteries suggests the diagnosis of subclavian steal syndrome.[1]

The skin examination is particularly helpful in alerting the physician to the presence of systemic illness. A number of the spondyloarthropathies cause dermatologic abnormalities: keratoderma blennorrhagicum, a rash over the palms and soles, is characterized by hyperkeratotic, yellowish, confluent plaques. Psoriasis causes erythematous raised plaques with overlying scales that occur on extensor surfaces (elbows and knees) and on the scalp, umbilicus, and perianal area. Erythema nodosum (erythematous raised nodules, particularly noted on the lower extremities) is associated with inflammatory bowel disease and sarcoidosis. Dermal plaques are also associated with sarcoidosis. Painful vesicles distributed in a dermatomal pattern are a telling sign of herpes zoster. Petechiae raise the possibility of thrombocytopenia, associated with a primary hematologic disorder (multiple myeloma), secondary metastatic tumor, or subacute bacterial endocarditis. The presence of small skin ulcers or needle marks raises the possibility of intravenous drug use, although the patient may deny substance abuse. Erythema chronicum migrans, a large raised erythematous skin lesion, is the cutaneous hallmark of Lyme disease.

The eye examination may reveal the presence of conjunctivitis (Reiter's syndrome) or iritis (ankylosing spondylitis). Asymmetric pupillary signs may indicate irritability of sympathetic nerves in the neck supplying the ciliary muscles. Complete paralysis of the sympathetic fibers (Horner's syndrome) is associated with miosis, vasomotor instability, increased perspiration, and ptosis. Examination of the oropharynx may reveal painless (Reiter's syndrome) or painful (Behçet's syndrome) oral ulcers. Examination of the neck may reveal thyromegaly, indicative of thyroid gland dysfunction. Lymphadenopathy may be associated with neoplastic processes (lymphoma), infectious processes (tuberculosis and subacute bacterial endocarditis), or idiopathic processes (sarcoidosis). Cervical ribs may be palpated in the supraclavicular area.

Excursion of the chest wall is important to measure. Arthritis of the costovertebral joints associated with a spondyloarthropathy limits motion, decreasing chest excursion and lung capacity. Chest excursion should be measured with the patient's arms held straight up over the head, with a tape measure pulled tight and placed at the fourth intercostal space in men and just below the breasts in women. The patient is then requested to take in a deep breath (normal excursion is ≤2.5 cm). Auscultation of the lung fields may result in discovery of abnormal breath sounds indicative of fibrosis. Pulmonary fibrosis is found in patients with spondyloarthropathies, sickle cell anemia, and sarcoidosis. Cardiac examination may demonstrate cardiomegaly, gallops, and murmurs. These abnormal findings may be associated with cardiac disease related to ankylosing spondylitis (aortic insufficiency), sickle cell disease (cardiomyopathy), and subacute bacterial endocarditis (valve insufficiency).

The abdominal examination is useful for documenting organomegaly. Hepatosplenomegaly is associated with individuals with hematologic or lymphoproliferative malignancies.

The musculoskeletal examination is helpful in identifying peripheral joint arthritis, which is often associated with cervical spine disease. For example, distal interphalangeal (DIP) joint arthritis is characteristic of psoriatic arthritis. Proximal interphalangeal joint disease in conjunction with DIP joint arthritis is commonly found in patients with osteoarthritis. Reiter's syndrome causes lower extremity arthritis in addition to sacroiliitis and spondylitis.

Ankle arthritis associated with erythema nodosum is associated with sarcoidosis. During the musculoskeletal examination it is appropriate to check for peripheral pulses, particularly in the upper extremities.

The lumbosacral spine examination is essential for evaluating cervical spine disorders. The axial skeleton works as a unit to support the head and maintain balance. Abnormalities in the lumbar spine in the form of a list, or loss of lordosis, result in mechanical alterations in the cervical spine that may cause pain. At a minimum, the lumbar spine should be moved through its full range of motion and palpated for any areas of tenderness and increased muscle tension.

EXAMINATION OF THE CERVICAL SPINE

Once the general examination is completed, the examination of the cervical spine should proceed. Common sense needs to be used in conducting the physical examination. Some patients who are in extreme pain do not tolerate an extensive general medical examination before evaluation of the cervical spine. In these patients an examination that concentrates solely on the cervical spine is appropriate. The remainder of the examination may be completed after evaluation of the cervical spine or on a subsequent visit.

The objective of the physical examination of the cervical spine is a demonstration of those physical abnormalities that help sort out the possible disease entities causing pain that were suggested from the medical history. Abnormalities of the cervical spine may be discovered while the spine is static or in motion. Unless the tests are done in orderly fashion, important observations may be missed. Therefore, it is helpful to evaluate the patient in a series of positions that test the function of musculoskeletal and neurologic structures of the cervical spine. In circumstances where involvement is unilateral, the uninvolved side should be compared to the affected side.

It is helpful to observe the patient disrobing. The head should move naturally with body movements. If the head is held stiffly to one side to protect or splint an area of pain, there may be a pathologic reason for such a posture. The neck region should then be inspected for normal characteristics as well as abnormalities, such as blisters, scars, and discoloration. Surgical scars on the anterior portion of the neck most often indicate previous thyroid surgery, and irregular pitted scars in the anterior triangle are likely events of previous tuberculous adenitis. Facial expression of the patient often gives the examiner an indication of the amount of pain the patient is experiencing.

The patient is initially examined standing. The patient should be undressed. Initially, gait is observed to detect any asymmetry or any list or limp. The patient can be asked to walk approximately 5 to 10 feet on the toes and then to return walking on the heels. This is a quick and cursory test of distal motor strength. Some of the earliest findings of cervical cord compression may be simply an abnormality in a patient's gait.

The spine is then viewed from behind, laterally, and anteriorly to see if the alignment is normal. From behind, the levels of the shoulders and any lateral spinal curves (scoliosis) should be noted. The patient stands with the head centered over the feet and the eyes level. Therefore, any deviation of the spine from the vertical is compensated by an opposite deviation elsewhere in the spine. The spine is compensated if the first thoracic vertebra is centered over the sacrum. A list occurs if that vertebra is not centered. The degree of list may be measured by dropping a perpendicular line from the first thoracic vertebra and measuring how far to the right or left of the gluteal cleft it falls. Pain in the neck may cause deviation that can be toward or away from the painful side.

The position of the scapulae should be noted. Asymmetry of the scapular height may be related to trapezius muscle weakness (spinal accessory nerve dysfunction), leg length discrepancy, or long thoracic nerve neuritis.

Laterally, any exaggeration or decrease of the normal cervical curvature is noted. Does the patient have a hyperlordosis (increased concavity) at the back of the neck or flattened cervical lordosis (lack of the normal curve in the posterior portion of the neck)? Is frank cervical kyphosis present as is seen with ankylosing spondylitis, whose severest form produces a chin-on-chest deformity? Torticollis causes the head to be tilted toward the side with the contracted sternocleidomastoid muscle.

During this portion of the examination, the examiner should engage the patient in some conversation. Typically, patients turn their head to speak to the physician. Discrepancies between ranges of motion should be noted.

The neck should be palpated while the patient is supine. Because muscles overlying in the deeper prominences of the neck are relaxed in that position, the bony structures become more sharply defined. To palpate the anterior bony structures of the neck, it is best to support the patient's neck from behind at the base with one hand and to examine with the opposite hand. The hyoid bone, a horseshoe-shaped structure, is situated above the thyroid cartilage. On a horizontal plane, it is opposite the C3 vertebral body. This can easily be palpated just above the thyroid cartilage—if the patient is asked to swallow, the movement of the hyoid bone becomes palpable.

Moving inferiorly in the midline allows the fingers to come in contact with the thyroid cartilage and its small, identifiable superior notch. The upper portion of the cartilage, commonly known as the Adam's apple, corresponds with the level of the C4 vertebral body, and the lower portion designates the C5 level.

The first cricoid ring is situated immediately inferior to a lower border of the thyroid cartilage and lies opposite C6. It is the only complete ring of the cricoid series that is an integral part of the trachea, and is immediately above the site for an emergency tracheostomy. This structure should be palpated gently as vigorous pressure may cause the patient to gag.

Moving laterally about 1 inch from the first cricoid ring, the examiner will come across the carotid tubercle, also known as Chassaignac's tubercle. The carotid tubercle is small and lies away from the midline, deep under the overlying muscles, but is palpable. The carotid tubercle of C6 should be palpated separately because simultaneous palpation can restrict the flow of blood in both carotid arteries, which run adjacent to the tubercles. The carotid tubercle is frequently used as an anatomic landmark for an anterior surgical approach to the C5–C6 level, and it is a site for the injection of the stellate cervical ganglion.

While exploring the anterior portion of the neck, it is possible to locate a small, hard bump of the C1 transverse process that lies between the angle of the jaw and the skull styloid process just behind the ear. As the broadest transverse process in the cervical spine, it is readily palpable and, although it has little clinical significance, it serves as an easily identifiable point of orientation.

The posterior landmarks of the neck are more accessible to palpation if the examiner stands behind the patient's head and cups the hands under the neck so that the fingertips meet at the midline. Because tense muscles can limit the palpation of the neck, the patient's head should be held in such a way that the neck muscles need not be used for support, and the patient should be encouraged to relax. Palpation of the posterior aspect of the cervical spine should begin at the occiput, the posterior portion of the skull. The inion, a dome-shaped bump, lies in the occipital region in the midline and marks the center of the superior nuchal line. As the examiner palpates laterally toward the end of the superior nuchal line, the rounded mastoid processes of the skull is felt. Next, the spinous processes of the cervical vertebrae lie along the posterior midline and should be palpated. Because no muscle tissue crosses the midline, these bony prominences are generally easily palpated. Beginning at the base of the skull, the C2 spinous process is the first one that is palpable, as the C1 spinous process is only a small tubercle and lies deep within the soft tissue. As the spinous processes are palpated from C2 through T1, the normal lordosis of the cervical spine should be noted. In some patients the spinous processes of C3 through C5 may be bifid (with two posterolateral projections rather than one midline projection of bone). The C7 and T1 spinous processes are larger than those above them, and the C7 spinous process is also known as the vertebrae prominens. The processes are normally in line with each other. A shift in the normal alignment may be due to a unilateral facet dislocation or to a fracture of the spinous process following trauma.

When the examiner moves laterally from the spinous processes approximately 1 inch, the joints of the vertebral facets that lie between the cervical vertebrae may be palpated. These joints often can cause symptoms of pain in the neck region. The joints feel like small domes and lie deep beneath the trapezius muscle. The facet joints are not always clearly palpable, and the patient must be completely relaxed to enable them to be palpated.

In general, when examining the cervical spine for posterior tenderness, it is important to determine whether the tenderness is midline, which is most often related to an intrinsic spinal problem, or whether it is paraspinal or off the midline and related to soft tissue pathology.

The remainder of the physical examination can be performed with the patient sitting. The sternocleidomastoid muscle extends from the sternoclavicular joint to the mastoid process and may be frequently stretched in hyperextension injuries of the neck that occur during automobile accidents. This muscle becomes more prominent when the patient turns the head to that side opposite the muscle to be examined. Palpable local swellings within the muscle may be due to hematoma and may cause the head to turn abnormally to one side (torticollis).

A chain of lymph nodes is situated along the medial border of the sternocleidomastoid muscle. In normal circumstances lymph nodes are either nonpalpable or only slightly so, and they are usually not tender. Lymph nodes may be palpable as small lumps that become tender to the touch when they are enlarged or inflamed.

The thyroid cartilage lies in a central position along the anterior midline of the neck anterior to the C4–C5 vertebrae. The thyroid gland lies superficial to the cartilage in a bilobed pattern, with a thin isthmus between them crossing the midline. A normal thyroid gland feels smooth and indistinct, whereas a gland with some pathologic changes may contain unusual local enlargements due to cysts or nodules that may also be tender to palpation. The thyroid gland is most easily felt from standing behind the patient.

The carotid artery is situated next to the carotid tubercle (C6). The carotid pulse is palpable if the examiner presses at this point with the tips of the index and middle fingers. As mentioned earlier, it is important to palpate only one side at a time to avoid an excessive decrease in flow to the brain. The pulses in each side of the neck should be approximately equal and both should be checked to determine the relative strengths.

The parotid gland overlies the sharp angle of the mandible. The gland is generally not palpable. If, however, the parotid gland is swollen (as in the case of mumps or Sjögren's syndrome), the angle of the mandible no longer feels sharp as it is covered by a larger soft tissue structure.

The supraclavicular fossa lies superior to the clavicle and lateral to the suprasternal notch. It is important to palpate this region for any unusual swellings or lumps. Although the platysma muscle crosses the fossa, it is not stretched tautly across it and therefore does change its concave shape. Swelling within the fossa may be caused by edema, secondary to trauma in the soft tissues about the shoulder as seen with a clavicular fracture. Small lumps in the fossa may be due to an enlargement of the lymph glands or may be an indicator of an apical disorder in the lung. If a cervical rib is present, it may be palpable in this fossa and can cause vascular or neurologic symptoms in the upper extremity.

In palpating the posterior aspect of the

neck, it is important to note the broad origin of the trapezius muscle from the ending of the skull to T12. The muscle's insertions must be palpated laterally under the clavicle, acromion, and spine of the scapula. It is most important to note any asymmetry from one side to the other when examining musculature. Any discrepancy in the size or shape on either side and any tenderness, unilateral or bilateral, should be noted. Tenderness most often is found in the superior-lateral portion of the muscle.

It is also important to feel for the exit point of the greater occipital nerves. This can be found by moving from the trapezius muscle to the base of the skull, probing both sides of the inion. If these nerves are inflamed, as may be the case following a whiplash injury, the nerves may be distinctly palpable. Inflammation of the greater occipital nerves may result in headache, with pain that radiates from the occipital ridge toward the apex of the skull.

The final structure to be palpated is the superior nuchal ligament, which arises from the inion at the base of the skull and extends to the C7 spinous process. Although this is not a distinctly palpable structure, the area in which it lies can be palpated to elicit tenderness. This structure runs between the tips of the spinous processes and the posterior aspect of the cervical spine. Tenderness at any one level may indicate either a stretched ligament as a result of a neck flexion injury or perhaps a defect within the ligament itself.

RANGE OF MOTION

The normal range of motion of the neck provides an extremely flexible mechanism for positioning the head in space to direct a wide scope of vision as well as an acute sense of balance. It is important to assess the range of motion in the cervical spine in all the basic planes (Fig. 5–1).

First, test active flexion-extension of the neck. Instruct the patient to nod forward and place the chin on the chest. The normal range of flexion should allow the chest to be touched with the chin. The patient is then asked to look directly at the ceiling; with a normal range of motion, this should be possible with extension of the cervical spine. As the patient's head moves, it is important to watch to see if the arc of motion is smooth rather than halting or jerking. An auto accident may cause soft tissue trauma around the cervical spine, which may result in limitation of the range of motion and a disruption of the normal smooth arc.

Next, rotation should be assessed. The patient should be able to move the head far enough to both sides so that the chin is almost in line with the shoulder. Again, the smoothness of the motion should be observed.

Active lateral bending can be tested by asking the patient to touch ear to shoulder, making sure the patient does not compensate for limited motion by lifting shoulder to ear. In normal circumstances the patient should be able to tilt the head approximately 45° toward each shoulder.

The physician should observe the patient carefully during active bending to identify any specific arcs of limited motion. The patient may repeat the range of motion while the physician palpates the neck muscles for increased muscle tension that may limit motion.

Testing for passive range of motion in the

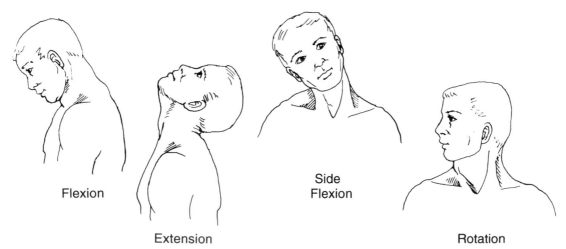

Flexion

Extension

Side Flexion

Rotation

Figure 5–1. Range of motion tests for examination of movement of the cervical spine.

TABLE 5–1. CERVICAL RADICULOPATHY SYMPTOMS AND FINDINGS

DISC LEVEL	NERVE ROOT	SYMPTOMS AND FINDINGS
C2–C3	C3	Pain: Back of neck, mastoid process, pinna of ear Sensory change: Back of neck, mastoid process, pinna of ear Motor deficit: None readily detectable except by EMG Reflex change: None
C3–C4	C4	Pain: Back of neck, levator scapulae, anterior chest Sensory change: Back of neck, levator scapulae, anterior chest Motor deficit: None readily detectable except by EMG Reflex change: None
C4–C5	C5	Pain: Neck, tip of shoulder, anterior arm Sensory change: Deltoid area Motor deficit: Deltoid, biceps Reflex change: Biceps
C5–C6	C6	Pain: Neck, shoulder, medial border of scapula, lateral arm, dorsal forearm Sensory change: Thumb and index finger Motor deficit: Biceps Reflex change: Biceps
C6–C7	C7	Pain: Neck, shoulder, medial border at scapula, lateral arm, dorsal forearm Sensory change: Index and middle fingers Motor deficit: Triceps Reflex change: Triceps
C7–T1	C8	Pain: Neck, medial border of scapula, medial aspect of arm and forearm Sensory change: Ring and little fingers Motor deficit: Intrinsic muscles of hand Reflex change: None

From Boden SD, Wiesel SW, Laws ER Jr, et al.: The Aging Spine: Essentials of Pathophysiology, Diagnosis, and Treatment. Philadelphia: WB Saunders Co, 1991, p 46.

cervical spine is seldom necessary. In fact, if the patient has an unstable cervical spine as a result of trauma, passive range of motion examination may cause neurologic damage.

Scapular and shoulder movements should also be tested. The following scapular movements are tested: a full shrug (trapezius and levator scapulae muscles); forward movement (pectoralis major and minor and serratus anterior muscles); backward movement (rhomboids and lower trapezius muscles); upward and lateral movements of arms over the head, palms together; and forward movement pressing against a wall (serratus anterior). Approximation of the scapulae stretches the dura mater through traction in the upper thoracic nerve roots, sometimes causing pain in the chest, suggesting a thoracic disc lesion.[2] These motions may also identify areas of joint disease in the shoulder or acromioclavicular joints. Paresthesias in the hands with arm elevation to 90° suggest thoracic outlet syndrome.

NEUROLOGIC EXAMINATION

There are three phases to a neurologic examination of the cervical spine (Table 5–1): motor strength testing, sensory examination, and reflex examination.

The first part of the motor portion of the neurologic examination concerns testing the intrinsic muscles of the neck, cervical spine, and functional groups. In this respect, muscle testing indicates the presence of any motor weakness that may affect the motion of the neck and, in addition, may demonstrate the integrity of the nervous supply. Muscles of the cervical spine are innervated by multiple levels (Fig. 5–2). Muscle strength may not be perceived to be diminished if only a portion of the segmental innervation to an individual muscle is disrupted. The primary flexors of the neck are the sternocleidomastoid muscles, innervated by the spinal accessory nerve, and the secondary flexors are the splenius muscles and the prevertebral muscles. Resistive muscle testing in the cervical spine is no different from that in any other area. Essentially, the patient is asked to perform a motion against a resistive force. In the case of cervical flexion, the examiner's palm is placed on the patient's forehead and the patient is asked to flex the neck slowly.

Primary extensors in the cervical spine consist of the paravertebral extensor muscles and the trapezius muscle, and the secondary extensors consist of the small intrinsic neck muscles. Resistive testing of extension is performed by placing the examiner's hand over the midline

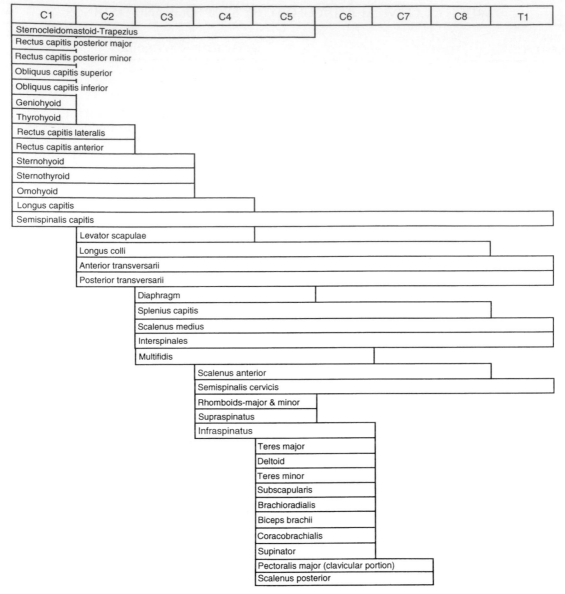

Figure 5–2. Segmental motor innervation of muscles supplied by C1 through T1 spinal nerves. The innervation of muscles from multiple (minimally two, and more commonly three) spinal cord levels is evident.

of the patient's upper posterior thorax and scapula, and the other hand is placed in the back of the skull. The patient is then asked to extend the neck actively.

The primary lateral rotators of the neck are the sternocleidomastoid muscles. The secondary rotators are the small intrinsic neck muscles. To test the strength of rotation, the examiner places one hand on the shoulder and the other hand on the opposite jaw, asking the patient to actively turn toward the side with the hand on the jaw. The strength of a resistive lateral motion should be compared from side to side.

The primary lateral benders in the neck are the three splenius muscles, which are innervated by the anterior primary divisions of the lower cervical nerves. The secondary lateral benders include some of the small intrinsic muscles in the neck. To test the strength of lateral bending, the examiner places one hand on the patient's shoulder and places the other hand on the superior lateral aspect of patient's skull on the same side. The patient is then asked to bend laterally toward that side and is resisted by the examiner's hand on the skull. In all these resistive muscle tests it is important to assess symmetry on both sides and get a

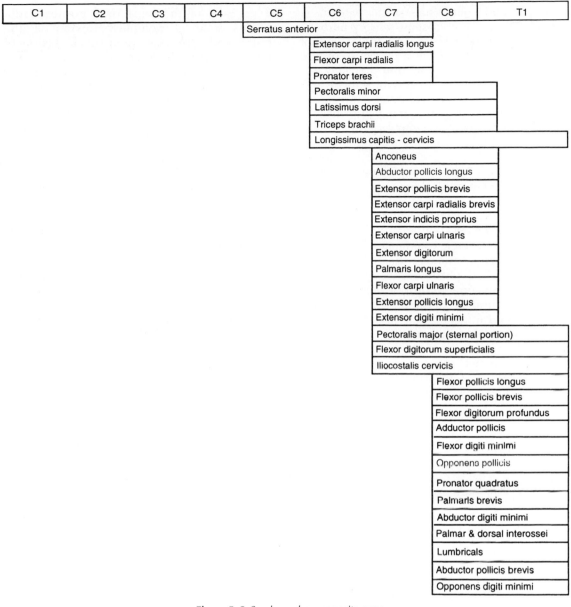

C1	C2	C3	C4	C5	C6	C7	C8	T1

Serratus anterior
Extensor carpi radialis longus
Flexor carpi radialis
Pronator teres
Pectoralis minor
Latissimus dorsi
Triceps brachii
Longissimus capitis - cervicis
Anconeus
Abductor pollicis longus
Extensor pollicis brevis
Extensor carpi radialis brevis
Extensor indicis proprius
Extensor carpi ulnaris
Extensor digitorum
Palmaris longus
Flexor carpi ulnaris
Extensor pollicis longus
Extensor digiti minimi
Pectoralis major (sternal portion)
Flexor digitorum superficialis
Iliocostalis cervicis
Flexor pollicis longus
Flexor pollicis brevis
Flexor digitorum profundus
Adductor pollicis
Flexor digiti minimi
Opponens pollicis
Pronator quadratus
Palmaris brevis
Abductor digiti minimi
Palmar & dorsal interossei
Lumbricals
Abductor pollicis brevis
Opponens digiti minimi

Figure 5–2 *See legend on opposite page*

sense of the maximal force that is attainable by the patient.

The second phase of the motor examination is designed to test motor strength of the muscles innervated by the nerve roots of the mid to lower cervical spine, which comprise the brachial plexus. Each nerve root, as it leaves the spinal canal through the neural foramen, is enclosed within a sleeve that contains spinal fluid and very small blood vessels about and within the nerve. This sac, referred to as the dural sleeve, provides nourishment to the nerve root. Any compression or traction to the dura will compress its contents and encroach upon the nerve and its blood supply. Secondary to compression, pain is perceived along the course of the peripheral nerve and is accompanied by dysesthesias, motor weakness, and decreased reflex function associated with the affected nerve root. The goal of many of the maneuvers done during this phase of the examination is to increase nerve compression to uncover neurologic dysfunction. One of the possible neurologic abnormalities, true muscle weakness, is one of the most reliable indicators of persistent nerve compression with loss of nerve conduction. In contrast, sensory changes are subjective and are easily affected by the emotional and energy state of the patient. As a patient fatigues, consistent sensory findings are difficult to reproduce. In addition, reflex changes may be lost from a previous episode of nerve root compression, and they may not return even with the recovery of sensory and motor function. With age, reflexes are more difficult to elicit even without any prior history of nerve compression. However, the loss of reflexes is generally symmetric with increasing age. Patients who lose reflexes in both lower extremities because of compression may have a central herniation of a disc.

In addition to nerve root lesions, upper motor neuron and peripheral nerve disease can cause abnormalities that may be discovered during the neurologic examination. Thus, it is also important to evaluate the cranial nerves and the brachial plexus. With upper motor neuron lesions, fine control of muscles is lost while the trophic effects of the peripheral nerves remain intact. Muscle strength is maintained initially, but patients develop spasticity of muscles (tonic contractions) and hyperreflexia. Patients also develop a positive Babinski's reflex (extension of the large toe and spreading of the other toes with stroking of the sole of the foot) or a positive Hoffmann's reflex (involuntary flexion of the thumb and fifth digit upon quick flexion of the DIP joint of the long finger).

Peripheral nerve injuries may cause sensory or motor abnormalities, depending on the damaged nerve. Peripheral nerves receive neurofibrils from a number of nerve root levels. The location of nerve roots and peripheral nerve lesions affecting cutaneous structures in the upper extremity are depicted in Figures 5–3 and 5–4. A lesion at one nerve root may cause a minor change in function if a structure is supplied by multiple spinal cord levels. However, if a peripheral nerve is injured, innervation in specific muscles and cutaneous areas is interrupted (Table 5–2). In this circumstance specific muscles may become paralyzed and areflexic or specific cutaneous areas anesthetized. The differentiation of upper motor neuron, nerve root, and peripheral nerve lesions is an important one. The locations of the abnormalities causing these neurologic manifestations are different. Also, the category of pathologic process causing upper motor neuron, nerve root, and peripheral nerve abnormalities may be different (multiple sclero-

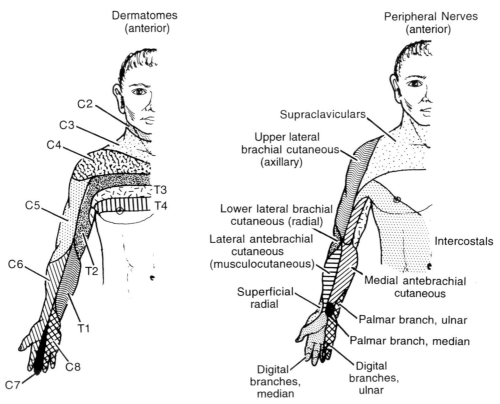

Figure 5–3. Anterior view of the upper extremities depicting skin areas innervated by nerve roots (*left*) and peripheral nerves (*right*).

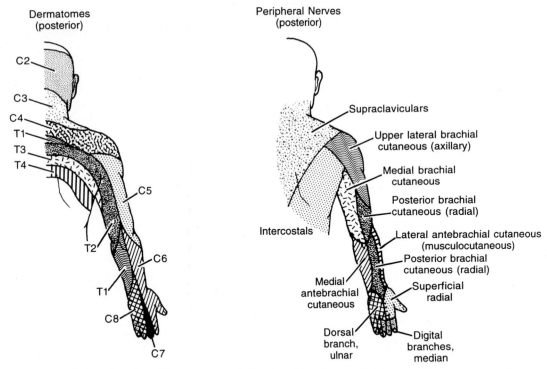

Figure 5–4. Posterior view of the nerve root *(left)* and peripheral nerve *(right)* areas of the upper extremities.

sis, disc herniation, and diabetes, respectively).

Although conceptually it is easiest to think about performing the neurologic examination of the upper extremities on a nerve root–level innervation basis, it is much more practical to perform an overall examination of the entire motor system, then the entire sensory distribution, and finally all the reflexes together (Fig. 5–5).

Motor strength quantification by physical examination is not precise, and some studies have suggested that as much as 30% to 40% of motor strength must be absent before any consistent detection of weakness on the basis

of a physical examination. In any case, one of the more common grading systems is a six-tier system, with 5 being normal strength, 4 being decreased strength against active resistance but ability to move against gravity; 3 being the ability to move only in the plane of gravity, not being able to move against gravity; 2 being the ability to contract the muscle but without purposeful motion; and 1 being the presence of muscle fibrillations. Grade 0 is the absence of any activity in the muscle group. When testing muscle power, it is important to test the muscles with the intervening joints in a neutral position. Pressure is applied to a nonarticular structure for a minimum of 5 sec-

TABLE 5–2. THE MAJOR PERIPHERAL NERVES

NERVE	MOTOR TEST	SENSATION TEST
Radial nerve	Wrist extension Thumb extension	Dorsal web space between thumb and index finger
Ulnar nerve	Abduction—little finger	Distal ulnar aspect—little finger
Median nerve	Thumb pinch Opposition of thumb Abduction of thumb	Distal radial aspect—index finger
Axillary nerve	Deltoid	Lateral arm—deltoid patch on upper arm
Musculocutaneous nerve	Biceps	Lateral forearm

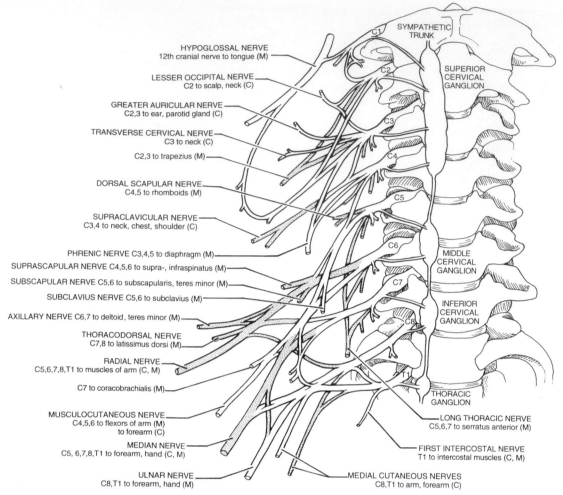

Figure 5–5. Nerves originating in the cervical spine. The plexus, roots, branches, divisions (anterior and posterior), terminal branches, and autonomic nervous system components of the brachial plexus are included. The cutaneous (C) and motor (M) components of the peripheral nerves are noted. The functions of muscles are listed under the associated nerves.

onds. When feasible, it is preferable to test both sides simultaneously.

An overlap of nerve innervation to muscles exists through the upper extremity. A general location of a lesion may be suspected with muscle weakness, but further evaluation is required to identify a specific location of nerve dysfunction. Testing the muscles innervated by the brachial plexus begins with the deltoid and biceps muscles, which are the two muscles with C5 innervation that are easily evaluated. Whereas the deltoid is innervated almost entirely by C5, the biceps has a dual innervation from both C5 and C6. The deltoid muscle has three parts: anterior, middle, and posterior. To test deltoid strength, resisted motion of the shoulder should be performed in flexion, adduction, and extension. The biceps acts as a flexor for the shoulder and elbow and as a supinator of the forearm. Biceps strength can

be tested relative to elbow flexion to determine the integrity of the C5 root. Because the brachialis muscle, the other main flexor of the elbow, is also innervated by the musculocutaneous nerve, a flexion test of the elbow should provide an adequate indication of C5 integrity. To test elbow flexion, the patient should flex the elbow slowly with the forearm supernated, as the examiner resists motion.

The next muscle group that should be tested is the wrist extensors. This muscle group does not have pure C6 innervation; it has partial innervation by C7. The wrist extensor group is composed of three muscles: the extensor carpi radialis longus (C6), the extensor carpi radialis brevis (C6), and the extensor carpi ulnaris (C7).

Next, the C7 nerve root can be evaluated by testing elbow extension, a function of the triceps, as innervated by the radial nerve, as well as the wrist flexor group innervated by C7 root, median, and ulnar nerves. The wrist flexor group is composed of two muscles, the flexor carpi radialis (median nerve) and the flexor carpi ulnaris (ulnar nerve). The flexor carpi radialis is the more significant of these two muscles because it powers most of the wrist flexion. Flexor carpi ulnaris (C8) is less powerful. Wrist flexion strength can be tested by asking the patient to make a fist and then flexing the wrist as the examiner resists against the palmar aspect of the fist. Finger extension is also a test of the C7 root and radial nerve innervation.

The next motor group to be tested is the finger flexors. The two muscles that flex the fingers are the flexor digitorum superficialis and the flexor digitorum profundus. The superficialis muscle receives innervation from the median nerve, and the profundus muscle receives half its innervation from the ulnar nerve and half from the median nerve. To test the strength of finger flexion, ask the patient to curl the fingers around the examiner's index and long finger, while the examiner tries to pull out of the grip.

The T1 neurologic level is tested by examining the intrinsic muscles of the hand. The finger abductors, innervated by the ulnar nerve and largely the T1 root, consist of the dorsal interossei and abductor digiti quinti. Finger abduction strength can be tested by asking the patient to abduct the fingers and then have the examiner attempt to squeeze them together at the level of the proximal phalanx of the index and little finger of the patient (Fig. 5–6).

REFLEX TESTING

The scapulohumeral reflex tests the integrity of the cord segments from C4 to C6. The reflex is elicited by striking the lower end of the medial border of the scapula. The response is adduction and lateral rotation of the arm. This reflex tests the supply of the suprascapular (axillary) nerve to the infraspinatus and teres minor.

The biceps reflex primarily indicates the neurologic integrity of the C5 nerve root. However, the reflex also has a C6 component. Because the muscle has two major levels of innervation, even a slightly diminished reflex in comparison with the opposite side indicates potential pathologic changes. The biceps reflex may be tested by the examiner placing a

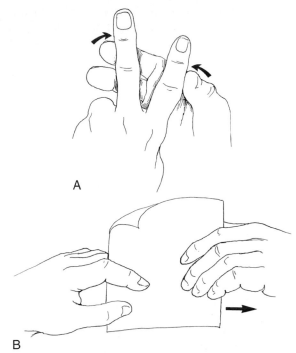

Figure 5–6. *A* and *B,* Motor examination of T1 nerve root, testing the strength of intrinsic hand muscles.

thumb over the biceps tendon and then tapping the reflex hammer on the examiner's thumb.

The brachioradialis reflex is tested proximal to the wrist where the muscle becomes tendonless just before it inserts into the radius. This tendon can be tapped directly with the blunt end of the reflex hammer and may result in wrist extension and elbow flexion. The primary innervation of this reflex is C6.

The triceps reflex is predominantly a C7 root reflex. To test the triceps reflex, it is necessary to tap the tendon of the triceps muscle where it crosses the olecranon fossa, just proximal to the elbow joint on the posterior aspect of the arm.

Because C8 has no reflex, muscle strength and sensory tests are used primarily to determine the integrity of the C8 nerve root. Similarly, T1, like C8, has no identifiable reflex, so it is evaluated for its motor and sensory components only.

It is also important to test for evidence of upper motor neuron lesions, and these can be detected through several additional reflexes. The Hoffmann's sign is the equivalent of the Babinski's sign in the lower extremity. This test can be performed by placing the patient's middle phalanx of the long finger over across the DIP joint of the examiner's long finger on their dominant hand, with the palm facing down. Next, by placing the patient's long finger in slight extension, the DIP joint is flicked downward by the examiner's thumb. An involuntary flexion of the DIP joints of the patient's thumb and little finger at the same time represents a positive Hoffmann's reflex. Another reflex that can be tested for upper motor neuron lesions is the jaw reflex, which can be tested by having the patient relax the open jaw. The examiner places a finger over the mental area of the chin and taps with the reflex hammer. The normal reflex should result in the jaw closing. A brisk reflex may be due to an upper motor neuron lesion somewhere along the course or above the level of the fifth cranial nerve (Fig. 5–7). If pathologic reflexes are present, motor examination should be expanded to determine signs of paralysis or weakness of voluntary motion, and increased muscle tone is indicative of an upper motor neuron lesion. Sensory examination may determine sensory loss on one side of the body with contralateral analgesia and thermesthesia a few segments below. These findings are compatible with the Brown-Séquard syndrome.

One final reflex is the Chvostek's sign. This can result from tapping over the facial nerve as it passes through the carotid gland, anterior to the ear. A hyperactive reflex in this area may result from hypocalcemia or other systemic metabolic abnormality.

SENSATION TESTING

The C5 neurologic level supplies sensation to the lateral aspect of the arm. The purest patch of axillary sensation is located on the lateral arm and the skin covering the lateral portion of the deltoid portion. This localized area is useful in diagnosing injuries to the axillary nerve or of general C5 nerve root injury.

Testing the sensation of the C6 nerve root can be performed by examining the sensory function to the lateral forearm, thumb, index, and half of the middle finger. An easy way to remember the sensation to the fingers of the hand, from the purist's standpoint, is that C6 innervates thumb and index finger, C7 the middle finger, and C8 the little finger. The ulnar side of the little finger is the purest area for ulnar nerve sensation (predominately C8).

Sensation is supplied to the medial side of the upper half of the forearm and the arm by T1. T2 supplies the axillary area, T3 supplies the anterior chest, and T4 supplies approximately at the level of the nipple on the anterior chest wall.

In general, sensory innervation can be tested in a cursory fashion by examining light touch in all the areas mentioned in this section. In addition, a pin can be used to test sensation to pinprick. Although posterior column function, position, and vibratory sense are not routinely tested, these sensory modalities become more relevant in patients who have any suggestion of cord compression or any posterior canal impingement.

If abnormalities are found in any component of the neurologic examination, additional tests should be completed, including tests of cranial nerves and thoracic nerve roots. These additional tests may be able to better define the location of a lesion in the upper spinal cord or thoracic spine that may be associated with neck pain.

Special Tests

Distraction Test. This test demonstrates the effect that neck traction might have in relieving a patient's neck pain. Distraction relieves

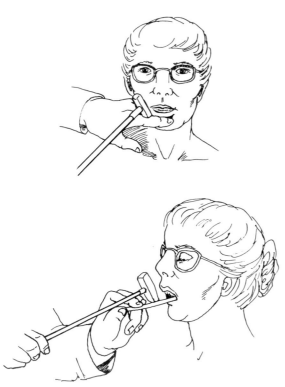

Figure 5–7. Jaw jerk obtained by alternative methods.

pain, which is caused by a narrowing of the neural foramen and resulting nerve root compression, by widening the foramen. Distraction also relieves pain in the cervical spine by decreasing pressure on the joint capsules around the facet joints. In addition, it may help alleviate muscle spasm by relaxing the contractive muscles, although this is less reliable.

To perform the cervical spine distraction test, the examiner places the open palm of one hand under the patient's chin and the other hand on the patient's occiput. The head is then gently lifted to remove its weight from the neck (Fig. 5–8A). Distraction is continued for 30 to 60 seconds.

Compression Test. A narrowing of the neural foramen, pressure on the facets, or muscle spasm can cause increased pain on compression. In addition, a compression test may reproduce pain referred to the upper extremity from the cervical spine and, in so doing, may locate the neurologic level of any existing pathologic problem, which may not be evident on routine examination without such a provocative test.

To perform the compression test, press down on the top of the patient's head while the patient is either sitting or lying down. If there is an increase in pain in either the cervical spine or in the extremity, it is important to note its exact distribution and whether it follows any of the previously described dermatomal pattern (Fig. 5–8B).

Valsalva's Test. This test increases the intrathecal pressure. If a space-occupying lesion, such as a herniated disc or tumor, is present in the cervical canal, the patient may develop pain in the cervical spine secondary to increased pressure. Pain may also radiate into the dermatome distribution that corresponds to the neurologic level of the intracanal pathology. Abnormalities in the supraclavicular fossa, such as enlarged lymph glands, may also become prominent with the Valsalva's test.[3]

To perform the Valsalva's test, the patient is instructed to hold breath and to bear down as if moving the bowels. The examiner asks if the patient feels any increase in pain and, if so, asks the patient to describe its character and location.

Spurling's Maneuver. This is a test of nerve root compression or irritation. This maneuver may be carried out by performing an extension and rotation movement of the head or extension and bending of the cervical spine to the right or left. A positive result is noted by reproduction of the patient's radicular pain.[4]

Lhermitte's Sign. This is the sensation of lightning-like paresthesias or dysesthesias in the hands or legs on cervical flexion. This

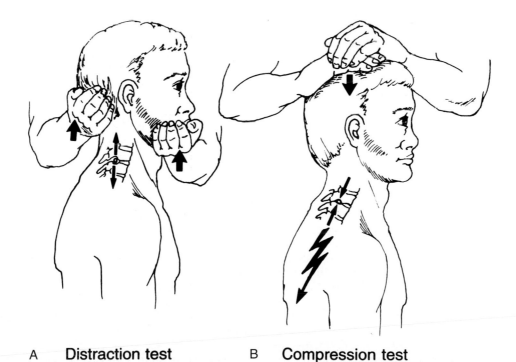

| A | **Distraction test** | B | **Compression test** |

Figure 5–8. Distraction test *(A)* is positive when radicular pain is relieved with upward traction on the neck. Compression test *(B)* is positive when radicular pain is increased with downward pressure on the cervical spine.

sensation is most often caused by a large disc herniation impinging the anterior spinal cord or by bony compression of the anterior cord in patients with a narrow canal diameter. This sign may also be associated with instability associated with rheumatoid arthritis. Similar sensations are reported in patients with multiple sclerosis affecting the spinal cord. Lhermitte's sign has also been associated with a variety of spinal cord lesions, including neoplasm, arachnoiditis, syringomyelia, and subacute combined degeneration.[5]

Shoulder Depression Test. This is a test of nerve root irritation. The neck is laterally flexed while downward pressure is placed on the shoulder. The test stretches nerve roots that cause radicular pain or paresthesias with lesions of the spinal nerve roots.

Shoulder Abduction Test. This test relieves pressure on nerve roots. The arm on the painful side is placed on top of the head. This shortens the distance between the cervical spine and coracoid process, releasing tension on the nerve roots. Some authors have suggested that the relief of pain is an indicator of cervical extradural compressive disease that may be related to disc herniation or osteophytes.[6] Others have suggested that relief of pain is related to cervical disc herniation. Pain associated with foraminal stenosis secondary to spondylosis is not improved with shoulder abduction.[7]

Adson's Test. This test is used to determine any potential compression of the subclavian artery, which may be caused by an extra cervical rib or by tightened scalene muscles. Compression may occur at the thoracic outlet where the artery passes between the chest and the upper extremity.

To perform the Adson's test, the patient's radial pulse is examined at the wrist. While the pulse is continuously palpated, the arm is then abducted, extended, and externally rotated. The patient is then instructed to take a deep breath and turn the head toward the arm being tested. If there is compression in the subclavian artery, there is a marked diminution or disappearance of the radial pulse. Auscultation, above and below the clavicle, may discover bruits that are only audible with critical narrowing of the subclavian artery by arm abduction.

Sharp-Purser Test. This test is accomplished by placing a hand on the patient's forehead and the thumb of the other hand on the tip of the spinous process of the axis. As the patient flexes the neck against the hand on the forehead, a sound may be appreciated as the atlantoaxial subluxation is reduced.[8] This test may exacerbate neurologic symptoms. The determination of subluxation may be better quantified by flexion and extension radiographs of the cervical spine.

PERIPHERAL NERVE ENTRAPMENT SYNDROMES

Peripheral nerves in the upper extremity may be compressed in predictable areas of disease, giving rise to upper extremity numbness, paresthesias, and sensory and motor loss. Although these radicular-type signs and symptoms may mimic cervical radiculopathy owing to pathologic problems of the cervical spine, concomitant neck pain may be noncontributory, simply occurring simultaneously. It is important to be able to differentiate peripheral nerve entrapment from more central root compression. The most reliable method of making this differentiation is through careful history and physical examination (Table 5–3).

Median Nerve. The median nerve may be compressed anywhere along its course. However, there are three common points. The most proximal level of compression may produce the pronator syndrome, which is associated with pain in the proximal volar forearm and sensory signs and symptoms in the radial 3 1/2 digits of the hand. Weakness of all median nerve–innervated muscles occurs because the compression is proximal to the branching of the anterior interosseous nerve. Symptoms are generally aggravated by flexion of the elbow against resistance from 90° to 135° of flexion and may be caused by compression from the ligament of Struthers or the lacertus fibrosus. Symptoms that are worsened by resistance to forced voluntary pronation of the forearm combined with simultaneous wrist flexion may indicate compression by the pronator teres muscle. This muscle may cause compression of the median nerve by hypertrophy or by the sharp aponeurotic edge of the deep head or reflected head muscle fascia forming fibrous bands. Symptoms elicited by resistive flexion of the long finger flexor digitorum superficialis muscle may be referable to compression from a deep tendinous aponeurotic arch of the muscle, underneath which the median nerve passes. Sensory symptoms and signs of the pronator syndrome typically mimic a C6 and C7 radiculopathy. Although the pronator syndrome may affect the function of the median nerve–innervated muscles in the C6 and C7 distribution, it spares the

TABLE 5–3. PERIPHERAL NERVE ENTRAPMENT SYNDROMES

NERVE	PAIN	SENSORY	WEAKNESS
Median Nerve			
Pronator syndrome (C6 + C7 mimic)	Proximal volar forearm	Radial 3½ digits	Pronator teres Flexor carpi radialis
Anterior interosseous syndrome (C8 mimic)	Proximal forearm	None	Flexor pollicus longus Pronator quadratus Flexor digitorum profundus (index)
Carpal tunnel syndrome (C6 + C7 sensory mimic) (T1 motor mimic)	Hand	Radial 3½ digits	Thenar muscles
Ulnar Nerve			
Cubital tunnel syndrome (C8 or T1 mimic)	Medial elbow	Ulnar 1½ digits	Flexor carpi ulnaris Flexor ditorum profundus (long + ring) Interossei Hypothenar muscles
Guyon's canal (C8 or T1 mimic)	Ulnar wrist	Volar, ulnar 1½ digits	Hypothenar muscles Interossei Abductor pollicis
Radial Nerve			
Posterior interosseous syndrome (C7 mimic)	Proximal forearm	None	Extensor digitorum communis Extensor carpi ulnaris Abductor pollicis longus Extensor pollicis longus

radial nerve–innervated muscles in the C6–C7 distribution (elbow, wrist, and finger extensors). In addition, it may induce abnormalities in muscles innervated by the median nerve, but not in the C6–C7 distribution (finger flexors and thenar muscles).

Since the anterior interosseous nerve is essentially a motor branch of the median nerve, anterior interosseous syndrome is not characterized by sensory abnormalities. Pain in the proximal forearm is typically aggravated by exercise and abates with rest. Motor abnormalities are manifested as weakness and are referable to those muscles innervated by this nerve (flexor pollicis longus, pronator quadratus, and flexor digitorum profundus of the index finger). This syndrome may mimic a C8 radiculopathy because this is the root through which they are all innervated. Other C8-innervated muscles unaffected by the anterior interosseous nerve syndrome include the flexor digitorum superficialis (median nerve proximal to anterior interosseus nerve), the flexor carpi ulnaris, and the flexor digitorum profundus to the ring and little fingers (ulnar nerve). Electrodiagnostic evaluation may also be helpful in differentiating a C8 radiculopathy from this syndrome.

Compression of the median nerve in the carpal tunnel typically causes sensory symptoms. Night pain, paresthesias, and numbness in the hand in the radial 3 1/2 digits are common and are caused by a thickened transverse carpal ligament. Carpal tunnel disease occurs most commonly in middle age and more frequently in women and those with occupations that require significant use and overuse of the hands and wrists. Symptoms may be referred proximally from the hand toward the forearm and even the elbow and may be reproduced or elicited by Phalen's maneuver or Tinel's sign. Thenar muscle weakness and atrophy represent advanced disease. Sensory symptoms may mimic C6 and C7 radiculopathy, but no C6 or C7 muscles demonstrate abnormalities because they are all innervated proximal to the carpal canal. Thenar motor weakness may mimic a T1 radiculopathy because of abnormalities of the opponens pollicis and the abductor pollicis brevis; however, other T1-innervated muscles are normal, including the hypothenar muscles and the first dorsal interosseus (ulnar nerve).

Ulnar Nerve. The ulnar nerve has two common areas of entrapment. The most common location of ulnar nerve entrapment is the elbow in the cubital tunnel. The most typical symptom of cubital tunnel syndrome is aching pain on the medial aspect of the elbow, although radiation of the pain and paresthesias may migrate distally on the ulnar forearm and into the ulnar 1 1/2 digits of the hand. Symptoms may be elicited by percussion of the nerve behind the medial epicondyle or by acute, prolonged flexion of the elbow. The weakness is manifested in muscles innervated by the ulnar nerve distal to the elbow (flexor carpi ulnaris, flexor digitorum profundus to the long and ring fingers, and the interossei and hypothenar muscles). All these muscles are innervated by the C8 and T1 nerve roots. However, because the sensory changes also occur in the distribution of the C8 and T1 roots, cubital tunnel syndrome may be difficult to differentiate from a C8 or T1 radiculopathy. Clinical tenderness and pain referable to the medial aspect of the elbow and electrodiagnostic studies demonstrating a significant conduction delay across the elbow may be useful in this regard. Furthermore, abnormalities in C8-innervated muscles or T1-innervated muscles that are not innervated by the ulnar nerve, such as the flexor pollicis longus, the thenar muscles, and the index and long finger flexors (median nerve), may signal a C8 or T1 radiculopathy rather than an ulnar nerve entrapment.

The ulnar nerve may also be compressed at the wrist in Guyon's canal. Compression at this level usually affects both the superficial and deep branches of the ulnar nerve. Therefore, sensory symptoms are referred to the volar aspect of the ulnar 1 1/2 fingers. The dorsal aspect of these digits remains unaffected because that area of skin is supplied by the dorsal sensory branch of the ulnar nerve, which originates proximal to the wrist and does not traverse Guyon's canal. The deep branch is essentially all motor, and the superficial branch is essentially all sensory. Therefore, motor symptoms, weakness, and atrophy are referable only to those muscles innervated by the deep branch of the ulnar nerve. These include the hypothenar muscles, the interossei, and the abductor pollicis. Because the sensory symptoms are in the C8 distribution and the abnormal muscles are innervated by T1 and C8, the syndrome may mimic a T1 and C8 radiculopathy. In this syndrome, however, sensation over the dorsum of the ulnar 1 1/2 fingers is normal. In addition, median nerve–innervated muscles in the T1 distribution (thenar) are normal.

Radial Nerve. The radial nerve is most commonly compressed at the elbow. Radial tunnel syndrome is a compression neuropathy of the radial nerve between the supinator muscle and the radial head just proximal to its entrance into the supinator muscle. The radial nerve gives motor branches to the brachioradialis, extensor carpi radialis longus and brevis, and supinator muscles, and then splits into a superficial sensory branch that does not enter the radial tunnel and the all-motor deep branch, the posterior interosseus nerve. Because only the motor branch is compressed, sensory symptoms are rare, although aching over the site of compression is felt and may be elicited by full extension of the elbow with the forearm in supination and the wrist in neutral. These symptoms may be aggravated by full flexion of the wrist with the forearm held in full pronation. Motor weakness may be seen in those muscles supplied by the posterior interosseus nerve (extensor digitorum communis, extensor carpi ulnaris, abductor pollicis longus, and extensor pollicis longus), all of which are supplied by the C7 root. A C7 radiculopathy may be ruled out by noting no abnormalities in median-innervated C7 muscles (flexor carpi radialis and pronator teres). In addition, the triceps (C7) muscle should be spared because it receives its radial nerve innervation in the upper arm, a significant distance proximal to the typical site of compression.

EXAMINATION OF RELATED AREAS

In most cases it is the cervical spine that refers pain to other areas of the upper extremity; however, it is possible for pathologic problems of the temporomandibular joint; infections of the lower jaw, teeth, or scalp; and pathologic problems of the intrinsic shoulder to refer pain to the neck.

The temporomandibular joint is the most frequently used joint in the body. This joint may be palpated by placing an index finger into the patient's external auditory canal, pressing anteriorly, and instructing the patient to open and close the mouth slowly. As the patient does so, the motion of the mandibular condyle becomes palpable to the tip of the examiner's finger. Both sides should be palpated simultaneously, and the motion should feel smooth and symmetric. A palpable crepitation or clicking may be due to a damaged meniscus in the temporomandibular joint or to synovial swelling secondary to trauma. Asymmetric dentition or poor occlusion can overload the joint and cause palpable clicking in the external auditory canal. Constant grinding or clenching of the teeth may also overload the joint and eventually cause clinical problems. Normal range of motion of this joint should allow the patient to open and close the mouth to admit a minimum of three fingers inserted between the incisor teeth (approximately 35 to 40 mm).

A tooth abscess of the lower jaw may refer pain to the temporomandibular joint and the neck but, more commonly, pathologic changes and dysfunction of the temporomandibular joint refer pain to the head and neck and cause headache or mandibular pain. In addition to pathologic problems about the jaw, intrinsic shoulder pathology and strain may cause pain that refers to the neck. The shoulder joint should be examined completely in any patients with lower cervical problems. This can be performed in a cursory fashion by principles similar for any physical examination. First, inspection of the shoulder joint from anterior to posterior is helpful. It is important to note any muscle atrophy. Second, the examiner should palpate all the joint complexes of the shoulder, including the sternoclavicular joint, the acromioclavicular joint, and the glenohumeral joint. Pain from biceps or rotator cuff tendinitis can also be detected by palpation of the biceps tendon in its groove. Shoulder tendinitis may be detected by a provocative movement, such as the palm-down shoulder abduction test, in which the shoulder is abducted to 90° and internally rotated maximally; or the forward flexed abduction test, in which the shoulder is externally rotated, flexed, and abducted anteriorly in an attempt to impinge the greater tuberosity on the acromial process. Production of pain in the shoulder on either of the provocative maneuvers may be an indication of rotator cuff tendinitis. It is particularly important to note whether motions of the shoulder reproduce, in total or in part, any of the pain that is associated with the person's cervical problems. It is a common error to mistake intrinsic shoulder pathology for radicular symptoms of the cervical spine. In such cases, management of the cervical spine may not result in resolution of the patient's shoulder problems.

In cases in which it is difficult to discern intrinsic shoulder pathologic changes from referred cervical pain, it is possible to do an intra-articular injection of xylocaine (with or without steroid). Within 10 to 15 minutes of injection, it is generally possible to eliminate the component of pain that is due to intrinsic shoulder pathologic changes. The patient can then be reexamined and a determination can be made whether or not the majority of the

pain is from within the shoulder joint or being referred from the cervical spine.

FUNCTIONAL DISORDERS

In some cases, objective findings associated with the neck problem do not match the subjective complaints. This is especially true in cases associated with psychogenic rheumatism, compensation, and litigation. These cases are termed functional, which is used medically in contradistinction to organic. For these functional cases, there is usually a psychological component as well as secondary gain involved.

Accentuation of symptoms for greater effect may be a sign of a patient with psychogenic difficulties. Lurching from one piece of office furniture to another, behavior associated with sudden paroxysms of twitching and pain in the cervical spine, is unusual for a patient with organic neck disease. Abrupt onset of total inability to move the head in any direction is suggestive of a psychogenic origin for neck dysfunction.[2]

To evaluate patients with these functional disorders, a list of physical signs was developed by Waddell and colleagues.[9] This provides a simple and rapid screen to help identify the few patients who require more detailed investigation. Although these signs were originally developed for patients with low back problems, many of them are applicable to cervical spine. Any of the individual signs count as one if positive. A finding of three or more of the five types is clinically significant. Isolated positive signs are ignored.

1. Tenderness—when related to physical disease, tenderness is usually localized to a particular skeletal or neuromuscular structure. Nonorganic tenderness is nonspecific and diffuse.
   a. Superficial—the skin is tender to light pinch over a wide area of cervical skin.
   b. Nonanatomic—deep tenderness is felt over a wide area and is not localized to one structure; it often extends to the arms, thoracic spine, and lumbar spine.
2. Simulation tests—these tests should not be uncomfortable; if pain is reported, a nonorganic influence is suggested.
   a. There is a complaint of thoracic or low back pain with vertical pressure on the skull of a patient who is standing. This is least applicable to the cervical spine because intrinsic neck pathologic changes may in fact be exacerbated by

axial loading. However, this should not cause pain in the low back in a patient with a cervical complaint.
   b. Rotation—neck pain should not be reported when the shoulders and pelvis are passively rotated in the same plane.
3. Distraction tests—first, a positive finding is demonstrated in the usual manner; next, this finding is rechecked while the patient's attention is distracted. Findings that are present only on formal examination and disappear at other times are considered positive. For example, the patient may describe an inability to use the hands because of muscular weakness but is able to lift off the examination table with the use of the wrists. Another example of a distraction test is the consistency of numbness in the forearm in the supinated and pronated positions.
4. Regional disturbances—findings that involve divergence from accepted neural anatomy.
   a. Weakness—nonanatomic (voluntary release) or unexplained (giving way) of muscle groups in the arms. Simultaneous strength testing of the hands may demonstrate equal strength (weak or strong) after finding weakness in one hand when tested one at a time. In true weakness, an antagonist muscle (triceps) should be relaxed when testing a weak agonist muscle (biceps). The tense antagonist muscle can be palpated while testing the weak agonist muscle.
   b. Sensory—sensory abnormalities fit a stocking rather than a dermatomal pattern.
5. Overreaction—this may take the form of disproportionate verbalization, jumping, cringing, excessive facial expression, and so on. Judgment should, however, be made with caution, as it is easy to introduce observer bias.

The preceding standardized group of nonorganic physical signs is easily learned and can be incorporated unobtrusively to add less than 1 minute to the routine physical examination. These tests are important, and when three are positive the findings should be followed up.

A distraction test may also be used for patients with a rigid neck.[10] The patient's range of motion is observed during the initial part of the examination. During the portion of the examination with the patient prone, a pillow is removed from under the patient's head. The head should have limited motion. Later in the examination with the patient supine, the pillow is replaced under the head. The range of motion should be noted.

SUMMARY

With conclusion of the history and physical examination, the examining physician should have the answers to important questions concerning prior surgery, preexisting neck injuries, the presence of malignancy or systemic illness, the presence of a nerve root irritation, and the possibility of a patient's being a malingerer. The physician should gather these facts and construct a list of diseases for the differential diagnosis. The diagnosis of neck pain of undetermined etiology is inadequate. Patients may have muscle strain, facet joint disease, discogenic disease with or without nerve root irritation, or systemic illness. In patients with mechanical abnormalities, no additional evaluation is necessary with the initial visit. Other patients with systemic symptoms and signs may require additional evaluation. Appropriate laboratory evaluation is useful in differentiating part of the myriad of systemic illnesses associated with neck pain. Laboratory evaluation is the subject of Chapter 6.

References

1. A neurovascular syndrome—the subclavian steal (editorial). N Engl J Med 264:912, 1961.
2. Bland J: Clinical methods. In: Bland JH (ed): Disorders of the Cervical Spine: Diagnosis and Medical Management, 2nd ed. Philadelphia: WB Saunders Co, 1994, p 120.
3. Keuper DH, Papp JP: Supraclavicular adenopathy demonstrated by the Valsalva maneuver. N Engl J Med 280:1007, 1969.
4. Spurling RG, Scoville WB: Lateral rupture of the cervical intervertebral discs. Surg Gynecol Obstet 78:350, 1994.
5. Brody IA, Wilkins RH: Lhermitte's sign. Arch Neurol 21:338, 1969.
6. Davidson RI, Dunn EJ, Metzmaker JN: The shoulder abduction test in the diagnosis of radicular pain in cervical extradural compressive monoradiculopathies. Spine 6:441, 1981.
7. Beatty RM, Fowler FD, Hanson EJ Jr: The abducted arm as a sign of ruptured cervical disc. Neurosurgery 21:731, 1987.
8. Sharp J, Purser DW: Spontaneous atlanto-axial dislocation in ankylosing spondylitis and rheumatoid arthritis. Ann Rheum Dis 20:47, 1961.
9. Waddell G, McCullogh JA, Kummel E, et al.: Nonorganic physical signs in low back pain. Spine 5:117, 1980.
10. Macnab I, McCulloch J: Neck Ache and Shoulder Pain. Baltimore: Williams & Wilkins, 1994, pp 121–139.

6

Laboratory Tests

The availability and expense of an ever-expanding variety of laboratory tests have complicated the professional life of the practicing physician. In the period when the laboratory evaluation was limited to blood counts, urinalysis, sedimentation rates, and serum chemistries, the physician obtained basic information about a patient for an inexpensive price. The present state of affairs is quite different. The number of available tests has grown at a great rate without corresponding increase in diagnostic accuracy but with an appreciable increment in cost. In fact, the results of tests done at an inappropriate time or interpreted incorrectly may only confuse the physician and may hide the true diagnosis. For example, a patient with cryoglobulinemia secondary to multiple myeloma will have an inappropriately "normal" erythrocyte sedimentation rate. Therefore, laboratory tests should be used in the situation in which a physician has developed a differential diagnosis by means of a history and physical examination for which laboratory data are needed to confirm or reject specific diagnoses.

In general, laboratory tests play a minor role in the diagnosis of neck pain. In the evaluation of neck pain, laboratory tests are required only on an emergent basis when a diagnosis of meningitis is considered. They do have a role in separating mechanical from systemic diseases. They are also useful in distinguishing metabolic-endocrinologic disorders from those with more inflammatory characteristics.

The vast majority of individuals with neck pain do not require laboratory studies with their initial evaluation. This is particularly true of a patient with a history of acute onset of pain related to physical activity. These patients may be given therapy for their neck pain without additional tests. They are candidates for laboratory evaluation if they fail to respond to neck pain therapy or develop a significant change in the character of their pain. The threshold for obtaining a laboratory evaluation at an initial visit is lowered for new-onset neck pain in an elderly individual. Since medical etiologies (infections and tumors) for neck pain occur commonly in older individuals, evaluation for systemic pathologic problems should be pursued earlier in the diagnostic process in this group. Occasionally, younger individuals present with severe, systemic symptoms (fever, chills, and eye inflammation) that strongly suggest a local (infection) or systemic (spondyloarthropathy) inflammatory process as the source of their neck pain. Laboratory evaluation during the initial evaluation may help confirm the inflammatory nature of their disease. Laboratory tests that are important in the study of disorders associated with neck pain include blood counts, blood chemistries, urinalysis, immunologic studies (cellular and humoral), body fluid analysis, cultures, and tissue biopsy. (For laboratory abnormalities associated with specific illnesses, refer to the relevant chapter in Section III and the appropriate listing in the Appendix.)

HEMATOLOGIC TESTS

Erythrocyte Sedimentation Rate (ESR)

The most useful test in helping to differentiate medical from mechanical neck pain is the erythrocyte sedimentation rate (ESR). The ESR mirrors the state of activity of the acute phase response. The acute phase response is a reaction by the body to tissue injury. With tissue necrosis, a systemic response is initiated that results in the increase in concentration of glycoproteins of hepatic origin that affect complement and coagulation cascades. The acute phase response has a beneficial effect of limiting the spread of tissue damage and facilitating wound healing. The increased concentration of plasma proteins causes an increased aggregation of erythrocytes, which forms stacks of discs (rouleaux). With rouleaux formation, erythrocyte mass is increased in relationship to cell surface area, resulting in an increased rate of fall of the cells.

The test is done by collecting blood from a patient and placing it in a specialized tube. The decrease in height of the column of erythrocytes is measured for 1 hour. The Wintrobe's method uses a tube 100 mm long and cannot measure ESR values greater than the patient's hematocrit.[1] The Wintrobe's method is most useful for mild elevations of ESR and may be more sensitive than the Westergren's method for minimal elevations.[2] The Westergren's method is the standard method for measuring ESR and involves diluting blood and using a tube that has a measuring length of 200 mm.[3] This method allows for the fall of erythrocytes to a distance greater than the packed height of the red blood cells (RBC). Greater ESRs are more accurately determined by the Westergren's method.

In general, an elevated ESR suggests the presence of inflammation in the body. The ESR is elevated with tissue injury, whatever the source (Table 6–1). The ESR is used to screen for inflammatory diseases and to follow the response to therapy. For example, the spondyloarthropathies (ankylosing spondylitis and Reiter's syndrome) produce an elevation of the ESR. The ESR is normal in mechanical neck pain (cervical muscle strain and osteoarthritis).

The ESR value must be interpreted according to the sex and age of the patient. The Westergren upper limits of normal are 15 mm/h for men younger than 50 years of age and 20 mm/h for men older than 50 years of age. The normal range is greater for women. The upper limit is 25 mm/h to 50 years of age and up to 30 mm/h after 50 years. The upper limit continues to rise as patients grow older. In patients older than 70 years of age, an ESR of 50 mm/h or higher may be normal.[4] The change in ESR may be more important than the absolute value when a patient is evaluated by a clinician. A 70-year-old patient who had a Westergren ESR of 10 mm/h who now has an ESR of 48 mm/h is worthy of additional evaluation despite the ESR value being in the normal range.

ESR may be "falsely" normal with any process that alters RBC morphology, inhibiting rouleaux formation and slowing the rate of fall of erythrocytes despite the presence of increased concentrations of acute phase reactants. Sickle cell anemia is associated with a normal ESR despite extensive tissue injury.

Markedly elevated ESR (100 mm/h or greater) is most commonly associated with malignancies, particularly those that are metastatic.[5] Other diseases associated with markedly increased ESR include connective tissue disease (polymyalgia rheumatica-temporal arteritis), acute bacterial infection (meningitis), and vertebral osteomyelitis with epidural abscess.

The ESR is the most valuable screening test for the detection of medical spinal pathologic conditions. In one series, an ESR of over 25 mm/h had a false positive rate of only 6%.[6]

The test has a number of flaws.[7] ESR is seldom the sole clue to systemic disease and is not a useful tool in asymptomatic individuals.[8] The ESR may be normal in patients with systemic diseases, including cancer. RBC morphology, a factor independent of the concentration of acute phase reactants, influences the rate of cell sedimentation. ESR is an indirect measure of the concentration of acute phase reactants. The activity of an illness is not always mirrored in the rise or fall of the ESR.[9] ESR may remain elevated for up to 3 to 5 weeks after spinal surgery, in the absence of infection.

TABLE 6–1. CONDITIONS ASSOCIATED WITH ELEVATED ERYTHROCYTE SEDIMENTATION RATE

RHEUMATIC DISEASES	ACUTE INFECTIONS
Spondyloarthropathies	Bacterial, including
Rheumatoid arthritis	endocarditis and
Rheumatic fever	pyelonephritis
Polymyalgia rheumatica	Tuberculosis
Systemic lupus	Meningitis
erythematosus	Discitis
	Vertebral osteomyelitis
MALIGNANT DISEASES	**TISSUE NECROSIS**
Multiple myeloma	Surgery
Solid tumors (colon,	Myocardial infarction
breast)	
Metastases	
GASTROINTESTINAL DISEASES	**MISCELLANEOUS**
Cholecystitis	Endocrinopathies
Peptic ulcer disease	Pregnancy
Inflammatory bowel	Vaccinations
disease	

Despite its shortcomings, ESR remains the most cost-efficient test for screening for systemic illness in patients with neck pain. The continued use of the test is based on its availability in a wide variety of office and hospital laboratories, its simplicity, and the broad experience with test results in a multitude of medical conditions.

C-Reactive Protein (CRP)

C-reactive protein (CRP) is an acute phase protein synthesized by hepatocytes first described in 1930.[10] CRP was named for its property of precipitating the somatic C-polysaccharide of the pneumococcus. The protein is an aggregate of five identical subunits that are arranged in a planar, cyclic pentagon.[7] CRP may recognize inflammatory tissue damage by binding to phosphocholine, a cell membrane–based compound. Phosphocholine is part of endogenous damaged tissues and exogenous tissues, such as bacteria. The exact function of CRP in acute phase response is not known. CRP does activate complement and interacts with phagocytic cells. CRP modulates neutrophils, suppressing superoxide production and degranulation and reducing phosphorylation of intracellular proteins. CRP also interacts with monocytes, platelets, and lymphocytes.

Levels of CRP in normal adult humans is less than 0.2 mg/dL. Slight variations occur with minor injuries. Concentrations of less than 1 mg/dL are regarded as normal or insignificant elevations. Concentrations between 1 and 10 mg/dL are moderate increases and those over 10 mg/dL are marked increases. CRP increases within hours of an inflammatory stimulus. CRP usually reaches a peak in 2 to 3 days and then recedes in 3 to 4 days. CRP may remain elevated in chronic inflammatory states such as rheumatoid arthritis and tuberculosis.

CRP may be measured to levels as low as 0.2 mg/dL by a number of methods, including laser nephelometry, enzyme immunoassay, radial immunodiffusion, and radioimmunoassay. Latex agglutination, a test that was the measurement standard in the past, is not adequately sensitive to be currently useful in the clinical setting. CRP is more accurate than ESR in detection of infections after spinal surgery because it returns to baseline more quickly than ESR.[11, 12] Serial determinations of CRP may also be helpful in following the course of acute and chronic inflammatory illnesses.[13] Elevated CRP after disc surgery has been associated with retrodiscal infection that has been detected with magnetic resonance evaluation.[14] With greater availability and accuracy of measurement techniques, CRP can be used more frequently in detecting inflammatory states in patients with neck pain.

Hematocrit (Hct)

The hematocrit level (Hct) is normal in mechanical neck pain, including herniated nucleus pulposus, spinal stenosis, and muscle strain. The presence of anemia suggests an inflammatory process of a systemic variety that has diminished erythrocyte production or hastened blood cell destruction. Rheumatologic disorders cause chronic inflammation and frequently cause so-called anemia of chronic disease, which is associated with inadequate production of RBCs. Malignancies, particularly those of hematologic origin (multiple myeloma), characteristically cause anemia. Hematologic disorders and hemoglobinopathies are also associated with decreased Hct levels.

Most laboratories determine Hct levels indirectly. Coulter machines measure erythrocyte volume (MCV) and hemoglobin (Hgb) concentration and derive the Hct level from these measurements. Changes in the MCV may have a significant effect on the Hct value. In serial determinations, the Hct level may vary widely, and the variation may be disconcerting to the physician. In these circumstances, following the measured Hgb concentration is helpful. A drop in Hgb level signifies a true change in the number of erythrocytes and requires further investigation.

Not all decreases in the Hct level are related to primary disorders of the cervical spine. Many patients ingest nonsteroidal anti-inflammatory drugs (NSAIDs) for neck pain. Many of these preparations are sold over the counter and contain aspirin. Patients may not mention these drugs to the physician, thinking that the medications are unimportant because they are nonprescription. However, these medications, as well as other NSAIDs, irritate the gastric mucosa, causing bleeding. In some patients, the amount of NSAID-associated bleeding is appreciable, causing a drop in the Hct level. Therefore, a falling Hct level may be more closely associated with therapy than the lesion causing the pain. A decreased Hct level should be evaluated with RBC indices, reticulocyte count, serum iron level, total iron binding capacity, haptoglobin level, and examination of the stool for occult blood.

In addition to the determination of the hematocrit level, levels of iron and transferrin saturation may be helpful in determining the cause of anemia. Low serum ferritin and low transferrin saturation suggest iron deficiency anemia. Elevated levels of ferritin above 400 µg/L and transferrin saturation of more than 55% are suggestive of hemochromatosis.[15] This determination may be useful in the patient with neck pain and chondrocalcinosis.

White Blood Cell (WBC) Count and Differential

The white blood cell (WBC) count is normal in mechanical neck pain. The WBC count is also normal in many forms of medical neck pain. An elevated WBC (leukocytosis) count suggests the presence of an infection, particularly if early forms of polymorphonuclear leukocytes (bands) are present. Increased numbers of WBCs are also seen in malignancies, particularly those of bone marrow or lymphatic origin. Elevations of WBC count occur less commonly in the spondyloarthropathies.

Drugs may alter the number and distribution of WBCs in the differential. Corticosteroids loosen the WBCs that line blood vessels (marginated pool). The pool is predominantly polymorphonuclear leukocytes. Corticosteroids are also lympholytic. Patients on corticosteroids have an increased WBC count in the 12,000 to 20,000 range (depending on the dose of medication). Polymorphonuclear leukocytes, as compared with lymphocytes, are present in greater number in the WBC differential. A rare toxicity of some of the drugs used in the treatment of neck pain is agranulocytosis or aplastic anemia (phenylbutazone). A WBC count obtained before the institution of therapy helps determine the patient's normal WBC level. A drop in WBC count after the institution of therapy requires close monitoring.

Platelets

Platelets are normal in mechanical neck pain and most medical causes as well. In malignancies, platelets are commonly abnormal and may be elevated (thrombocytosis).[16] Platelets are frequently decreased (thrombocytopenia) in bone marrow and lymphatic tumors. Platelet counts may also be modified by drug therapy. A complete blood count obtained at the initiation of drug therapy will establish the patient's usual platelet count.

Blood Chemistry Tests

Blood chemistries are usually obtained as a battery of 12 or more tests (SMA 12). There is nothing mysterious about the selection of tests included in the chemistry profile other than the fact that they are frequently ordered and the process for their measurement is automated. Although the groupings of tests seem haphazard, combinations of tests help identify abnormalities associated with dysfunction in specific organ systems.[17] Disorders may be associated with specific tests as follows: renal—blood urea nitrogen, uric acid, creatinine, and glucose; hepatic—total bilirubin, alkaline phosphatase, lactic dehydrogenase, and serum glutamic oxaloacetic transaminase (SGOT); parathyroid—calcium and phosphorus; bone—calcium; tumor—total protein, albumin, and lactic dehydrogenase; and hematologic—lactic dehydrogenase and total protein.

Serum Calcium and Phosphorus

An increase in serum calcium and decrease in serum phosphorus reflect activity of parathormone on bone and kidney. Patients with primary hyperparathyroidism have this relationship of calcium to phosphorus. Malignancies are associated with hypercalcemia. Malignancies with elevated serum calcium levels include those with parathormone activity (parathyroid adenoma and oat cell carcinoma of the lung), bone metastases, and multiple myeloma.

Metabolic bone disease may be associated with altered serum calcium and phosphorus concentrations. Osteomalacia (diminished vitamin D effect on bone) results in decreased serum calcium level and a range of changes in phosphorus levels. Phosphorus levels may be elevated in renal disease and acromegaly or diminished as in hereditary disorders, including hypophosphatemia. Osteoporosis is not associated with any serum alterations of serum calcium or phosphorus concentrations. Calcium and phosphorus levels are also unaltered in osteoarthritis and mechanical causes of neck pain.

Serum Alkaline Phosphatase (ALP)

Alkaline phosphatase (ALP) is produced to the greatest extent by osteoblasts. Any condition that increases osteoblastic activity increases ALP.[18, 19] Disorders associated with ALP elevations include Paget's disease, metastatic carcinoma, hyperparathyroidism, osteomalacia, fractures during healing phase, and hypophosphatasia. Of the illnesses that cause neck pain, metastatic tumors and Paget's disease cause the greatest increases (2 to 30 times normal). Up to 86% of patients with metastatic prostate carcinoma and 77% with metastatic breast cancer to bone have ALP elevations.[20] Not all bone tumors cause ALP elevations. Multiple myeloma, which causes little osteoblastic activity, is associated with increased ALP activity in less than 20% of patients. The ALP abnormalities in these myeloma patients may reflect healing bone fractures and may persist for several weeks.

The increase in ALP associated with Paget's disease is proportional to the activity of osteoblasts that are activated by increased osteoclastic resorption of bone. The extent of enzyme elevation is proportional to the extent of skeletal involvement. ALP increases with time in patients who are untreated. A rapid and marked elevation of enzyme activity is indicative of sarcomatous degeneration of a Paget's lesion.

Metabolic bone disease, particularly osteomalacia, is associated with abnormal levels of ALP. Osteomalacia is associated with increased enzyme levels with accompanying low normal or decreased serum calcium concentration. Hyperparathyroidism is associated with increased ALP levels if the disease has caused bone disease. Radiographic changes of hyperparathyroidism may be present in the hands before serum elevations of ALP occur.[20]

Decreased levels of ALP are associated with an inherited deficiency of the enzyme (hypophosphatasia). The disease clinically resembles osteomalacia.

Not all elevations of ALP are associated with bone disease. Disease of the hepatobiliary system may be associated with marked increases of ALP activity. This is particularly evident in patients with obstructive lesions in the biliary system who may have concomitant abnormalities in other serum parameters of liver damage (gamma glutamyl transpeptidase, SGOT, serum glutamic pyuric transaminase (SGPT), bilirubin, and cholesterol). Women who are pregnant may develop increased ALP levels of placental origin during the second and third trimesters. Diseases of the intestinal mucosa, peptic ulcer, or ulcerative colitis may also cause enzyme elevations.

Serum Uric Acid

Uric acid determination is normal in the vast majority of patients with neck pain. Serum uric acid may be elevated in patients with tophaceous gout affecting the cervical spine.[21] These patients usually have extensive gouty disease in peripheral joints. The diagnosis of gout is documented by the demonstration of sodium urate crystals in synovial fluid or from a tophus. Hyperuricemia alone is insufficient to make a diagnosis of gout. Increased uric acid concentrations are also associated with any process that causes rapid cell turnover. Lactate dehydrogenase may also be increased in these circumstances. These disease states include myeloproliferative and lymphoproliferative disorders, psoriasis, hypothyroidism, hyperparathyroidism, and Paget's disease. Chronic renal failure as well as a variety of drugs, including thiazide diuretics, furosemide, low-dose salicylate, phenothiazine, phenylbutazone, and corticosteroids, cause hyperuricemia.

Serum Glucose

The serum glucose determination obtained on a chemical profile has significance only if obtained when the patient is in a fasting state. Elevations of glucose in the fasting state require formal testing of glucose metabolism, including a 2-hour glucose tolerance test. A number of drugs may increase or decrease serum glucose concentrations. The drug history of the patient may help clarify abnormalities of glucose concentration observed with screening chemical evaluations.

Total Protein and Serum Albumin

Total protein and serum albumin concentrations are determined in most screening chemistry profile tests. In most patients with neck pain, these tests are normal. However, in patients with chronic, systemic inflammatory diseases, the total protein concentrations may be altered. With chronic inflammation or infection (tuberculosis), the total globulins of the total protein may be increased. Marked increase in total protein associated with elevated globulin levels should raise the possibility of multiple myeloma.

Patients with increased total protein should be evaluated with a serum protein electrophoresis. An increase in gamma globulins requires a serum immunoelectrophoresis test. An increase in globulins requires serum immunoelectrophoresis to characterize the increased component. Increased monoclonal immunoglobulins may occur with benign (monoclonal gammopathies) or malignant (multiple myeloma) disorders. A diffuse elevation of gamma globulins (polyclonal increase) suggests the presence of a chronic inflammatory process.

Blood Urea Nitrogen and Serum Creatinine

Elevations in blood urea nitrogen and serum creatinine are associated with decreased renal function. Patients with visceral back pain of genitourinary origin may have elevations of these parameters. Additional evaluations, in the form of 24-hour urine collection for creatinine clearance and radiographic or sonographic examination, are helpful in defining the parenchymal or obstructive origin of the renal impairment. The drug history is important in a patient with abnormalities of blood urea nitrogen and creatinine. A number of drugs, including corticosteroids and NSAIDs, may cause elevations of these tests.[22, 23]

IMMUNOLOGIC TESTS

Histocompatibility Typing

The human leukocyte antigens (HLA) are present on all human nucleated cells.[24] HLA typing determines A, B, C, and D antigens. Specific haplotypes are associated with a wide variety of disorders. In regard to disorders of the lumbosacral spine, class IB antigens are most closely associated with the spondyloarthropathies. The histocompatibility antigen, HLA B27, is present in more than 90% of patients with ankylosing spondylitis and 80% of patients with Reiter's syndrome, compared with 8% of the normal white and 4% of the normal black population. The HLA B27 test is performed in vitro, using the patient's lymphocytes and antisera directed against specific HLA antigens. The presence of HLA B27

is not diagnostic for any specific spondyloarthropathy. In general, the majority of patients with ankylosing spondylitis are more readily diagnosed on the basis of history, physical examination, and roentgenographic findings of sacroiliitis. HLA B27 is a superfluous test. The test is most helpful for the young woman who presents with neck pain and equivocal changes of vertebral body squaring on plain radiographs. HLA B27 positivity in a patient with neck pain and equivocal radiographs is additional evidence for the diagnosis of ankylosing spondylitis.

Four percent to 8% of normal people in the United States are HLA-B27–positive. The presence of HLA B27 in a patient with noninflammatory back pain of bone or muscle origin is of no consequence.[25]

The HLA class II molecules are encoded in the HLA-D region. DR, DQ, and DP are the three major subregions of the D region. HLA class II molecules are expressed on a limited number of cells in the immune system, such as B lymphocytes and macrophages. Class II molecules play a central role in antigen recognition and effective collaboration between immunocompetent cells for an efficient immune response.[26] Histocompatibility testing for class II molecules is primarily used for research purposes. Like class I antigens, class II antigens are not found exclusively in patients with specific illnesses. A proportion of normal individuals have certain class II antigens.

Rheumatoid Factor (RF)

Rheumatoid factors (RF) are a group of autoantibodies to human immunoglobulin G (IgG). RF may be of IgM, IgG, IgA, IgD, and IgE varieties. The classic RF is IgM antibody. RF occur in a wide range of autoimmune and chronic infectious diseases (Table 6–2). The disease most closely associated with RF is rheumatoid arthritis. Approximately 80% of patients with rheumatoid arthritis are seropositive for RF. The cervical spine is commonly involved in patients with rheumatoid arthritis. Patients with cervical spine disease usually have joint inflammation in other locations, such as the wrists, fingers, and toes, that precedes neck involvement. The RF status of the patient is frequently known when the patient becomes symptomatic with neck pain.

The presence of RF activity may be important in the evaluation of patients with musculoskeletal pain secondary to subacute bacterial endocarditis. Patients with chronic endocarditis de-

TABLE 6–2. DISEASES ASSOCIATED WITH RHEUMATOID FACTOR

RHEUMATIC DISEASES	VIRAL INFECTIONS
Rheumatoid arthritis	AIDS
Systemic lupus erythematosus	Mononucleosis
	Hepatitis
Sjögren's syndrome	Influenza
Systemic sclerosis	
Mixed connective tissue disease	
CHRONIC BACTERIAL INFECTIONS	**PARASITIC INFECTIONS**
Tuberculosis	Trypanosomiasis
Subacute bacterial endocarditis	Kala-azar
Salmonellosis	Malaria
Brucellosis	Schistosomiasis
Syphilis	Filariasis
Leprosy	
HYPERGLOBULINEMIC STATES	**NEOPLASMS**
Hypergammaglobulinemic purpura	Post-therapy radiation or chemotherapy
Cryoglobulinemia	
Chronic liver disease	
Sarcoidosis	

velop RF after 6 weeks of infection in the setting of hypocomplementemia and immune complex deposition manifested by glomerulonephritis.[27] RF titers play a greater role in following the response therapy than in diagnosing endocarditis. RF diminishes in titer as the patient's infection responds to antibiotic therapy.

RF in low titer may also be identified in an increasing proportion of normal individuals as they grow older. More than 40% of healthy individuals who are 75 years of age have detectable RF.[28] Therefore, RF determinations add little information to the evaluation of the patients with mechanical pain and should not be included in the laboratory examination of these individuals.

RF may also appear as part of a panel of tests combined to facilitate more accurate diagnosis when screening patients with musculoskeletal complaints. The three tests most commonly offered are the RF, antinuclear antibody, and uric acid level. The predictive value of these tests is only 35% in a population of individuals with joint disease and an estimated combined prevalence of the three illnesses of 10%.[29] Therefore, 65% of individuals with a positive test would not have one of these illnesses. The use of panels of tests in the evaluation of neck pain patients is not useful.

URINALYSIS

Abnormalities detected during a routine urinalysis are most helpful in identifying those individuals with viscerogenic-referred back pain of genitourinary origin. They are not usually helpful in the evaluation of neck pain. The presence of protein in the urine may be indicative of a dysproteinemic state, multiple myeloma. The presence of proteinuria on a dipstick determination requires further evaluation. If the concentration of urinary protein is small, repeat urinalysis may detect no additional protein. If proteinuria persists, quantification of a 24-hour collection of urine is necessary. If multiple myeloma is suspected, a negative dipstick protein does not rule out the diagnosis because myeloma proteins are not detected by dipstick methods. The presence of myeloma proteins in urine is detected by adding sulfasalicylic acid to urine (nonspecific test for protein that turns urine turbid) or immunoelectrophoresis of urine, which identifies the specific protein present in increased concentration.

Twenty-four-hour urine collections may be helpful in patients with metabolic bone disease. Urine collection for calcium helps determine calcium excretion, degree of calcium absorption, and patient compliance with ingestion of calcium supplements. The value of the test result is only as good as the completeness of the collection. Partial collections are of no clinical value.

MISCELLANEOUS TESTS

The most crucial diagnostic procedure for bacterial meningitis is lumbar puncture for examination of cerebrospinal fluid (CSF). If the neurologic examination reveals meningismus and signs of increased intracranial pressure (papilledema), imaging of the central nervous system may be required to document the status of intracranial structures. Timely evaluation is essential to establishing the diagnosis of meningitis so that antibiotic therapy can be initiated quickly.[30]

CSF is clear, colorless fluid that fills the subarachnoid space. The volume of CSF is 125 to 150 mL. Approximately 500 mL to 600 mL is produced by the choroid plexus each day.[31] The normal characteristics of CSF are listed in Table 6–3.

Abnormalities in CSF cells, glucose, protein, or pressure are noted in patients with infec-

TABLE 6–3. NORMAL CSF VALUES

PRESSURE

65–195 mm H_2O

CELL COUNT

Mononuclear cells 0–5
   Borderline 5–10
   Abnormal >10

PROTEIN

0–45 mg/dL

GLUCOSE

Ratio of CSF to blood glucose ≥0.6
If blood glucose concentration is high, then ratio
   decreases (0.4)
If blood is present in CSF, correction for cells and
   protein:
   True CSF WBC = measured CSF WBC − blood WBC
     × CSF RBC/blood RBC
   True CSF protein = serum protein × CSF RBC/
     blood RBC

Modified from Van Scoy RE: Evaluation of cerebrovascular fluid. In: Schlossberg D (ed): Infections of the Nervous System. New York: Springer-Verlag, 1990.

tion, tumors, or other inflammatory lesions of the spinal cord or nerve roots. Subarachnoid bleeding may cause a centrifuged fluid to be xanthochromic for 2 to 4 weeks. CSF pressure may be increased by congestive heart failure, superior vena caval obstruction, thrombosis of the intracranial venous sinus, impaired resorption of CSF, or intracranial mass lesion. Low CSF pressure may occur in patients with dehydration, hypotension, subdural hematomas, spinal subarachnoid block, and barbiturate intoxication. The Queckenstedt's test is used to evaluate CSF pressure but is rarely used in the emergency setting of meningitis. The test is performed by occluding the jugular veins bilaterally for 10 seconds. Normal findings include an increase of pressure to 150 mm H_2O that returns to baseline in 15 to 20 seconds. No increase in pressure is associated with a positive test. Herniated discs, vertebral fractures, extradural abscesses, and neoplastic adhesions are associated with a positive test.[32] Decreased CSF glucose levels are most frequently associated with infections of the central nervous system, including meningitis, neurosyphilis, neoplasms, subarachnoid hemorrhage, sarcoidosis, and hypoglycemia. CSF protein levels are increased in a wide variety of disorders, including infections, multiple sclerosis, vasculitis, cerebrovascular accidents, encephalitis, and Guillain-Barré syndrome. Increased leukocyte count is most frequently associated with bacterial meningitis when the predominant cell is neutrophil. Lymphocytosis is most fre-

quently associated with tuberculosis; fungal, viral meningitis; Guillain-Barré syndrome; vasculitis; and multiple sclerosis. Cultures for bacteria, tuberculosis, fungi, virus, and anaerobes should be obtained when adequate fluid is available. CSF should be examined with a Gram's stain, India ink stain, or acid-fast stain. The detection of bacterial antigens is increased with the use of counterimmunoelectrophoresis. The organisms most frequently detected by this technique include *Haemophilus influenzae, Neisseria meningitidis,* and *Streptococcus pneumoniae.*[33]

BIOPSY SPECIMENS

In certain patients with neck pain, the diagnosis cannot be determined without histologic examination of tissue from the cervical spine. Evaluation of biopsy specimens is most helpful in identifying benign and malignant tumors as well as obtaining bone, disc, or other tissues for culture to confirm the presence of infection. Tissue biopsy is indicated after noninvasive tests have been completed, the cause of the patient's pain remains in doubt, and examination of tissue becomes necessary to establish the diagnosis. Close cooperation is needed among the clinicians, radiologists, and surgeons to choose the appropriate site and method of biopsy. Some lesions are accessible to needle biopsy and do not require an operation. Other lesions, particularly those in the anterior portion of cervical vertebrae, are inaccessible to the biopsy needle and require an open biopsy. Careful handling of the biopsy material is necessary so the greatest amount of information is obtained from the invasive procedure.

SUMMARY

Laboratory test results should never replace a careful history and physical examination in the evaluation of the patient with neck pain. In the majority of circumstances, the laboratory results help separate patients into categories (inflammatory versus noninflammatory, bone versus liver) but rarely establish specific diagnoses, except in the setting of infection. The clinician may place too much significance on laboratory findings, which results in inaccurate diagnoses. Laboratory tests are helpful when used appropriately. If their relative importance is kept in mind, the clinician will not be misled.

References

1. Wintrobe MM, Landsberg JW: A standardized technique for the blood sedimentation test. Am J Med Sci 189:102, 1935.
2. Pepys MB: Acute phase phenomena. In: Cohen AS (ed): Rheumatology and Immunology. Orlando, Florida: Grune & Stratton, 1979, p 85.
3. International Committee for Standardization in Hematology: Recommendation for measurement of erythrocyte sedimentation rate of human blood. Am J Clin Pathol 68:505, 1977.
4. Hayes GS, Stinson IN: Erythrocyte sedimentation rate and age. Arch Ophthalmol 94:939, 1976.
5. Zacharski LR, Kyle RA: Significance of extreme elevation of erythrocyte sedimentation rate. JAMA 202:264, 1967.
6. Waddell G: An approach to backache. Br J Hosp Med 28:187, 1982.
7. Ballou SP, Kushner I: Laboratory evaluation of inflammation. In: Kelley WN, Harris ED Jr, Ruddy S, Sledge CB (eds): Textbook of Rheumatology, 4th ed. Philadelphia: WB Saunders Co, 1993, 671–679.
8. Sox HC Jr, Liang MH: The erythrocyte sedimentation rate: Guidelines for rational use. Ann Intern Med 104:515, 1986.
9. Malkiewitz A, Kushner I: Biochemical markers of inflammation in spondylitis. Spine State Art Rev 3:553, 1991.
10. Tillet WS, Francis T Jr: Serological reactions in pneumonia with a non-protein somatic fraction of pneumococcus. J Exp Med 52:561, 1930.
11. Thelander U, Larsson S: Quantitation of C-reactive protein levels and erythrocyte sedimentation rate after spinal surgery. Spine 17:400, 1992.
12. Mustard RA Jr, Bohnen JMA, Haseeb S, Kasina R: C-reactive protein levels predict postoperative septic complications. Arch Surg 122:69, 1987.
13. Okamura JM, Miyagi JM, Terada K, Hokama Y: Potential clinical applications of C-reactive protein. J Clin Lab Anal 4:231, 1990.
14. Schulitz KP, Assheuer J: Discitis after procedures on the intervertebral disc. Spine 19:1172, 1994.
15. Edwards CQ, Kushner JP: Screening for hemochromatosis. N Engl J Med 328:1616, 1993.
16. Levin H, Conley CL: Thrombocytosis associated with malignant disease. Arch Intern Med 114:497, 1964.
17. Ward PCJ: Chemical profiles of disease. Orthop Clin North Am 10:405, 1979.
18. Van Lente F: Alkaline and acid phosphatase determinations in bone disease. Orthop Clin North Am 10:437, 1979.
19. Schwartz MK: Enzymes in cancer. Clin Chem 19:10, 1973.
20. Goldsmith RS: Laboratory aids in the diagnosis of metabolic bone disease. Orthop Clin North Am 3:545, 1972.
21. Sequeira W, Bouffard A, Salgia K, Skosey J: Quadriparesis in tophaceous gout. Arthritis Rheum 24:1428, 1981.
22. Galen RS: The effects of drugs on laboratory tests. Orthop Clin North Am 10:465, 1979.
23. Clive DM, Stoff JS: Renal syndromes associated with nonsteroidal anti-inflammatory drugs. N Engl J Med 310:563, 1984.
24. Brenner MB, Glass DN: HLA polymorphisms and rheumatic disease. In Cohen AS (ed): Laboratory Diagnostic Procedures in the Rheumatic Diseases, 3rd ed. Orlando, Florida: Grune & Stratton, 1985, pp 249–271.
25. Kahn MA, Khan MI: Diagnostic value of HLA-B27 testing in ankylosing spondylitis and Reiter's syndrome. Ann Intern Med 90:70, 1982.
26. Strominger JL: Biology of the human histocompatibility leukocyte antigen (HLA) system and a hypothesis regarding the generation of autoimmune disease. J Clin Invest 77:1411, 1986.
27. Williams RC Jr, Kunkel HG: Rheumatoid factor, complement, and conglutinin aberrations in patients with subacute bacterial endocarditis. J Clin Invest 41:666, 1962.
28. Heimer R, Levin FM, Rudd E: Globulins resembling rheumatoid factor in serum of the aged. Am J Med 35:175, 1963.
29. Lichtenstein MJ, Pincus T: How useful are combinations of blood tests in "rheumatic panels" in diagnosis of rheumatic diseases? J Gen Intern Med 3:436, 1988.
30. Martin JB, Tyler KL, Scheld WM: Bacterial meningitis. In: Tyler KL, Martin JB (eds): Infectious Diseases of the Central Nervous System. Philadelphia: FA Davis Co, 1993, pp 176–187.
31. Van Scoy RE: Evaluation of cerebrovascular fluid. In: Schlossberg D (ed): Infections of the Nervous System. New York: Springer-Verlag, 1990, pp 381–388.
32. Dougherty JM, Roth RM: Cerebral spinal fluid. Emerg Med Clin North Am 4:516, 1986.
33. Feldman WE: Relation of concentrations of bacteria and bacterial antigen in cerebrospinal fluid to prognosis in patients with bacterial meningitis. N Engl J Med 296:433, 1977.

Radiographic Evaluation

7

Evaluation of patients with neck or arm pain frequently includes the use of radiographic techniques to visualize the structures of the cervical spine. When obtained at the appropriate time in the diagnostic evaluation, and when interpreted correctly in the setting of the patient's clinical history and physical examination, the radiographic images of the spine are extremely helpful in suggesting the possible location and source of a patient's pain (vertebral fracture, tumor, or osteoarthritis). On the other hand, radiographic images that are obtained too soon in the diagnostic process or are interpreted incorrectly may delay the determination of the true diagnosis. For example, the presence of degenerative disc disease on a radiograph may dissuade the clinician from fully evaluating a patient with new onset neck pain. The physician may ascribe the patient's pain to radiographic changes found in the cervical spine associated with degenerative disc disease. The patient may not respond to therapy, and pain may persist. Does the physician continue therapy or take another radiograph? The patient may not like being exposed to additional radiation and may be resistant to reevaluation. Only the persistence of pain persuades the patient to undergo radiographic evaluation again at a later date. At this time the process (infection, tumor, or joint inflammation) has destroyed enough bone for its presence to be detected with a plain radiograph. In this scenario, a radiograph taken between the initial and subsequent examination may have detected the lesion at an earlier stage of development. Unless certain risk factors are present, which would suggest an infection or tumor, radiographs should be reserved until the patient has documented that they are refractory to conservative management. Not only does this avoid unnecessary x-rays for those who respond to the usual maneuvers, it also increases the chances that the source of the pathologic changes may be visible on a radiograph in patients who do not respond.

The underlying fact that complicates the relationship of neck pain, particularly of a mechanical nature, and radiographic findings is the progressive anatomic changes that occur naturally in the cervical spine over time and are not associated with pain. While radiographic evidence of chronic disc degeneration is common in middle age, it is almost universal in the elderly. Degenerative disc disease of the cervical spine is not seen as an isolated finding. Rather, it is part of a process that affects the structure of the entire cervical spine. DePalma and Rothman reported gross microscopic and radiographic studies of aging cervical spine specimens.[1] Severe disc degeneration was seen in 72% of the specimens older than 70 years of age. The most commonly affected level was C5–C6, with 86% of specimens having observable abnormalities. The C6–C7 level was the next most frequently affected, and the C2–C3 level was least often involved in chronic disc degeneration.[1, 2]

The radiographic and morphologic findings of cervical spondylosis are as readily observed in asymptomatic patients. Gore and colleagues reported that by age 65, 95% of men and 70% of women had at least one degenerative change on their radiographs.[3] Anterior osteophyte formation and disc space narrowing were common findings. Anterior osteophyte formation was the only component of cervical spondylosis that occurred as an isolated finding. A similar study comparing groups of symptomatic and asymptomatic individuals found no difference between the two groups in the incidence of degenerative changes at the joints of Luschka, the intervertebral foramen, or the posterior articular processes.[4] In a study of asymptomatic patients ranging in age from 30 to 70 years, Friedenberg and Miller found that 35% had radiographic evidence of spondylosis.[4] Thus, it is important to remember that just because anatomic change is present and identifiable on radiographs, it is not necessarily the cause of any particular component of a patient's pain.

On the other hand, radiographic evaluation of the cervical spine can be helpful in detecting specific abnormalities (lytic or blastic bone lesions, expansive spinal cord tumors, disc space infections, and metabolic bone disease) that may be directly related to a patient's clinical symptoms and signs. Radiographic techniques are available to identify anatomic abnormalities associated with local destructive processes or systemic inflammatory illnesses that affect the skeletal system in general. The closest correlation between anatomic changes discovered with radiographic techniques and clinical symptoms occurs with medical diseases of the cervical spine. The physician must not make the mistake of assuming the same close correlation between anatomy and symptoms when evaluating mechanical lesions in the cervical spine.

The poor correlation between anatomic changes and clinical symptoms has also been found with more advanced imaging modalities, including computerized tomography (CT) and magnetic resonance (MR) imaging. This introduction is presented with the hope that physicians who evaluate patients with neck pain will temper their enthusiasm for radiographic evaluation as an easy way to diagnose the cause of pain. Radiographic studies of the cervical spine play an important role in evaluation of neck and arm pain, but the limitations of the technique must be considered. Presence of degenerative disease in the cervical spine may or may not be the cause of the patient's symptoms. Radiographic changes associated with systemic illnesses have greater diagnostic importance.

PLAIN RADIOGRAPHS OF THE CERVICAL SPINE

Plain radiographs remain the initial step in diagnostic imaging of the cervical spine because of their availability, speed, relatively low exposure of tissue to radiation, and reasonable costs. Conventional radiographs offer good spatial and contrast resolution of bony struc-

tures, but they are unable to image soft tissue structures clearly. The initial evaluation should consist of an anteroposterior (AP), lateral, oblique, and open-mouth odontoid view of the cervical spine. Other views, such as flexion-extension views, may be obtained later to confirm specific clinical suspicions of subluxation.

The lateral view of the cervical spine is the single most important in evaluating degenerative conditions, and it provides a wealth of information (Fig. 7–1). It is important that in a good-quality radiograph the bone and soft tissue, all seven cervical vertebrae, and the top of the first thoracic vertebra are visible. In a true lateral radiograph, the lateral masses should be superimposed so that these paired structures appear as a single posterior cortical line. Similarly, the facet joints should also be superimposed so that a single facet joint is seen on the lateral radiograph. The same is true for the posterior cortical margin of the body and the apophyseal joints. Even the slightest change in rotation of the patient will disrupt this relationship and make findings on the radiograph difficult to interpret.

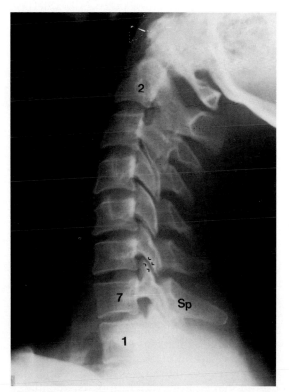

Figure 7–1. Lateral radiograph of a normal cervical spine shows all seven cervical vertebrae as well as the C7–T1 interspace. Also seen are the facet joints *(arrows)* and the spinous process (Sp), which is most prominent at C7 and is also known as the vertebra prominens.

When interpreting radiographs, an organized and orderly process should be used by the physician to avoid missing subtle findings. It is generally recommended to look at the area of highest interest last. Thus, the soft tissues should be examined first, to be sure there are no abnormal soft tissue calcifications, masses, or swellings anterior or posterior to the cervical spine. The upper limits of normal radiologic width for the prevertebral space are 7 mm for C2–C4 and 20 mm for C5–C7.[5] Next, the outline of all the bony structures should be examined to be sure there are no lytic or blastic lesions or fractures. In addition, the overall alignment of the cervical spine should be noted, including the normal lordosis and that there are no anterior or posterior translations of the cervical vertebrae relative to each other. This can be judged by looking at the anterior and posterior cortical margins of the cervical vertebra as well as at the smooth curve formed by the posterior spinolaminar line. The presence of osteophytes or syndesmophytes should be noted, and the heights of the disc spaces relative to each other should be observed.

The finding of disc space narrowing is facilitated by a comparison of the disc in question with the adjacent disc spaces. Disc space narrowing is the most constant feature of cervical spondylosis and is best seen on the lateral view in the lower portion of the cervical spine. Disc space narrowing can lead to relative loss of lordosis as the disc spaces decrease in height. Disc space narrowing is not pathognomonic of degenerative disc changes in the cervical spine and may be seen in other conditions, including rheumatoid disease, neuropathic joints, disc space infection, and traumatic disc herniation. The disc space is often spared with neoplastic involvement in contrast with an infectious process that generally involves the disc. The disc space should also be examined for the vacuum disc phenomenon, which is thought to be an accumulation of nitrogen in the center of a severely degenerative disc, because this is one of the findings that is strongly suggestive of spondylosis. In contrast, erosive changes of the discs and end plates are more suggestive of inflammatory lesions.

In examining the lateral radiographs for osteophytes, several types may be seen. Anterior osteophytes are the largest and may alter the overall shape of the vertebral body. Such large anterior osteophytes may be seen in diffuse idiopathic skeletal hyperostosis. On occasion, these anterior osteophytes may cause dysphagia. In contrast, posterior osteophytes or chondro-osseous spurs are smaller but more important clinically because these hypertrophic changes can project posteriorly into the ventral aspect of the spinal cord and nerve roots. As a general rule, on a standard lateral cervical spine film, the spinal canal as measured from the posterior aspect of the vertebral body to the narrowest point on the spinolaminar line should be about 17 mm. If this distance is narrowed by a posterior osteophyte to a diameter of 13 mm or less, it is likely that there is spinal cord compression. Such a narrowing would prompt further evaluation of this area with neurodiagnostic imaging study (CT or MR).

Spondylosis is the term used to designate bone production in the spine associated with disc space narrowing and more advanced degenerative changes. This is most commonly manifested as the production of osteophytes occurring as a result of a breakdown in the outer annulus fibrosis of the intervertebral disc. This process must be distinguished from the formation of syndesmophytes in ankylosing spondylitis, Reiter's disease, and psoriatic arthritis. It is commonly felt that the formation of osteophytes is due to the pressure of disc material stretching and displacing the posterior annular fibers, causing stress at the ligament attachments and leading to ossification extending first horizontally, then vertically from the edges of the vertebra. In essence, this is an attempt by the disc to eliminate abnormal motion or to autostabilize.

Another component of degenerative disease of the cervical spine that can be evaluated on radiographs is the development of osteoarthritis in the synovial apophyseal joints. This predominates in the middle and lower cervical spine and is thought to be induced by excessive stress across these joints. In most instances, it is felt that changes in the disc space predate any facet joint changes. These facet changes result in joint space narrowing, marginal osteophytosis, bone fragmentation and, less commonly, capsular laxity with subluxation.

Uncovertebral joint arthrosis involves what are also known as the joints of Luschka, extending from C3 through C7. As loss in disc space height occurs, the bony ridges known as the uncinate processes can make contact at the back of the vertebral body resulting in central clefts and a rounding off of the articular surface. Osteophytes that form in this area may project into the disc space or posteriorly into the intervertebral foramen, compressing nerve roots and producing radicular symp-

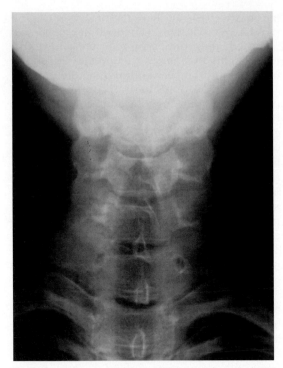

Figure 7–2. Anteroposterior view of a normal cervical spine shows C3 through T1 vertebral bodies. The lateral masses appear as a continuous pillar with a smooth undulating outline on either side. The spinous processes can be seen in the midline and are bifid on C5 and C6.

toms. Less commonly, osteophytes can encroach on the vertebral artery and cause vertebrobasilar insufficiency.

Although these entities—spondylosis, disc space degeneration, facet arthritis, and uncovertebral joint arthritis—have been described as separate processes, they generally progress

together at variable rates to produce a continuing range of changes in the cervical spine. Thus, the term cervical spondylosis is generally used to include all of these degenerative aspects. Each entity produces radiographically identifiable changes that are easily detected on plain films and can help to confirm the diagnosis of cervical degenerative disease.

The AP view of the cervical spine shows the cervical vertebrae from C3 through T1 (Fig. 7–2). The first two cervical vertebrae are generally hidden from view by the superimposed mandible/occiput and must be evaluated separately on an open-mouth odontoid view. In the AP projection the disc spaces, the uncinate processes, and the uncovertebral joints are easily seen. In a correctly positioned AP view, the apophyseal or facet joints are generally not seen secondary to superimposed articular masses. The lateral margins of the articular masses should form what appears to be a continuous undulating pseudocortex at the lateral margin of the cervical spine. In addition, the spinous processes should be linear in the midline and without rotation.

The open-mouth odontoid view is useful for evaluating the relationship of the occiput, atlas, and axis; in addition, any erosive changes can be detected in the inflammatory arthropathies. In addition, this view is most useful for detecting arthritis between the articulations of the occiput and atlas or the atlantoaxial joint complex (Fig. 7–3). An abnormal relationship between the upper cervical spine and the base of the skull, resulting in basilar invagination, may be detected by this view.

Oblique views are used to evaluate the intervertebral foramina, the pedicles, the lateral

Figure 7–3. Open-mouth odontoid view shows the lateral masses of C1 (1) and the odontoid process (2) of the dens. The C1–C2 articulations are also clear.

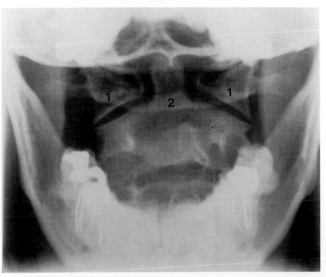

masses, and apophyseal joints (Fig. 7–4). In addition, the relative relationship of the laminae can be evaluated. The oblique view is taken with the patient rotated approximately 45° from the AP position. A recent study suggests that better visualization occurs with a 55° oblique view of the lower cervical spine neural foramina.[6] The foramina viewed on the radiograph are on the side opposite to the side of rotation of the chin. It is preferable that the entire body be rotated rather than just the head and neck. With a properly positioned oblique view, the intervertebral foramina become readily apparent, and any osteophytes that may be encroaching on their margins can be seen. The oblique views also allow the laminae to be viewed and seen as an oval-shaped structure, which should be normally aligned like shingles on a roof.

Other views of the cervical spine, including flexion-extension views and the swimmer's views, can be obtained if specific areas need to be evaluated (Fig. 7–5). In general, flexion-extension views add little to the routine evaluation of the patient for cervical spondylosis, except in situations in which subluxation or instability is suspected on the basis of history or on the basis of static displacements on a standard radiograph. The swimmer's view is obtained with one arm elevated above the head.[7] The swimmer's view is preferred for investigating the cervicothoracic junction.

Normal variations in the configuration of the cervical spine may be identified on plain radiographs of the cervical spine.[8] Pointed configuration of the superior aspect of the tip of the odontoid process should not be confused with an erosive change. Fusion of posterior cervical elements may be produced with superimposed projections of the vertebral laminae. Rotation of the spine may also simulate posterior spinal ligament calcification. The superior articular surfaces of the fifth to seventh cervical vertebrae may show a groove or depression, which should not be confused with inflammatory changes.[9]

In summary, plain radiography of the symptomatic degenerative cervical spine remains a beneficial, relatively inexpensive, and readily available diagnostic tool (Table 7–1). Plain radiographs can clearly exclude deformities, congenital anomalies, infection, and tumor. The standard views recommended for routine evaluation for degenerative problems in the neck include the AP, lateral, open-mouth odontoid, and 45° oblique radiographs. Flexion-extension views are not routinely recommended. Although the clinical symptoms of patients with neck pain, referred pain, or arm pain frequently correlate poorly with degenerative changes on plain radiographs of the cervical spine, the use of plain films still represents the best initial confirmatory test to direct further and more expensive radiographic evaluation in conjunction with history and physical findings.

RADIONUCLIDE IMAGING (BONE SCAN)

Radionuclide imaging addresses function and tissue metabolism of organs by delivering to target structures a small dose of radioisotope material. This tracer emits radiation in proportion to its attachment to the target structure. This imaging is not invasive or associated with high risk, but it is relatively expensive. Radionuclide imaging is a good technique for the detection of bone abnormalities. Bone is a living tissue containing osteoblasts and osteoclasts. Normally the activities of these cells are balanced. Any process that disturbs the normal balance of bone production and resorption can produce an abnormality on

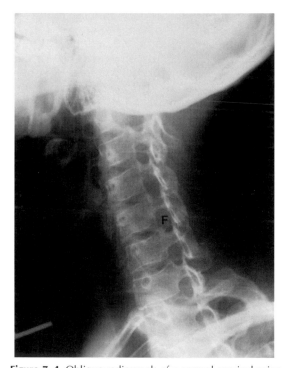

Figure 7–4. Oblique radiograph of a normal cervical spine shows the intervertebral foramina (F) and the facet joints just posterior to them, which have a normal shingling appearance. Spurs from the uncovertebral joints are frequently seen in this view, encroaching on the foramina where the nerve roots exit.

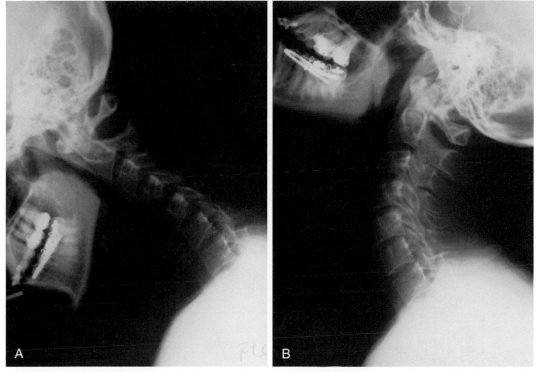

Figure 7–5. *A,* Lateral flexion view of a normal cervical spine. *B,* Lateral extension view of a normal cervical spine. These views show the normal range of motion with flexion and extension and can be useful in detecting instability at one or multiple levels when it is present. Instability can be noted either as a translation of one vertebra on another or an increase in the posterior angular interspace distance between the spinous processes.

bone scan. Increased osteoblastic activity is associated with greater concentration of radionuclide tracer on the bone scan. Interruption of blood flow to the bone results in the absence of tracer on the scan (cold spot). Interruption of metabolic activity also results in decreased activity on the bone scan. In addition to blood flow to the bone, a number of other factors affect the distribution of radionuclide in the normal adult skeleton. Bone turnover is an important factor. In children, the epiphyseal and metaphyseal growth plates are sites of active bone turnover in areas of increased radionuclide concentration. In adults, the metaphyses of long bones may show more activity than the diaphysis. Other factors, including the surface adsorption to bone, diffusion of tracer within bone tissue, and ion exchange between ionic tracers and the ions within the bone, also play a role.

The most commonly used radiopharmaceutical for bone scanning is technetium 99m (^{99m}Tc). This radiopharmaceutical is ideal for bone scans. It has a half-life of 6 hours, emits gamma rays, but has low radiation exposure, approximately 150 mrads.[10] The ^{99m}Tc compounds used for bone imaging are phosphates (inorganic compounds) or phosphonates (organic compounds). The phosphates have a greater propensity for protein binding, whereas diphosphonates are chemically more stable.[11] Examples of these compounds are methylene diphosphate or ethylene hydroxydiphosphonate. Pertechnetate may also be attached to technetium and may be used for radionuclide angiographic studies of bone. ^{99m}Tc pertechnetate binds primarily to serum albumin and is taken up rapidly by organs with increased blood flow.[12] Bone scan images must be taken within 5 to 15 minutes after injection of pertechnetate to allow this effect to be seen.

Bone scan images should be taken at variable times following injection of radionuclide. The most useful study is a form of three-phase scan that involves an immediate blood pool image that is obtained by sequential images 3 to 5 seconds apart. Images are then obtained after several minutes, at 2 to 4 hours after injection, and occasionally at 24 hours to detect residual increase of bone activity.

The normal bone scan image depends on the response of normal bone to mechanical pressure, the thickness of bone, and the excre-

TABLE 7–1. RADIOGRAPHIC STUDIES AND DISEASE CATEGORIES OF THE CERVICAL SPINE

RADIOGRAPHS	HERNIATED NUCLEUS PULPOSUS	SPINAL STENOSIS (OSTEOARTHRITIS)	SPONDYLOLISTHESIS	SPONDYLOARTHROPATHY	INFECTION	TUMOR	ENDOCRINOLOGIC DISORDER	TRAUMA	OTHER**
Plain radiation: 2.6 rads Cost: $125	1	1	1 (Motion)	1 (Syndesmophytes)	1	1	1 (Gout)	1	1
Tomogram radiation: 5 rads Cost: $300					4				
Bone scan radiation: 0.15 rads Cost: $600				2	3	2* (Metastatic)	2 (CPPD)	4 (Old)	2
Computerized tomography radiation: 3–5 rads Cost: $890	2	2	2	3		4 (Myeloma)	3 (Mineral quantification)	2* (Intraspinal)	
Magnetic resonance imaging Radiation: None Cost: $1,250	1*	3			2*	3*		3	
Myelogram Radiation: 6–7 rads Cost: $1,025	2	2				4 (Cord compression)			
Discography radiation: 2 rads (variable) Cost: $500	+/– (Disc degeneration)								
(Normal background) Radiation: 0.6 rads/y									

*Best method.
Numbers indicate sequence of radiographic studies used for diagnosis.
CPPD = Calcium pyrophosphate dihydrate disease
**Other = Paget's disease, vertebral sarcoidosis

tion of 50% of the radionuclide in the kidney and bladder (Fig. 7–6). On the anterior view, normal concentrations of radionuclide are visible over the calvarium, facial bones, sternum, humeral heads, acromioclavicular joints, pelvis (particularly iliac wings), bladder and, to a lesser degree, the knees and ankles. On the posterior view the calvarium, axial spine, kidneys, and sacroiliac joints are prominent. Bone scans of reduced quality may occur secondary to dehydration, marked obesity, therapeutic agents (such as corticosteroids), increased age (patients older than 30 years of age have pro-

gressively diminished uptake), and defective radionuclide preparations.[13]

In the clinical situation, radionuclide imaging is a useful technique for screening the entire skeletal system for abnormal activity. A bone scan is particularly useful in circumstances of radiographic changes lagging behind increased bone activity. The bone scan has been used most commonly for detecting metastatic disease. Approximately 80% of metastatic lesions are found in the axial skeleton.[14] From 10% to 40% of patients with metastatic disease with normal radiographs have abnor-

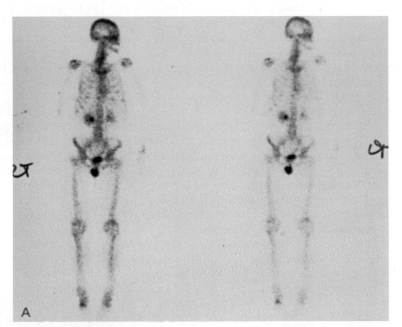

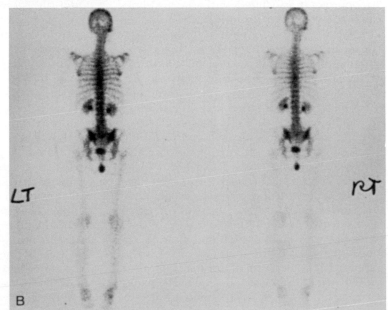

Figure 7–6. Normal bone scan using ⁹⁹ᵐTc methylene diphosphate. *A,* Anterior view—early image *(right),* late image *(left). B,* Posterior view—early image *(right),* late image *(left).*

malities on bone scan, including areas that are painless.[15] One notable exception to early detection of metastatic bone lesions by bone scan is multiple myeloma. The neoplastic plasma cells do not induce an osteoblastic response by bone. Therefore, the lytic lesions of myeloma do not cause increased activity on bone scan until a fracture occurs.[16]

A lack of correlation between radiographic findings and bone scan activity also occurs in osteomyelitis. Radiographs may not be positive for 10 to 14 days after the onset of the disease, whereas the bone scan may be abnormal within the first day.[17] Radionuclide bone imaging is also useful for detecting the early stages of septic arthritis. The bone scan images demonstrate increased activity in blood flow, and delayed static scans before radiographs show changes in infection other than capsular distension.

Trauma to bone, particularly stress fractures, may be difficult to detect by conventional radiography. Bone scintigraphy can detect lesions within 3 days of fracture. Activity at the fracture site may remain increased for an extended period but with a diminishing level of intensity on scan. The older the fracture, the milder the increase in uptake. This fact may be useful in determining the age of compression fractures of the spine.[18]

Generalized bone disease associated with metabolic abnormalities is often associated with diffuse increased uptake on bone scan. Bone scan is more sensitive than radiography in the detection of primary hyperparathyroidism, renal osteodystrophy, and osteomalacia. Osteoporosis is associated with a normal bone scan, unless a compression fracture has occurred.[19]

Arthritis may be detected by bone scan. Noninflammatory joint disease (osteoarthritis) is associated with osteoblastic activity in the form of sclerosis and osteophyte formation. Inflammatory arthropathies are associated with increased blood flow and increased activity on bone scan. The bone scan can quantitate increased activity in portions of the sacroiliac joints in patients with spondyloarthropathies.[20]

Other diseases associated with abnormal bone scans include Paget's disease, hemoglobinopathies, and aseptic necrosis of bone. Paget's disease is a generalized disease of bone associated with increased blood flow to the bone. The correlation between plain radiographs and bone scan abnormality is close. The activity of disease is reflected in the extent of bone scan intensity of the bone lesions. Patients with sickle cell anemia have positive bone scans. In patients with acute infarcts of bone, the bone scan may demonstrate a cold spot. Within a few days, blood flow is restored and increased uptake appears.

Aseptic necrosis of bone is associated with bone death, which may occur by a number of different mechanisms. Interruption of blood flow occurs secondary to disruption of vessels, increased pressure, or intraluminal occlusion. Early in the course of this lesion, blood flow is halted and an absence of radionuclide is noted on the scan. With revascularization, reparative processes are initiated, and increased blood flow is noted.

In general, radionuclide imaging is a useful technique for the evaluation of bone abnormalities in patients with neck pain. Although the bone scan is a highly sensitive test, the resolution of the image is relatively low. It also has less specificity than other radiographic techniques for diagnosing pathologic processes affecting the cervical spine. With the advent of single photon emission CT, three-dimensional localization of increased activity on bone scans may be more readily possible. This technique is under investigation.

MYELOGRAPHY

The myelogram is the benchmark for evaluating neural compression within the spinal canal. The technique of cervical myelography consists of injecting radiopaque contrast media into the subarachnoid space and maneuvering this material into the cervical region under fluoroscopic guidance. Radiographs are then taken with the dye in the cervical spine in the AP lateral and oblique planes. The flow characteristics and defects in the dye column of contrast material are observed fluoroscopically and then permanently recorded on images, using spot film techniques.

There are several contrast media available for myelography. When the technique was first developed, Pantopaque, an oil-based dye, was used. The oil-based dyes, however, were associated with a significant rate of long-term complications, including foreign body granulomas and chronic adhesive arachnoiditis.[21] Water-soluble contrast media, such as metrizamide, essentially eliminated the long-term complications but are associated with a few short-term side effects, including seizure activity.[22] Nonionic water-based contrast agents, such as iohexol, are associated with the fewest numbers of side effects and are being used routinely, often on an outpatient basis.[23]

The contrast material may be instilled into the subarachnoid space by either lumbar or lateral C1–C2 puncture. The lateral cervical route allows direct injection of contrast media into the cervical spinal canal; as a result, lower concentrations and a lower total dose of iodine may be used. The lateral C1–C2 puncture is somewhat more painful and hazardous than lumbar puncture.[24–26] For these reasons fluoroscopic-guided lumbar puncture is frequently recommended, using a 22-gauge needle and 10 mL of contrast media in 200 to 300 mg of iodine/mL concentration. The radiographs generally need to be completed within 20 to 30 minutes after the injection of dye to avoid dilution.

Certain precautions are necessary before and after myelography. Any drugs that lower seizure thresholds (such as phenothiazine derivatives) should be discontinued for 48 hours before the procedure. Patients with epilepsy should be maintained on their anticonvulsants. Patients should not eat for 4 hours before the procedure.

After the procedure patients should be in a semisitting position in bed for several hours. After that initial period the patient may lie down in bed, with the head raised 10°. This helps prevent contrast material reaching the upper subarachnoid space. The most common complication is headache in 68% of patients. Nausea and vomiting occur in 38%, back pain in 26%, and seizures in 0.4%.[27] The complications with iohexol are less frequent, but if they occur they may be treated with analgesics along with caffeine, antiemetics, intravenous fluids, and intravenous diazepam for acute seizures.

Neural compression shows up as a defect in the dye column. The possible locations for lesions are extradural, intradural-extramedullary, or intramedullary. A prime example of an extradural lesion is a herniated nucleus pulposus (Fig. 7–7). Other extradural lesions include osteophytes, abscesses, tumors, and hematomas. Neurofibromatosis causes intradural-extramedullary lesions, as do arachnoiditis and infection. Intramedullary lesions include spinal cord tumors, vascular malformations, and syringomyelia. Extradural lesions push the cord and subarachnoid space away from their normal course and interrupt the column of contrast material. Intradural-extramedullary lesions push the cord away from the dura. Intramedullary tumors cause expansion of the cord with symmetrical obliteration of the subarachnoid space.

Like all diagnostic studies in the spine, the myelogram should be employed as a confirmatory study. An abnormal myelogram without substantiating historical and physical findings is not meaningful. It has been shown that 21% of asymptomatic people have an abnormal cervical myelogram (with Pantopaque contrast material).[28] The experienced spine surgeon usually reserves the myelogram for preoperative assurance to confirm the location of the damaged disc or to check for congenitally anomalous nerve root tumor or double disc. If the myelogram is used as a screening test in the absence of objective clinical findings, exploratory surgery and disaster are the frequent results. Furthermore, patients who undergo a myelogram without positive physical findings (nerve root tension sign, motor weakness, or sensory deficit) are reported to have a significantly higher chance of developing side effects from the procedure itself (nausea, vomiting, or increased pain). A particular advantage of the myelogram is that in addition to evaluating the cervical spine it can also evaluate the upper thoracic spine. Whereas the major advantage of myelography is that it provides visualization of the entire length of the cervical canal up to the level of the foramen magnum, as well as the remainder of the spine if necessary, the major disadvantage is its invasive nature and, to some extent, its lack of diagnostic specificity. Accuracy rates for water-soluble nonionic cervical myelography in the diagnosis of nerve root compression range between 67% and 92%.[29–32] Difficulties in diagnostic accuracy can occur with small central disc protrusions. In addition, making the distinction between hard discs (bony spurs) and soft discs (herniations) can be difficult with the use of myelography alone. The use of myelography in combination with CT provides increased visualization of neural compression and its relation to the bony elements of the spine.

COMPUTERIZED TOMOGRAPHY (CT)

CT has become extremely useful for evaluating abnormalities of the cervical spine where the spatial anatomy is complex. CT creates cross-sectional images of the internal structure of the spine at various levels and, with reformatting, one can also obtain coronal and sagittal sections. The CT scan assesses not only the bony configuration and structure-space relationship but also the soft tissue in graded shadings so that ligaments, nerve roots, free

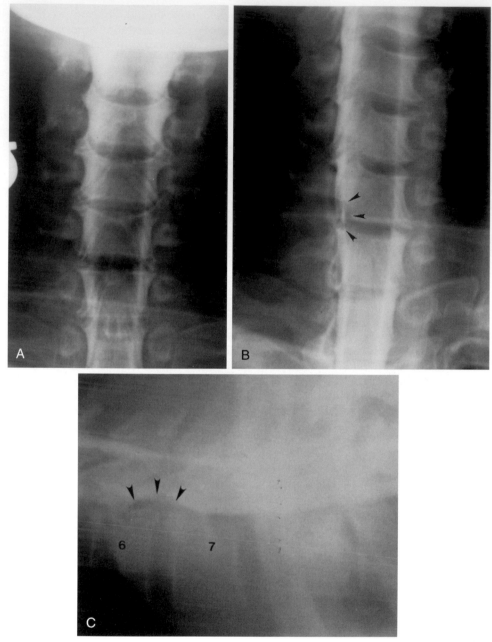

Figure 7–7. *A,* Anteroposterior view of cervical myelogram shows central dye column with exiting nerve roots that appear as linear filling defects in the dye column. *B,* Oblique view of a cervical myelogram shows a filling defect *(arrows)* on the left side at the C6–C7 disc level. *C,* Lateral cervical myelogram shows a ventral filling defect *(arrows)* at the C6–C7 disc level, which represents the typical appearance of a herniated cervical disc.

fat, and intervertebral disc protrusions can be evaluated as they relate to their bony environment in a single scan. CT also permits excellent visualization of paraspinal soft tissues.

A CT image is produced by passing a tightly collimated beam of x-rays produced in a x-ray tube through the patient's body, which absorbs or attenuates portions of the beam to varying degrees, depending on the initial in-

tensity of the beam and the density of the structures encountered. The attenuated beam is then picked up by a detector, amplified, and quantitated as electric signals that are then manipulated by a computer to produce the resulting image.

A CT/myelogram is a CT examination of the cervical spine performed after intrathecal instillation of contrast media. The presence of radiopaque contrast media in the subarachnoid space significantly improves the diagnostic value of the CT examination, which can be performed either as an adjunct to standard myelography or as the primary procedure using lower dosages (3 to 5 mL) and lower concentrations (170 to 180 mg of iodine/mL) of contrast material. Using lower dosages of contrast media provides a safer method of studying patients on an outpatient basis. Although it has been shown that the anatomy of the cervical neural foramina and contents may be demonstrated by conventional high-resolution CT, the addition of intrathecal contrast material allows the demonstration of swollen nerve roots and quantitative analysis of cord compression, which increases the specificity of this diagnostic modality.[33, 34]

As opposed to bone scintigraphy, which generates a survey of the entire skeleton on one view, the CT scan is able to assess only one cross-sectional cut of the skeleton per view. Lesions that are not contained in the plane will not be viewed by the CT scanner. The scanner can be programmed to make axial cuts at varying distances. The usual amount required for the cervical spine is 2 to 3 mm in thickness because of the small size of the cervical anatomic structures.

A CT section of the cervical spine contains different anatomic structures, depending on the level of the cross section (Fig. 7–8). A scan through the superior portion of the vertebral body shows the transverse and spinous processes, laminae, inferior articular process of the cephalad vertebra, superior articular process of the caudad vertebra, pedicles, and vertebral body. A view in the middle of the vertebral body demonstrates cancellous bone in the center of the vertebral body along with pedicles and laminae—a complete bony ring of the spinal canal. The intervertebral foramina are shown in a view of the lower third of the vertebra. A section through the intervertebral disc demonstrates the inferior articular process of the cephalad vertebra and superior articular process of the caudad vertebra, the spinous process, and the intervertebral disc.

The significant advantage of the CT scan over the myelogram as a radiographic technique in evaluation of the cervical spine is not its resolution of structures but its ability to define the spatial relationships of the anatomic structures. CT is helpful in evaluation of spinal stenosis, infections with paraspinal abscesses, postsurgical epidural scarring, facet and uncovertebral joint arthritis, primary metastatic tumors of the cervical spine, and

trauma to the spinal column. Degenerative enlargement of facet joints and uncovertebral joints may produce symptoms of foraminal stenosis. The facet joints and the size of the spinal canal are readily examined. CT can also visualize the medullary portion of the vertebral body and detect bone destruction before changes are visible on plain radiographs.

CT is particularly useful in the diagnosis and assessment of trauma as the patient is stationary during the procedure, limiting the hazards of moving the patient. Small fragments of bone that may not be detectable by plain radiograph are easy to localize on CT scan. Furthermore, evaluation of the craniocervical and cervicothoracic junctions is difficult on a plain radiograph but becomes quite clear on the CT examination.

The clinical significance of CT/myelographic findings in cervical spondylosis was studied by Penning and colleagues.[35] A 100% correlation was found between the site of disc herniation with an occlusion of the intervertebral foramen and the site of nerve root symptoms. Long tract signs were noted after the cross-sectional area of the spinal cord had been reduced by 30% to a value of about 60 mm^2 or less. Penning and colleagues also noted that in the presence of a normal conventional plain film myelogram, postmyelographic CT studies were superfluous. CT investigations in these cases may lead to false-positive interpretation of clinically irrelevant findings.

Reported accuracy rates for CT range from 72% to 91%.[29, 31, 32, 36–38] Agreement rates between contrast-enhanced CT and myelography have been reported to range from 75% to 96%.[31, 37, 38] When a discrepancy exists between myelographic and CT findings, postcontrast CT is invariably the more accurate study.

Despite the diagnostic accuracy of the CT scan in the cervical spine, one must not make clinical decisions based on CT scan findings isolated from the patient's clinical picture. Although the analogous study has not been performed in the cervical spine, a significant number of asymptomatic patients have abnormalities on CT scans of the lumbar area, and there is every reason to believe that this would occur in the cervical spine as well. Thus, this diagnostic test, as with all others, should be used to confirm clinical suspicions and not used as a screening test.

MAGNETIC RESONANCE (MR) IMAGING

MR imaging is a new diagnostic technique that displays small differences in tissue density

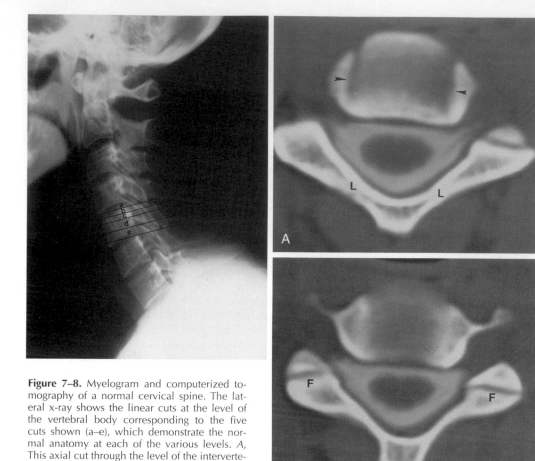

Figure 7–8. Myelogram and computerized tomography of a normal cervical spine. The lateral x-ray shows the linear cuts at the level of the vertebral body corresponding to the five cuts shown (a–e), which demonstrate the normal anatomy at each of the various levels. *A,* This axial cut through the level of the intervertebral disc space shows the spinal cord surrounded by the dye in the subarachnoid space anteriorly. The uncovertebral joints can be seen *(arrows)* posterior to the spinal canal. The lamina (L) can be seen. *B,* This axial cut just distal to the intervertebral joint space shows the top of the vertebral body and the beginning of the transverse processes. In addition, the facet joints (F) can be seen on each side as well as the foramen and exiting nerve roots.

with sharp contrast without exposing the patient to radiation or contrast material. MR has been clinically available since the middle 1980s. Since then, MR has been used increasingly for evaluation of the musculoskeletal system, including low back and neck pain. MR has become the diagnostic imaging procedure of choice for certain disorders, including infection, disc herniations, and intramedullary tumors of the spinal cord. MR technology, owing to both hardware and software algorithmic manipulations, continues to be refined to decrease acquisition time of the scans and increase the spatial resolution.

The basic principle behind MR imaging involves the generation of a magnetic field by the nuclei of atoms with an odd number of protons. When placed between the poles of a strong magnet (up to 20,000 times the earth's magnetic field), the protons line up between the magnetic poles and vibrate at a frequency specific to each type of atom. Transmitting radio waves equal to the specific frequency of the target atoms and directed at a right angle to the static magnetic field causes the atoms to vibrate at an angle away from the vertical orientation. When the transmission of the radio waves is discontinued, the protons return to a state of relaxation (vertical position) by releasing radio waves. The radio waves generated by the atoms are detected by radio antennas, and the information is analyzed by computer to generate cross-sectional images of the body. Variations in proton density, radio frequency, and the time to return to a state of relaxation (relaxation time) modify the image produced by the MR scanner.

Proton density refers to the number of nuclei per unit volume of the structure to be examined. The most commonly measured

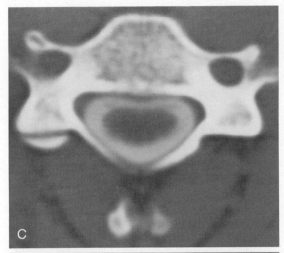

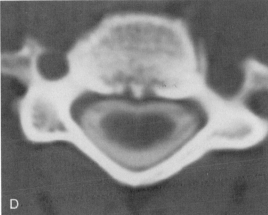

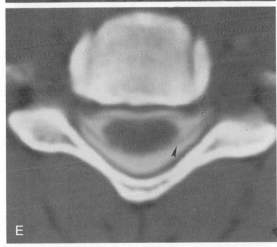

Figure 7–8 *Continued C,* This axial cut through the midportion of the vertebral body shows the transverse process and the foramen transversarium, which contain the vertebral arteries on either side. *D,* This cut is at the lower third of the vertebral body and shows the inferior portion of the transverse process. *E,* This cut is at the inferiormost portion of the vertebral body bordering on the intervertebral disc space, again showing the uncovertebral joints. On this image the exiting spinal rootlets, both anterior and posterior, can be seen as a linear filling defect in the subarachnoid dye column *(arrow).*

atom is hydrogen. The hydrogen in water generates a different amplitude of MR image if it is loosely bound to tissue molecules than if tightly bound to specific molecules. Therefore, the amount and binding of water in the target tissue have a direct effect on the image generated by the MR scanner.

The proton relaxation times also play a major role in the generation of the MR image. When the aligned protons are deflected by the radio wave, they achieve a level of increased excitation by their axes spinning in the shape of a cone. The time it takes for the proton to regain its magnetization in its vertical position is the T_1 relaxation time. The time it takes for the proton to lose its magnetization in the horizontal plane is the T_2 relaxation time. It is possible to change the pulse sequences of radio waves to accentuate differences in T_1 and T_2 relaxation times. The weighting of the images to T_1 or T_2 relaxation time has a marked effect on the appearance of the MR image. With T_1-weighted images, nerve tissue is white and cerebrospinal fluid (CSF) is gray. CSF is white and nerve tissue is gray in T_2-weighted images.

The MR scan includes a sagittal and axial view of the cervical spine, frequently with T_1 and T_2 or some equivalent weighted image. Patients who are on life-support systems (metal machines) or who have cardiac pacemakers or metal clips on intracranial aneurysms are not suitable candidates for MR imaging. Pacemakers may revert from the demand mode to a fixed-rate mode of operation. Metal clips may twist or loosen. Although nonferromagnetic implants, such as stainless steel appliances, are not attracted to the magnets, these objects cause artifacts that degrade the MR image. Claustrophobic individuals may have great difficulty in the closed space on the scanner and may need to be sedated with medications such as oral diazepam to complete the study.

The normal MR image of the cervical spine visualizes the vertebral column, intervertebral discs, spinal canal, spinal cord, and CSF in the sagittal view (Fig. 7–9). The axial views generally show the paravertebral soft tissue structures, the disc or vertebral body, the spinal canal, and the spinal cord (Fig. 7–10). The choice of relaxation times (T_1 or T_2) and pulse sequences as well as other parameters may be modified to highlight specific structures or produce contrast that accentuates abnormalities associated with certain pathologic states.

MR imaging is an excellent technique for viewing the spinal cord within the spinal canal. It is the preferred imaging modality for syrin-

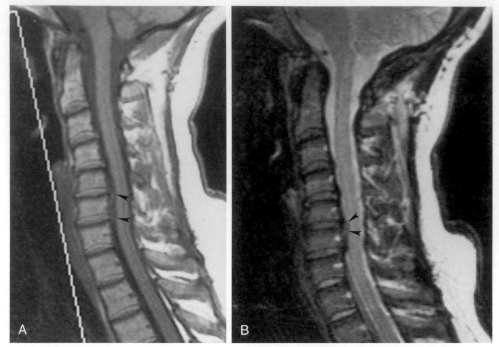

Figure 7–9. Magnetic resonance image of the cervical spine. *A,* T₁-weighted sagittal image shows the vertebral bodies, intervertebral discs, spinal cord, and subarachnoid space. Small disc herniations are seen at C3–C4 and C4–C5. A larger disc herniation is seen at C5–C6 and C6–C7 *(arrows).* *B,* T₂-weighted sagittal image shows similar findings of a moderate herniated disc at C5–C6 *(arrows).* Cerebrospinal fluid appears white instead of gray.

gomyelia, cord atrophy, cord infarction, traumatic injury to the cord, and intramedullary tumors or multiple sclerosis affecting the spinal cord. MR imaging is likely to be more accurate than CT at characterizing extramedullary tumors. MR imaging delineates the extent of extradural tumor invasion of the spinal canal as well as compression or displacement of the spinal cord. It can identify the vertebral bodies in which bone marrow has been replaced with tumor.[39] It also shows early changes in discs and vertebral end plates with infectious discitis.[40] Most clinicians believe that CT scanning continues to offer better definition of the bony architecture of the spinal canal than does MR imaging (Fig. 7–11).

MR images may be obtained through traditional two-dimension imaging or with more advanced three-dimension acquisition techniques. Two-dimension imaging may include the traditional spin-echo images or gradient echo imaging techniques with partial flip angle. The difficulty, in general, with two-dimension techniques in identifying foraminal disease is due to long echo times, thick image cuts, and the inability to view the course of the exiting nerve roots and planes other than axial. Although overall examination time tends to decrease with gradient echo imaging, the length of examination continues to be problematic. One potential solution may be found in gradient echo volume imaging (3D), which would allow short echo times with thin contiguous cuts and the ability to reformat the data in a desired viewing plane. Three-dimension imaging techniques include fast low-angle shot (FLASH) and spoiled gradient recall acquisition in the steady state. Turbo-FLASH or magnetization-prepared rapid acquisition gradient echo is a technique that uses short relaxation times and low flip angles for very rapid volume imaging. Another technique is fast imaging with steady precession, which can produce a hyperintense CSF signal (and a myelogram effect). In addition to providing new acquisition modalities, improved surface coils continue to increase the signal-to-noise ratio and improve the overall image quality.

Many of the early-generation MR scanners that are still used produce what are considered to be inferior MR images. Such suboptimal images can both be misleading in terms of false positive diagnoses and can fail to detect more subtle problems. In general, a poor MR scan is worse than no MR scan, and the patient is better served with a standard myelogram followed by a high-resolution CT scan.

Two studies have documented the preva-

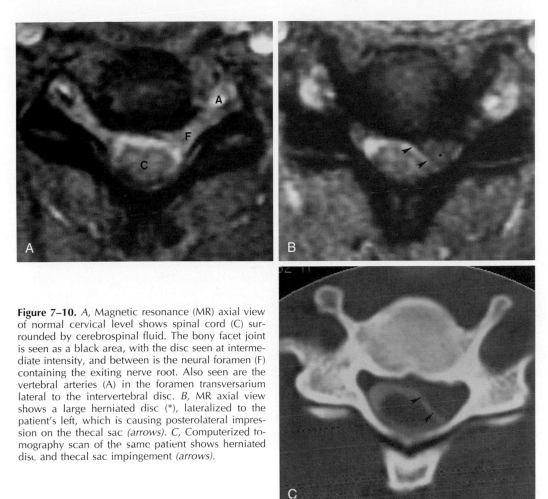

Figure 7–10. *A,* Magnetic resonance (MR) axial view of normal cervical level shows spinal cord (C) surrounded by cerebrospinal fluid. The bony facet joint is seen as a black area, with the disc seen at intermediate intensity, and between is the neural foramen (F) containing the exiting nerve root. Also seen are the vertebral arteries (A) in the foramen transversarium lateral to the intervertebral disc. *B,* MR axial view shows a large herniated disc (*), lateralized to the patient's left, which is causing posterolateral impression on the thecal sac *(arrows). C,* Computerized tomography scan of the same patient shows herniated disc and thecal sac impingement *(arrows).*

lence of degenerative changes in the cervical spine in asymptomatic subjects studied with MR imaging.[41, 42] A wide variety of abnormalities were displayed in more than 20% of the asymptomatic subjects. Disc protrusion was seen in about 10% to 15% of subjects and may have increased frequency in older individuals. The prevalence of disc narrowing, disc degeneration, and spurs increased from 25% in subjects younger than 40 years of age to 60% in those older than 40 years of age.[41] Foraminal stenosis was present in 7% of subjects younger than 40 years of age and in 23% of those older than 40 years of age. Spinal cord impingement was seen in 10% to 15% of younger subjects and in 20% to 25% of older subjects. Spinal cord compression was seen in fewer than 5% and was due solely to disc protrusion. Cord area reduction averaged 7% and never exceeded 16%.[42] Thus, the cord appears to tolerate a certain amount of volume loss without demonstrating symptoms. In another study, degenerative disc disease of the cervical spine was noted to be more common in older individuals who were examined by MR imaging.[43] Degenerative disc disease begins at a later age in the cervical spine than in the lumbar region. Although asymptomatic anatomic abnormalities may be detected with MR evaluation, this technique remains the most sensitive for detecting bony and soft tissue changes in the cervical spine.[44]

DISCOGRAPHY

Since its introduction by Smith and Nichols in 1957, cervical discography has remained controversial.[45] Many authors believe the procedure has diagnostic value,[46–50] and others maintain that it is useless and misleading and should be discontinued altogether.[51–59] Advocates of the procedure state that a normal disc

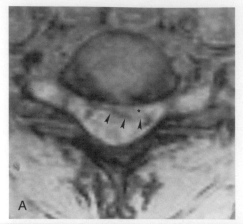

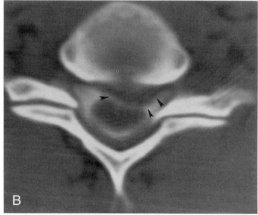

Figure 7–11. *A,* Magnetic resonance view shows axial posterolateral herniated disc (*) causing compression of the thecal sac and exiting nerve rootlet on the left *(arrows).* *B,* Computerized tomography/myelogram shows the same herniated disc and compression *(arrows)* of the exiting nerve rootlet on the left.

accepts no contrast material or at most 0.1 to 0.2 mL. Injection of a normal disc infrequently produces pain at the base of the neck. Injection of an abnormal disc, however, generally reproduces the type of pain and discomfort from which the patient is suffering. Injection of a local anesthetic promptly relieves this pain, which is confirmatory for the level of involvement. More than one disc is generally studied, and at least one level considered to be normal should not elicit pain and serve as a negative control level. Cervical discography may be useful in patients who present with chronic neck or radicular pain and shoulder and upper extremity pain, after noninvasive imaging has been inconclusive.[54]

The technique is performed by placing a fine-gauged spinal needle into the disc space, followed by injection of radiopaque dye. The amount of dye accepted into the disc, the injection pressure, the radiographic appear-

ance of the dye, and the reproduction of the patient's pain are important data generated during the test. Although a variety of complications are possible, disc space infection is the most common.

Although some reports have suggested a close correlation among abnormal discograms, degenerative disc disease, and chronic neck pain, other studies have reported little correlation between abnormal discograms and the local source of the patient's pain. Although a discographic study may reproduce a patient's cervical pain, the results of surgery for relief of neck pain alone without radicular symptoms have been unpredictable. Therefore, reliance on data generated regarding the status of cervical discs by noninvasive radiographic techniques, such as MR and CT, is usually adequate to define the integrity of the intervertebral disc space. Discograms are rarely indicated.

SUMMARY

The problem in patients with cervical pain is the identification of the level or levels that are productive of the symptomatology. The accuracy of the diagnostic tools that are employed is commonly compared to surgical findings. Although the surgeon can confirm or disprove the radiologic assessment of the anatomic status within the spinal canal, the surgeon is no more able than the radiologist to unequivocally ascertain that the patient's symptoms are etiologically related to the morphologic status of the canal. In other words, both the radiologist and the surgeon are capable of describing the morphologic features of cervical spondylosis, but neither can tell with certainty whether these features are responsible for the patient's symptoms. Accordingly, the results of an operation can provide an indication of the accuracy of these imaging modalities, but they are by no means conclusive. The importance of strict correlation of positive diagnostic studies with the patient's signs and symptoms cannot be overstressed. This is particularly important in light of the fact that a significant percentage of asymptomatic subjects have radiographic abnormalities on any of the imaging modalities that have been tested. In conclusion, imaging studies are useful for confirming a clinical diagnosis suggested by the history and physical examination, but they should never be interpreted in isolation from the overall clinical picture, and they should never be used as general screening tests.

References

1. DePalma AF, Rothman RH: The Intervertebral Disc. Philadelphia, WB Saunders Co, 1970.
2. Friedenberg ZB, Ediken J, Spenser N, et al.: Degenerative changes in the cervical spine. J Bone Joint Surg Am 41:61, 1959.
3. Gore DR, Sepie SB, Gardner GM: Roentgenographic findings of the cervical spine in asymptomatic people. Spine 11:521, 1986.
4. Friedenberg ZB, Miller WT: Degenerative disc disease of the cervical spine. J Bone Joint Surg Am 45:1171, 1963.
5. Penning L: Prevertebral hematoma in cervical spine injury: incidence and etiological significance. Neuroradiology 1:557, 1980.
6. Marcelis S, Seragini FC, Taylor JA, et al.: Cervical spine: comparison of 45 degrees and 55 degrees anteroposterior oblique radiographic projections. Radiology 188:253, 1993.
7. Scher A, Vambeck V: An approach to the radiological examination of the cervicodorsal junction following injury. Clin Radiol 28:243, 1977.
8. Keats TE: Plain film radiography: Sources of diagnostic errors. In: Resnick D (ed): Diagnosis of Bone and Joint Disorders, 3rd ed. Philadelphia: WB Saunders Co, 1995, pp 41–43.
9. Keats TE, Johnstone WH: Notching of the lamina of C7: a proposed mechanism. Skeletal Radiol 7:233, 1982.
10. Davis M, Jones A: Comparison of ^{99m}Tc-labeled phosphate agents for skeletal imaging. Semin Nucl Med 7:19, 1976.
11. Pendergrass HP, Potsaid MS, Costronovo FP Jr.: The clinical use of ^{99m}Tc-diphosphonate (HEDSPA). Radiology 109:557, 1973.
12. Weiss TE, Shuler SE: I. New techniques for identification of synovitis and evaluation of joint disease. II. Joint imaging as a clinical aid in diagnosis and therapy. Bull Rheum Dis 25:786, 1974.
13. Wilson MA: The effect of age on the quality of bone scans using ^{99m}Tc-pyrophosphate. Radiology 139:703, 1981.
14. McNeil BJ: Rationale for the use of bone scans in selected metastatic and primary bone tumors. Semin Nucl Med 8:336, 1978.
15. De Nardo GL, Jacobson SJ, Raventos A: ^{85}Sr bone scan in neoplastic disease. Semin Nucl Med 2:18, 1972.
16. Woolfenden JM, Pitt MJ, Durie BGM, Moon TE: Comparison of bone scintigraphy and radiography in multiple myeloma. Radiology 134:723, 1980.
17. Handmaker H, Leonards R: The bone scan in inflammatory osseous disease. Semin Nucl Med 6:95, 1976.
18. Marty R, Denney J, McKamey MR, Rowley MJ: Bone trauma and related benign disease: assessment by bone scanning. Semin Nucl Med 6:107, 1976.
19. Fogelman I, Bessent RG, Turner JG, et al.: The use of whole-body retention of Tc-99m diphosphonate in the diagnosis of metabolic bone disease. J Nucl Med 19:270, 1978.
20. Goldberg RP, Genant HK, Shimshak R, Shames D: Applications and limitations of quantitative sacroiliac joint scintigraphy. Radiology 128:683, 1978.
21. Skalpe IO: Adhesive arachnoiditis following lumbar myelography. Spine 3:61, 1978.
22. Ratcliff G, Sandler S, Latchaw R: Cognitive and affective changes after myelography: a comparison of metrizamide and iohexol. AJR 147:777, 1986.
23. Vezina JL, Fontaine S, Laperriere J: Outpatient myelography with fine-needle technique: an appraisal. AJNR 10:615, 1989.
24. Hinck VC, Sachdev NS: Developmental stenosis of the cervical spinal canal. Brain 89:27, 1966.
25. Orrison WW, Eldevik OP: Lateral C1–2 puncture for cervical myelography: part III: historical, anatomic, and technical considerations. Radiology 146:401, 1983.
26. Orrison WW, Sackett JF, Amundsen P: Lateral C1–2 puncture for cervical myelography: part II: recognition of improper injection of contrast material. Radiology 146:395, 1983.
27. Baker RA, Hillman BJ, McLennan JE, et al.: Sequelae of metrizamide myelography in 200 examinations. AJR 130:499, 1978.
28. Hitselberger WE, Witten RM: Abnormal myelograms in asymptomatic patients. J Neurosurg 28:204, 1968.
29. Coin CG: Cervical disk degeneration and herniation: diagnosis by computerized tomography. South Med J 77:979, 1984.
30. Hitselberger WE, Witten RM: Abnormal myelograms in asymptomatic patients. J Neurosurg 28:204, 1968.
31. Modic MT, Ross JS, Masaryk TJ: Imaging of degenerative disease of the cervical spine. Clin Orthop 239:109, 1989.
32. Sobel DF, Barkovich AJ, Munderloh SH: Metrizamide myelography and postmyelographic computer tomography: comparative adequacy in the cervical spine. AJNR 45:385, 1984.
33. Pech P, Daniels DL, Williams AL, Haughton VM: The cervical neural foramina: correlation of microtomy and CT anatomy. Radiology 155:143, 1985.
34. Badami JP, Norman D, Barbaro NM, et al.: Metrizamide CT myelography in cervical myelopathy and radiculopathy: correlation with conventional myelography and surgical findings. AJR 144:675, 1985.
35. Penning L, Wilmink JT, van Woerden HH, et al.: CT myelographic findings in degenerative disorders of the cervical spine: clinical significance. AJNR 7:119, 1986.
36. Dorwart RH, LaMasters DL: Applications of computed tomographic scanning of the cervical spine. Orthop Clin North Am 16:381, 1985.
37. Landman JA, Hoffman JC, Braun IF, et al.: Value of computed tomographic myelography in the recognition of cervical herniated disk. AJNR 5:391, 1984.
38. Nakagawa H, Okumura T, Sugiyama T, et al.: Discrepancy between metrizamide CT and myelography in diagnosis of cervical disk protrusions. AJNR 4:604, 1983.
39. Porter BA, Shields AF, Olson DO: Magnetic resonance imaging of bone marrow disorders. Radiol Clin North Am 24:269, 1986.
40. Modic MT, Pflanze W, Feiglin DHI, Belhobek G: Magnetic resonance imaging of musculoskeletal infections. Radiol Clin North Am 24:247, 1986.
41. Boden SD, McCowin PR, Davis DO, et al.: Abnormal cervical spine MR scans in asymptomatic individuals: a prospective and blinded investigation. J Bone Joint Surg Am 72A:1178, 1990.
42. Teresi LM, Lufkin RB, Reicher MA: Asymptomatic degenerative disk disease and spondylosis of the cervical spine: MR imaging. Radiology 164:83, 1987.
43. Lehto IJ, Tertti MO, Komu ME, et al.: Age-related MRI changes at 0.1 T in cervical discs in asymptomatic subjects. Neuroradiology 36:49, 1994.
44. Bell GR, Ross JS: The accuracy of imaging studies of

the degenerative cervical spine: myelography, myelo-computed tomography, and magnetic resonance imaging. Semin Spine Surg 7:9, 1995.

45. Smith GW, Nichols P Jr: The technique of cervical discography. Radiology 68:163, 1963.

46. Cloward RB: Cervical discography: a contribution to the etiology and mechanism of neck, shoulder, and arm pain. Ann Surg 150:1052, 1959.

47. Massare C, Bard M, Tristant H: Cervical discography: speculation on technique and indications from our own experience. J Radiol 55:395, 1974.

48. Roth DA: Cervical analgesic discography: a new test for the definitive diagnosis of the painful-disk syndrome. JAMA 235:1713, 1976.

49. Simmons EH: An evaluation of discography in the localization of symptomatic levels in discogenic diseases of the spine. Clin Orthop 108:57, 1975.

50. Whitecloud TS, Seago RA: Cervical discogenic syndrome: results of operative intervention in patients with positive discography. Spine 12:313, 1987.

51. Collins HR: An evaluation of cervical and lumbar discography. Clin Orthop 107:133, 1975.

52. Hirsch C, Schajowicz F, Galante J: Structural changes in the cervical spine. Acta Orthop Scand Suppl 109:1, 1967.

53. Holt EP: Fallacy of cervical discography. JAMA 188:799, 1964.

54. Holt EP: Further reflections on cervical discography. JAMA 231:613, 1975.

55. Klafta LA Jr, Collins JS Jr: The diagnostic inaccuracy of the pain response in cervical discography. Cleve Clin Q 36:35, 1969.

56. Meyer RR: Cervical diskography: a help or hindrance in evaluating neck, shoulder, arm pain? AJR 90:1208, 1963.

57. Shapiro R: Myelography, 4th ed. Chicago, Year Book Medical Publishers, 1984.

58. Sneider SE, Winslow OP, Pryor TH: Cervical discography: is it relevant? JAMA 185:163, 1963.

59. Taveras J: Is discography a useful diagnostic procedure? J Canad As Radiol 18:294, 1967.

8

Miscellaneous Tests

ELECTRODIAGNOSTIC STUDIES

Electrodiagnostic studies are commonly used in the evaluation of disease affecting the peripheral nervous system. These studies are extensions of the neurologic examination and provide an objective measure of nerve damage. They can confirm the clinical impression of nerve root compression, define the severity and distribution of involvement, and document or exclude other illnesses of nerves or muscles that could contribute to the patient's symptoms and signs. Electrodiagnostic tests measure the integrity of the nerve-muscle relationship and do not, by themselves, offer a specific etiologic diagnosis or quantify the degree of nerve damage. For patients with neck and arm pain, electrodiagnostic studies are helpful in documenting radiculopathy (disease located at the level of the spinal roots). These studies are also useful in differentiating abnormalities associated with entrapment neuropathies, distal peripheral neuropathies, myopathies, and myelopathies.[1]

Electrodiagnostic studies include evaluation of electrical activity generated by muscle fibers at rest and during contraction (electromyogram) and speed of conduction of impulses electrically generated in peripheral nerves (nerve conduction studies). Studies of the integrity of the neuromuscular junction are not done in the evaluation of patients with spinal disease but are reserved for patients with neuromuscular abnormalities, such as myasthenia gravis.

Electromyography (EMG) is the study of the action potentials of muscle fibers. The EMG machine consists of an amplifier, oscilloscope, audio system, and recording electrodes. The recording electrodes are needles, ranging from 18-gauge to 26-gauge, that are inserted into muscles. The procedure consists of inserting needle electrodes through the skin to varying depths of each muscle to be studied. Each muscle is examined at two or more locations and in three or more directions. The multiple locations and directions are needed because abnormalities are focal in distribution. The test is painful but usually does not require sedation or analgesics. The test takes over an hour to complete and may cost up to $600.

Nerve conduction studies of motor and sensory nerves may also be done as part of an electrodiagnostic study of a patient with neurologic symptoms. Surface electrodes are attached to the skin over a hand muscle, and electric shocks of increasing voltage are generated until the largest electrical potential response of the muscle is recorded. A point distal in the nerve is tested and is termed the distal latency. Latency is determined by stimulation of the same nerve at a proximal site. The distance between the points of stimulation is divided by the difference between the proximal and distal latencies to compute the conduction velocity of the tested peripheral nerve. Conduction is measured in the fastest-conducting fibers only. Conduction in slower fibers is masked by the faster velocity in the fast fibers. Sensory conduction velocities have low amplitude and are difficult to detect.

EMG and nerve conduction studies are unable to detect the location of spinal cord lesions or sensory radiculopathy. Evoked potentials are electrical responses of the nervous system to external sensory stimuli.[2] Testing of evoked potentials demonstrates abnormalities of the sensory system when clinical signs and symptoms are ambiguous. Evoked potentials may identify the location of unsuspected lesions in the central nervous system and may monitor the response of the lesion to therapy.

Evoked potentials generate low amplitude electrical activity from 0.1 to 20 microvolts (μV). These low amplitude potentials are obscured by the background noise produced by muscle artifact, electroencephalogram activity, and environmental interference. The evoked potential occurs at the same time interval following a stimulus. Averaging of the signal response after repeated stimulation identifies the evoked potential that can be separated from background noise. The evoked response is characterized by peaks and waves that are identified by their polarity, latency, amplitude, and configuration. Normal values are influenced by patient factors, including gender, age, body size, and temperature.[3]

Somatosensory evoked potentials (SEPs) are a means to determine the conduction of potentials generated by stimulation of peripheral structures to the spinal cord or cerebral cortex. A stimulus is generated peripherally, travels through the dorsal root ganglion, and ascends in the ipsilateral dorsal column. The stimulus then ascends to the contralateral ventroposterolateral nucleus of the thalamus and then to the primary sensory cortex. The stimulus can be measured over the spinal cord or scalp overlying the cortex. A computer is able to average the small potentials generated by peripheral stimulation and determine the latency associated with the peripheral site. SEPs may test large mixed nerves, such as the median and ulnar nerves; small sensory nerves; or a single dermatome.[4]

To understand the significance of abnormal electrodiagnostic findings, a review of basic EMG and nerve conduction concepts is worthwhile.

EMG Studies

1. *Motor unit.* The motor unit includes an anterior horn cell, axon terminal arborization, myoneural junction, and all the muscle fibers supplied by that single nerve cell.

2. *Motor unit potential.* The motor unit potential is a summation of electrical activity associated with the fibers in one motor unit. Motor unit fiber size varies from a few to thousands of fibers. Therefore, motor unit potentials vary in amplitude and duration. Normal motor unit potentials have two to four spikes, an amplitude up to 4.0 millivolts (mV), and a duration up to 15 milliseconds (ms).

In a partially denervated muscle (commonly the circumstance with disc herniations) the remaining normal axons grow to innervate more of the muscle fibers than composed the original motor unit (Fig. 8–1). The increase in the number of muscle fibers per motor unit results in a longer duration and asynchronous depolarization of muscle fibers. The result is a motor unit potential of increased amplitude and longer duration. The slightly different time intervals of stimulation result in a polyphasic response with multiple spikes. The amplitude may vary up to 20 mV or greater.

Fibrillations are action potentials of small clusters of denervated, healthy muscle fibers awaiting reinnervation. Fibrillations have an amplitude of 20 to 300 μV and a short duration of less than 5.0 ms. They may fire up to 30 times per second. Fibrillations are abnormal but are a nonspecific finding (myopathies are also associated with fibrillations). Positive sharp waves are thought to come from denervated, healthy muscle fibers injured by the entry of the electrode needle. The amplitude of these waves is 4.0 mV or greater with a duration of 10 ms. Like fibrillations, positive waves are abnormal but a nonspecific finding (Fig. 8–2). Giant motor unit potentials are extremely high-voltage and long-duration motor unit potentials. In patients with denervated muscles, these potentials appear after reinnervation.

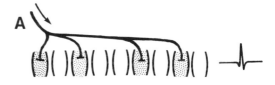

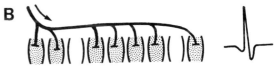

Figure 8–1. Schematic of a motor unit. The shaded muscle fibers are functional members of one motor unit with an axon that branches terminally to innervate the appropriate muscle fibers. The action potential produced by each motor unit is seen on the right. The unshaded muscle fibers belong to other motor units. *A,* A normal motor unit with four innervated muscle fibers, with corresponding action potential. *B,* Fibers that belonged to other motor units and had been denervated have been reinnervated by terminal sprouting from a normal, undamaged axon. The corresponding action potential has greater amplitude and duration.

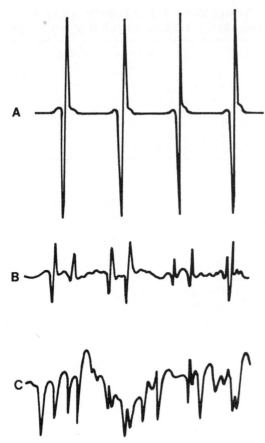

Figure 8–2. Electromyographic signals. *A,* Normal motor unit potential with four spikes, amplitude of 4.0 mV and duration of 15 ms. *B,* Fibrillations consisting of small clusters of spikes with diminished amplitude and duration (200 μV). *C,* Positive sharp waves (250 μV).

creased insertional activity is a subjective evaluation dependent on observer criteria. This abnormality becomes significant only with other supporting EMG evidence.

A normal EMG, with the muscle relaxed, generates normal insertional activity only with electrode movement. Background fasciculations may be present. Motor unit potentials are normal in size, shape, and number. Maximum intensity of muscle contraction results in an interference pattern that observes individual action potentials.

Nerve Conduction Studies

1. *H-reflex.* An H-reflex is an electrically elicited analog of the tendon reflex (Fig. 8–3). By electrically stimulating large afferent fibers in a mixed nerve that synapses with alpha motor neurons, a monosynaptic reflex is evoked. The H-reflex is commonly used in the evaluation of S1 root lesions. The H-reflex is also used in the evaluation of C7 root lesions affecting the flexor carpi radialis.[5] The time latency (the period from time of stimulation until the impulse has traveled through the spinal cord to produce the reflex in the associated muscle) is standardized for the age and length of the limb or height of the patient. The difference between latencies of the upper extremities is 1 ms or less.

3. *Interference.* As muscle contraction increases, greater numbers of individual motor units come into play, resulting in generation of greater numbers of unit potentials. The potentials observe individual patterns on the screen, resulting in a blur of activity near the baseline level. This is normal and is referred to as interference.

4. *Insertional activity.* The insertion of the needle electrode damages nerve fibers, which results in electrical activity. The activity is present only with movement of the needle. In normal fibers, action potential generation ceases once the needle electrode comes to rest.

In radiculopathies, the insertional activity persists with decreased intensity for a number of seconds. This phenomenon is termed prolonged insertional activity and may be the only indication of an abnormality. However, in-

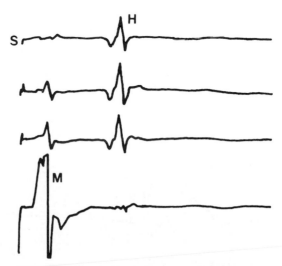

Figure 8–3. The H-reflex. The H wave (H) appears and becomes maximum as the stimulus (S) intensity increases, and it disappears at supraphysiologic levels of stimulation when the M wave is maximum.

2. *F response.* Antidromic activation of motor neurons following supramaximal stimulation of a peripheral nerve gives rise to an F response (Fig. 8–4). The F response travels along the motor nerve that supplies the innervation of the muscle. It is not a reflex because it does not involve sensory fiber. It is dependent on integrity of the motor unit only. Unlike the H-reflex, the F response is variable in the latency, and a number of repeated responses must be recorded. The most commonly reported result of the F response is the minimum response time or latency. The difference in the minimal latency between two extremities is usually less than 2 ms.

Sensory nerve action potential (SNAP) abnormalities do not occur with usual radiculopathy without dorsal root ganglion damage. However, discrepancies between latencies of SNAP of the two arms help differentiate plexopathy from radiculopathy. Plexus lesions cause damage at a location distal to the dorsal root ganglion. Therefore, SNAP is abnormal. Bilateral abnormalities suggest a diffuse process affecting nerves, such as peripheral polyneuropathy.

Electrodiagnostic Abnormalities Associated with Nerve Root Compression

In the first 3 days after compression, a decreased number of motor unit action potentials are noted during muscle contraction (Ta-

TABLE 8–1. ELECTROPHYSIOLOGIC ABNORMALITIES IN NERVE ROOT LESIONS

Day 3	Reduced muscle action potentials
	H-reflex delayed (C7)
	F-response delayed (C7)
Day 7	Paraspinal fibrillations
Day 14	Paraspinal positive waves
	Associated proximal limb muscle positive waves
Day 21	Positive waves in entire myotome
Day 28	Fasciculations
Day 42	Prolonged polyphasic motor unit potentials

ble 8–1). Also within the first week, H-reflex latency differences may appear before EMG changes are noted.[6] At day 7 to 10, the paraspinous muscles show the presence of positive waves. Changes in the paraspinous muscles occur before changes in the extremities supplied by the same nerve root.[7] In about one third of patients, EMG abnormalities were found solely in the paraspinous muscles. Soon after the appearance of positive waves and fibrillations an increasing proportion of polyphasic waves is noted in muscles supplied by the corresponding nerve root.

Evaluation of the paraspinous muscles is helpful in localizing the area of nerve impingement. The paraspinous muscles are supplied by the posterior primary rami, which branch off the mixed peripheral nerve soon after its formation by the coalescence of the dorsal and ventral nerve root. There is marked anatomic segmental overlap in the superficial erector spinae muscles. The deepest layer, the multifidus layer, has the least degree of overlap. EMG studies done with electrodes placed 3 to 5 cm within the paraspinal muscle mass test the multifidus. Lesions of a single nerve root have abnormalities at one level only. Lesions that affect the anterior primary ramus, plexus, or peripheral nerve, distal to the division of the spinal root, have no effect on the paraspinous muscles.

Lesions that occur proximal to the branching of the primary rami result in abnormalities in both anterior and posterior divisions. Abnormalities may be limited to the paraspinous muscles in nerve root disease without anterior division abnormalities.

The most frequent abnormality found on an EMG for radiculopathy is the presence of positive waves. This is followed by an increased proportion of polyphasics and fibrillation potentials and a decreased number of motor units per contraction.[8]

By the third week, paraspinous muscle fi-

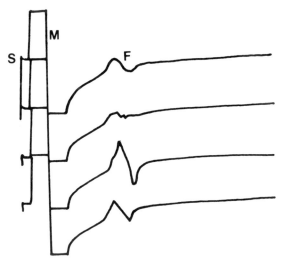

Figure 8–4. The F response. The F wave (F) is recorded after supraphysiologic stimulation (S). The amplitude, shape, and latency change with each stimulation.

brillation potentials are noted along with the emergence of positive waves in nerve root–associated limb muscles. With continued injury of 2 months or longer, motor unit amplitude and duration increase. In many patients, electrical signs of nerve damage do not appear until 21 days after the initial insult. EMG examination done too quickly in the course of events misses the lesion. An experienced electromyographer should be aware of this occurrence and should counsel the attending clinician on the appropriate time for electrodiagnostic studies.

EMG may not be helpful in chronic radiculopathies. Muscles may become reinnervated and not show spontaneous fibrillation potentials noted in acute radiculopathies. The severity of nerve dysfunction cannot be accurately determined by EMG. The cause of abnormal EMG findings cannot be specified by electrodiagnostic testing. Nerve root compression caused by a tumor, osteophyte, or herniated disc has similar findings. The level of a radicular injury can be localized to within one or two segments by EMG. The exact disc level can only be estimated.[9] EMG may also be of limited benefit after posterior spine surgery.

Relative contraindications for EMG examination are a patient with a bleeding tendency (hemophilia and thrombocytopenia) and a patient on anticoagulant therapy. The placement of needles through the skin may increase the possibility of cellulitis in those individuals particularly susceptible to infection. An EMG should be limited to one side of the body if a muscle biopsy is considered, as inflammation is associated with needle placement. The pathologic changes associated with needle examination may be confused with an acute inflammatory myositis.

Electrodiagnostic Results

Motor nerve conduction and sensory nerve conduction velocities are normal in nerve root disease because peripheral nerves contain fibers from several roots, and root lesions from disc disease rarely produce complete loss of conduction through the involved roots. Damage to sensory nerves proximal to the dorsal root ganglia, as would occur in intervertebral disc herniation, produces no change in the peripheral sensory fibers. Conduction studies are of value in patients with suspected root disease because they exclude peripheral nerve disease as a potential cause of denervation changes.

H-reflexes are most sensitive to lesions of the sensory fibers in the S1 roots. H-reflexes are also useful in evaluation of cervical radiculopathies, particularly those affecting the C7 segment.[5] Unilateral reduction of H-reflexes may be the sole electrophysiologic abnormality in some patients with C7 radiculopathy. H-reflex has an advantage over EMG in that H-reflex is abnormal almost immediately. Because both motor and sensory pathways are tested, lesions limited to sensory fibers may be detected. Both extremities must be tested to detect abnormalities.[10] These abnormalities may be missed by the experienced electromyographer. An abnormal H-reflex is sensitive but not specific in determining the site of the lesion. Any abnormality of spinal cord, sensory roots, motor roots, brachial plexus, or peripheral nerves demonstrates similar abnormalities. The H-reflex is not positive in all radiculopathies. If large fibers are spared, the H-reflex may be normal. Once affected, the H-reflex tends to remain abnormal indefinitely, making it a less sensitive test for suspected radiculopathy.

One benefit of the F response is that it may become abnormal almost immediately after injury. However, the F response is relatively insensitive in detecting radiculopathy.[11] The F response tests a peripheral nerve served by several nerve roots. An abnormality in one nerve root may be overshadowed by normal function in the surrounding spinal nerves. The reliance on motor fibers alone may play a role in the relative insensitivity of F responses. Sensory tracts may play a significant role in radiculopathy. F waves evaluate the block or slow conduction through a few motor fibers at a time. The long distance tested may dilute the differences that may be detected side to side. Like the H-reflex, an abnormal F response is not synonymous with radiculopathy. Any lesion along the length of the affected nerve results in an abnormal F response. Acute and chronic radiculopathies cannot be distinguished by F responses.

A normal electrophysiologic examination does not exclude the possibility of a radiculopathy causing neurologic symptoms, but a definite abnormality points toward an organic origin of a patient's symptoms. This may be of particular importance in patients claiming disability or workers' compensation.

Electrodiagnostic studies may be helpful in detecting cervical spinal stenosis.[12] These tests may be particularly helpful in differentiating anterior motor horn cell disease from myelopathy. A number of findings, including upper and motor neuron signs, decreased reflexes in the arms and increased reflexes in the legs, fasciculations, and muscle atrophy, may be found in both groups. However, patients with cervical spinal stenosis should not have electrodiagnostic abnormalities above the foramen magnum, whereas anterior horn cell disease affects muscles in the head, including the tongue.

Electrodiagnostic studies may also be used to differentiate individuals with shoulder and neck pain associated with upper extremity entrapment syndromes (carpal tunnel syndrome) from those with neck pain associated with cervical radiculopathy.[13, 14] In some individuals, a double crush syndrome (median nerve compression and cervical nerve root compression) may explain the occurrence of neck, arm, and hand pain.[15] Electrodiagnostic testing is able to help detect the presence of two separate lesions.

Some nonneurologic disorders may be associated with EMG abnormalities. Metabolic disorders, particularly diabetes, may cause diffuse paraspinal abnormalities with no evidence of radiculopathy. Patients may improve with control of their diabetes. Paraspinal fibrillation and positive waves have been reported with metastatic disease.[16] EMG examination demonstrating marked segmental compromise of the posterior primary ramus distal to the spinal root with relative sparing of the anterior ramus may be the earliest evidence of paraspinal muscle metastases. Although computerized tomography (CT) scan may be unable to identify the presence of metastases, magnetic resonance (MR) imaging is able to detect paraspinal lesions. Although a pattern of posterior primary ramus segmental compromise is not diagnostic of metastases, the abnormal EMG pattern may suggest MR examination.[17] Patients with arachnoiditis have also been associated with abnormal paraspinal electrophysiologic studies.[18] Mechanical abnormalities like muscle strains, ligamentous injury, and degenerative disc disease without nerve root compression should be associated with a normal EMG.

The role of serial EMG determinations in the management of patients is not well established compared with therapy decisions based on patients' symptoms and clinical findings. Once EMG changes of reinnervation occur, they may persist indefinitely. Denervation changes may also persist for many years following injury to the motor nerve, even when there is no evidence of continuing injury. It is difficult to determine the age or activity of a lesion once reinnervation changes appear. In addition, the extent of EMG abnormalities does not necessarily correlate with the extent of nerve damage.

Electrophysiologic studies obtained after laminectomy present particular difficulty in interpretation because of the injury associated with ischemia from retractors during surgery. In addition, patients may develop a recurrent cervical herniated disc after surgery. In 25% of all patients with lumbar root lesions from disc disease, denervation changes persist after surgery even in the absence of persistent impingement.[19] EMG abnormalities, particularly in the paraspinous muscles, are significant for a new lesion in a postlaminectomy patient if the patient has acute recurrence of symptomatology and EMG abnormalities at a level different from the level affected during the previous episode of radiculopathy.

Somatosensory Evoked Potentials

Somatosensory evoked potentials (SEPs) of large mixed nerves measure the function of motor nerves and the sensory function of peripheral nerves. The most common nerves stimulated in the upper extremity are the median and ulnar nerves (Fig. 8–5). Theoretically, SEPs have advantages over peripheral nerve conduction studies for the diagnosis of cervical radiculopathies.[20] However, mixed nerve SEPs are not helpful for detecting single-level sensory radiculopathies because large mixed nerves carry nerves from multiple nerve roots. The findings from studies of SEPs in patients with cervical radiculopathies have been too inconsistent to be helpful in replacing any other test as a means of detecting spinal root dysfunction.[21] A more reliable method of detecting radiculopathies may be obtained with those of spinal rather than cortical somatosensory potentials.[22] However, mixed nerve SEPs are sensitive in detecting spinal cord abnormalities that affect cord pathways. Spinal cord tumors and multiple sclerosis are two types of pathologic pathways that result in abnormal mixed nerve SEPs. Cervical spondylodegenerative myelopathies may be detected by abnormal mixed nerve SEPs. A normal test does not exclude the possibility of a cord lesion, particularly affecting motor function.[23]

A dermatomal somatosensory evoked potential (DSEP) is generated by direct stimulation of skin and recording of cortical responses. The accuracy of the test depends on the placement of stimulating electrodes. In the upper

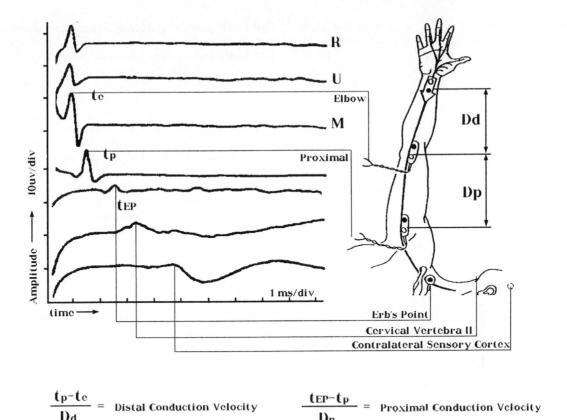

$$\frac{t_p - t_c}{D_d} = \text{Distal Conduction Velocity} \qquad \frac{t_{EP} - t_p}{D_p} = \text{Proximal Conduction Velocity}$$

Figure 8–5. Sensory evoked potentials, median nerve stimulation. The top three traces (t), labeled R, U, and M, reflect activity at electrodes placed at the elbow over the expected course for the radial, ulnar, and median nerves, respectively. Each of these traces contains a negative (that is, upward) potential at the latency t_c. The potential measured at R and U reflects volume conduction. The larger potential at M reflects the proximity of the median nerve action potential. The fourth trace shows a peak at t_p. This electrode is positioned in the biceps groove. Median and ulnar nerve stimulations result in a potential recorded in this electrode pair, but radial nerve stimulation does not because of its course on the far side of the humerus. The fifth tracing shows the latency as the potential passes the electrode at Erb's point (t_{EP}) over the brachial plexus. The sixth tracing is derived from the electrode over C2 in the neck. The seventh tracing shows negative potential (that is, upward) at the time that the cortex is activated. The methods for calculating the distal and proximal conduction velocities are shown. The position of radial and ulnar pickup electrodes is not shown to avoid confusion. They are located lateral to the biceps tendon and just below the olecranon groove. (Courtesy of Elizabeth Tidman.)

extremity, C6 is tested by stimulating the thumb, C7 by testing the middle finger, and C8 by testing the little finger. The recording of DSEPs is technically demanding, requiring an experienced technician. A DSEP is complementary to other electrodiagnostic tests. A DSEP does not evaluate motor nerve function and is not as sensitive as EMG for the diagnosis of nerve root lesions.[23]

SEPs have been used during surgical procedures to determine the integrity of the function of components of the nervous system. The monitoring is used for procedures that correct spinal deformities, decompress spinal stenosis lesions, repair spinal fractures, resect spinal tumors, and assess spinal cord injuries.[24]

Quantitative somatosensory thermotest is another form of somatosensory testing that

measures the function of small afferent fibers in the peripheral nervous system.[25] The test is accomplished through the use of a Peltier device that supplies a controlled, progressively increasing or decreasing range of temperatures to the skin. The patient is asked to respond to the signal the instant of first sensation of cold, warmth, cold pain, or heat pain by pressing a switch that immediately returns the stimulator to baseline temperature. A recorder allows visual analysis of the temperatures associated with these sensations. Normal control values are available for rates of temperature change and standard stimulus area.[26] The function of different caliber sensory fibers is associated with different temperature sensations. Cold sensation is associated with small A-delta myelinated afferents, warm sensation with unmyelinated fibers, and cold and heat pain with unmyelinated C-fiber polymodal nociceptors and A-delta nociceptors. Abnormalities with each temperature modality are associated with a specific pattern (Fig. 8–6). For example, heat hyperalgesia (reduced threshold for heat pain) is associated with sensitization of C-unmyelinated nociceptors. The site of the test, distal or proximal in a limb, may be associated with a variety of findings. A distal site with more severe denervation may demonstrate warm, cold, and thermal hypoesthesia, whereas a more proximal lesion reveals sensitization of the remaining functioning afferent fibers with hyperalgesia to temperatures. The test measures function from the peripheral nerve endings to sensorium in the cerebral cortex. The test is reproducible in patients with organic neuropathic lesions. The test may be used to detect psychogenic disorders associated with thermal complaints of pain. Psychogenic pain patterns tend to be less consistent.

In summary, although they are not tests that pinpoint specific diagnoses, electrodiagnostic studies are helpful in the evaluation of patients with neurologic dysfunction. The procedure is performed in the outpatient department. These studies may identify a specific nerve root lesion when clinical symptoms suggest abnormalities at two levels. MR imaging tends to be more closely associated with electrodiagnostic abnormalities than myelograms. However, EMG tests may be abnormal when corresponding radiographic results are normal. An abnormal EMG is corroborative evidence of organic disease and helps the surgeon select patients who are candidates for surgery. EMG changes may recede after resolution of nerve impingement. Nonneurologic disorders have normal EMG findings. Electrodiagnostic tests help differentiate peripheral nerve lesions from radiculopathy. When used in the appropriate setting and with the limitations of the tests in mind, the clinician may rely on these procedures to supply information that is useful in the diagnosis and management of patients with neck and arm pain.

THERMOGRAPHY

Thermography is a noninvasive procedure that images the infrared radiation (heat) emitted from the body surface. Thermography is based on the principle that alterations in a variety of body functions alter the cutaneous vascular supply that heats the skin. Postganglionic sympathetic cell bodies involved in the control of the cutaneous vessel are located in the sympathetic chain ganglia, which are connected to the spinal nerves distal to the dorsal root ganglia by the rami communicantes. The postganglionic nerve fibers from these cells travel to the cutaneous blood vessels by

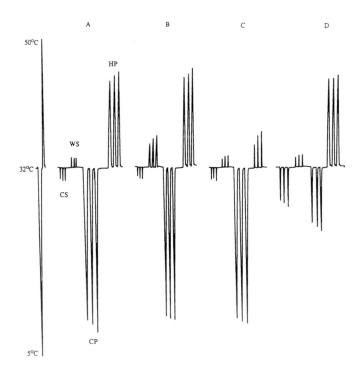

Figure 8–6. Quantitative somatosensory thermotest. Each peak represents one thermal stimulus ramp. A, Normal pattern, B, pure warm hypoesthesia, C, heat hyperalgesia, D, cold hypoesthesia associated with cold hyperalgesia. WS = warm sensation; CS = cold sensation; CP = cold pain; HP = heat pain. (From Verdugo RJ, Ochoa JL: Use and misuse of conventional electrodiagnosis, quantitative sensory testing, thermography, and nerve blocks in the evaluation of painful neuropathic syndromes. Muscle Nerve 16:1058, 1993. By permission of Oxford University Press.)

way of the peripheral nerves. Since the post-ganglionic nerves travel with peripheral nerves composed of multiple root fibers, sympathetic abnormalities spread beyond a single dermatome. Irritation of peripheral sensory nerves may affect sympathetic nerve fibers at the same segment level, resulting in alterations of blood flow to the skin. Factors that are associated with sensory activation of nociceptive fiber stimulation (substance P) may also have an effect on cutaneous blood flow. However, pain is a complex phenomenon that cannot be simplified to a direct correlation with cutaneous heat production. Thermography does not take a picture of pain itself; it does reveal pathophysiologic conditions associated with neurovascular, soft tissue, circulatory, and musculoskeletal disorders.

The two types of thermography are liquid crystal (contact) and electronic (noncontact) thermography. Contact thermography uses cholesterol crystals that change color with variations of surface temperature. The crystals are placed inside inflatable transparent boxes with one flexible, thermosensitive side that is applied to the body. Each box has a limited temperature range. An examination with liquid crystals requires selection of a box with the appropriate temperature range. A picture is taken of the box to record the patterns of surface temperature. The box is chosen by trial and error. The advantages of contact thermography include the absence of radiation exposure, ease of use, and lower cost than electronic thermography.

Electronic thermography uses an infrared radiation sensor that converts heat reading to electrical signals that are displayed on a black-and-white or color monitor. A picture can be taken of the video screen or can be stored on computer discs. This system has the advantage of viewing large areas of the body during a single examination.

The examination must be performed in an air-conditioned, draft-free room. The ambient temperature must be between 68° and 72°F. The patient should have refrained from smoking for the day of the test. In addition, the patient should refrain from pain medications, physical therapy, and exposure to strong sunlight for at least 24 hours. The patient must disrobe and be in equilibrium with room temperature for 30 to 60 minutes before the examination is started. The patient's temperature must be normal. If the patient is febrile, the examination must be postponed.

Examination of the cervical spine and arms with liquid crystals consists of separate images of the posterior neck and superior shoulders; lateral oblique shoulders; lateral upper arms; posterior, lateral, anterior, and medial forearms; and dorsal and ventral aspects of the hands.[27] The examination requires 1 to 2 hours to complete.

The assessment of a thermogram is based on the distribution and temperature range of the skin. Both sides of the body have a temperature within 0.17° to 0.45° C in the healthy state.[28] The extent of thermal asymmetry between opposite sides of the body varies in different locations but remains less than 0.5°. Values are reproducible for as long as 5 years. A thermogram is abnormal if a side-to-side difference of 1° C involving 25% of its evaluated area is present. Alterations in the physiologic temperature distribution patterns also indicate abnormalities.[29]

Acute pain is associated with increased heat, whereas chronic pain is linked with decreased temperatures. Increased temperature is found over areas involved with an inflammatory process. Increased muscle metabolism associated with spasm or tonic contraction can be detected as increased heat conveyed to the surface by circulation.

Artifacts are common. Skin folds conserve heat and appear "hot" on a thermogram. Sunburn alters the skin pattern. Alterations of the skin associated with injections, tattoos, or vaccinations change the normal thermographic patterns as well.[30]

Thermographic Abnormalities Associated with Neck Pain

Thermographic diagnosis of neck pain syndromes includes evaluation of the cervical spine and upper extremities. Thermal asymmetry in patients with neck pain is associated with a decrease in the affected limb's temperature. In one study of the lumbar spine, when the asymmetry of temperature exceeded one standard deviation from the mean temperature of homologous regions measured in 90 normal subjects, the positive predictive value of detecting root impingement was 94.7% and the specificity was 87.5%.[31]

Whereas a number of studies of thermography in the evaluation of lumbar spine pain and radiculopathy have been reported, cervical spine studies are fewer in number.[32–35] The thermogram had 60% specificity and 100% sensitivity in detecting lumbar nerve root lesions. Thermographic accuracy in detecting nerve root irritation has also been reported to be greater than electromyographic accuracy. This difference in sensitivity was thought to be related to thermographic ability to detect sensory nerve abnormalities.[31] Comparison of thermography and EMG in the diagnosis of cervical radiculopathy was not favorable.[36] In a study of 20 normal controls and 14 patients with cervical radiculopathy, thermography was abnormal in 43%, and EMG was abnormal in 71%. Thermographic abnormalities were seen only in the hands and fingers, and the pattern did not follow the dermatome of the affected cervical root. In contrast, others have reported a higher frequency of positive thermographic tests in patients with cervical radiculopathy.[37] Hubbard and colleagues have suggested that a normal thermogram would negate the necessity for a CT scan for a patient with neck pain.[37] In the majority of circumstances, the thermogram has no diagnostic or predictive value in the evaluation of cervical radiculopathy. In another study, liquid crystal thermography was compared with nerve conduction studies for the evaluation of carpal tunnel syndrome. Thermography identified 0 of 9 patients with mild entrapment and 7 of 14 patients with marked entrapment. The sensitivity of thermography was significantly less than nerve conduction tests for the evaluation of carpal tunnel syndrome.[38] In a study of whiplash injury, Mahoney and colleagues found no significant difference in 28 symptomatic individuals when compared with 50 control subjects. In the two groups, only 1 of 28 whiplash subjects and 4 control subjects had abnormal thermograms.[39]

Psychogenic or functional neck pain is difficult to differentiate from structural disease. Hendler and associates tried to differentiate psychogenic pain and malingering from true organic pain syndromes.[40] Forty-three (19%) of 224 patients referred with a diagnosis of psychogenic pain had abnormal thermograms corresponding to the symptomatic area. The thermogram was positive when other diagnostic tests, including an EMG, were normal.

Although a number of studies have reported on the usefulness and accuracy of thermography in musculoskeletal conditions, the procedure has not won acceptance by many physicians. The reasons for this lack of acceptance may be the need for special rooms in which to do the test, the array of equipment needed to do the examination, and the necessity of extensive experience with the technique to evaluate test results. However, the most important factor is that the exact role of the thermogram in diagnosis of neck pain problems remains to be determined. Large prospective studies including control patients must be completed before the scientific merit of this diagnostic technique can be determined.

At present thermograms are not recommended for use in making routine decisions for diagnosis of patients with neck pain. Thermograms detect autonomic dysfunction in different parts of the body. In the majority of individuals, determination of autonomic function is not necessary to adequately treat patients for their neck pain. Interpretation of thermograms needs to be standardized. Additional prospective studies must be conducted to correlate the findings of thermography with the most sensitive radiographic techniques. The specificity and sensitivity of the thermogram need further definition. The value and role of thermography will be clarified as well-designed studies are completed that demonstrate diagnostic significance and effects on therapy. The technique will become more significant as it becomes more widely available and well-trained physicians can interpret thermographic results. Recent articles in Australia and a position paper by the American Medical Association's Council on Scientific Affairs question the use of thermography in the clinical setting at this time.[41, 42]

DIFFERENTIAL NERVE BLOCKS

In patients who have intractable and chronic neck pain, identification of the source of pain, whether somatic, sympathetic, or psychogenic, is essential in planning an appropriate treatment regimen. Differential nerve blocks are an invasive means for examining the central and peripheral components of a patient's pain. They are particularly helpful in localizing the source of pain in patients who have undergone multiple operations on their cervical spine and continue to experience neck pain.

The different susceptibilities of sensory fibers to anesthesia is the physiology on which differential blocks are based.[43] The different peripheral sensory fibers are classified into A (alpha and delta), B (preganglionic autonomic), and C (unmyelinated) groups. Different concentrations of local anesthetics have selective sensitivity for these fibers.[44] Fiber sensitivity in decreasing order is B, C, and A.[45] The sensitivity is related in part to the amount of myelination of the fibers. Unmyelinated fibers have exposure of the entire surface of the axon membrane to local anesthetics. In myelinated nerves, the membrane is exposed only at Ranvier's nodes because the myelin layer insulates the rest of the axon. Higher concentrations of local anesthetics are needed to penetrate the nerve to block transmission. Alternative explanations have suggested that large, fast-conducting fibers are more susceptible to conduction blockade than smaller, slower-conducting fibers.[46] The study concluded that conduction velocity is directly proportional to distance between Ranvier's nodes. The fastest fibers with the longest internodal distances should be affected before fibers with small diameters. The discrepancy between these conflicting findings may be explained by the location of nerve fibers in neural bundles. Small-diameter fibers are more superficial and surround large-diameter fibers in dorsal spinal roots. Anesthetics injected as part of a spinal block reach the small fibers first and affect their function before the large fibers.

Anesthetics may also be given that block sensory fibers but leave motor function intact. The local anesthetics with rapid onset, short duration of action, and ability to selectively block sympathetic, sensory, and then motor fibers with increasing concentrations are lidocaine and mepivacaine. Fiber size, degree of myelination, nerve fiber location, length of nerve fiber exposed to anesthetic, neuropathologic state of the nerve, and concentration and lipid solubility of the anesthetic all play a role in the effects of anesthetic blockade on nerve function.[47]

Differential Block Procedure

Differential nerve blocks may be able to differentiate pain of somatic and sympathetic nerve origin. Pain in the neck, upper extremity, and upper chest may be relieved with an injection of the stellate ganglion. Normal saline would be injected as the placebo. Relief of pain would be associated with a placebo effect. If there is no effect, a block with 10 to 15 mL of a local anesthetic is given. A successful sympathetic block would be manifested by the development of a Horner's syndrome, including ptosis, miosis, and anhydrosis. If no pain relief is noted, a somatic block to the painful areas is completed. A successful somatic block is associated with peripheral motor and sensory loss. In the upper neck a block of the cervical plexus would be appropriate, whereas upper extremity pain would be helped by a brachial plexus injection.

Subarachnoid and epidural injections are used more commonly for differential spinal blockade in the evaluation of lumbar spine pain. Subarachnoid blockade is usually confined to the thoracic or lumbar spine. Blockade in the cervical spine would have the potential of affecting the function of the phrenic nerve, resulting in decreased breathing capacity. The effects of epidural blockade in the cervical spine are not useful in diagnosing the source of neck pain. Bilateral effects of epidural injection usually occur, and controlled manipulation of the area of action of the anesthetic is difficult. The epidural fluids do not flow freely or predictably. For these reasons, these techniques are not used for diagnosing the source of cervical spine pain.

Patients who do not experience any pain relief from differential nerve blockade may have pain of central or psychogenic origin. Techniques that affect central neurologic function are used to differentiate origins of pain central to the level of spinal blockade and those of psychogenic origin.[47] The tests are based on the assumption that patients in a light plane of sleep respond to pain in a pattern similar to when fully awake. Conversely, if the neck pain resolves and the individual responds to other painful stimuli over other body locations, such as the anterior tibia, the implication is that the pain is of psychogenic origin. Sodium pentothal is slowly infused until the patient falls into a light plane of sleep. The infusion is stopped and the patient is allowed to wake up while being periodically tested for typical pain responses in areas other than the neck. When the patient responds to the pain stimulus, a stimulus that causes the typical neck pain is given. If the stimulus does not cause typical neck pain, the origin of the pain is psychogenic. Intravenous lidocaine at a dose of 1.2 to 2.0 mg/kg is given until tingling is reported by the patient. Two minutes later the patient's pain is assessed. A relief of pain that has been resistant to peripheral injections suggests a central origin. No relief suggests a psychogenic origin of pain. Few studies have been completed proving the validity of these intravenous tests for determining the source of neck pain.[48, 49]

Nerve blocks are invasive procedures with the potential for significant morbidity. The spread of injected materials is unpredictable. The exact site of the injection may not be known unless radiographic techniques document the site of the needle.[50] The complexity of the central nervous system makes discovering the source of neck pain difficult. A positive response to a placebo injection does not absolutely demonstrate a central or psychogenic source of pain. Nerve blocks should be undertaken by experienced anesthesiologists in the evaluation of pain in patients with complicated symptomatology. In those difficult patients, the risks of surgery outweigh the risks associated with differential nerve block. The blocks should be undertaken if an unnecessary surgical procedure can be prevented based on the results of the procedure. Otherwise, the potential complications of the injections outweigh their benefits.

References

1. American Association of Electrodiagnostic Medicine: Guidelines in electrodiagnostic medicine. Muscle Nerve 15:229, 1992.
2. Chiappa KH (ed): Evoked Potentials in Clinical Medicine, 2nd ed. New York: Raven Press, 1990.
3. Waldman HJ: Evoked potentials. In: Raj PP (ed): Practical Management of Pain, 2nd ed. St Louis: Mosby-Year Book, 1992, pp 155–167.
4. Glantz RH, Haldeman S: Other diagnostic studies: Electrodiagnosis. In: Frymoyer JW, Tucker TB, Hadler NM, et al. (eds): The Adult Spine: Principles and Practice. New York: Raven Press, 1991, pp 541–548.
5. Sabbahi MA, Khalil M: Segmental H-reflex studies in upper and lower limbs of patients with radiculopathy. Arch Phys Med Rehabil 71:223, 1990.
6. Schuchmann JA: Evaluation of H-reflex latency in radiculopathy. Arch Phys Med Rehabil 58:560, 1976.
7. Johnsson B: Morphology, innervation and electromyographic study of the erector spinae. Arch Phys Med Rehabil 50:638, 1969.
8. Johnson EW, Melvin JL: Value of electromyography in lumbar radiculopathy. Arch Phys Med Rehabil 52:239, 1971.
9. Haldeman S: The electrodiagnostic evaluation of nerve root function. Spine 9:42, 1984.
10. Deschuytere J, Rosselle N, DeKeyser C: Monosynaptic reflexes in the superficial forearm flexors in man and their clinical significance. J Neurol Neurosurg Psychiatry 39:555, 1976.
11. Eisen A, Schomer D, Melmed C, et al.: The application of F-wave measurements in the differentiation of proximal and distal upper limb entrapments. Neurology 27:662, 1977.
12. Stark RJ, Kennard C, Swash M: Hand wasting in spondylotic high cord compression: an electromyographic study. Ann Neurol 9:58, 1981.
13. Watson R, Waylonis GW: Paraspinal electromyographic abnormalities as a predictor of occult metastatic carcinoma. Arch Phys Med Rehabil 56:216, 1975.
14. Cherington M: Proximal pain in carpal tunnel syndrome. Arch Surg 108:69, 1974.
15. Dawson DM: Entrapment neuropathies of the upper extremities. N Engl J Med 329:2013, 1993.
16. Massey EW: Coexistent carpal tunnel syndrome and cervical radiculopathy (double crush syndrome). South Med J 74:957, 1981.
17. LaBan MM, Tamler MS, Wang AM, Meerschaert JR: Electromyographic detection of paraspinal muscle metastasis: correlation with magnetic resonance imaging. Spine 17:1144, 1992.
18. Grue BL, Pudenz RH, Sheldon CH: Observations on the value of clinical electromyography. J Bone Joint Surg 39A:492, 1957.
19. Blom S, Lemperg R: Electromyographic analysis of the lumbar musculature in patients operated on for lumbar rhizopathy. J Neurosurg 26:25, 1967.
20. Siivola J, Sulg I, Heiskari M: Somatosensory evoked potentials in diagnostics of cervical spondylosis and herniated disc. Electroencephalogr Clin Neurophysiol 52:276, 1981.
21. Schmid U, Hess C, Ludin H: Somatosensory evoked potentials following nerve and segmental stimulation do not confirm cervical radiculopathy with sensory deficit. J Neurol Neurosurg Psychiatry 51:182, 1988.
22. Seyal M, Palma G, Sandhu L, et al.: Spinal somatosensory evoked potentials following segmental stimulation: a direct measure of dorsal root function. Electroencephalogr Clin Neurophysiol 69:390, 1988.
23. Glantz RH, Haldeman S: Other diagnostic studies: Electrodiagnosis. In: Frymoyer JW (ed): The Adult Spine: Principles and Practice. New York: Raven Press, 1991, pp 541–548.
24. Brown RH, Nash CL Jr: Intra-operative spinal cord monitoring. In: Frymoyer JW (ed): The Adult Spine: Principles and Practice. New York: Raven Press, 1991, pp 549–562.
25. Verdugo RJ, Ochoa JL: Use and misuse of conventional electrodiagnosis, quantitative sensory testing, thermography, and nerve blocks in the evaluation of painful neuropathic syndromes. Muscle Nerve 16:1056, 1993.
26. Verdugo RJ, Ochoa JL: Quantitative somatosensory thermotest: a key method for functional evaluation of small calibre afferent channels. Brain 115:893, 1992.
27. Pochaczevsky R: The value of liquid crystal thermography in the diagnosis of spinal root compression syndromes. Orthop Clin North Am 14:271, 1983.
28. Uematsu S, Edwin DH, Jankel WR, et al.: Quantification of thermal asymmetry. Part 1: Normal values and reproducibility. J Neurosurg 69:552, 1988.
29. Pochaczevsky R, Wexler CE, Myers PH, et al.: Liquid crystal thermography of the spine and extremities. J Neurosurg 56:386, 1982.
30. LeRoy PL, Bruner WM, Christian CR, et al.: Thermography as a diagnostic aid in the management of chronic pain. In: Aronoff GM (ed): Evaluation and Treatment of Chronic Pain. Baltimore: Urban and Schwarzenberg, 1985, pp 232–250.
31. Uematsu S, Edwin DH, Jankel WR, et al.: Quantification of thermal asymmetry. Part 2: Application in low-back pain and sciatica. J Neurosurg 69:556, 1988.
32. Thomas D, Cullum D, Siahamis G, Langlois S: Infrared thermographic imaging, magnetic resonance imaging, CT scan and myelography in low back pain. Br J Rheumatol 29:268, 1990.
33. Chafetz N, Wexler CE, Kaiser JA: Neuromuscular thermography of the lumbar spine with CT correlation. Spine 13:922, 1988.
34. Harper CM Jr, Low PA, Fealev RD, et al.: Utility of thermography in the diagnosis of lumbosacral radiculopathy. Neurology 41:1010, 1991.
35. So YT, Aminoff MJ, Olney RK: The role of thermography in the evaluation of lumbosacral radiculopathy. Neurology 39:1154, 1989.
36. So YT, Olney RK, Aminoff MJ: A comparison of thermography and electromyography in the diagnosis of cervical radiculopathy. Muscle Nerve 13:1032, 1990.
37. Hubbard J, Maultsby J, Wexler C: Lumbar and cervical thermography for nerve fiber impingement: a critical review. Clin J Pain 2:131, 1986.
38. Meyers S, Cros D, Sherry B, Vermeire P: Liquid crystal

thermography: quantitative studies of abnormalities in carpal tunnel syndrome. Neurology 39:1465, 1989.

39. Mahoney L, Wiley M, McMiken D: Thermography in whiplash injuries of the neck. Advocates Q 10:1, 1988.

40. Hendler W, Uematsu S, Long D: Thermographic validation of physical complaints in "psychogenic pain" patients. Psychosomatics 23:283, 1982.

41. Awerbuch MS: Thermography—its current diagnostic status in musculoskeletal medicine. Med J Aust 154:441, 1991.

42. Cotton P: AMA's council on scientific affairs takes a fresh look at thermography. JAMA 267:1885, 1992.

43. Gasser HS, Erlanger J: Role of fiber size in establishment of nerve block by pressure or cocaine. Am J Physiol 88:581, 1929.

44. Nathan PW, Sears TA: Some factors concerned in differential nerve block by local anesthetics. J Physiol (Lond) 157:565, 1961.

45. McCollum DE, Stephen CR: Use of graduated spinal anesthesia in the differential diagnosis of pain of the back and lower extremities. South Med J 57:410, 1964.

46. Gissen AJ, Covino BG, Gregus J: Differential sensitivities of mammalian nerve fibers to local anesthetic agents. Anesthesiology 53:467, 1980.

47. Nehme AE, Warfield CA: Diagnostic measures. In: Warfield CA (ed): Principles and Practice of Pain Management. New York: McGraw-Hill Book Co, 1993, pp 53–61.

48. Boas RA, Covino BG, Shahnarian A: Analgesic responses to I.V. lignocaine. Br J Anaesth 54:501, 1982.

49. Schoichet RP: Sodium amytal in the diagnosis of chronic pain. Can Psychiatr Assoc J 23:219, 1978.

50. Purcell-Jones G, Pither CE, Justins DM: Paravertebral somatic nerve block: a clinical, radiographic, and computed tomographic study in chronic pain patients. Anesth Analg 68:32, 1989.

9

A Standardized Approach to the Diagnosis and Treatment of Neck Pain

A patient with neck pain presents to a physician with a set of symptoms and signs. At presentation, these clinical complaints are unassociated with any specific diagnosis. The task of the physician is to integrate patient complaints and physical findings into an accurate diagnosis and to prescribe appropriate therapy. The primary objective for the physician is to return patients to their normal level of function as quickly as possible. In this physician-patient interaction, there must be concern for the efficient and precise use of diagnostic studies, minimization of ineffectual medical and surgical treatments, and monetary cost to the patient and society in general. Achievement of these goals depends on the accuracy of the physician's decision-making process. Although specific information is not available for every aspect of neck pain, there is a large body of data to guide the handling of these patients, such as that presented in Section II.

Using the available knowledge, an algorithm for the diagnosis and treatment of neck pain has been designed (see the Neck Pain Algorithm immediately following this chapter). The algorithm is a sequence of clinical decisions and thought processes found to be useful in approaching the universe of patients with cervical spine problems. The algorithm follows well-delineated rules, established from the consensus of a broad segment of qualified physicians who diagnose and treat patients with neck pain. The algorithm does not include all cervical spine diagnoses, and there are exceptions to the rule. Not all patients fit easily into

the categories to be discussed. Common sense helps the examining physician individualize the evaluation of the unusual patient. The diagnostic process may also be presented in the format of a table (see the Appendix).

DIAGNOSTIC AND TREATMENT PROTOCOL

The diagnostic and treatment protocol begins with the evaluation of patients who are initially seen for neck pain with or without arm or shoulder pain. Patients with major trauma to the cervical spine, including fractures and dislocations, are not included because these individuals are treated primarily in emergency rooms that have specific neck trauma protocols. After an initial medical history and physical examination are completed, and on the assumption that the patient's symptoms are originating from the cervical spine, the first major decision is to rule in or out the presence of cervical myelopathy.

Cervical Myelopathy

Cervical myelopathy occurs secondary to compression of the neural elements (spinal cord and nerve roots) in the cervical spinal canal.[1, 2] Progressive and profound neurologic deficits, including weakness, spasticity, and gait abnormalities, are clinical manifestations of myelopathy. The etiology of the compression

140

is usually a combination of osteoarthritis associated with osteophytes and degenerative disc disease that leads to a decrease in the volume of the spinal canal. If the canal becomes too small, the spinal cord may be compromised, resulting in neurologic dysfunction.

The character and severity of the problem depend on the size, location, and duration of the lesion. Ventrolateral lesions encroach on the nerve roots and lateral aspects of the spinal cord, producing all the manifestations of nerve root compression. The main radicular signs are weakness with loss of tone and volume of the muscles in the upper extremity. Pressure on the spinal cord may produce pyramidal tract signs and spasticity in the lower extremities. The most frequent presentation of myelopathy is a combination of arm and leg dysfunction.[3]

Midline lesions intrude on the central aspect of the anterior spinal cord. They generally do not produce signs of nerve root compression. Both lower extremities are usually involved, and the most common problem relates initially to gait disturbances. As the problem progresses, bowel and bladder control may be affected.

Although the natural history of cervical spondylitic myelopathy is one of gradual progression, severe myelopathy rarely develops in patients who do not demonstrate it when they first present to the physician. Once the diagnosis of cervical myelopathy is made, surgical intervention should be considered quickly. The best results are attained in patients with one or two motor units involved and with a myelopathy of relatively short duration. A cervical myelogram or magnetic resonance (MR) image should be obtained to define the neural compression precisely, and an adequate surgical decompression should be performed as soon as possible to achieve the best results. After surgical intervention, many individuals require rehabilitation to return to an improved functional status.

Systemic Medical Illness

The patients who do not have cervical myelopathy should be evaluated for acute, severe symptoms suggestive of an underlying medical illness as the cause of their neck pain. These individuals should be asked five questions that identify patients at increased risk of medical causes of neck pain. These groups include individuals with constitutional symptoms of fever or weight loss suggestive of an infection or tumor. Patients with pain that is increased with recumbency or at night may have a spinal cord infiltrative process or a tumor of the vertebral column. Patients with prolonged morning stiffness may have spondyloarthropathy. Localized cervical bone pain may be secondary to a systemic process that replaces bone (Paget's disease) or a local tumor (osteoblastoma). Patients with viscerogenic pain (angina, thoracic outlet syndrome, and esophageal disorders) have symptoms that affect structures beyond the cervical spine and recur in a regular pattern. Patients with constitutional symptoms should receive a medical evaluation that is specific for the corresponding symptom or sign. Patients with acute neck pain who are older than 60 years of age (malignant tumor) or younger than 15 years of age (benign bone tumor) should be considered for plain roentgenograms of the cervical spine and determination of erythrocyte sedimentation rate. These tests have a greater probability of showing abnormalities in this group of patients. If these tests are unrevealing, patients should be treated with conservative therapy for 3 to 6 weeks.

Nonoperative Management

After a cervical myelopathy and acute systemic medical disorders have been ruled out, the remainder of patients with neck pain, who constitute the majority, should be started on a course of conservative (nonoperative) management. Initially, a specific diagnosis, such as a herniated disc, cervical spondylosis, or neck strain, is not required to start therapy because the entire group is treated in a similar fashion.

Short-term immobilization is useful in therapy for acute episodes and exacerbations in patients with chronic cervical intervertebral disc disease. A soft felt collar should fit properly and usually provides comfort for the patient. The collar initially should be worn continuously, day and night. The patient must understand that the collar protects the neck from awkward positions and movements during sleep and is therefore important. Soft collars play a lesser role in conservative management of patients with other causes of neck pain, such as whiplash and osteoarthritis. The use of collars is limited so that motion of the cervical spine is gradually increased to its baseline status.[4] The other major component of the initial treatment program is drug therapy. Anti-inflammatory drugs, analgesics, and muscle relaxants usually improve patient comfort and should supplement appropriate position of the cervical spine. Medication is not a substitute for proper support and mobilization.

Most patients respond to this short-term immobilization and pharmacotherapy in the first 10 days. The patients who improve should be encouraged to increase their activities gradually and begin a program of exercises directed at strengthening the paravertebral musculature rather than at increasing the range of motion. For patients with intervertebral disc problems, use of the soft collar is decreased over the next 2 to 3 weeks. The unimproved group of patients with disc herniation should continue with full-time collar immobilization and anti-inflammatory medication.

If there is not a significant improvement in symptoms in 3 to 4 weeks in patients with local neck pain, a local injection into the area of maximum tenderness in the paravertebral musculature and trapezii should be considered. Marked relief of symptoms is often achieved dramatically by infiltration of these trigger points with a combination of 3 to 5 mL of lidocaine (Xylocaine) and 10 mg of a corticosteroid preparation. If the trigger point injection is not successful at 4 to 5 weeks after the onset of symptoms, a trial of cervical traction may be instituted for cervical disc herniation and radiculopathy. A home traction device with light weights is preferred. Isometric strengthening exercises should be instituted as the patient returns to full activity.

The remaining patients should be treated conservatively for up to 6 weeks. The majority of cervical spine patients get better and return to a normal life pattern within 2 months. If the initial conservative treatment fails, symptomatic patients may be separated into two groups. The first group consists of patients with neck pain as a predominant complaint, with or without interscapular radiation. The second group consists of those who complain primarily of arm pain (brachialgia).

Neck Pain Predominant

If no symptomatic improvement is achieved by 6 weeks of conservative therapy, plain roentgenograms, including lateral flexion-extension motion films, should be taken and carefully examined. Roentgenograms before this point are usually not helpful because of the lack of significant differences between symptomatic and asymptomatic patients, except in individuals older than 60 years of age or younger than 15 years of age. Nonspecific radiographic de-

generative changes in the cervical spine are almost universal by age 60. Careful examination of roentgenograms in older individuals is necessary to be sure that lesions, in addition to spondylosis, are identified.

Some patients may have objective evidence of instability on the motion films. In the lower cervical spine (C3–C7), instability is defined as horizontal translation of one vertebra on another of more than 3.5 mm or as an angulatory difference of adjacent vertebrae of more than 11°.[5] The majority of patients with degenerative (nontraumatic) instability respond to further nonoperative measures, including a thorough explanation of the problem and some type of bracing. In severe cases, segmental spinal fusion may be necessary.

Other patients who complain mainly of neck pain show degenerative disease on their plain films. The roentgenographic findings include loss of height of the intervertebral disc space, osteophyte formation, secondary encroachment of the intervertebral foramina, and osteoarthritic changes in the zygapophyseal joints.[6] The diagnostic difficulty is not in identifying these abnormalities but in determining their clinical significance. Degeneration in the cervical spine can be a normal part of aging. Many asymptomatic patients show roentgenographic, myelographic, and MR imaging evidence of abnormal degenerative disease.[7] The most significant finding relevant to symptomatology is narrowing of the intervertebral disc space, particularly at C5–C6 and C6–C7. Changes at the zygapophyseal joints, foramina, and posterior articular processes do not correlate well with clinical symptoms. These patients should be treated with anti-inflammatory medications, cervical support, and trigger-point injections as required. In the quiescent stages, they should be placed on isometric exercises. Finally, they should be reexamined periodically because some may develop myelopathy.

The majority of patients with neck pain have normal roentgenograms. The preliminary diagnosis for this group is neck strain.[8] However, in the absence of objective findings as well as failure to improve with appropriate conservative management, other problems must be considered.

Without x-ray findings of degenerative spine disease, the evaluation of the patient with neck pain limited to the neck must start with a review of the patient's history and physical examination. Symptoms may have appeared or changed in intensity since the initial evaluation. The histories of patients with neck pain may be divided according to symptoms into five groups (see the algorithm): fever and weight loss, pain at night or with recumbency, morning stiffness, acute localized bone pain, and visceral pain. The medical evaluation of each group differs. It is helpful to identify the patient's symptoms at the initial visit so that a specific evaluation can be completed thoughtfully and expeditiously.

Fever and Weight Loss. Patients with neck pain and fever should be evaluated for any change in mental status or severe headache. These individuals should have their cerebrospinal fluid (CSF) examined for inflammatory cells, increased protein, or decreased glucose concentration compatible with meningitis. These patients require immediate broad-spectrum antibiotic therapy while cultures are incubated from the CSF examination. Antibiotic therapy is altered as the causative organism is determined and antibiotic sensitivity identified. Plain roentgenograms of the patients with fever and weight loss should be reviewed for alterations in bone integrity. Because a significant portion of bone calcium must be lost before lesions are identified, bone scan is a useful screening test to discover increased bone cell activity. A normal bone scan does not eliminate the possibility of a tumor. An MR image or computerized tomography (CT) scan identifies the patients with a destructive lesion without osteoblastic response (multiple myeloma) (Fig. 9–1). These radiographs locate the lesion for appropriate biopsy and culture. Determining erythrocyte sedimentation rate (ESR) or C-reactive protein (CRP) identifies those individuals with an inflammatory lesion of the cervical spine. Antibiotics are the treatment of choice for osteomyelitis and discitis. Surgical excision is preferred if tumors, particularly benign lesions, are accessible for total removal. In postsurgical patients who develop fever, determining CRP or ESR is useful to identify infections. CRP is the more sensitive indicator.[9]

Pain at Night or with Recumbency. Infiltrative lesions of the spinal cord and tumors of the spinal column are associated with nocturnal increase in pain. Patients with neurologic signs and nocturnal or recumbency pain should undergo MR evaluation of the central nervous system. The presence of multiple lesions compatible with plaques is compatible with a demyelinating disease such as multiple sclerosis. A spinal cord tumor appears as a single mass lesion. Such a lesion requires biopsy for diagnosis. Those patients without neurologic signs and nocturnal pain may have a bone tumor as the cause of symptoms. A plain roentgenogram of the cervical spine should be reviewed for the presence of benign or malignant tumors. Benign tumors tend to involve the posterior elements of vertebrae, and malignant tumors affect vertebral bodies. Plain roentgenograms may be unable to detect lesions because inadequate calcium has been lost. Bone scan is a more sensitive test in detecting increased bone turnover. A CT scan is better than an MR image for bone detail in identifying bone tumors. These lesions require biopsy and lesion-specific therapy.

Morning Stiffness. Morning stiffness of the neck lasting for hours is a common symptom of patients with spondyloarthropathy or rheumatoid arthritis. Patients with this symptom should have a flexion-extension view of the cervical spine to detect subluxation (Fig. 9–2). On occasion, a patient with rheumatoid arthritis may have mild peripheral joint disease and more significant cervical spine involvement. A positive rheumatoid factor may identify these unusual patients. Women with spondyloarthropathy may have neck disease without significant low back pain. Occasional patients with spondyloarthropathy do not have back pain despite the presence of sacroiliitis. Therefore, a Ferguson's view of the pelvis is a useful test to identify the presence of sacroiliitis if neck films are unrevealing for squaring of vertebral bodies or syndesmophytes. Patients with spondyloarthropathy with increased neck pain require radiographic evaluation to eliminate the possibility of fracture (Fig. 9–3). A bone scan and ESR are useful tests to identify those individuals with inflammatory polyarthritis. If the bone scan is normal and the ESR is abnormal and the patient is older than 60 years, a diagnosis of polymyalgia rheumatica should be considered. Patients with polyarthritis are treated with nonsteroidal anti-inflammatory drugs and stabilization of the cervical spine. Patients with polymyalgia rheumatica are treated with daily low-dose corticosteroids.

Acute Localized Bone Pain. Acute localized bone pain is usually associated with either fracture or expansion of bone. Any condition that replaces bone with abnormal cells (tumor or sarcoidosis) or increases mineral loss from bone (hyperparathyroidism) weakens bone to the point at which fracture may occur spontaneously or with minimal trauma (Fig. 9–4). Patients with acute fractures experience acute onset of pain in the area of the neck that corresponds to the fractured bone. Physical examination will identify the maximum point of tenderness. A plain roentgenogram should be reviewed with special attention to the pain-

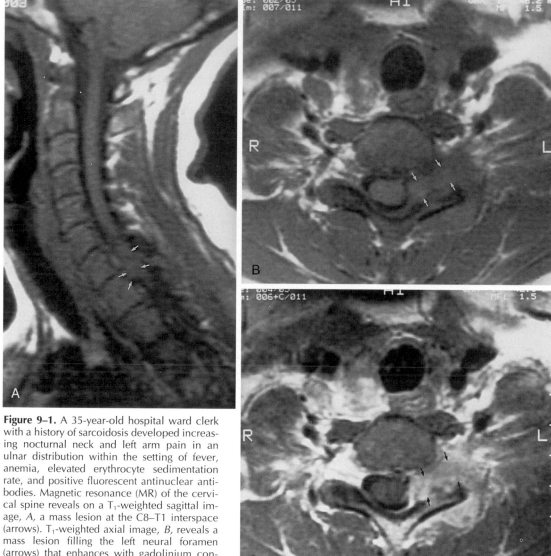

Figure 9–1. A 35-year-old hospital ward clerk with a history of sarcoidosis developed increasing nocturnal neck and left arm pain in an ulnar distribution within the setting of fever, anemia, elevated erythrocyte sedimentation rate, and positive fluorescent antinuclear antibodies. Magnetic resonance (MR) of the cervical spine reveals on a T_1-weighted sagittal image, *A,* a mass lesion at the C8–T1 interspace (arrows). T_1-weighted axial image, *B,* reveals a mass lesion filling the left neural foramen (arrows) that enhances with gadolinium contrast media (arrows) in *C.*

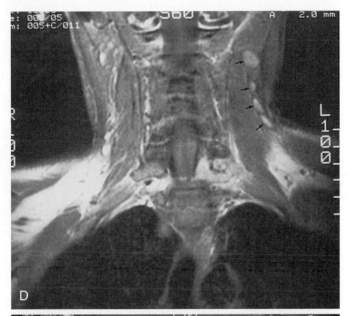

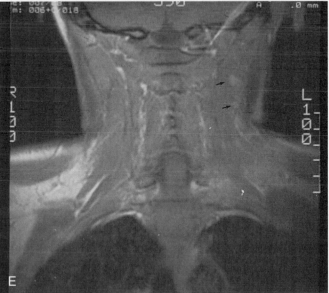

Figure 9–1 *Continued* MR T$_1$-weighted contrast coronal view, *D,* reveals enhancement of left cervical lymph glands *(arrows).* Biopsy of the mass lesion revealed caseating granulomas and culture grew M. tuberculosis. The patient received five anti-tuberculous drugs. After 5 months of therapy with resolution of neck and arm pain, T$_1$-weighted contrast coronal view, *E,* reveals resolution of the enhancement of cervical lymph nodes *(arrows).*

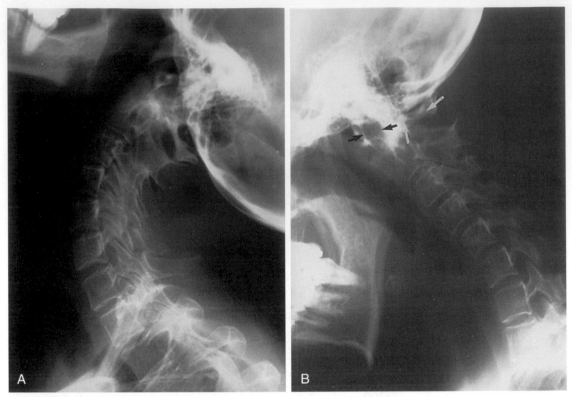

Figure 9–2. A 30-year-old woman with rheumatoid arthritis for 10 years complained of increased neck discomfort without any neurologic deficit. Flexion, *A*, and extension, *B*, views of the cervical spine demonstrate atlantoaxial subluxation with anterior measurement of 10 mm *(black arrows)* and posterior measurement of 15 mm *(white arrows)*. Flexion view reveals minimal anterior subluxation at the C3–C4 and C5–C6 levels. The patient is being followed for the appearance of headache or neurologic symptoms that would require evaluation for stabilization.

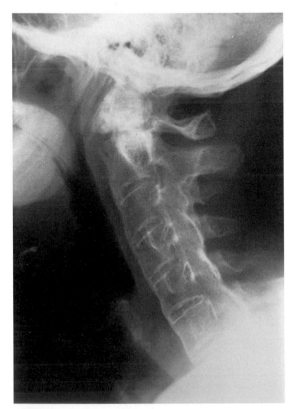

Figure 9–3. A 67-year-old man with a 20-year history of ankylosing spondylitis had increased neck pain without increased movement. Lateral view of the cervical spine reveals anterior and posterior syndesmophytes, fusion of zygapophyseal joints, and no evidence of fracture. Neck pain improved with an increase in nonsteroidal therapy and the addition of a muscle relaxant.

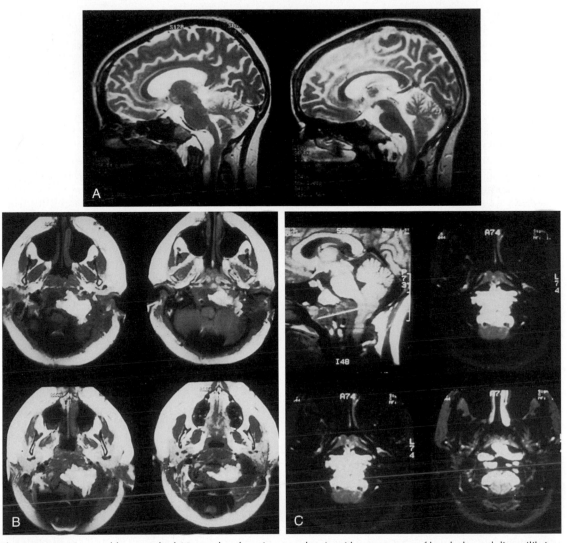

Figure 9–4. A 15-year-old woman had 18 months of persistent neck pain with recent onset of headache and disequilibrium. A T_2-weighted sagittal magnetic resonance scan, *A*, reveals a mass lesion affecting the clivus and atlas, with posterior displacement of the brainstem. Computerized tomography (CT) scan, *B*, reveals replacement of clival bone. Postoperative CT, *C*, reveals a decrease in the size of the mass with decompression of the brain stem. Pathologic examination of the mass revealed cells compatible with a chordoma. (Courtesy of Laligam N. Sekhar, M.D., and Donald Wright, M.D.)

ful area to identify a fracture. A bone scan is useful to detect increased bone activity soon after a fracture when a plain roentgenogram is normal. A CT scan is capable of detecting fractures that are located by a bone scan. If the bone scan is normal, an MR scan can identify the presence of malignant or inflammatory cells that do not stimulate osteoblasts (myeloma). An ESR test and chemistry profile can detect inflammatory and metabolic abnormalities associated with alteration of bony architecture. The diagnostic evaluation and therapeutic regimen for each disease are reviewed in Section III.

Visceral Pain. Patients with visceral pain have neck pain secondary to disorders in the cardiovascular, gastrointestinal, or neurologic systems. Patients may complain of neck and arm pain that occur with exertion. If chest pain occurs in conjunction with arm pain, evaluation for coronary artery disease is indicated. These patients should have an electrocardiogram and stress test. If these tests show abnormalities, referral to a cardiologist for angina therapy is required. If the exertional pain is limited to the arm alone, an evaluation for thoracic outlet syndrome is indicated. Adson's test identifies those patients with scalenus anterior syndrome; the hyperabduction test identifies compression of the neurovascular bundle between the costocoracoid membrane and the pectoralis minor. These individuals may improve with postural exercises. If the arm pain is persistent, a chest roentgenogram with particular attention to the apices is indicated.

Pancoast's tumors invade the inferior portions of the brachial plexus. These patients have malignant lesions that require palliative radiation therapy. Episodic neck or arm pain may be secondary to a transient ischemic attack. These individuals should have Doppler's ultrasonography to evaluate vascular narrowing. An angiogram identifies constriction or dissection of the carotid or vertebral arteries. Therapy may include drugs to prevent thrombosis or surgical correction of the lesion. Esophageal disorders should be considered if neck pain occurs in association with eating. Lesions in the posterior esophagus may affect the prevertebral space, causing neck pain. An esophagram identifies abnormalities of function as well as stricture. Esophagoscopy may be required to identify mucosal abnormalities. Patients with multiorgan system abnormalities in addition to neck pain should be asked about exposure to tick bites. If these individuals have erythema migrans, or Bell's palsy, a diagnosis of Lyme disease should be considered. The diagnosis of Lyme disease is considered in the patient with tick exposure and appropriate clinical symptoms and signs. Positive Lyme antibody titers are confirmatory but not diagnostic. Oral antibiotic therapy for 4 weeks is adequate for many patients with Lyme disease.

If the medical evaluation is normal, the patient should be evaluated for the presence of tender points or trigger points. An elevated ESR and muscle tenderness suggest a diagnosis of polymyalgia rheumatica. A normal ESR is compatible with fibromyalgia (tender points) or myofascial syndrome (trigger points). Patients with fibromyalgia improve with aerobic exercise and antidepressants; myofascial patients may benefit from injection at the maximum point of tenderness with a combination of an anesthetic and corticosteroid. If the patient does not have muscle tenderness, the patient should have a complete psychosocial evaluation and receive treatment when appropriate for depression or substance dependence, which are frequently seen in association with neck pain.

If the psychosocial evaluation proves normal, the patient is considered to have chronic neck pain. These patients require encouragement, patience, and education. They especially need to be detoxified from narcotic drugs and placed on an exercise regimen for the neck and an aerobic exercise program. Many respond to antidepressant drugs, such as amitriptyline hydochloride (Elavil). Regardless, these patients need to be periodically reevaluated to avoid missing any new problems.

Occasionally, it is difficult to distinguish those patients who have a true neck problem from those individuals using their neck as an excuse to miss work and collect compensation or because of pending litigation. The outcome of treatment of cervical disc disease has been shown to be adversely affected by litigation. Frequently with hyperextension neck injuries, there are no objective findings to substantiate the subjective complaints. The best solution to this dilemma in the compensation setting is to recommend an independent medical examination early in the course of treatment. In general, compensation and noncompensation patients respond to therapy in similar ways.[10] Patients should be encouraged to remain functional in spite of pain and other symptoms.[11]

ARM PAIN PREDOMINANT (BRACHIALGIA)

Extrinsic pressure on the vascular structures or peripheral nerves is the most likely imitator of brachialgia and must be ruled out. Problems in the chest and shoulder must also be considered. A careful physical examination, including Adson's test, shoulder evaluation, and a test for Tinel's sign at the ulnar and carpal tunnels, should be conducted. If these tests are equivocal, appropriate radiographs and an electromyogram (EMG) should be obtained.

In addition to spinal nerve root encroachment, diseases that directly affect the brachial plexus may result in a variety of upper extremity symptoms that must be distinguished from cervical root syndromes. Although trauma is the most common cause of brachial plexus injury, compression by vascular structure, cervical ribs, muscular or fibrous bands, or tumors may result in a plexus neuropathy. Apical carcinoma of the lung may encroach on the brachial plexus and may be seen in Horner's syndrome.

The patients with arm pain predominant (brachialgia) refractory to nonoperative management may have symptoms owing to mechanical pressure from a herniated disc or hypertrophic bone and secondary inflammation of the involved nerve roots.[12] The single best imaging test to confirm the diagnosis is MR. If the MR image is equivocal, a CT myelogram is then recommended. If the patient's pain, neurologic deficit, and imaging study abnormalities correlate, surgical decompression of the involved nerve root or spinal cord has an excellent success rate.

Peripheral nerve compression occasionally manifests patterns of arm pain that exceed the expected regional involvement of the specific peripheral nerve. Although peripheral nerve entrapment can usually be identified by motor and sensory loss pattern and by EMG studies, these peripheral lesions may coexist with cervical root compression. The double-crush hypothesis maintains that axons compressed in one region may become more susceptible to impairment at a distant site.

If there is unequivocal evidence of nerve root compression (neurologic deficit, abnormal EMG, and abnormal CT myelogram or MR image) consistent with the physical findings, surgical decompression should be considered. Some studies suggest that patients with radicular symptoms seem to do better with surgery. Although conservative management of patients with radicular symptoms has shown that this problem rarely progresses to cervical myelopathy, persistent symptoms are common.

Patients who have no specific diagnosis and have pain that is resistant to a 12-week trial of conservative therapy are considered to have chronic neck pain. The primary goal for therapy with chronic neck pain is maximum function, not pain relief. Patients with chronic pain require multimodality therapy. Exercises, nonsteroidal anti-inflammatory drugs, tricyclic antidepressants, physical interventions (heat or cold), and psychological support are among the modalities to be considered for patients with chronic pain. These patients should be consistently encouraged to maximize their function and to return to some form of work. The appearance of new symptoms or marked exacerbation of preexisting complaints should be reevaluated.

Immediately following the Neck Pain Algorithm are the Medical Evaluation Algorithm and a clinical evaluation form for neck pain, including historical, physical, laboratory, and radiographic components of the diagnostic examination. All or part of this form, as the physician thinks appropriate, may be used in the evaluation of the patient with neck pain.

An additional aid for differential diagnosis is in the Appendix, which includes a table of differential diagnosis of neck pain and clinical data associated with specific disease entities that cause neck pain.

References

1. LaRocca H: Cervical spondylitic myelopathy: natural history. Spine 13:854, 1988.
2. Clark CR: Cervical spondylitic myelopathy: history and physical findings. Spine 13:847, 1988.
3. Bernhardt M, Hynes RA, Blume HW, White AA III: Cervical spondylotic myelopathy. J Bone Joint Surg 75:119, 1993.
4. Spitzer WO, Skovron ML, Salmi LR, et al: Scientific monograph of the Quebec Task Force on whiplash-associated disorders: redefining "whiplash" and its management. Spine 20:1, 1995.
5. White AA, Panjabi MM, Posner I, et al.: Spinal stability: evaluation and treatment. American Academy of Orthopaedic Surgeons Instructional Course Lectures 30:457–483, 1981.
6. Friedenberg ZB, Miller WT: Degenerative disease of the cervical spine. J Bone Joint Surg 45:1171, 1963.
7. Gore DR, Sepic SB, Gardner GM: Roentgenographic findings of the cervical spine in asymptomatic people. Spine 11:521, 1986.
8. Greenfield J, Ilfeld FW: Acute cervical strain. Clin Orthop 122:196, 1977.
9. Thelander U, Larsson S: Quantification of C-reactive protein levels and erythrocyte sedimentation rate after spinal surgery. Spine 17:400, 1992.
10. Shapiro AP, Roth RS: The effect of litigation on recovery of whiplash. Spine 7:531, 1993.
11. Carette S: Whiplash injury and chronic neck pain. N Engl J Med 330:1083, 1994.
12. Dillin W, Booth R, Cuckler J, et al: Cervical radiculopathy: a review. Spine 11:988, 1986.

NECK PAIN ALGORITHM

0 WEEKS

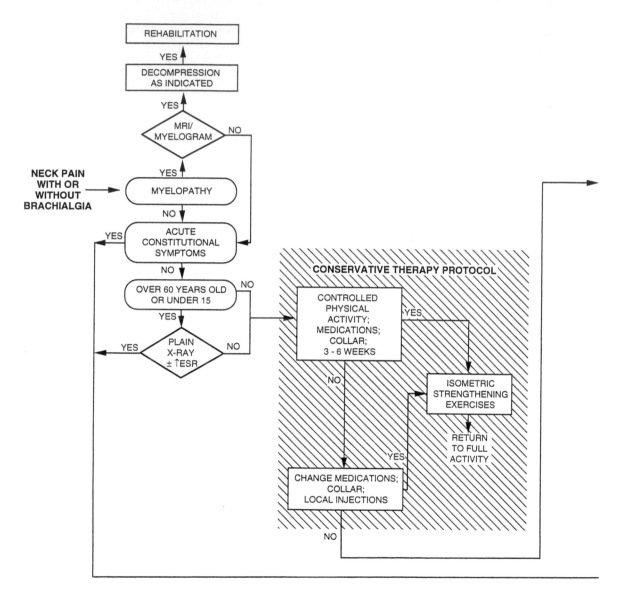

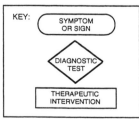

A

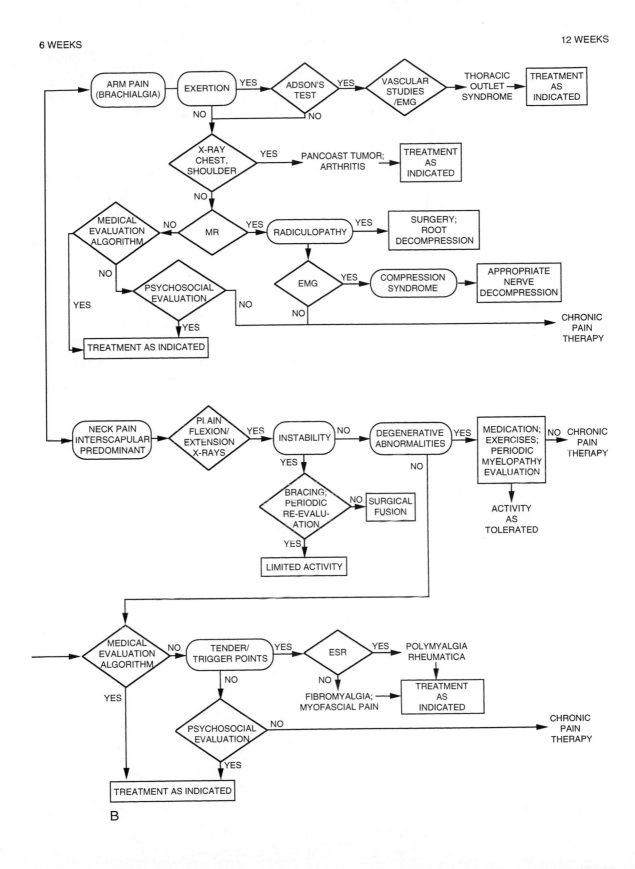

MEDICAL EVALUATION ALGORITHM FOR NECK PAIN

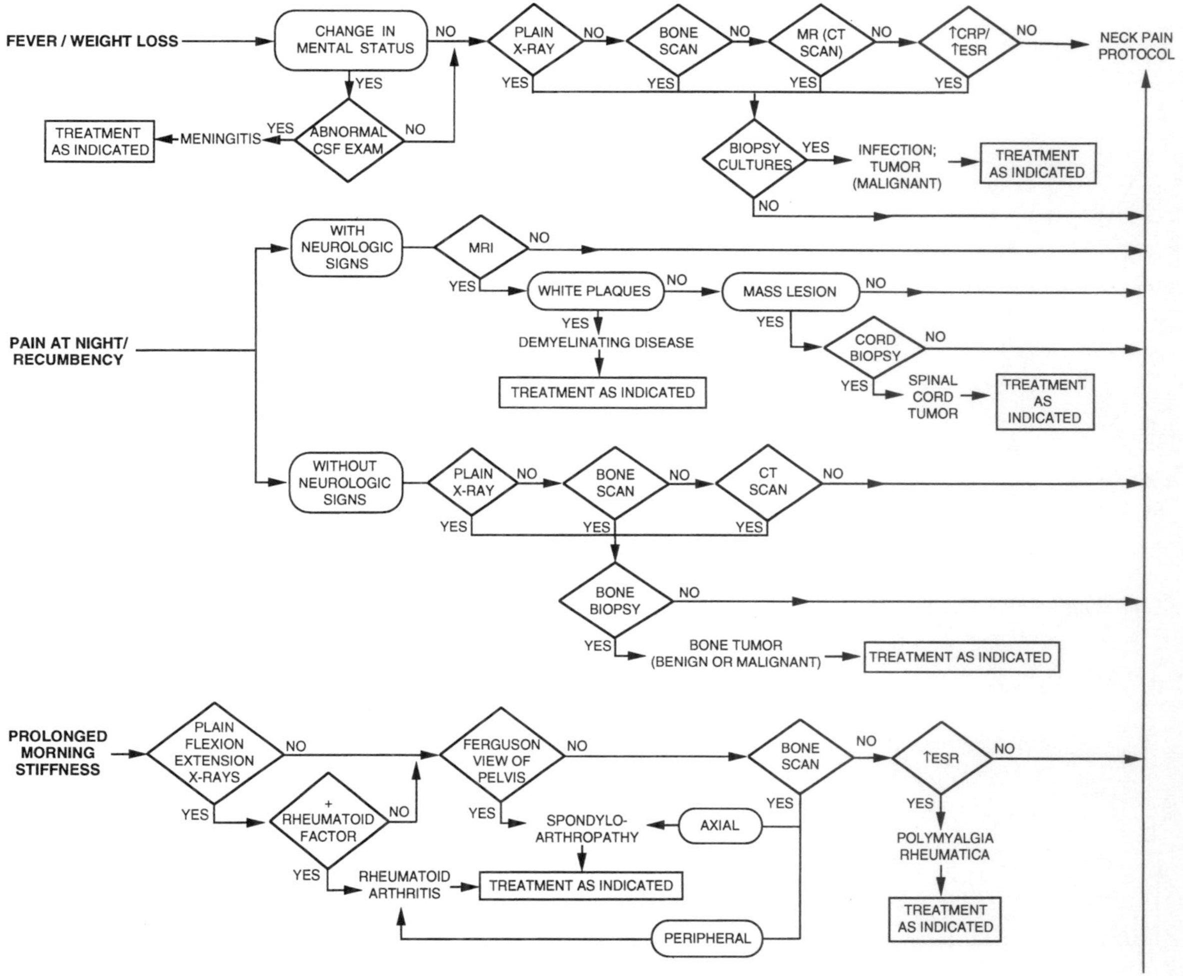

FEVER / WEIGHT LOSS

CHANGE IN MENTAL STATUS → YES → ABNORMAL CSF EXAM → YES → MENINGITIS → TREATMENT AS INDICATED

ABNORMAL CSF EXAM → NO

CHANGE IN MENTAL STATUS → NO → PLAIN X-RAY → YES → BONE SCAN → YES → MR (CT SCAN) → YES → ↑CRP/↑ESR → NO → NECK PAIN PROTOCOL

BIOPSY CULTURES → YES → INFECTION; TUMOR (MALIGNANT) → TREATMENT AS INDICATED

BIOPSY CULTURES → NO

↑CRP/↑ESR → YES

PAIN AT NIGHT/ RECUMBENCY

WITH NEUROLOGIC SIGNS → MRI → YES → WHITE PLAQUES → YES → DEMYELINATING DISEASE → TREATMENT AS INDICATED

WHITE PLAQUES → NO → MASS LESION → YES → CORD BIOPSY → YES → SPINAL CORD TUMOR → TREATMENT AS INDICATED

MASS LESION → NO

CORD BIOPSY → NO

WITHOUT NEUROLOGIC SIGNS → PLAIN X-RAY → YES → BONE SCAN → YES → CT SCAN → YES

PLAIN X-RAY → NO

BONE SCAN → NO

CT SCAN → NO

BONE BIOPSY → YES → BONE TUMOR (BENIGN OR MALIGNANT) → TREATMENT AS INDICATED

PROLONGED MORNING STIFFNESS

PLAIN FLEXION EXTENSION X-RAYS → YES → RHEUMATOID FACTOR → + → RHEUMATOID FACTOR → YES → RHEUMATOID ARTHRITIS → TREATMENT AS INDICATED

PLAIN FLEXION EXTENSION X-RAYS → NO

RHEUMATOID FACTOR → NO → FERGUSON VIEW OF PELVIS → YES → SPONDYLO-ARTHROPATHY → AXIAL → BONE SCAN → YES → PERIPHERAL

FERGUSON VIEW OF PELVIS → NO → BONE SCAN → NO → ↑ESR → YES → POLYMYALGIA RHEUMATICA → TREATMENT AS INDICATED

↑ESR → NO

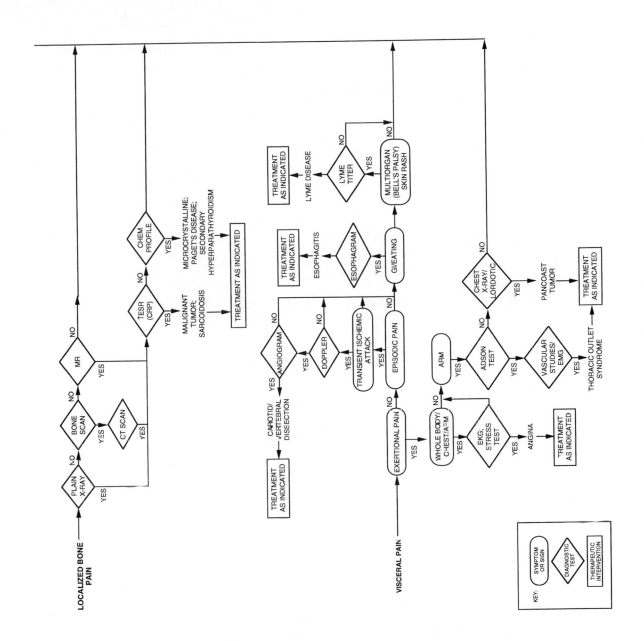

LOCALIZED BONE PAIN

PLAIN X-RAY — YES
NO → BONE SCAN — YES → CT SCAN — YES
NO → MR — YES
NO → ↑ESR (CRP) — YES → MALIGNANT TUMOR; SARCOIDOSIS → TREATMENT AS INDICATED
NO → CHEM PROFILE — YES → MICROCRYSTALLINE; PAGET'S DISEASE; SECONDARY HYPERPARATHYROIDISM → TREATMENT AS INDICATED

VISCERAL PAIN

EXERTIONAL PAIN — NO
YES → WHOLE BODY/CHEST/ARM — YES → EKG; STRESS TEST — YES → ANGINA → TREATMENT AS INDICATED
NO → ARM — YES → ADSON TEST — YES → VASCULAR STUDIES/EMG — YES → THORACIC OUTLET SYNDROME
NO → CHEST X-RAY/LORDOTIC — YES → PANCOAST TUMOR → TREATMENT AS INDICATED

EPISODIC PAIN — NO
YES → TRANSIENT ISCHEMIC ATTACK — YES → DOPPLER — YES → ANGIOGRAM — YES → CAROTID/VERTEBRAL DISSECTION → TREATMENT AS INDICATED
NO → GI/EATING — YES → ESOPHAGRAM — YES → ESOPHAGITIS → TREATMENT AS INDICATED
NO → MULTIORGAN (BELL'S PALSY) SKIN RASH — YES → LYME TITER — YES → LYME DISEASE → TREATMENT AS INDICATED
NO →

KEY:
SYMPTOM OR SIGN
DIAGNOSTIC TEST
THERAPEUTIC INTERVENTION

NECK/SPINE PAIN EVALUATION

MEDICAL HISTORY

Name: _____   Sex: M ____ F ____   Date _____

Address: _____   Date of Birth: _____

Occupation: _____   Workmen's Compensation: Y ____ N___

Self-employed: Y ____ N___

FAMILY HISTORY

Family members with spine pain: Y____ N ____

Describe:

Other familial illness:

SOCIAL HISTORY

Working: Y ____ N _____   Labor: Heavy _____ Moderate _____ Sedentary _____ Light _____

Smoking: Alcohol: Recreational Drugs:

Leisure time activities: Hobbies: Sports:

Education:

PAST MEDICAL HISTORY

Current Medical Illnesses: Diabetes _____   Vascular/Hypertension _____

Arthritis _____   Cancer _____   Other _____

Current Medications:

Severe Injuries: Hospitalizations/Operations:

REVIEW OF SYSTEMS

Constitutional:	Fever _____	Weight loss _____
	Anorexia _____	Severe fatigue _____
Skin:	Psoriasis _____	Nail changes _____	Nodules _____
Head/Neck:	Conjunctivitis_____	Iritis _____
	Oral ulcers _____	Thyroid _____
Cardiopulmonary:	Dyspnea _____	Cough _____
	Hemoptysis _____	Chest pain _____
Gastrointestinal:	Abdominal pain_____	Blood in stool _____
	Nausea/Vomiting _____	Change in	Ulcers _____
		bowel habits _____
Genitourinary:	Frequency _____	Burning _____	Hematuria _____
	Hesitancy _____	Sexual dysfunction_____	Menses _____
Hematologic:	Anemia _____	Bleeding disorder_____
Neurologic:	Mental status _____	Muscle weakness_____	Sensation _____
Personality:	Obsessive _____	Passive _____
	Depressive _____	Anxious _____
Musculoskeletal:	Arthritis _____

CHIEF COMPLAINT:

A

NECK/BACK PAIN:

Onset:
Acute _____ Gradual _____ With activity _____
Twist _____ Fall _____ Bending _____
Lifting _____ Pulling/pushing _____
Increasing _____ Decreasing _____ Same _____
Direct blow/trauma _____

Duration: Days _____ Weeks _____ Months _____

Frequency: Daily _____ Episodic _____
Weekly _____ Continuous _____
Monthly _____ Other _____

Location and Radiation:

Trapezius R _____ L _____
Paraspinous R _____ L _____
Sacroiliac R _____ L _____
Buttocks R _____ L _____
Thighs Anterior _____ Posterior_____
Lower leg R _____ L _____
Leg paresthesias _____ Leg weakness _____

Time of day: AM_____ PM _____

AGGRAVATING FACTORS: Standing _____ Walking _____ Sitting _____ Driving _____
Recumbency: Supine _____ Prone _____
AM stiffness: Y _____ N _____ Duration _____
Movements: Flexion _____ Extension _____
Other: Coughing _____ Valsalva _____ Sneezing _____

ALLEVIATING FACTORS: Standing _____ Walking _____ Sitting _____
Recumbency: Supine _____ Prone _____
Movements: Flexion _____ Extension _____
Medications: Antiinflammatories _____ Narcotics _____
Muscle relaxants _____
Supports: Brace _____

VISUAL PAIN SCALE

Severe |————————————————————————————————| None

☐ Numbness
⊞ Burning
■ Dull

▨ Pins & Needles
⊠ Stabbing

B

PHYSICAL EXAMINATION

Vital signs: T _____ P _____ R_____ BP _____ Weight _____ Height _____

General Description

Skin: Rash_____   Nodules_____

           Vesicles _____   Petechiae _____   Ulcers _____

Head/Neck: Conjunctivitis _____   Iritis _____

            Fundi _____   Oral ulcers _____   Thyromegaly _____

Lymph: Lymphadenopathy _____

Lungs: Chest expansion _____ cm   Breath sounds_____

Heart: Cardiomegaly _____   Gallops _____   Murmurs _____

Abdomen: Quadrant tenderness _____   Organomegaly _____   Masses–pulsatile _____

            Bowel sounds_____   Hernia _____   CVA tenderness _____

Vessels: Pulses: Dorsalis pedis _____   Posterior tibial _____   Other _____

Bone/Muscle:

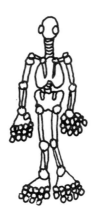

NECK

Motion: Flexion _____ ⁰   Extension _____ ⁰

            Lateral bend: R _____ L _____   Rotation: R _____ L _____

Tenderness: Axial loading _____

Reflexes: (scale 0–4, 2=normal)

            Biceps   R _____   L _____

            Triceps   R _____   L _____

            Brachioradialis   R _____   L _____

            Finger flexors   R _____   L _____

            Hoffman's   R _____   L _____

C

Cranial nerves: (Check if intact)

CN I _____ II _____ III _____ IV _____ V _____ VI _____

VII _____ VIII _____ IX _____ X _____ XI _____ XII _____

Pupils: R _____ L _____

Motor: (0–5, 5=normal)

Neck flexion _____

Neck extension _____

Lateral bend _____

Elbow flexion (C5, C6)   R _____   L _____

Elbow extension (C6, C7, C8)   R _____   L _____

Wrist extension (C6, C7, C8, radial nerve)   R _____   L _____

Finger abduction (C8, T1, ulnar nerve)   R _____   L _____

Thumb opposition (C8, T1, median nerve)   R _____   L _____

Sensory:

Shade affected area

Other:

Ptosis   R _____   L _____

Autonomic signs (sweat, temperature, flushing, blanching) _____

Circulation (pulses, capillary blush, bruit) _____

Integument (birthmarks, scars, lesions) _____

Tinel's sign   R _____   L _____

Phalen's sign   R _____   L _____

Spurling's sign   R _____   L _____

Lhermitte's sign   R _____   L _____

Neck traction test   R _____   L _____

Adson's maneuver   R _____   L _____

Muscle atrophy   R _____   L _____

(describe)

Fasciculations   Tongue _____

Upper extremities   R _____   L _____

(describe)

D

LUMBOSACRAL SPINE

STANDING:

Posterior view: Pigmentation_____ Hair tufts _____

Scoliosis _____ Bone prominence_____

Sacroiliac joint motion R _____ L _____

Trendelenburg's sign R _____ L _____

Lateral view: Lordosis: Normal _____ Decreased _____ Increased _____

Kyphosis: Normal _____ Decreased _____ Increased _____

Anterior view: Pelvic tilt _____

Motion: Flexion _____ Hair tufts _____

Extension _____ Bone prominence _____

Lumbosacral rhythm Normal _____ Reversed _____

Lateral bending R _____ ^{0} L _____ ^{0}

Rotation R _____ ^{0} L _____ ^{0}

Toe walking Heel walking _____ Squat _____

Tenderness: Midline _____ Paraspinous _____ Iliac crest _____

Posterior iliac spine _____ Greater trochanter_____

KNEELING: Ankle reflex R _____ L _____

Forward flexion _____ ^{0}

SEATED IN CHAIR: Foot dorsiflexor strength R _____ L _____

BENT FORWARD OVER

EXAM TABLE: Gait: Normal _____ Abnormal _____

Antalgic _____ Shuffling _____ Wide−based_____

Sacroiliac tenderness R _____ L _____

SEATED - LEGS DANGLING:

Tripod sign R _____ L _____

Knee reflex R _____ L _____

Thigh pain _____ Knee pain _____

SUPINE: Leg lengths R _____ L _____

Passive straight leg R _____ L _____

Lasèque's test R _____ ^{0} L _____ ^{0}

Bilateral straight leg R _____ L _____

Hip motion Flexion R _____ ^{0} L _____ ^{0}

Extension R _____ ^{0} L _____ ^{0}

Abduction R _____ ^{0} L _____ ^{0}

Adduction R _____ ^{0} L _____ ^{0}

Internal /rotation R _____ ^{0} L _____ ^{0}

External Rotation R _____ ^{0} L _____ ^{0}

Patrick's test R _____ ^{0} L _____ ^{0}

Hoover's test _____

E

Pelvic compression: Inward _____   Outward _____

         Posterior upper leg (S1– S2)   R _____   L _____

         Posterior lower leg (S3–S4)   R _____   L _____

         Perianal (S4– S5)   R _____   L _____

Reflexes:

         Abdominal (T12–L2)   R _____   L _____

         Cremasteric (L1–L2)   R _____   L _____

         Adductor (L2)   R _____   L _____

         Patellar (L4)   R _____   L _____

         Ankle (S1)   R _____   L _____

         Bulbocavernosus (S2–S3)   R _____   L _____

Sensory:

         Medial thigh (L4)   R _____   L _____

         First web space (L5)   R _____   L _____

         Posterior calf (S1)   R _____   L _____

         Lateral foot (S1)   R _____   L _____

         Perineum (S2–S3)   R _____   L _____

Motor strength: (0–5, 5=normal)

         Hip flexion (L2–L3)   R _____   L _____

         Hip extension (L4–L5)   R _____   L _____

         Knee flexion (L3–L4)   R _____   L _____

         Knee extension (L5–S1)   R _____   L _____

         Ankle dorsiflexion (L4–L5)   R _____   L _____

         Ankle plantar flexion (S1–S2)   R _____   L _____

         Ankle inversion (L4)   R _____   L _____

         Ankle eversion (L5–S1)   R _____   L _____

Long tract signs:

         Babinski's sign   R _____   L _____

         Oppenheim's sign   R _____   L _____

         Clonus   R _____   L _____

PRONE:

         Femoral stretch test (L2–L4)   R _____   L _____

         Gluteus maximus strength (L5–S1)   R _____   L _____

         Sensory:

      Rectal exam: Rectal tone _____   Rectal masses _____

                    Testicles _____   Pelvic organs _____

OTHER TESTS:

      Schober's test _____cm   Voluntary release _____

      Well leg straight leg raising _____   Bow-string sign _____

      Naffziger's test _____   Valsalva's test _____

      Milgram's test _____   Kneeling bench test _____   Stoop test _____

F

Waddell's test: Appropriate   Inappropriate
   1. Tenderness   _____   _____
   2. Simulation: axial loading   _____   _____
             rotation _____   _____
   3. Distraction: seated   _____   _____
             straight leg _____   _____
   4. Regional disturbances   _____   _____
   5. Overreaction   _____   _____

DIAGNOSTIC TESTS

CBC: HCT _____ WBC _____ Platelets _____ Differential _____

ESR: _____mm/h (Wintrobe or Westergren)

SMA-12: Ca _____ P _____ Uric acid _____ Cholesterol _____ T Protein _____ Albumin _____
       Bilirubin _____ Alkaline Phosphatase _____ LDH _____
       SGOT _____ Acid Phosphatase _____

URINALYSIS: Sp Gr _____ Blood _____ Bilirubin _____ Acetone _____ Glucose _____
         Protein _____ pH _____ Microscopic _____

RADIOGRAPHS:
    Plain Roentgenograms _____
    Bone Scan   _____
    CT Scan   _____
    MRI Scan   _____

ELECTRODIAGNOSTIC STUDIES:
    Electromyogram   _____
    Nerve conduction   _____
    Pain quality: Superficial somatic _____ Deep somatic _____ Radicular _____
                Visceral-Referred _____ Psychogenic _____

DIAGNOSIS:

THERAPY:
    Rest   _____
    Drugs   _____
    Physical therapy   _____
    Injection   _____
    Surgical consultation _____

G

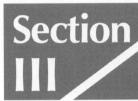

Section III

DISEASES ASSOCIATED WITH NECK PAIN

Section III is a review of illnesses associated with neck pain. The discussion of each illness opens with a capsule summary that lists the frequency, location, and quality of neck pain; the associated symptoms, signs, laboratory data, and radiographic findings; and the forms of therapy that are effective. The specifics of therapy are contained in the body of the associated chapter and in Section IV.

The frequency of neck pain associated with each illness is quantified by the terms very common, common, uncommon, and rare. The percentage of patients with neck pain associated with each term is as follows:

Very common—76% or greater
Common—51% to 75%
Uncommon—26% to 50%
Rare—25% or less

Each chapter contains data concerning prevalence and pathogenesis, clinical history, physical examination, laboratory data, radiographic evaluation, differential diagnosis, treatment, and prognosis for each disease.

The emphasis of each chapter is geared toward a review of neck pain as it pertains to each illness. The chapter should not be considered a complete listing of all clinical characteristics associated with each disease. Those factors that help the clinician recognize the underlying cause of the patient's neck pain and make the appropriate diagnosis are the ones listed.

The section is divided into chapters according to primary disease processes, which include the following:

Mechanical disorders
Rheumatologic disorders
Infections
Tumors and infiltrative lesions
Endocrinologic and heritable disorders
Neurologic and psychiatric disorders
Referred Pain
Miscellaneous

Discussion of diseases that are only very rarely associated with neck pain and are not included under the subheadings of these chapters may be found in the differential diagnosis section under each subheading. For example, hyperparathyroidism is included in the differential diagnosis section of microcrystalline diseases.

Referred pain, although not in itself a primary disease process, is another major source of patients' complaints of neck pain. Chapter 16, Referred Pain, includes disorders of vascular and gastrointestinal origin that are associated with neck pain.

10

Mechanical Disorders of the Cervical Spine

Mechanical disorders of the cervical spine are the most common cause of neck pain. Mechanical neck pain may be defined as pain secondary to overuse of a normal anatomic structure (muscle strain) or pain secondary to injury or deformity of an anatomic structure (herniated nucleus pulposus). Mechanical disorders are local disorders of the spine. That is, the processes that cause pain are limited to structures of the cervical spine. Mechanical disorders are truly musculoskeletal diseases. Systemic complications with involvement of other organ systems (except the nervous system) are not associated with mechanical disorders. The presence of systemic illness (e.g., fever, weight loss, or anemia) should make the clinician look for a disease other than a mechanical disorder as the cause of the patient's symptoms and signs.

Mechanical disorders are characteristically exacerbated by certain activities and relieved by others. The pattern of aggravating and alleviating factors helps localize the disorder to particular portions of the cervical spine; for example, neck flexion exacerbates disc disease but alleviates apophyseal joint disorders. The physical examination helps identify those individuals with neurologic dysfunction and significant muscle damage but is not sufficient to pinpoint the exact location of the injury. Laboratory data, in the form of electrophysiologic tests, can confirm the clinical suspicion of nerve impingement. By radiologic evaluation of a patient with a mechanical disorder, the physician may be able to identify anatomic alterations in the cervical spine but not necessarily be able to correlate those changes with the patient's symptoms. The physician must take all of the clinical data together and formulate a working diagnosis that is reasonable, based on the collected information.

Mechanical disorders, for the most part, are self-limited in duration such that the majority of these patients will improve, given enough time. The physician, however, needs to be constantly alert to the possibility of a serious complication like a myelopathy with resultant paralysis that is associated with cervical spondylosis. Common sense and an ever-present vigilance is required in the evaluation and therapy of these patients. Most patients improve with controlled physical activity, nonaddictive nonsteroidal anti-inflammatory drugs and, in appropriate patients, muscle relaxants. Surgical intervention is reserved for those patients who have not shown improvement on conservative therapy and have definitive symptoms and signs associated with a mechanical disorder.

NECK STRAIN

Capsule Summary

Frequency of neck pain—very common
Location of neck pain—neck, between scapula, top of shoulders
Quality of neck pain—ache, spasm, intermittent sharp twinges
Symptoms and signs—pain increased with any motion of the neck, headache, decreased range of motion
Laboratory and x-ray tests—none
Treatment—controlled physical activity and neck collar, medications

Prevalence and Pathogenesis

Neck strain can be defined as nonradiating neck pain associated with a mechanical stress or a prolonged abnormal position (sleeping with the neck twisted) of the cervical spine.[1] It is really a clinical condition describing a nonradiating discomfort or pain about the neck area associated with a concomitant loss of neck motion (stiffness). The exact number of patients with neck strain is unknown. It is a very common occurrence and presents with a range of severity. Almost 85% of neck pain results from acute or repetitive neck injuries or chronic stresses and strain.[2]

The etiology of neck strain is usually not clear but may be related to ligamentous or muscular problems secondary to either a specific traumatic episode or continuous mechanical stress. The major biomechanical function of the cervical spine is to support the skull and provide movement in flexion, extension, and rotation. Injury to the anatomic structures (facet joints, muscles, and ligaments) that provide these motions can easily occur because the supporting structures are relatively unprotected. Except for a traumatic injury to a particular structure, the specific abnormality in neck strain can almost never be identified.

Trauma to the cervical muscles that results in a strain may occur from mere elongation of muscle fibers with subsequent edema to rupture of muscle and secondary hemorrhage.[3] The response of the muscle to injury is contraction with reflex recruitment of surrounding muscles for protection. This protective spasm is an autonomic reflex. The contracted state decreases blood flow and produces relative anaerobic conditions in the injured muscle. The buildup of by-products of anaerobic metabolism causes nociceptive nerves to signal pain messages to the central nervous system.

The contracted state may occur secondary to environmental trauma, posture, or increased muscle tension. Environmental trauma (whiplash and subluxation) is discussed later in this chapter. Normal posture is effortless and painless. Abnormal forward posture of the head results in chronic strain on the posterior structures of the neck, including the paracervical muscles. The position of the head results in a drooping of the shoulders and a decrease in vital lung capacity. Postural tension is related to tonic isometric contraction of the extensor neck muscles. A variety of activities of daily living may result in chronic abnormal postures, such as the prolonged use of a computer with a screen below eye level, a faulty sitting position, or the use of bifocal glasses.

The tension of muscles is controlled by the interaction of spindle organs, Golgi's tendon organs, and extrafusal nerve fibers. The Golgi's organs or neurotendinous endings are large myelinated group IB afferent axons that lie in the musculotendinous junction and are stimulated by tension applied to the tendon during muscle contraction or, to a lesser extent, by passive stretching. The sensory endings are arranged in series with the muscle extrafusal fibers. Stimulation of these Golgi's nerves results in an inhibition of alpha motor neuron discharges to the corresponding muscle.[4] Muscle spindles have up to eight muscle fibers in a fluid-containing connective tissue capsule and are present in voluntary muscles. The contractile portion of the intrafusal muscle fibers is supplied with gamma efferent nerves, and the noncontractile portion is supplied with group IA afferent nerves (annulospiral endings) and group II flower-spray nerve endings that are arranged in parallel with the extrafusal fibers. Both types of nerves are tonic receptors that are depolarized by stretch. Stretching of extrafusal fibers applies tension to the spindle afferents, whereas extrafusal contraction relaxes the spindle fibers.

A balance exists between the impulses from the Golgi's apparatus stimulated by tendon stretch and the activity of the spindle fibers and muscle tension. This system coordinates muscular length, rate of contraction, tension, and relaxation of opposing muscles. This sensor feedback system allows for the generation of appropriate muscle power for the physical task. When the muscle is contracted, the Golgi organ is stimulated and the spindle system is unstimulated. When the muscle is stretched, nerve impulses from the Golgi's organs and spindle system are generated. With contraction of the extrafusal fibers, the intrafusal fibers (spindle system) record the change in muscle length and the Golgi's organs record muscle force and tension. The gamma neurons that set the tension of the spindle fibers also affect the system. Increased stimulation of the gamma fibers affects the sensory fibers, resulting in increased sensitivity of the muscle to tension. Passive stretching of the muscle when obtaining a tendon reflex produces afferent discharges that result in alpha neuron stimulation causing the muscle to contract to regain its original length, a monosynaptic reflex. In contrast, persistent muscle stretch produces stimulation of all afferent receptors, resulting in a polysynaptic reflex, eliciting alterations in gamma fiber stimulation and tonic or continuous muscle contraction.[4] Postural tone is the state of partial contraction of muscles needed to maintain a particular posture of the body, including the neck. The extent of gamma fiber stimulation sets the level of tone in the skeletal muscle system. With increased tone, the skeletal muscle may demonstrate rigidity or spasticity. Coordinating systems in the spinal cord and the cerebral cortex influence the setpoint of the balance between the two systems. Nerves from the reticulospinal tract have an inhibitory effect on the stretch reflex. Multisynaptic reflex arcs from the cerebellum, basal ganglia, and brainstem influence the level of excitability of the reticulospinal tract. The control of tone of muscles is a multifactorial process. Thought processes in the cerebral cortex can be manifested by alterations in function of other components of the nervous system, resulting in stress and increased muscle tone.[4]

Between contractions the muscle is able to relax. Relaxation is important for maintenance of muscle function. Relaxation allows for restoration of internal blood flow, removal of metabolic by-products, and influx of nutrients. Chronically contracted muscles develop subsequent ischemia and pain. In addition to direct effects on paracervical muscles, sustained muscle contraction may cause sustained intervertebral disc compression. Disc degeneration may result from persistent contraction because intervertebral discs are less able to imbibe nutrients when contracted.

Muscles may undergo isotonic or isometric contractions. Isotonic contractions occur with the same tension through the range of motion of the muscle while moving a constant load. Isometric contractions occur with increased tension without shortening of the muscle. Most contractions are hybrids, involving both load-bearing and shortening. Eccentric contractions occur when muscles are stretched while generating tension. Walking downstairs requires eccentric contractions.

A variety of factors extraneous to the muscles affect muscle tension. Factors such as fatigue, pain, anger, emotional stress, anxiety, and depression affect the level of muscle tension.[2] Spasm in the cervical muscles can cause pain in the occipital area that may radiate into the temples and frontal area.[5] Discrepancies exist between electromyography studies measuring the degree of muscle contraction and the degrees of pain.[4] A cycle of pain and spasm may result in persistence of symptoms from relatively insignificant events. During the evaluation it may be difficult to ascertain whether pain or spasm was the initiating factor causing the patient's symptoms and signs.[6]

Clinical History

Pain is the most common presenting symptom, although the associated complaint of a headache is not unusual. The pain is usually located in the middle to lower part of the posterior aspect of the neck. The area of pain can be limited to a small local point (unilateral) or can cover a diffuse area (bilateral). The pain may not radiate into the arms but may radiate toward the shoulders. A history of injury is rarely obtained but the pain may commence after a night's awkward sleep, turning the head rapidly, or coughing or sneezing.

The pain associated with a neck sprain is most often a dull, aching pain that is exacerbated by neck motion. The pain is usually abated by rest or immobilization. The pain may be referred to other mesenchymal structures derived from a similar sclerotome during embryogenesis. Common referred pain patterns include the scapular area, the posterior shoulder, the occipital area, or the anterior chest wall (cervical angina pectoris). Those referred pain patterns do not indicate a true radicular pain pattern and are not usually mechanical (nerve compression) in origin.

Physical Examination

Physical examination of patients with neck strain usually reveals nothing more than a locally tender area(s) just lateral to the spine. The intensity of pain is variable, and the loss of cervical motion correlates directly with the pain intensity. The presence of true spasm, defined as a continuous muscle contraction, is rare except in severe cases in which the head may be tilted to one side (torticollis). Muscles most commonly affected include the sternocleidomastoid and the trapezius. Active motion of the cervical spine against any type of resistance causes an increase in pain. Slow passive movement of the neck may allow for a greater arc of motion than determined during the active motion portion of the examination.

Other than the preceding abnormalities, the remainder of the physical examination is normal. Specifically the neurologic examination as well as the shoulder examination is normal.

Laboratory Data

Laboratory tests are normal in patients with neck strain.

Radiographic Evaluation

Radiographic evaluation of patients with neck strain is normal. On occasion, muscle spasm may be great enough to cause some straightening of the normal lordosis of the cervical spine (Fig. 10–1). This is a nonspecific finding and only indicates that there is significant muscle spasm secondary to pain. The presence of straightening of the cervical spine may be related as frequently to the positioning of the patient as to the presence of acute or chronic neck pain.[7] Thus, if the physician feels confident of the diagnosis of mechanical neck strain, a roentgenographic evaluation during the initial evaluation is not necessary. However, if the pain has not markedly resolved after 2 weeks or the patient develops other

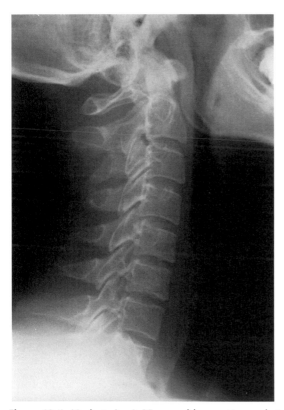

Figure 10–1. Neck strain. A 35-year-old computer analyst with a 4-month history of neck pain and muscle contraction of the trapezius and paracervical muscles. Lateral view of cervical spine demonstrates straightening of the cervical spine with loss of lordosis and normal intervertebral disc spaces.

TABLE 10–1. CONGENITAL ABNORMALITIES OF THE CERVICAL SPINE

CRANIO-OCCIPITAL DEFECTS	**INCREASED RISK OF INJURY**
Basilar impression[11]	Sharp clivoaxial angle
Hypoplasia of the occiput[12]	Atlanto-occipital subluxation
Occipitalization of the atlas[13]	Constriction of foramen magnum
ATLANTOAXIAL DEFECT	Arnold-Chiari malformation (cerebellar tonsil ectopy)
Os odontoideum[14]	
Aplasia—arch of atlas[15]	
Aplasia—arch of axis[16]	**ATLANTOAXIAL INSTABILITY**
Laxity transverse atlantal ligament[8]	
LOWER CERVICAL SPINE	**MYELOPATHY**
Klippel-Feil syndrome[17]	
Spondylolisthesis[18]	
Spina bifida[9]	

physical findings, then a cervical spine roentgenogram should be obtained to rule out other serious etiologies, such as neoplasia and instability.

Unlike in the lumbar spine, congenital abnormalities are rare in the neck. The most common is block vertebrae, in which two bodies are congenitally fused together. The term Klippel-Feil syndrome is used to identify all patients with congenital fusion of the cervical vertebrae that involve two segments, block vertebrae, or the entire cervical spine.[8] Individuals with extensive fusions have a recognizably abnormal appearance and severe disability during childhood. These individuals also have anomalies in other parts of the body, including renal abnormalities, scoliosis, Sprengel's deformity (undescended scapula), and facial anomalies (Apert's syndrome).[9] On physical examination they have a short neck, low hairline, and limited range of motion of the neck. Individuals with an autosomal dominant trait may have another form of Klippel-Feil syndrome associated with cervical fusion (block vertebrae) with segmental abnormalities in the thoracic and lumbar spine. The patients with the most benign form of Klippel-Feil syndrome are those with a single segment fusion.[10] Theoretically this abnormality could cause instability (increased motion) above or below the fused vertebrae because of increased stress. Although lateral flexion and extension x-ray films should be taken to determine the extent of motion, there is rarely an associated problem (Table 10–1).

Other congenital abnormalities may be confused with fracture on roentgenograms or may predispose to clinical symptoms because of anatomic relationships that increase the risk of damage from minor trauma, for example, accessory ossicles around the odontoid; overlying shadows from the pinna or teeth; Mach effect from overlapping shadows of the posterior arch of C1, the tongue, or occiput; or persistence of odontoid synchondrosis may simulate a pathologic process.[19, 20]

Differential Diagnosis

The diagnosis of neck strain is based on the history of localized neck pain and a compatible physical examination demonstrating localized pain, muscle spasm, and a normal neurologic examination. The symptoms of neck strain, however, may be components of the list of complaints mentioned by patients with a wide variety of disease processes, including spondyloarthropathies and tumors. Muscle spasm is a reflex that occurs in response to bone or joint inflammation and is a very nonspecific finding. The age of the patient, the presence of constitutional symptoms, or the persistence of pain should alert the physician to a cause other than a strain.

Trauma to the cervical spine can result in major neural damage with paralysis. If a history of significant trauma is obtained, a thorough evaluation including x-ray films should be performed. Because of the significant consequences of potential damage to the spinal cord, it is recommended that the expertise of an orthopedic surgeon or neurosurgeon be sought for the evaluation of patients with cervical spine trauma.

A variety of mechanical disorders cause neck and arm pain. These disorders may be differentiated by factors that exacerbate and alleviate neck and arm symptoms (Table 10–2).

Torticollis. Torticollis is associated with severe muscle contracture of the neck. The neck is fixed in side flexion with the chin rotated away from the painful side. Torticollis can be congenital or acquired. Congenital torticollis is associated with anatomic or neurologic abnormalities including Klippel-Feil syndrome, atlantoaxial subluxation, congenital absence of cervical muscles, Arnold-Chiari malformation, and syringomyelia.[21] Acquired torticollis may occur in the setting of trauma, muscle injury, fracture, or atlantoaxial subluxation; infection such as upper respiratory infection, cervical adenitis, osteomyelitis, and fasciitis; postinfections, influenza, or diphtheria; neoplasm; scar; vascular abnormalities with compression; drugs such as phenothiazines; nerve disorders; syringomyelia; dystonia; or herniated disc.[22, 23] Spasmodic torticollis occurs equally in both sexes, in the fourth or fifth decades, and may be considered a form of segmental dystonia. Early in the course of the movement, the tilt may be corrected with pressure on the chin. When the process becomes chronic, the contracture becomes painful with tonic spasm of sternocleidomastoid and secondary cervical osteoarthritis. The evaluation of the patients with torticollis includes radiography, computerized tomography, or magnetic resonance imaging, to determine the presence of anatomic abnormalities associated with congenital or acquired torticollis. Therapy of torticollis includes local trigger-point injections (lidocaine and corticosteroids), cooling spray and stretching, range-of-motion exercises, or drug therapy (benztropine, amantadine, and haloperidol).[22] In severe cases, botulinum toxin injection is indicated.[24] Surgical denervation is indicated in patients resistant to all medical therapy.[25] In patients with spasmodic torticollis who respond to botulinum toxin therapy, selective peripheral denervation of the posterior branches of the cervical roots may be helpful, as it was helpful for 76% of patients reported

TABLE 10–2. MECHANICAL NECK PAIN

	NECK STRAIN	HERNIATED NUCLEUS PULPOSUS	OSTEOARTHRITIS	MYELOPATHY	WHIPLASH
Age (years)	20–40	30–50	>50	>60	30–40
Pain pattern					
Location	Neck	Arm	Neck	Arm/Leg	Neck
Onset	Acute	Acute	Insidious	Insidious	Acute
Flexion	+	+	−	−	+
Extension	−	+/−	+	+	+
Plain x-ray	−	−	+	+	−

+ present
− absent

by Braun and Richter.[26] Torticollis is occasionally associated with psychopathology (hysteria). These individuals require biofeedback or psychotherapy. Patients with spasmodic torticollis of any etiology require therapy. In a study of 116 patients, only 14 patients (12%) had a spontaneous remission.[27]

Treatment

The mainstay of treatment of neck strain includes controlled physical activity and immobilization in a soft cervical orthosis. It is important that the patient wear the collar at night. During sleep, the neck is at greatest risk of undergoing abnormal movements or assuming unnatural positions. Convincing the patient to limit activities is a primary goal of therapy. Decreased activity allows the injured tissues to heal. The time spent by the physician explaining the rationale for controlled physical activity to the patient is well worth the effort.

Nonnarcotic analgesics in the form of nonsteroidal anti-inflammatory drugs are helpful in making patients comfortable. These drugs may be continued until the patient's symptoms have resolved. Muscle relaxants may be helpful in the patient who has palpable spasm on physical examination or has difficulty sleeping at night. Physical therapy modalities may take the form of cold (ice) initially or heat (warm bath) subsequently. Intermittent lightweight cervical traction may decrease pain and diminish spasm. Patients with localized pain and severe spasm limiting mobility may benefit from an injection of anesthetic with or without the addition of corticosteroids. The injection relieves pain and blocks reflex spasm. These injections are indicated after 2 to 4 weeks of rest and medication without significant improvement. Finally, once the patient starts to improve, a course of isometric exercises should begin. Neck pain and mobility are improved with physiotherapy.[28] Modification of the position of the patient while at work may help decrease neck pain. Relief of chronic muscle contraction is associated with pain relief.[29]

Prognosis

The course of patients with neck strain is one of progressive improvement with complete resolution of the symptoms over several weeks. The recovery is total without any lasting impairment. A small percentage of patients may continue to experience neck pain in spite of adequate treatment. Pain may continue for months or years. These patients must be evaluated and treated in a manner that takes into account the special difficulties of individuals with chronic pain. The goal of therapy is to maximize function of the cervical spine. These patients may receive drugs, physical therapy, psychiatric support, and vocational rehabilitation as part of their therapeutic regimen.

The preceding discussion does not include patients who have associated compensation or litigation cases. These patients have special problems and needs with different projected outcomes. The broad topic of occupational injuries is in Chapter 20. Hyperextension (whiplash) injuries are discussed in the final section of this chapter.

References

NECK STRAIN

1. DePalma AP, Rothman RH: The Intervertebral Disc. Philadelphia, WB Saunders Co, 1970, pp 58–92.
2. Jackson R. Cervical trauma: not just another pain in the neck. Geriatrics 37:123, 1982.
3. Cailliet R: Neck and Arm Pain, 3rd ed. Philadelphia: FA Davis Co, 1991, pp 55–80.
4. Walton J: Brain's Diseases of the Nervous System, 9th ed. New York: Oxford University Press, 1985, pp 27–29.
5. Kunkel RS: Muscle contraction (tension) headache. Clin J Pain 5:39, 1989.
6. Ashton-Miller JA, McGlashen KM, Herzenberg JE, Stohler CS: Cervical muscle myoelectric response to acute experimental sternocleidomastoid pain. Spine 15:1006, 1990.
7. Helliwell PS, Evans PF, Wright V: The straight cervical spine: does it indicate muscle spasm? J Bone Joint Surg 76B:103, 1994.
8. Hensinger RN: Congenital anomalies of the cervical spine. Clin Orthop 264:16, 1991.
9. Sherk HH, Whitaker LA, Pasquariello PS: Facial malformations and spinal anomalies: a predictable relationship. Spine 7:526, 1982.
10. Bland JH: Congenital anomalies. In: Bland JH (ed): Disorders of the Cervical Spine, 2nd ed. Philadelphia: WB Saunders Co, 1994, pp 417–431.
11. DeBarros MC, Farias W, Ataide L, Lins S: Basilar impression and Arnold-Chiari malformation: a study of 66 cases. J Neurol Neurosurg Psychiatry 31:596, 1968.
12. Sherk HH: Lesions of the atlas and axis. Clin Orthop 109:33, 1975.
13. Bharucha EP, Dastur HM: Craniovertebral anomalies: a report on 40 cases. Brain 87:469, 1964.
14. Fielding JW, Hensinger RN, Hawkins RJ: Os odontoideum. J Bone Joint Surg 62A:376, 1980.
15. Dubousett J: Torticollis in children caused by congenital anomalies of the atlas. J Bone Joint Surg 68A:178, 1986.
16. Hanson EC, Shook JE, Wiesseman GJ, Wood VE: Congenital pedicle defects of the axis vertebra: report of a case. Spine 15:236, 1990.
17. Hensinger RN, Lang JR, MacEwen GD: The Klippel-

Feil syndrome: a constellation of related anomalies. J Bone Joint Surg 56A:1246, 1974.

18. Charlton DP, Gehweileer JA, Morgan CL, et al.: Spondylolysis and spondylolisthesis of the cervical spine. Skeletal Radiol 3:79, 1978.
19. Keats TE: Atlas of Normal Roentgen Variants that May Simulate Disease, 5th ed. St Louis: Mosby-Year Book, 1992, pp 143–229.
20. Kim KS, Rogers LF, Regenbogen V: Pitfalls in plain film diagnosis of cervical spine injuries: false positive interpretation. Surg Neurol 25:381, 1986.
21. Kiwak K: Establishing an etiology for torticollis. Postgrad Med 75:129, 1984.
22. Gilbert RL, Warfield CA: Neck Pain. In: Warfield CA (ed): Principles and Practice of Pain Management. New York: McGraw-Hill Book Co, 1994, pp 109–121.
23. Shima F, Fukui M, Matsubara T, Kitamura K: Spasmodic torticollis caused by vascular compression of the spinal accessory root. Surg Neurol 26:431, 1986.
24. Jankovic J, Brin MF: Therapeutic uses of botulinum toxin. N Engl J Med 324:1186, 1991.
25. Duvoisin RC: Spasmodic torticollis: the role of surgical denervation. Mayo Clin Proc 66:433, 1991.
26. Braun V, Richter H: Selective peripheral denervation for the treatment of spasmodic torticollis. Neurosurgery 35:58, 1994.
27. Shoen RP: Soft tissue cervical spine syndromes. In: Bland JH (ed): Disorders of the Cervical Spine, 2nd ed. Philadelphia: WB Saunders Co, 1994, pp 365–372.
28. Koes BW, Bouter LM, van Mameren H, et al.: The effectiveness of manual therapy, physiotherapy, and treatment by the general practitioner for nonspecific back and neck complaints: a randomized clinical trial. Spine 17:28, 1992.
29. Harms-Ringdahl K, Ekholm J: Intensity and character of pain and muscular activity levels elicited by maintained extreme flexion position of the lower-cervical–upper-thoracic spine. Scand J Rehabil Med 18;117, 1986.

ACUTE HERNIATED NUCLEUS PULPOSUS

Capsule Summary

Frequency of neck pain—common

Location of neck pain—neck to distal arm and hand

Quality of neck pain—sharp, shooting, burning with paresthesias in the hand

Symptoms and signs—positive compression test, weakness in the arms and hands, asymmetric reflexes

Laboratory and x-ray tests—computerized tomography, magnetic resonance imaging, myelogram

Treatment—controlled activity, medication, cervical collar, injection, surgical excision of disc on failure of conservative therapy

Prevalence and Pathogenesis

A herniated disc can be defined as the protrusion of the nucleus pulposus through the fibers of the annulus fibrosus.[1] The description of disc herniation was initially lesions in the lumbar spine. In the early 1940s, a number of reports appeared describing cervical intervertebral disc herniation with radiculopathy.[2–4] There is a direct correlation between the anatomy of the cervical spine and the location and pathophysiology of disc lesions.[5] The eight cervical nerve roots exit via intervertebral foramina that are bordered anterormedially by the intervertebral disc and posterolaterally by the zygopophyseal joint. The formina are largest at C2–C3 and decrease in size until C6–C7. The nerve root occupies 25% to 33% of the volume of the foramen. The C1 root exists between the occiput and the atlas (C1). All lower roots exit above their corresponding cervical vertebrae (the C6 root at the C5–C6 interspace), except C8, which exits between C7–T1. A differential growth rate affects the relationship of the spinal cord and nerve roots and the cervical spine. The lower cervical vertebrae are at the same level as the next lower cord segment.[5] The C5–C6 interspace is opposite the C7 cord level where the C7 nerve root arises and the C6 root exits. The sinuvertebral nerve (SVN) is the primary innervation of the intervertebral disc.[6] The SVN originates from both the ventral primary ramus (somatic) and gray rami communicantes (autonomic) at each segmental level. The nerve runs back into the neural foramen and branches to supply innervation to structures in a variety of patterns, including one segment above and below the foramen, multiple levels above and below, and on the or contralateral side.[7] Nerve fibers supply the periosteum of the pedicle, vertebral body, epidural veins, dura mater, and the annulus fibrosus.[8] The innervation of the annulus runs parallel and perpendicular to the fibers of the annulus fibrosus. The nerves are most numerous in the middle third of the disc. The nerve receptors have Pacini's corpuscles, Golgi tendon organs, and free nerve endings.[9] These nerve endings mediate proprioception, tension, and pain.

Most acute disc herniations occur posterolaterally and in patients around the fourth decade of life when the nucleus is still gelatinous. The most common areas of disc herniation are C6–C7 and C5–C6. The C7 nerve root is affected in 37% to 75.6% of individuals reported in large studies with cervical radiculopathy.[10–13] The same studies reported frequency of C6 radiculopathy of 15.8% to 48%. C7–T1 and C3–C4 disc herniations are infrequent (less than 15%). Disc herniation of C2–C3 is rare. Unlike the lumbar herniated disc, the cervical herniated disc may cause myelopathy in addition to radicular pain because of the spinal cord in the cervical region.[14] The uncovertebral prominences play a role in the location of ruptured disc material. Pure nerve root compression occurs if extruded disc material enters into the nerve root canal. The uncovertebral joint tends to guide extruded disc material medially where cord compression may also occur.

The disc herniation usually affects the nerve root numbered most caudally for the given disc level; for example, C3–C4 disc affects the fourth cervical nerve root, C4–C5 the fifth cervical nerve root, C5–C6 the sixth cervical nerve root, C6–C7 the seventh cervical nerve root, and C7–T1 the eighth cervical nerve root. Individual disc herniations do not involve other roots but more commonly present some evidence of upper motor neuron findings secondary to spinal cord compression.

Not every herniated disc is symptomatic. The presence of symptoms depends on the spinal canal reserve capacity, the presence of inflammation, the size of the herniation, as well as the presence of concomitant disease such as osteophyte formation. In disc rupture, protrusion of nuclear material results in tension on annular fibers and compression of the dura or nerve root causing pain.

Cervical radiculopathies have been divided into two categories according to the hardness of the disc lesion. Individuals usually younger than 45 years of age have soft disc lesions associated with herniation of the nucleus pulposus, resulting in nerve root or cord compression. Hard disc lesions, produced by disc calcifications or osteophytes, occur in individuals older than 45 years of age. Soft disc lesions resolve more frequently than hard disc lesions. Hard discs are more closely associated with cord compression.

Clinical History

Clinically, the patient's major complaint is arm pain, not neck pain. The pain is often perceived as starting in the neck area and then radiating from this point down the shoulder, arm, and forearm, and usually into the hand. The onset of the radicular pain is often gradual, although there can be a sudden onset associated with a tearing or snapping sensation. As time passes, the magnitude of the arm pain clearly exceeds that of the neck or shoulder pain. The arm pain may also be variable in intensity, precluding any use of the arm without a range from severe pain to a dull, cramping ache in the arm muscles. The pain is usually severe enough to awaken the patient at night. Additionally, a patient may complain of associated headaches as well as muscle spasm, which can radiate from the cervical spine to below the scapulae. The pain may also radiate into the chest, mimicking angina (pseudoangina), or the breast.[15, 16] Symptoms including back pain, leg pain, leg weakness, gait disturbance, or incontinence suggest compression of the spinal cord.

Physical Examination

Physical examination of the neck usually shows some limitation of motion, and on occasion the patient may tilt the head in a cocked-robin position (torticollis) toward the side of the herniated cervical disc. Extension of the spine often exacerbates the pain as the intervertebral foramina are narrowed further (Spurling's sign). Axial compression, Valsalva's maneuver, and coughing may also exacerbate or re-create the pain pattern.

A neurologic examination that shows abnormalities is the most helpful aspect of the diagnostic workup, although the examination may remain normal despite a chronic radicular pattern. Even when a deficit exists it may not be related temporarily to the present symptoms but to a prior attack at a different level. To be significant, the examination must show objective signs of reflex diminution, motor weakness, or atrophy. Manual muscle testing has greater specificity than reflex or sensory abnormalities.[13] The presence of atrophy helps document the location of the lesion as well as its chronicity. The presence of subjective sensory changes is often difficult to interpret and requires a coherent and cooperative patient to be of clinical value. Paresthesias are poorly localized because a number of nerve roots may result in a similar pain distribution. The presence of sensory changes alone is usually not enough to confirm the diagnosis.

Compression of individual spinal nerve roots results in alterations in motor, sensory, and reflex functions (Table 10–3). When the third cervical nerve root is compressed, no reflex change or motor weakness can be identified. The pain radiates to the back of the neck and toward the mastoid process and pinna of the ear.

Involvement of the fourth cervical nerve root leads to no readily detectable reflex changes or motor weakness. The pain radiates

TABLE 10–3. MOTOR, SENSORY, AND REFLEX DISTRIBUTION OF CERVICAL ROOTS

INTERSPACE	ROOT	MOTOR WEAKNESS	SENSORY	REFLEXES
C4–C5	C5	Deltoid, biceps Shoulder abduction External rotation	Axillary patch, Proximal arm	Biceps (brachioradialis)
C5–C6	C6	Biceps, wrist extensors Elbow flexion (scapular winging)	Thumb, Index finger	Brachioradialis
C6–C7	C7	Triceps Elbow extension Wrist and finger extension, pronation	Long finger, Ring finger	Triceps
C7–T1	C8	Finger flexors Wrist flexors Thumb opposition Finger abduction	Little finger Hypothenar Medial forearm	Finger flexors

into the back of the neck and into the superior aspect of the scapula. Occasionally, the pain radiates into the anterior chest wall. The pain is often exacerbated by neck extension.

Unlike the third and fourth cervical nerve roots, the fifth through the eighth cervical nerve roots have motor functions. Compression of the fifth cervical nerve root is characterized by weakness of shoulder abduction usually above 90° and weakness of shoulder extension. The biceps reflexes are often depressed and the pain radiates from the side of the neck to the top of the shoulder. Decreased sensation is often noted in the lateral aspect of the deltoid, representing the autonomous innervation area of the axillary nerve.

Involvement of the sixth cervical nerve root produces biceps muscle weakness as well as a diminished brachioradialis reflex. The pain again radiates from the neck down the lateral arm and forearm into the radial side of hand (index finger, long finger, and thumb). Numbness occurs occasionally in the tip of the index finger, the autonomous area of the sixth cervical nerve root.

Compression of the seventh cervical nerve root produces reflex changes in the triceps jerk with associated loss of strength in the triceps muscles, which extend the elbow. The pain from this lesion radiates from the lateral neck down the middle of the area into the middle finger. Sensory changes occur often in the tip of the middle finger, the autonomous area for the seventh nerve. Patients should also be tested for scapular winging that may occur with C6 or C7 radiculopathy.[17]

Finally, involvement of the eighth cervical nerve root by a herniated C7–T1 disc produces a significant weakness of the intrinsic musculature of the hand. This involvement can lead to a rapid atrophy of the interosseous muscles

because of the small size of these muscles. Loss of the interossei leads to significant loss in fine hand motion. No reflexes are easily found, although the flexor carpi ulnaris reflex may be decreased. The radicular pain from the eighth cervical nerve root radiates into the ulnar border of the hand and the ring and little fingers. The tip of the little finger often demonstrates a diminished sensation.

Nerve root sensitivity can be elicited by a method that increases the tension of the nerve root. Radicular arm pain is often increased by the Valsalva's maneuver or by directly compressing the head. Radicular pain secondary to a herniated cervical disc may be relieved with abduction of the affected arm.[18] Although these signs are helpful when present, their absence alone does not rule out a nerve root lesion.

Laboratory Data

All of the serum laboratory blood tests are normal in patients with a herniated disc. Electromyelography (EMG) findings may be positive in patients with nerve root impingement. Evidence of positive waves, giant potentials, and insertional irritability suggest radiculopathy associated with significant nerve root impingement.[19] EMG findings become much more significant in the presence of historical and physical findings consistent with herniation of a disc. EMG and myelography correlate with the level of disc herniation in from 77% to 90% of cases studied.[20, 21]

EMG is an electronic extension of the physical examination. The primary use of EMG is to diagnose radiculopathy in cases of questionable neurologic origin. Although it is 80% to 90% accurate in establishing cervical radiculopathy as the cause of pain, false negative results do occur. If cervical radiculopathy affects the sensory root only, EMG will be unable to demonstrate an abnormality. A false negative examination also occurs if the patient with acute symptoms is examined early (4 to 28 days from onset of symptoms). A normal study should be repeated in 2 to 3 weeks if symptoms persist.

Radiographic Evaluation

Plain radiographs may be entirely normal in a patient with an acute herniated cervical disc. Conversely, 70% of asymptomatic women and 95% of asymptomatic men between the ages of 60 and 65 years have evidence of degenerative disc disease on plain roentgenogram.[22] Views to be obtained include anteroposterior, lateral, flexion, and extension. Oblique views are optional because they increase the cost and radiation exposure without supplying significant additional information.[5] Plain roentgenograms may be used as an initial screening test for those individuals who have failed conservative therapy, who have sustained trauma to the cervical spine, or who are 60 years of age or older with new symptoms of neck pain.

Additional radiographic studies are indicated for individuals with myelopathic signs, progressive neurologic deficit, treatment failure, and consideration for surgical intervention. Myelography identifies neural compression indirectly by the changes in the contour of structures outlined by water-soluble contrast agents, such as iohexol and iopamidol. This invasive procedure requires the introduction of dye through a lateral cisternal puncture at C1–C2. Myelography is able to visualize the entire length of the cervical spine and identify unsuspected abnormalities.[23] Myelography is useful for identifying the exact level of nerve root impingement. In a study of 53 patients with surgical confirmation of nerve compression, myelography accurately identified disc abnormalities in 85% of them.[24] Diagnostic inaccuracies occur secondary to small central disc protrusions and bone spurs. Cervical myelograms have been shown to be abnormal in 21% of asymptomatic individuals without neck or arm pain.[25]

Computerized tomography (CT) permits direct visualization of compression of neural structures and therefore is more precise than myelography. The advantages of CT over myelography include better visualization of lateral abnormalities such as foraminal stenosis

and of abnormalities caudal to the myelographic block, less radiation exposure, and no hospitalization. From the surgical perspective CT is best at distinguishing soft disc compression from hard bony compression.[26] Disadvantages of CT include length of time to complete the study and changes in spinal configuration between motion segments. Myelographic dye may be injected and CT images obtained. The combination of the two studies gives excellent differentiation of bone and soft tissue lesions and allows direct demonstration of the spinal cord and the spinal canal dimensions. The CT-myelogram is accurate in 96% of cervical lesions.

Magnetic resonance (MR) imaging allows excellent visualization of soft tissues, including a herniated disc in the cervical spine (Fig. 10–2). The test is noninvasive. In the cervical spine, in a study of 34 patients with cervical lesions, MR imaging predicted 88% of the surgically proven lesions, compared with 81% for myelography-CT, 58% for myelography, and 50% for CT alone.[27] Not all MR imaging disc abnormalities are symptomatic. In a study of 63 asymptomatic individuals, 19% had MR imaging abnormalities, including disc protrusion, that were identified by independent readings by three neuroradiologists.[28] This study highlights the importance of the correlation of clinical symptoms and signs with radiographic abnormalities. Exploratory MR imaging has a significant opportunity to find anatomic abnormalities that have no correlation with clinical symptoms. MR imaging is the radiographic technique of choice for the evaluation of cervical radiculopathy to confirm the presence of anatomic changes that explain clinical findings. MR imaging acquisition techniques (magnetization transfer) that allow for better delineation of disc herniation, foraminal stenosis, and intrinsic cord lesions continue to improve.[29]

Differential Diagnosis

The provisional diagnosis of a herniated cervical disc is made by the history and physical examination. Individuals who frequently lift heavy objects on the job, smoke, or frequently dive from a diving board are at increased risk for cervical disc herniation.[30] The plain roentgenogram is usually nondiagnostic, although occasionally disc space narrowing at the suspected interspace or foraminal narrowing on the oblique films is seen. The value of the roentgenograms is to exclude other causes of

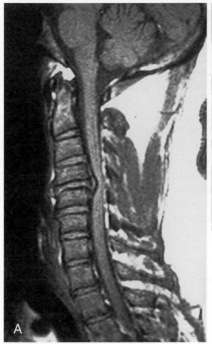
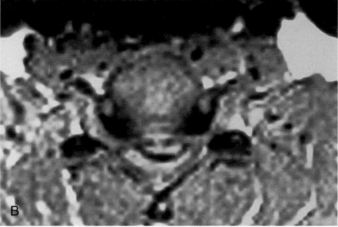

Figure 10–2. Herniated cervical disc. A 35-year-old man with left upper arm pain and decreased biceps reflex. Magnetic resonance scan of cervical spine. *A,* Sagittal T_1-weighted image demonstrates a large disc herniation compressing the spinal cord. The spinal cord is reduced to a 3 mm anteroposterior diameter. *B,* Axial T_1-weighted image demonstrates central disc material compressing the spinal cord.

neck and arm pain, such as an infection and a tumor. MR imaging and CT-myelogram are the best confirmatory examinations for disc herniation.

Cervical disc herniations may affect structures other than nerve roots. Disc herniation may cause vessel compression (vertebral artery) associated with vertebrobasilar artery insufficiency, manifested by blurred vision and dizziness.[31] Nerve root compression secondary to disc herniation may be mimicked by anomalous vessels. Expansion of vertebral arteries in transverse foramina may compress contiguous nerve roots.[32]

Other mechanical causes of arm pain should be excluded. The most common is some form of compression on a peripheral nerve. This can occur at the elbow, forearm, or wrist. An example is compression of the median nerve by the carpal ligament, leading to carpal tunnel syndrome. The best diagnostic test to rule out these peripheral neuropathies is EMG. Excessive traction on the arm secondary to heavy weights may cause radicular pain without disc compression of nerve roots.[33] Spinal cord abnormalities must be considered if signs of myelopathy are present in combination with radiculopathy. Spinal cord lesions such as syringomyelia are identified by MR imaging, and motor neuron disease is identified by EMG. Multiple sclerosis should be considered in a patient with radiculopathy if physical signs in-

dicate lesions above the foramen magnum (optic neuritis).[34]

Treatment

The treatment for most patients with a herniated cervical disc is nonoperative because most patients respond to conservative treatment for 2 to 3 months. The efficacy of the nonoperative approach depends heavily on the physician-patient relationship. If a patient is well informed, insightful, and willing to follow instructions, the chances for a successful nonoperative outcome are greatly improved.

The cornerstone to the management of a herniated cervical disc is rest and immobilization. The use of a cervical orthosis greatly increases the likelihood that the patient will rest. Initially, the patient should remain at home resting in bed except for necessary trips to the bathroom.[5] Controlled physical activity should be maintained for at least 2 weeks and the patient should wear the cervical orthosis at all times. After the acute pain begins to abate, the patient should gradually increase activity and decrease the use of the orthosis. Most people are able to return to work in a month in a light-duty capacity.

Drug therapy is an important adjunct to controlled physical activity and immobilization. Anti-inflammatory medications, analgesics, and muscle relaxants have been used in the acute management of these patients. Because it is commonly believed that radicular pain is in part secondary to inflammation of the nerve root, the use of aspirin or other nonsteroidal anti-inflammatory drug (NSAID) is appropriate.[35] All these medications have gastrointestinal side effects but are generally well tolerated for brief periods. Medications, such as prostaglandin analogues, are available to protect the gastrointestinal tract in individuals who have had prior history of gastric ulcers, if NSAIDs are required for longer periods. Oral systemic corticosteroids administered in a tapering dosage for 7 days may provide relief in more refractory cases but should not be used routinely.[5] A trigger-point injection may give dramatic relief of referred muscle pain. Epidural corticosteroid injections have shown to improve cervical radicular pain. In a study of 16 patients, improvement of pain occurred in 12, with 6 of the same patients developing improvement of neurologic signs.[36] Cervical epidural injections are most helpful for those individuals with radicular pain in contrast to those with axial pain.[37] Epidural corticosteroid injections may also be helpful in decreasing pain in patients with cervical radicular pain lasting 12 months or longer.[38]

Analgesic medication is only rarely needed if the patient is compliant and approaches full bed rest with near total immobility; however, if the pain is severe enough, a brief course of oral codeine may be prescribed. If the patient is resistant to oral narcotic therapy, inpatient hospitalization for intramuscular narcotic may be required in rare circumstances. The muscle relaxants and the benzodiazepines have tranquilizing and central nervous system–depressant properties. As such, they have at best a limited role in the management of the acute herniated disc patients. Although it is true that the benzodiazepines help the patient relax and ensure rest, the potential for additive effect on the patient's psychosocial problems is not worth the long-term risk for the short-term gain.

Cervical traction is used to distract the interspace associated with disc herniation. Weights of up to 50 pounds are applied for periods of up to 60 seconds with the head flexed. Traction instruction is usually given by a physical therapist, and the traction may be applied by the patient at home. Traction is used up to 3 times a day for 15-minute sessions for 4 to 6 weeks. Although the efficacy of traction has not been proven, it is commonly used and thought to be of benefit.[5]

Prognosis

The majority of patients respond to nonoperative treatment. Even patients with MR-documented herniated cervical discs may have regression of the disc with conservative therapy.[39] Once these patients improve, they should be maintained on a graduated isometric neck exercise program. One in five patients fail conservative measures and require a surgical procedure. If performed with good surgical technique and for the correct clinical indications, surgery is successful for more than 90% of surgical patients. Anterior discectomy with fusion results in excellent outcomes in 94% of patients.[40]

References

ACUTE HERNIATED NUCLEUS PULPOSUS

1. Mixter WJ, Barr JS: Rupture of the intervertebral disc with involvement of the spinal canal. N Engl J Med 211:210, 1934.
2. Semmes RE, Murphey MF: The syndrome of unilateral rupture of the sixth cervical intervertebral disk with compression of the seventh cervical nerve root: a report of four cases with symptoms simulating coronary disease. JAMA 121:1209, 1943.
3. Spurling RG, Scoville WB: Lateral rupture of the cervical intervertebral discs: a common cause of shoulder and arm pain. Surg Gynecol Obstet 78:350, 1944.
4. Michelsen JJ, Mixter WJ: Pain and disability of shoulder and arm due to herniation of the nucleus pulposus of cervical intervertebral disks. N Engl J Med 231:279, 1944.
5. Ellenberg MR, Honet JC, Treanor WJ: Cervical radiculopathy. Arch Phys Med Rehabil 75:342, 1994.
6. Bogduk N, Windsor M, Inglis A: The innervation of the cervical intervertebral discs. Spine 13:2, 1988.
7. Groen GJ, Baljet B, Drukker J: Nerves and nerve plexuses of the human vertebral column. Am J Anat 188:282, 1990.
8. Chabot MC, Montgomery DM: The pathophysiology of axial and radicular neck pain. Semin Spine Surg 7:2, 1995.
9. Mendel T, Wink CS, Zimny ML: Neural elements in human cervical intervertebral discs. Spine 17:132, 1992.
10. Odom GL, Finney W, Woodhall B: Cervical disk lesions. JAMA 166:23, 1958.
11. Lundsford LD, Bissonette DJ, Jannetta PJ, et al.: Anterior surgery for cervical disc disease. Part 1: treatment of lateral cervical disc herniation in 253 cases. J Neurosurg 53:1, 1980.
12. Honet JC, Puri K: Cervical radiculitis: treatment and results in 82 patients. Arch Phys Med Rehabil 57:12, 1976.
13. Yoss RE, Corbin KB, McCarthy CS, Love JG: Significance of symptoms and signs of localization of involved root in cervical disc protrusion. Neurology 7:673, 1957.
14. Hunt WE, Miller CA: Management of cervical radiculopathy. Clin Neurosurg 33:485, 1986.
15. Booth RE Jr, Rothman RH: Cervical angina. Spine 1:28, 1976.

16. LaBan MM, Meerschaert JR, Taylor RS: Breast pain: a symptom of cervical radiculopathy. Arch Phys Med Rehabil 60:315, 1979.

17. Makin GJV, Brown WF, Ebers GC: C7 radiculopathy: importance of scapular winging in clinical diagnosis. J Neurol Neurosurg Psychiatry 49:640, 1986.

18. Beatty RM, Fowler FD, Hanson EJ Jr: The abducted arm as a sign of ruptured cervical disc. Neurosurgery 21:731, 1987.

19. Wilbourn AJ, Aminoff MJ: The electrophysiologic examination in patients with radiculopathies. Muscle Nerve 11:1099, 1988.

20. Marinacci AA: A correlation between the operative findings in cervical herniated discs with the electromyograms and opaque myelograms. Bull Los Angeles Neurol Soc 30:118–130, 1965.

21. Negrin P, Lelli S, Fardin P: Contribution of electromyography to the diagnosis, treatment and prognosis of cervical disc disease: a study of 114 patients. Electromyogr Clin Neurophysiol 31:173, 1991.

22. Gore DR, Sepic SB, Gardner GM: Roentgenographic findings of the cervical spine in asymptomatic people. Spine 11:521, 1986.

23. Sobel DF, Barkovich AJ, Munderloh SH: Metrizamide myelography and postmyelographic computed tomography: comparative adequacy in the cervical spine. AJNR 45:385, 1984.

24. Bell GR, Ross JS: The accuracy of imaging studies of the degenerative cervical spine: myelography, myelo-computed tomography, and magnetic resonance imaging. Semin Spine Surg 7:9, 1995.

25. Hitselberger WE, Witten RM: Abnormal myelograms in asymptomatic patients. J Neurosurg 28:204, 1968.

26. Coin CG: Cervical disc degeneration and herniation: diagnosis by computerized tomography. South Med J 77:979, 1984.

27. Brown BM, Schwartz RH, Frank E, Blank NK: Preoperative evaluation of cervical radiculopathy and myelopathy by surface coil MR imaging. AJNR 9:859, 1988.

28. Boden SD, McCowin PR, Davis DO, et al.: Abnormal magnetic-resonance scans of the cervical spine in asymptomatic subjects: a prospective investigation. J Bone Joint Surg 72A:1178, 1990.

29. Finelli DA, Hurst GC, Karaman BA, et al.: Use of magnetization transfer for improved contrast on gradient-echo MR images of the cervical spine. Radiology 193:165, 1994.

30. Kelsey JL, Githens PB, Walter SD, et al.: An epidemiological study of acute prolapsed cervical intervertebral disc. J Bone Joint Surg 66A:907, 1984.

31. Budway RJ, Senter HJ: Cervical disc rupture causing vertebrobasilar insufficiency. Neurosurgery 33:745, 1993.

32. Duthel R, Tudor C, Motuo-Fotso M, Brunon J: Cervical root compression by a loop of the vertebral artery: case report. Neurosurgery 35:140, 1994.

33. LaBan MM, Braker AM, Meerschaert JR: Airport induced "cervical traction" radiculopathy: the OJ syndrome. Arch Phys Med Rehabil 70:845, 1989.

34. Ramirez-Lassepas M, Tulloch JW, Quinones MR, Snyder BD: Acute radicular pain as a presenting symptom in multiple sclerosis. Arch Neurol 49:255, 1992.

35. Rubin D: Cervical radiculitis: diagnosis and treatment. Arch Phys Med Rehabil 41:580, 1960.

36. Warfield CA, Biber MP, Crews DA, Dwarakanath GK: Epidural steroid injection as a treatment for cervical radiculitis. Clin J Pain 4:201, 1988.

37. Ferrante FM, Wilson SP, Iacobo C, et al.: Clinical classification as a predictor of therapeutic outcome after cervical epidural steroid injection. Spine 18:730, 1993.

38. Castagnera L, Maurette P, Pointillart V, et al.: Long-term results of cervical epidural steroid injection with and without morphine in chronic cervical radicular pain. Pain 58:239, 1994.

39. Krieger AJ, Maniker AH: MRI-documented regression of a herniated cervical nucleus pulposus: a case report. Surg Neurol 37:457, 1992.

40. Herkowitz HN, Kurz LT, Overholt DP: Surgical management of cervical soft disc herniation: a comparison between the anterior and posterior approach. Spine 15:1026, 1990.

CERVICAL SPONDYLOSIS

Capsule Summary

Frequency of neck pain—very common
Location of neck pain—confined to cervical spine
Quality of neck pain—ache
Symptoms and signs—pain increased with activity, especially rotation of the neck
Laboratory and x-ray tests—osteophytes and decreased disc space height on plain x-rays and magnetic resonance imaging
Treatment—medications, bracing, and controlled physical activity

Prevalence and Pathogenesis

Cervical spondylosis was formerly known as cervical degenerative disc disease.[1] Cervical spondylosis is a chronic process defined as the development of osteophytes and other stigmata of degenerative arthritis as a consequence of age-related disc disease. This process may produce a wide range of symptoms. However, a patient may have significant spondylosis and be asymptomatic. In an evaluation of 400 spine specimens, Nathan found 100% involvement with anterior osteophytes in individuals 40 years of age and older.[2] The severity of involvement increases with age. The location of frequent involvement corresponds to areas of maximum activity. In the cervical area, the C5–C6 area is maximally affected. In the cervical spine, the inferior border of the vertebral body is more commonly affected, in contrast to the superior border in the lumbar spine.[2]

Cervical spondylosis is believed to be the direct result of age-related changes in the intervertebral disc.[3] These changes include desiccation of the nucleus pulposus, loss of annular elasticity, and narrowing of the disc space with or without disc protrusion or rupture. In turn, fibers of the annulus fibrosus produce periosteal traction through the anterior and posterior longitudinal ligaments, thereby inducing bone formation at the insertion of Sharpey's fibers.[4] Loss of vascular supply to the area may also contribute to degeneration. In the early stage of disc degeneration, the involved segment becomes unstable and the movement of the surrounding vertebrae becomes excessive and irregular. The segment becomes vulnerable to local trauma with damage to the surrounding ligaments and corresponding facet joints. Once initiated, the early damage is amplified over time with increasing instability and associated tissue damage. The result is secondary changes including overriding of facet joints, increased motion of the spinal segments, osteophyte formation in the uncovertebral and zygapophyseal joints, local inflammation of synovial joints, and microfractures. These macroscopic and microscopic changes can result in various clinical syndromes (spondylosis, ankylosis, central or foraminal spinal stenosis, radiculopathy, myelopathy, or spinal segmental instability).

As humans achieved erect posture, the cervical spine evolved to obtain a remarkable degree of mobility and flexibility. Although subjected to loads of less magnitude than the lumbar spine, the cervical spine manifests degenerative changes of aging with exceptional regularity. It may be because of this remarkable mobility that degenerative changes are so consistently seen during the process of aging. The radiographic and pathologic consequences of the aging process begin to manifest themselves in the third decade of life. Because the natural history of cervical spondylosis parallels the aging process, it is often difficult to determine whether these morphologic changes are the result of the aging process or of disease states. Indeed, the anatomic and radiographic expressions of cervical spondylosis become significant only when etiologically related to distinct clinical syndromes.

Cervical spondylosis may present in several ways: cervical spondylosis alone; cervical spondylosis with radiculopathy; cervical spondylosis with myelopathy; and cervical spondylosis with myeloradiculopathy. Cervical radiculopathy due to a soft herniated nucleus pulposus is discussed in the preceding section. Cervical spondylosis alone is presented in this section and with myelopathy in the following section.

Clinical History

The usual patient with symptomatic cervical spondylosis is older than 40 years of age and complains of neckache with an occasional associated headache.[5] Headache that is suboccipital with radiation to the base of the neck or vertex is reported in about one third of patients.[6] Osteoarthritis in the atlantoaxial central or atlantoaxial lateral joints may be associated with severe headaches in individuals older than 40 years of age.[7, 8] The pain in the neck is poorly localized and is exacerbated with movement. Not infrequently though, these patients have very little neck pain symptoms but present with referred pain patterns: shoulder area, suboccipital area, occipital headaches, intrascapular areas, and anterior chest wall; or other vague symptoms suggestive of anatomic disturbances affecting vascular structures or the sympathetic nervous system, such as blurring of vision, vertigo, and tinnitus. About 15% of patients have vertigo or tinnitus, and 5% have vertebrobasilar vascular insufficiency with syncope.[9] Arthritis in the cervical zygapophyseal joints causes referred pain in the occiput (C2–C3), upper neck (C3–C4), base of neck (C4–C5), trapezius (C5–C6), or scapula (C6–C7).[10] In patients with predominantly referred pain, a history of neck pain is usually obtained.

Physical Examination

Physical examination of the patient with cervical spondylosis is often associated with a dearth of objective findings. The patient usually has some limitation of neck motion associated with midline tenderness. Not infrequently, palpation of the referred pain areas also produces local tenderness and should not be confused with local disease. The neurologic examination is normal.

Laboratory Data

Patients with straightforward cervical spondylosis have normal laboratory findings.

Radiographic Evaluation

Roentgenograms (anteroposterior, lateral, oblique) of the cervical spine in cervical spondylosis show a continuum of abnormalities. Initially, loss of disc hydration results in a loss of disc height and the development of vacuum phenomena secondary to gas (nitrogen) forming in the nuclear clefts.[11] Reactive sclerosis of the end plates and the occasional appearance of Schmorl's nodules represents intraosseous disc displacements. Subsequent to these early changes, osteophytes with osteoarthritis of the apophyseal joints, foraminal narrowing, or segmental instability with degenerative spondylolisthesis may occur. Bony ankylosis occurs in advanced disease. Involvement of the uncovertebral processes results in hypertrophy of the ridges, with the development of osteophytes that may project into the foraminal space or the spinal canal causing nerve impingement. Spondylosis deformans is the term used to designate bone production in the spine associated with more advanced degenerative disease (Fig. 10–3). Roentgenographic evidence of cervical spine disease occurs in more than 70% of individuals older than 70 years of age.[12] As previously discussed, these findings do not correlate with symptoms.[13–15] However, patients with degenerative joint disease of the cervical spine may experience greater paracervical muscle fatigue as measured by electromyogram than do control subjects.[16] In large part, the roentgenogram serves to rule out other more serious causes of neck and referred pain such as tumors. Further diagnostic testing in the form of computerized tomography or magnetic resonance (MR) imaging is usually not warranted unless greater detail of bony structures is required. In a population of 89 asymptomatic individuals, MR imaging identified degenerative cervical discs in 62% of individuals 40 years of age or older. No abnormalities were seen in those younger than 30 years of age.[17]

Differential Diagnosis

Cervical spondylosis is diagnosed by exclusion of other possible causes of localized neck pain. The patient's age and a clinical history of neck pain of long duration that increases with mechanical stresses and is documented by characteristic changes on roentgenograms support this diagnosis.

The radiographic changes of cervical spondylosis, including loss of disc space height and osteophytes, occur as patients age. These changes, as already indicated, do not necessarily produce neck pain. Most patients with symptoms are in the same age groups as patients with primary or metastatic tumors of the cervical spine. The physician must be aware of these complicating illnesses and feel confident about excluding the possibility of a more ominous cause of neck pain before ascribing the patient's complaints to spondylosis.

Treatment

Cervical spondylosis alone is treated by nonoperative measures. The mainstay of treatment for the acute pain superimposed on the chronic problem is rest (controlled physical activity) and immobilization in a neck brace. In addition, oral nonsteroidal anti-inflammatory drugs are beneficial. Often these medications need to be administered on a chronic basis. The same drugs may be given intermit-

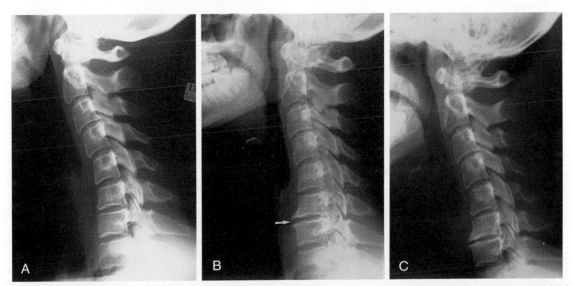

Figure 10–3. Cervical spondylosis. A 33-year-old physician was involved in a motor vehicle accident and developed left neck and trapezial pain. Lateral view of cervical spine. *A,* 4/11/89: Reversal of normal cervical lordosis with angulation at C5–C6 level. *B,* 1/16/92: Straightening of cervical spine with narrowing at C6–C7 level with anterior osteophytes *(arrow).* *C,* 11/18/93: Further disc space narrowing and enlargement of osteophytes.

tently for those patients who have pain only with acute exacerbations. Trigger-point injections with local anesthetics (lidocaine) and corticosteroids (triamcinolone) may be therapeutic for those patients with associated muscle pain. Referred pain in the shoulder and trapezius may be improved with zygapophyseal joint injections.[18] These injections are indicated only if other components of conservative therapy are ineffective. Once the pain abates, the immobilization (usually a soft cervical collar) should be discontinued and the patient maintained on a series of cervical isometric exercises. Further counseling about sleeping position, automobile driving, and work is in order. Manipulation and traction are rarely needed and may in fact be deleterious to the patient.

Prognosis

The majority of patients with cervical spondylosis have a relapsing course with recurrent episodes of neck pain. The severity can vary and treatment is an ongoing process. The natural history is for continued gradual deterioration of spinal structures.

References

CERVICAL SPONDYLOSIS

1. Rothman RH, Simeone FA: The Spine, 3rd ed. Philadelphia, WB Saunders Co, 1992, pp 547–597.
2. Nathan H: Osteophytes of the vertebral column. J Bone Joint Surg 44A:243, 1962.
3. DePalma AF, Rothman RH, Levitt RL, et al.: The natural history of severe cervical disc degeneration. Acta Orthop Scand 43:392, 1972.
4. Jones MD, Pais MJ, Omiya B: Bony overgrowths and abnormal calcifications about the spine. Radiol Clin North Am 26:1213, 1988.
5. Nurick S: The natural history and the results of surgical treatment of the spinal cord disorder associated with cervical spondylosis. Brain 95:101, 1972.
6. Heller JG: The syndromes of degenerative cervical disease. Orthop Clin North Am 23:381, 1992.
7. Star MJ, Curd JG, Thorne RP: Atlantoaxial lateral mass osteoarthritis: a frequently overlooked cause of severe occipitocervical pain. Spine 17:71, 1992.
8. Zapletal J, Hekster REM, Straver JS, Wilmink JT: Atlanto-odontoid osteoarthritis: appearance and prevalence at computed tomography. Spine 20:49, 1995.
9. Brain L: Some unresolved problems of cervical spondylosis. Br Med J 1:771, 1963.
10. Dwyer A, Aprill C, Bogduk N: Cervical zygapophyseal joint pain patterns I: a study in normal volunteers. Spine 15:453, 1990.
11. Rahim KA, Stambough JL: Radiographic evaluation of the degenerative cervical spine. Orthop Clin North Am 23:395, 1992.
12. Fenlin J: Pathology of degenerative disease of the cervical spine: symposium on disease of the intervertebral disc. Orthop Clin North Am 2:371, 1971.
13. Edward WC, LaRocca SH: The developmental segmental sagittal diameter in combined cervical and lumbar spondylosis. Spine 10:43, 1985.
14. Friedenberg ZB, Miller WT: Degeneration disc disease of the cervical spine. J Bone Joint Surg 45A:1171, 1963.
15. Gore DR, Sepic SB, Gardner GM: Roentgenographic findings of the cervical spine in asymptomatic people. Spine 11:521, 1986.
16. Gogia PP, Sabbahi MA: Electromyographic analysis of neck muscle fatigue in patients with osteoarthritis of the cervical spine. Spine 19:502, 1994.
17. Lehto IJ, Tertti MO, Komu ME, et al.: Age-related MRI changes at 0.1 T in cervical discs in asymptomatic subjects. Neuroradiology 36:49, 1994.
18. Aprill C, Dwyer A, Bogduk N: Cervical zygapophyseal joint pain patterns II: a clinical evaluation. Spine 15:458, 1990.

CERVICAL SPONDYLOSIS WITH MYELOPATHY/SPINAL STENOSIS

Capsule Summary

Frequency of neck pain—uncommon
Location of neck pain—neck, head, between scapulae
Quality of neck pain—ache
Symptoms and signs—headaches, difficulty walking associated with clumsiness and weakness of arms
Laboratory and x-ray tests—plain x-rays demonstrate degenerative changes and the magnetic resonance image reveals compression of the spinal cord
Treatment—surgery

Prevalence and Pathogenesis

When the secondary bony changes of cervical spondylosis encroach on the spinal cord, a pathologic process called myelopathy develops. When this involves both the spinal cord and nerve roots, it is called myeloradiculopathy. Radiculopathy, regardless of its cause, causes shoulder or arm pain.[1–3]

Myelopathy is the most serious and difficult sequelae of cervical spondylosis to treat effectively. Brain and colleagues were the first to describe the syndrome in 1952.[2] Less than 5% of patients with cervical spondylosis develop myelopathy, and they usually range from 40 to 60 years of age. Cervical spondylotic myelopathy (CSM) is the most common cause of spinal cord dysfunction in individuals older than 55 years of age.[4] The changes of myelopathy are most often gradual and associated with posterior osteophyte formation (called spondylitic bone or hard disc) and spinal canal narrowing (spinal stenosis). The pathogenesis of this condition begins extrinsic to the spinal cord. Deterioration of the intervertebral disc results in reactive hyperostosis. Osteophytes project posteriorly into the spinal canal, compressing the spinal cord and its vascular supply. Other potential sources of osteophytes are the uncovertebral joints and zygapophyseal joints. The onset of symptoms may occur in the static and dynamic states. The size of the canal is the important static component. Congenital narrowing of the canal increases the risk of myelopathy.[5] Stenosis has been associated with a midsagittal (anteroposterior) diameter of 10 mm or less. Space-occupying bodies such as the foreshortened and thickened ligamentum flavum and posterior longitudinal ligament, bulging of disc material, and loss of cervical lordosis add to the risk of static stenosis. Dynamic stenosis may occur secondary to segment instability causing compression of different portions of the spinal cord with flexion or extension.

Compression of the spinal cord results in a consistent pattern of nerve degeneration in the posterior and lateral white-matter columns.[6, 7] The anterior columns are relatively spared. Pressure on the spinal cord causes a blockage of axoplasmic flow, distortion of the tissue of the cord, and stretching of the intrinsic transverse terminations of the anterior spinal artery.[4] Persistent pressure causes demyelination. Pressure on the anterior spinal artery in the lower cervical region is another mechanism of tissue damage.[8] Acute myelopathy is most often the result of a central soft disc herniation producing a high-grade block.

Clinical History

The clinical picture of CSM varies considerably. The onset of symptoms is usually after 50 years of age and males are more often affected. Onset is usually insidious, although there is occasionally a history of trauma. The natural history is that of initial deterioration followed by a plateau period lasting several months. The resulting clinical picture is often one of an incomplete spinal lesion with a patchy distribution of deficits. Disability varies with the number of vertebrae involved and the degree of involvement at each level.

CSM may be divided into five distinct clinical syndromes (Table 10–4). The lateral syndrome is associated with radicular pain. The medial syndrome causes myelopathy associated with long-tract signs. The combined syndrome includes both radicular and myelopathic signs and is the most common presentation of CSM. The least common syndrome is vascular, associated with variable symptoms and signs associated with ischemia of the spinal cord. The anterior syndrome is associated with painless upper extremity weakness. This syndrome occurs secondary to pressure affecting only the anterior horns containing motor neurons in the spinal cord.

The characteristic stooped, wide-based, and somewhat jerky gait of the aged summarizes the chronic effects of cervical spondylosis with myelopathy on ambulation. The spinal cord changes may develop at single or multiple levels and as such do not present in a standard manner. A typical clinical presentation of chronic myelopathy begins with the gradual onset of a peculiar sensation in the hands, associated with clumsiness and weakness. The patient may also note lower extremity symptoms that may antedate the upper extremity findings, including walking difficulty, peculiar sensations, leg weakness, and spontaneous leg movements indicative of hyperreflexia, spasticity, and clonus. Older patients may describe leg stiffness, shuffling of their feet, with associated fear of falling. The upper extremity findings may start out unilaterally and include hyperreflexia, brisk Hoffmann's sign, and muscle

TABLE 10–4. CERVICAL SPONDYLOTIC MYELOPATHY CLINICAL SYNDROMES

SYNDROME	PAIN	EXTREMITY INVOLVEMENT	GAIT ABNORMALITY	LOCATION
Lateral (radicular)	Yes	Arm	Occasional	Unilateral
Medial (myelopathic)	No	Leg	Yes	Bilateral
Combined	Occasional	Both	Yes	Unilateral/upper Bilateral/lower
Vascular	No	Both	Yes	Bilateral
Anterior (weakness in arms)	No	Arm	No	Unilateral

Modified from Bernhardt M, Hytes RA, Blume HW, White AA III: Cervical spondylotic myelopathy. J Bone Joint Surg Am 75:119, 1993.

atrophy (especially hand muscles). Neck pain per se is not a prominent feature of myelopathy. In a study of 199 patients with CSM, radicular pain and paresthetic pain were reported in 39% and 34% of patients, respectively. In contrast, 98% reported spasticity.[9] Sensory changes can evolve at these levels and are often a less reliable index of spinal cord disease. Bladder incontinence is uncommon.

Physical Examination

For the clinician treating patients with CSM, the most critical problem is identification of the level (or levels) responsible for the clinical symptoms. The patient's gait should be observed, and the extent of motor disability, which may vary from mild to severe, should be ascertained. Pyramidal tract weakness and atrophy are more commonly seen in the lower extremities and are the most common abnormal physical signs. The usual clinical findings in the lower extremities are spasticity and weakness. Weakness and wasting of the upper extremities and hands along with fasciculations may also be the result of combined CSM syndrome including myelopathy and radiculopathy. Hands that are clumsy and numb may be caused by a myelopathic lesion in the upper cervical cord at C3–C5.[10] Decreased adduction and extension of the ulnar digits and inability to open and close the hand quickly may have their source in a lesion affecting the pyramidal tract at or above the C7 cord level.[11, 12] A diminished or absent upper extremity deep tendon reflex, often the triceps reflex, can indicate compressive radiculopathy superimposed on spondylitic myelopathy.

Sensory deficits in spinothalmic (pain and temperature) and posterior column (vibration and proprioception) function should be documented. Alterations of sensation may include numbness, loss of temperature on the contralateral side, loss of proprioception, or decreased dermatomal sensation.[13] Usually there is no gross impairment of sensation; rather, a patchy decrease in light touch and pinprick is seen. Hyperreflexia, clonus, and positive Babinski's sign are seen in the lower extremities. Hoffmann's sign and hyperreflexia may be observed in the upper extremities.

The physical findings may be confusing when cervical and lumbar spinal stenosis coexist.[14] Lumbar compression may hide upper motor neuron signs. Both upper and lower extremity reflexes should be tested in stenosis patients. Abnormal physical findings in the lower extremities may be elicited by having the patient assume an extended, upright position or by walking. The finding of jaw hyperreflexia suggests a lesion above the foramen magnum or a systemic process, such as hyperthyroidism.

Laboratory Data

Serum laboratory tests are normal in patients with CSM. Patients with CSM may have abnormalities in somatosensory and motor-evoked potentials. Change in the position of the neck may result in abnormalities in somatosensory potentials.[15] An experienced electromyographer may have greater success in identifying these abnormalities in complicated patients.

Radiographic Examination

Roentgenographic evaluation may include anteroposterior, lateral, flexion-extension, atlanto-occipital, and oblique views. Roentgenograms of the cervical spine in these patients often reveal advanced degenerative disease, including spinal canal narrowing with prominent posterior osteophytosis, variable foraminal narrowing, disc space narrowing, facet joint arthrosis, and instability (Fig. 10–4). These findings are usually more prominent in the lower cervical spine. Lumbar disc disease frequently coexists in the setting of cervical spondylosis.[16] Congenital canal narrowing may be detected if the ratio of Pavlov is a value of 0.8 or less.[17] The ratio is determined by dividing the anteroposterior diameter of the canal by the anteroposterior diameter of the corresponding vertebral body. The ratio is usually 1.0. Although plain roentgenograms are able to detect bony alterations of the vertebrae, the technique is unable to determine the extent of damage of soft tissues in the cervical spine. Other radiographic techniques, such as myelography, computerized tomography (CT), or MR imaging, are required.

Myelography is a diagnostic technique that introduces dye into the spinal canal to exhibit the presence of posterior or anterior defects compressing neural elements. Posterior defects are secondary to facet arthrosis and buckling of the ligamentum flavum. Anterior defects are secondary to changes in the posterior longitudinal ligaments and intervertebral discs.[18] MR imaging is the noninvasive examination of choice for the evaluation of CSM.

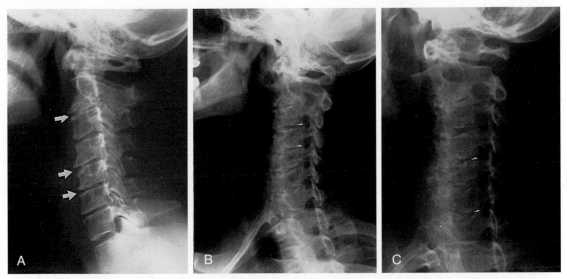

Figure 10–4. Cervical spondylosis. A 64-year-old woman with generalized osteoarthritis and decreased motion of the cervical spine without neurologic signs. Lateral view, *A,* and oblique views, *B* and *C,* reveal loss of lordosis, diffuse narrowing of disc spaces C2–C7 *(large arrows),* and moderate encroachment by osteophytes of neural foramina *(small arrows).*

The spinal cord is visualized in sagittal and axial planes. MR imaging is able to detect the extent of spinal cord compression and alterations of the spinal cord proper[19] (Fig. 10–5). CT is superior to MR imaging for the identification of osteophytes. CT/myelography is useful for distinguishing disc tissue from osteophytes.[20]

Differential Diagnosis

The diagnosis of CSM is based on the clinical symptoms and signs and is confirmed by abnormalities detected on MR or CT evaluation. A variety of disorders that affect the spinal cord, peripheral nerves, and skeletal muscles or that cause narrowing of the spinal canal need to be considered in the patient with myelopathic symptoms. The most common problem is an intradural tumor (primary or metastatic) compressing the spinal cord. Other disorders to be considered include multiple sclerosis, cerebrovascular disease, hydrocephalus (normal pressure), intracranial tumor, syringomyelia, amyotrophic lateral sclerosis, Arnold-Chiari malformation, vascular ischemia of the cord, tabes dorsalis, myopathies, and neuropathies. Many of these abnormalities may be discovered by MR image evaluation of the head and spine.[21] MR imaging may also identify the effects of radiation therapy on the spinal cord resulting in myelopathic syndrome.[22] Syphilis can be diagnosed by sero-

logic tests. Peripheral neuropathies and myopathies can be identified by electromyography and by muscle and nerve biopsy. Disorders that increase bone growth may also cause stenosis. For example, acromegalic patients may develop cervical myelopathy.[23] As well, chest and shoulder abnormalities need to be excluded.

Treatment

Patients with CSM may improve in 50% of instances with nonoperative therapy.[24] Other studies have reported greater disability in those individuals who do not undergo surgical decompression.[25, 26] Conservative therapy should be attempted in those individuals without severe neurologic compromise or those who are poor surgical risks. Conservative therapy includes immobilization with a firm cervicothoracic orthosis, intermittent bed rest, nonsteroidal anti-inflammatory drugs, muscle relaxants, epidural corticosteroid injections, and physical therapy.[4]

In general, myelopathy is a surgical disease. Myelopathy is not an absolute indication for surgical decompression. The goal of surgery in the myelopathic patient is to decompress the spinal canal to prevent further spinal cord compression and vascular compromise. If the myelopathy is progressive despite a trial of conservative treatment, surgery is clearly indicated. In rare circumstances, prompt surgical

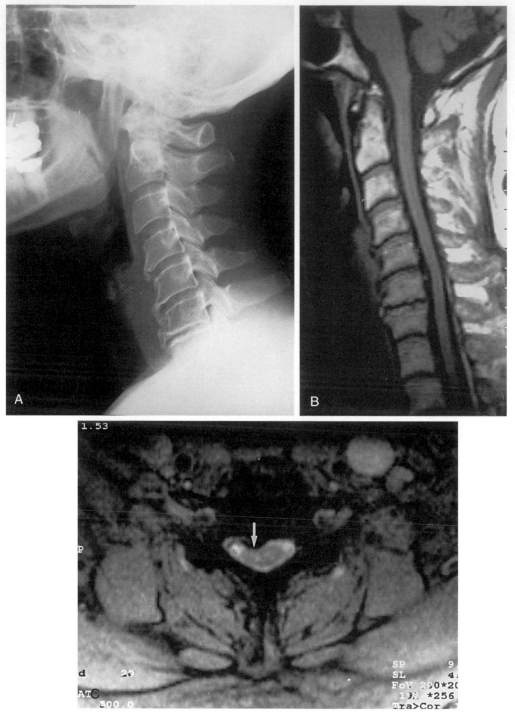

Figure 10–5. Cervical spondylotic myelopathy. A 65-year-old woman had bilateral carpal tunnel syndrome documented by electromyography and developed right shoulder pain and arm heaviness. *A,* Lateral view of cervical spine reveals cervical spondylosis with anterior osteophytes at C4–C6. Magnetic resonance T_1-weighted sagittal, *B,* and axial, *C,* views reveal diffuse spondylosis with spondylitic bar at C4–C5 causing moderate canal stenosis *(arrow).*

decompression is indicated for the individual with rapid onset of myelopathic symptoms and signs associated with spinal cord compression.[27] These indications may vary slightly from surgeon to surgeon because of the lack of absolute or definitive clinical data. Surgical therapy works best in the early stages of disease. Elderly patients with long-standing disease and profound neurologic deficits are poor candidates. A number of surgical procedures are available for decompression of neural elements. Among these procedures are anterior cervical discectomy with interbody arthrodesis, anterior cervical corpectomy and strut graft arthrodesis, posterior cervical laminectomy, and posterior cervical laminaplasty.[28] Each procedure has its potential benefits and complications. Anterior decompression is recommended for anterior compression at one or two levels. Posterior approach is indicated for compression at multiple levels. An experienced spine surgeon should be able to choose the appropriate procedure for the specific clinical characteristics of the patient.

Prognosis

The natural history of CSM was described by Clarke and Robinson in 120 patients.[29] Most patients have progressive deterioration between episodes of increased symptoms. Twenty percent of patients had slow progression without remission and 5% had rapid onset with long periods of no progression. Another study of 44 patients described only 5 of 15 patients with symptoms for 10 years or longer who had improvement.[30] Symon and Lavender reported that only 18% of patients had improvement from the time of presentation.[25]

Patients with congenital narrowing of the spinal canal are at risk of developing transient neuropraxia in the absence of spondylosis. These patients may develop transient quadriplegia with hyperflexion or hyperextension of the neck. These people are usually athletes who undergo direct pressure on the head. These patients should be evaluated for the presence of spinal stenosis, which would preclude participation in contact sports.[31]

Patients with overt signs of a myelopathy have a guarded future. Surgery may bring some relief, but they will continue to have intermittent difficulty. Okada and colleagues reported that shorter duration of disease, greater preoperative spinal cord area, and normal intramedullary signal intensity on MR evaluation were associated with better surgical outcome in CSM patients.[32]

References

CERVICAL SPONDYLOSIS WITH MYELOPATHY/SPINAL STENOSIS

1. Bohlman HH: Cervical spondylosis with moderate to severe myelopathy. Spine 2:151–162, 1977.

2. Brain WR, Northfield D, Wilkinson M: The neurological manifestations of cervical spondylosis. Brain 75:187–225, 1952.
3. The Cervical Spine Research Society: The Cervical Spine. Philadelphia: JB Lippincott Co, 1989, pp 388–430.
4. Bernhardt M, Hynes RA, Blume HW, White AA III: Cervical spondylotic myelopathy. J Bone Joint Surg 75A:119, 1993.
5. Kessler JT: Congenital narrowing of the cervical spinal canal. J Neurol Neurosurg Psychiatry 38:1218, 1975.
6. Veidlinger OF, Colwill JC, Smyth HS, et al.: Cervical myelopathy and its relationship to cervical stenosis. Spine 6:550, 1981.
7. Nurick S: The pathogenesis of the spinal cord disorder associated with cervical spondylosis. Brain 95:87, 1972.
8. Doppman JL: The mechanism of ischemia in anteroposterior compression of the spinal cord. Invest Radiol 10:543, 1975.
9. Crandall PH, Batzdorf U: Cervical spondylotic myelopathy. J Neurosurg 25:57, 1966.
10. Good DC, Couch JR, Wacaser L: Numb, clumsy hands and high cervical spondylosis. Surg Neurol 22:285, 1984.
11. Ono K, Ebara S, Fuji T, et al.: Myelopathy hand: new clinical signs of cervical cord damage. J Bone Joint Surg 69B:215, 1987.
12. Heller JG: The syndromes of degenerative cervical disease. Orthop Clin North Am 23:381, 1992.
13. Clark CR: Cervical spondylotic myelopathy: history and physical findings. Spine 13:847, 1988.
14. Epstein NE, Epstein JA, Carras R, et al.: Coexisting cervical and lumbar spinal stenosis: diagnosis and management. Neurosurgery 15:489, 1984.
15. Yiannikas C, Shahani BT, Young RR: Short-latency somatosensory-evoked potentials from radial, median, ulnar, and peroneal nerve stimulation in the assessment of cervical spondylosis: comparison with conventional electromyography. Arch Neurol 43:1264, 1986.
16. Jacobs B, Ghelman B, Marchisello P: Coexistence of cervical and lumbar disc disease. Spine 15:1261, 1990.
17. Pavlov H, Torg JS, Robie B, Jahre C: Cervical spinal stenosis: determination with vertebral body ratio method. Radiology 164:771, 1987.
18. Penning L, Wilmink JT, van Woerden HH, Knol E: CT myelographic findings in degenerative disorders of the cervical spine: clinical significance. AJR 146:793, 1986.
19. Nagata K, Kiyonaga K, Ohashi T, et al.: Clinical value of magnetic resonance imaging for cervical myelopathy. Spine 15:1088, 1990.
20. Brown BM, Schwartz RH, Frank E, Blank NK: Preoperative evaluation of cervical radiculopathy and myelopathy by surface-coil MR imaging. AJR 151:1205, 1988.
21. Arlien-Soborg P, Kjaer L, Praestholm J: Myelopathy, CT, and MRI of the spinal canal in patients with myelopathy: a prospective study. Acta Neurol Scand 87:95, 1993.
22. Wang P, Shen W, Jan J: MR imaging in radiation myelopathy. AJNR 13:1049, 1992.
23. Mikawa Y, Watanabe R, Nishishita Y: Cervical myelopathy in acromegaly. Spine 17:1542, 1992.
24. LaRocca H: Cervical spondylotic myelopathy: natural history. Spine 13:854, 1988.
25. Symon L, Lavender P: The surgical treatment of cervical spondylotic myelopathy. Neurology 17:117, 1967.
26. Phillips DG: Surgical treatment of myelopathy with cervical spondylosis. J Neurol Neurosurg Psychiatry 36:879, 1973.

27. Wilberger JE Jr, Chedid MK: Acute cervical spondylytic myelopathy. Neurosurgery 22:145, 1988.
28. Kurz LT, Herkowitz HN: Surgical management of myelopathy. Orthop Clin North Am 23:495, 1992.
29. Clarke E, Robinson PK: Cervical myelopathy: a complication of cervical spondylosis. Brain 79:483, 1956.
30. Lees F, Turner JWA: Natural history and prognosis of cervical spondylosis. Br Med J 2:1607, 1963.
31. Torg JS, Pavlov H, Genuario SE, et al.: Neuropraxia of the cervical spinal cord with transient quadriplegia. J Bone Joint Surg 68A:1354, 1986.
32. Okada Y, Ikata T, Yamada H, et al.: Magnetic resonance imaging study on the results of surgery for cervical compression myelopathy. Spine 18:2024, 1993.

CERVICAL HYPEREXTENSION INJURIES (WHIPLASH)

Capsule Summary

Frequency of neck pain—very common
Location of neck pain—neck, head, between scapulae, shoulders
Quality of neck pain—ache, soreness
Symptoms and signs—headaches, neck pain with movement of the head
Laboratory and x-ray tests—normal
Treatment—medications, physical therapy

Prevalence and Pathogenesis

Hyperextension injuries of the neck occur most often when the driver of a stationary car is struck from behind by another vehicle.[1] The driver is usually relaxed and unaware of the impending collision. The sudden acceleration of the struck vehicle pushes the back of the car seat against the driver's torso. This force pushes the driver's torso (shoulders) forward and the head remains static but moves posteriorly, causing hyperextension of the neck. This occurs quickly after impact. If no head rest is present, the driver's head is hyperextended past the normal limit of stretch of the soft tissues of the neck. This injury is called whiplash because of the hyperextension of the head. Neck pain may also be the result of lateral and frontal collisions. Whiplash is an acceleration-deceleration mechanism of energy transfer to the neck. The impact may result in bony or soft-tissue injuries that in turn may lead to a variety of clinical manifestations.[2] The sternocleidomastoid, scalene, and the longus coli muscles may be mildly or severely stretched or, at worst, torn. Muscle tears of the longus coli muscles might involve injury to the sympathetic trunk unilaterally or bilater-

ally, resulting in a Horner's syndrome, nausea, or dizziness. Further hyperextension may injure the esophagus, resulting in temporary dysphagia and injury to the larynx, causing hoarseness. Tears in the anterior longitudinal ligament may cause hematoma formation with resultant cervical radiculopathy (arm pain) and injury to the intervertebral disc. In the recoil forward flexion that occurs when the car stops accelerating, the head is thrown forward. This forward flexion of the head is usually limited by the chin striking the chest and does not usually cause significant injury. However, if the head is thrown forward and strikes the steering wheel or the windshield, a head injury can occur. If the head is in slight rotation, additional stresses are placed on the capsules of the zygapophyseal joints, intervertebral discs, and alar ligaments. In motor vehicle accidents (MVAs), the neck is subject to forced flexion, extension, and lateral flexion as well as shear forces parallel to the direction of impact. Muscles do not have time to react to protect the structures of the neck. A variety of potential injuries may occur corresponding to the type of injury.[3] Autopsy studies have detected injuries to the cervical intervertebral discs. Clefts in the cartilage plates of the intervertebral discs of neck trauma patients are distinctly different from those associated with spondylosis.[4]

Whiplash-type injuries were first recognized in World War I pilots in airplanes without head supports who were catapulted on takeoff. In 1928, Crowe introduced the term whiplash to describe hyperextension injuries from an indirect force.[5] In 1953, Gay and Abbott redefined the whiplash injury and the term has been used extensively in the medical literature and as a diagnostic code for insurance reimbursement.[6]

The prevalence of whiplash injury has not been measured prospectively. Of those individuals involved in a rear-end MVA, approximately 20% develop neck pain.[7] In data collected by the Quebec Task Force on Whiplash-Associated Disorders, the incidence rate was 131 whiplash injuries per 100,000 vehicles per year in 1987.[2] In Australia, an annual incidence rate of 80 per 100,000 has been reported.[3]

Clinical History

Usually, the driver is often unaware of having been injured. The driver suffers little discomfort at the scene of the accident and often does not wish to go to the hospital. Later, 12 to 14 hours after the accident, the driver begins to feel stiffness in the neck. Pain at the base of the neck increases and is made worse by head and neck movements. Soon any movement of the head or neck causes excruciating pain. Headaches are the second most common symptom associated with whiplash injury.[8] The anterior cervical muscles are often tender to the touch. The patient may have pain on opening the mouth or chewing, hoarseness, or difficulty swallowing, and seeks medical care. Other symptoms associated with whiplash injuries include visual disturbances manifested by accommodative problems and oculomotor dysfunction mediated through increased sympathetic tone.[9] Dizziness may occur secondary to damage to the vestibular apparatus, with perilymph fistulas causing disequilibrium.[10] Whiplash patients may develop paresthesias in the arms, particularly in the ulnar nerve distribution. One proposed mechanism of injury is compression of the lower nerve roots of the inferior portion of the brachial plexus as it passes under the scalene muscles, a form of thoracic outlet syndrome.[11] Other patients may have dysesthesias of the face below the ear, associated with traction injuries to the great auricular nerve and superficial branches of the cervical plexus as they are stretched winding around the sternocleidomastoid muscle. Cognitive functions, such as concentration, memory, and attention span are decreased in whiplash patients.[12] Psychological factors have been suggested as playing a role in the symptom complex and delaying resolution of whiplash injuries.[13] However, recent studies have refuted this notion, demonstrating the lack of correlation between psychological stress and personality traits with the outcome of a whiplash injury.[14] Psychological stress that whiplash patients experience is similar to that associated with chronic pain of any source.[15] The primary reason for psychological dysfunction in association with whiplash injuries is the trauma itself.

Physical Examination

The physical examination must be detailed and complete to rule out other significant problems. If the patient only has a hyperextension injury, the neurologic examination is normal. The only finding, which is subjective, is decreased range of motion and, on occasion, persistent muscle contraction.

Laboratory Data

Laboratory tests are normal for patients with a hyperextension neck injury.

Radiographic Evaluation

Plain roentgenograms may demonstrate on the lateral view some loss of the normal lordotic curve due to muscle spasm. A recent study suggests that loss of lordosis is not a specific finding in whiplash patients and may occur in normal individuals.[16] Otherwise, there are no abnormalities found on the plain radiographs or other examinations such as magnetic resonance (MR) imaging. The association of clinical symptoms and signs and abnormalities on MR scan in patients with hyperextension injuries is poor.[17]

Differential Diagnosis

Considering other abnormalities to account for the patient's complaints is the most important aspect of the diagnostic process for the treating physician. One does not want to be in the situation of treating a patient for a hyperextension injury when, in fact, there is a significant traumatic abnormality, such as a subdural hematoma, to account for the patient's symptom complex.

Each patient requires a thorough examination with particular attention given to neurologic function. Abrasions on the forehead suggest forward flexion of the head resulting from impact on the steering wheel or windshield. A dilated pupil might suggest a Horner's syndrome secondary to the injury of the sympathetic chain along the longus coli muscles or be a sign of significant intracranial injury if the patient's level of consciousness is altered. Point tenderness in front of the ear is suggestive of injury to the temporomandibular joint, and tenderness to touch in the suboccipital area suggests impact of the head on the back of the seat.

The Quebec Task Force on Whiplash-Associated Disorders proposed a classification of whiplash injuries (Table 10–5). A complete neurologic examination is crucial to differentiate the extent of damage. Any evidence of objective neurologic deficit merits immediate diagnostic tests to determine the cause. Although, by definition, hyperextension cervical injury causes damage only to the soft-tissue structures of the neck, plain roentgenograms

TABLE 10–5. WHIPLASH-ASSOCIATED DISORDERS CLASSIFICATION

GRADE	NECK PAIN, STIFFNESS, TENDERNESS	PHYSICAL SIGNS	MUSCULO-SKELETAL SIGNS	NEUROLOGIC SIGNS	FRACTURE DISLOCATION
0	−	−	−	−	−
I	+	−	−	−	−
II	+	+	+	−	−
III	+	+	+/−	+	−
IV	+	+	−	+/−	+

Modified from Spitzer WO, Skovron ML, Salmi LR, et al.: Scientific monograph of the Quebec Task Force on whiplash-associated disorders: redefining "whiplash" and its management. Spine 20:1, 1995.

of the cervical spine should be obtained in all instances of neurologic dysfunction.[3] Unsuspected fracture—dislocations of the cervical spine, facet fractures, odontoid fractures, or spinous process fractures—might otherwise be missed in the neurologically intact patient. The Quebec study suggests that patients with injuries grade II or greater should have plain roentgenograms of the cervical spine.[2] Cervical spondylosis is demonstrated on plain roentgenograms as well. Of course, if objective neurologic deficits are present, then further diagnostic aids are necessary, including computerized tomography (CT) of the head or spine, myelogram, or MR scan.

Treatment

A great deal of controversy is involved in the treatment of whiplash injuries because few scientific studies exist demonstrating definite efficacy of a number of treatment modalities.[2] A reasonable medical routine, as the majority of patients have no neurologic deficit, is based on the premise of resting the involved injured soft tissues.[18] Soft cervical collars have been used with the thought that they relieved muscle spasm and prevented quick movements of the head. Collars were worn for no more than 2 to 4 weeks, lest the recovering muscles start weakening from nonuse.[19] Recommendations from the Quebec Task Force suggest restricting the use of collars to a minimal period. They suggest that prolonged use of a collar is detrimental.[2] Cervical soft collars do not limit motion of the cervical spine. Other braces, such as the Philadelphia collar or four-poster brace, are needed to restrict neck motion significantly.

Heat is helpful and should be applied by a heating pad, hot showers, or hot tub soaks. If neck pain is severe, a short period of bed rest may be necessary. Mild analgesics, non-steroidal anti-inflammatory drugs, and muscle relaxants are helpful and are generally indicated. Narcotic analgesics should be avoided if at all possible. Activity should be encouraged as determined by the severity of the symptoms. Generally, driving should be avoided for the acute symptomatic period. After approximately 2 weeks of this regimen, significant improvement should be noted. If not, 2 more weeks of continued conservative care with the addition of some light home cervical traction should be employed. If symptoms persist at 4 weeks post-injury, some further testing is necessary before emotional overlay complicates the clinical course of the patient. If headaches persist, a cranial CT scan should be done. If normal at 4 weeks, the patient can be assured that no intracranial abnormality is present. If arm or shoulder pain persists, then a spine CT scan or MR image should be performed. If these tests are normal, the patient can be assured that no compression of neural structures is present and be strongly encouraged to increase activities.

Manual therapy has not been shown to be of particular benefit greater than placebo in the treatment of neck pain.[20] Corticosteroid injections of the cervical facet joints are not helpful in patients with chronic whiplash pain.[21]

Prognosis

Most patients with whiplash injuries resolve over a period up to 12 weeks. Most individuals, particularly those with lower-grade lesions, improve rapidly from 7 to 14 days. Patients with finger paresthesias have a greater likelihood of persistent neck pain for 6 months.[14] Patients with preinjury headaches are at risk for persistent headache at 6 months.[22] For those individuals with persistent neck pain, few patients experience significant improvement of symptoms present for a period of 2 years.[3] A misconception exists that litigation tends to prolong symptoms in patients with whiplash injuries. The likelihood of chronicity is independent of litigation. Compensation and noncompensation patients respond to therapy in similar ways.[23]

References

CERVICAL HYPEREXTENSION INJURIES (WHIPLASH)

1. McNab I, McCulloch J: Neck Ache and Shoulder Pain. Baltimore: Williams & Wilkins, 1994, 140–159.
2. Spitzer WO, Skovron ML, Salmi LR, et al.: Scientific monograph of the Quebec Task Force on whiplash-associated disorders: redefining ''whiplash'' and its management. Spine 20:1, 1995.
3. Barnsley L, Lord S, Bogduk N: Whiplash injury. Pain 58:283, 1994.
4. Taylor JR, Twomey LT: Acute injuries to cervical joints: an autopsy study of neck sprain. Spine 18:1115, 1993.
5. Crowe HE: Injuries to the cervical spine. Paper presented at the meeting of the Western Orthopaedic Association, San Francisco, 1928.
6. Gay JR, Abbott KH: Common whiplash injuries of the neck. JAMA 152:1698, 1953.
7. States JD, Korn MW, Masengill JB: The enigma of whiplash injuries. NY State J Med 70:2971, 1970.
8. Maimaris C, Barnes MR, Allen MJ: ''Whiplash injuries'' of the neck: a retrospective study. Injury 19:393, 1988.
9. Hildingsson C, Wenngren BI, Toolanen G: Eye motility dysfunction after soft-tissue injury of the cervical spine. Acta Orthop Scand 64:129, 1993.
10. Chester JB Jr: Whiplash, postural control, and inner ear. Spine 16:716, 1991.
11. Capistrant TD: Thoracic outlet syndrome in whiplash injury. Ann Surg 185:175, 1977.
12. Radanov BP, Di Stefano G, Schnidrig A, et al.: Cognitive functioning after common whiplash: a controlled follow-up study. Arch Neurol 50:87, 1993.
13. Pearce JM: Whiplash injury: a reappraisal. J Neurol Neurosurg Psychiatry 52:1329, 1989.
14. Radanov BP, Stefano G, Schnidrig A, Ballinari P: Role of psychological stress in recovery from common whiplash. Lancet 338:712, 1991.
15. Merskey H: Psychological consequences of whiplash injuries. Spine 7:471, 1993.
16. Helliwell PS, Evans PF, Wright V: The straight cervical spine: does it indicate muscle spasm? J Bone Joint Surg 76B:103, 1994.
17. Pettersson K, Hildingsson C, Toolanen G, et al.: MRI and neurology in acute whiplash trauma: no correlation in prospective examination of 39 cases. Acta Orthop Scand 65:525, 1994.
18. Greenfield J, Ilfeld FW: Acute cervical strain: evaluation and short-term prognostic factors. Clin Orthop 122:196, 1977.
19. Pennie BH, Agambar LJ: Whiplash injuries: a trial of early management. J Bone Joint Surg 72B:277, 1990.
20. Koes BW, Bouter LM, Mameren H, et al.: The effectiveness of manual therapy, physiotherapy, and treatment by the general practitioner for nonspecific back and neck complaints: a randomized clinical trial. Spine 17:28, 1992.
21. Barnsley L, Lord SM, Wallis BJ, Bogduk N: Lack of effect of intra-articular corticosteroids for chronic pain in cervical zygapophyseal joints. N Engl J Med 330:1047, 1994.
22. Radanov BP, Sturzenegger M, Di Stefano G, et al.: Factors influencing recovery from headache after common whiplash. Br Med J 307:652, 1993.
23. Shapiro AP, Roth RS: The effect of litigation on recovery of whiplash. Spine 7:531, 1993.

11

Rheumatologic Disorders of the Cervical Spine

Rheumatologic disorders of the cervical spine are common causes of neck pain. These disorders affect the bones, joints, ligaments, tendons, and muscles that are anatomic components of the cervical spine. Whereas mechanical disorders, such as muscle strain, disease of the intervertebral discs, and osteoarthritis of the cervical spine, are frequent causes of neck pain, there are a number of other inflammatory and noninflammatory disorders associated with pain in the cervical spine. The most important rheumatic disorders that cause inflammation of the joints of the axial skeleton are rheumatoid arthritis and the seronegative spondyloarthropathies. Rheumatoid arthritis, a disease that causes chronic inflammation of the synovial lining of the joints, affects the cervical spine at the atlantoaxial junction and the subaxial apophyseal joints. These changes occur in patients with diffuse disease of long duration. Cervical spine involvement in rheumatoid arthritis is associated with a wide range of symptoms and signs, from mild neck pain and headaches to severe neurologic dysfunction consisting of radiculopathy, paresthesias, incontinence, quadriplegia, and sudden death.

The seronegative spondyloarthropathies are characterized by disease and the absence of rheumatoid factor. The seronegative spondyloarthropathies include ankylosing spondylitis, Reiter's syndrome, psoriatic arthritis, and enteropathic arthritis. They are closely associated with genetic factors that predispose patients to these illnesses. Environmental factors play a role as the triggers of the inflammatory response in genetically predisposed individuals. Among the environmental factors that have been suggested but unproven are bacterial infection and trauma. Neck pain usually occurs in a patient who has developed arthritis in the lumbosacral portion of the axial skeleton.

In rheumatoid arthritis and the seronegative spondyloarthropathies, joint pain is most severe in the morning and improves with activity. Physical examination demonstrates localized tenderness with palpation and limitation of motion in all planes of motion of the cervical spine. Laboratory abnormalities are consistent with systemic inflammatory disease but are nonspecific, except for the presence of rheumatoid factor in 80% of patients with rheumatoid arthritis. Radiographic evaluation is useful in identifying characteristic changes in the cervical spine and peripheral joints that may help in the differential diagnosis of the patient with neck pain.

A noninflammatory lesion affecting the bone in the cervical spine is diffuse idiopathic skeletal hyperostosis. Muscle syndromes associated with neck pain include polymyalgia rheumatica and fibromyalgia.

In addition to drug therapy, treatment for these rheumatologic disorders involves a number of therapeutic modalities that include patient education and physical and occupational therapies. Although there are no cures for these illnesses, medical therapy can be effective in controlling symptoms.

The prognosis and course of these rheumatic conditions are rarely related to the extent of cervical spine disease alone. Occasionally, atlantoaxial subluxation secondary to rheumatoid arthritis or the spondyloarthropathies may result in catastrophic neurologic dysfunction. In most circumstances, the status of disease in other areas of the musculoskeletal system and the severity of constitutional symptoms have a greater effect on the patient's daily existence.

RHEUMATOID ARTHRITIS

Capsule Summary

Frequency of neck pain—very common
Location of neck pain—cervical spine, occiput
Quality of neck pain—ache
Symptoms and signs—joint disease of long duration, cervical spine tenderness
Laboratory and x-ray tests—anemia, rheumatoid factor, atlantoaxial subluxation, subaxial subluxation
Treatment—nonsteroidal anti-inflammatory drugs, antirheumatics, corticosteroids

Prevalence and Pathogenesis

Rheumatoid arthritis (RA) is a chronic, systemic, inflammatory disease that causes pain, heat, swelling, and destruction in synovial joints. The joints characteristically affected by RA are small joints of the hands and feet, wrists, elbows, hips, knees, ankles, and cervical spine. A majority of RA patients have cervical spine disease manifested as neck pain, headaches, or arm numbness. Signs of cervical spine disease include decreased neck motion with stiffness, undue prominence of the spinous process of the axis (C2), and neurologic dysfunction including paresthesias, spasticity, incontinence, and quadriplegia. The diagnosis of RA is made in the setting of a history of persistent joint inflammation in the appropriate joints and the presence of specific serum antibodies (rheumatoid factor). The degree of cervical spine destruction in RA does not always correlate with patient complaints and is detected by radiographic evaluation. RA of the cervical spine responds to the same therapy that is effective for the peripheral joints. Surgical intervention with stabilization of the cervical spine is required for persistent neurologic abnormalities.

The prevalence of RA is approximately 1% to 3% of the United States population.[1] RA is found in all racial and ethnic groups. The condition occurs in all age groups. The male-to-female ratio is approximately 1:3. Symptoms of cervical spine disease occur in 40% to 80% of RA patients.[2, 3] Radiographic evidence of cervical spine involvement is found in up to 86% of RA patients, whereas neurologic symptoms from cervical spine disease occur less frequently in 10% of patients with radiographic changes.[4, 5] Cervical spine disease usually occurs in the setting of active peripheral disease; however, on occasion, neck symptoms may be the initial or predominant symptom without clinical signs of RA in other locations.[6, 7]

The causes of RA are probably multifactorial and are mediated through environmental and genetic factors. The combination of these factors produces an imbalance in immune function that results in the inflammation of synovial joints.[4, 8] RA is a chronic immune-mediated disease whose initiation and perpetuation are dependent on T lymphocyte response to unknown antigens.[9] A possible environmental factor that may initiate RA is a virus.[10] After an initial flurry of scientific interest associating in the presence of Epstein-Barr virus (EBV) as a source of infection in RA, subsequent investigations have not found convincing evidence of a cause-and-effect relationship between the two processes.[11] Cross-reactivity may exist between EBV nuclear antigens and autoantigens, including collagen, actin, and cytokeratin, and synovial membrane antigens.[12] Cellular immunity is altered in RA. T-cell stimulation produces lymphokines (interferon-gamma) that activate macrophages to release monokines (interleukin-1), tumor necrosis factor-alpha, granulocyte-macrophage colony-stimulating factor, and other growth factors. Fibroblasts and endothelial cells proliferate, new blood vessels form, and osteoclasts are stimulated to erode bone. Increased numbers of T4 lymphocytes that activate B lymphocytes to produce immunoglobulin are frequently found in synovium from RA patients.[13] Many of the B and T lymphocytes and monocytes in rheumatoid synovium express histocompatibility antigens (DR and DQ), indicating increased cellular activity of these cells.[14] Lymphocytes from RA patients demonstrate sensitity to collagen present in the joints and eyes (types II and III).[15] Collagen and chondrocytes may present antigens that help perpetuate the illness.[16, 17]

These unspecified environmental antigens are presented to antigen-presenting cells bearing major histocompatibility complex class II antigens.[18] The haplotypes associated with RA include human leukocyte antigen (HLA)-DR4 and HLA-DR1.[19] Subtypes of DR4 associated with RA include DRB*0401, DRB*0404/08, and DRB1*0405.[20] The appropriately presented antigen located in the peptide-binding groove formed by the HLA molecule activates lymphocytes that attract macrophages into synovium. The activation of macrophages results in the production of monokines. These factors attract additional lymphocytes and neutrophils. T lymphocytes accumulate in the synovial membrane. Helper-inducer T lymphocytes adhere better to the endothelial adhesive proteins than do suppressor-inducer subsets and gain access more easily to the extracellular matrix of the synovial membrane. There is a relative absence of suppressor-inducer T cells. Angiogenesis factors result in the growth of new capillaries. Activated metalloproteinases, including procollagenase and progelatinase, are released by synovial cells and cause tissue destruction. Arachidonic acid metabolites are produced and affect components of the inflammatory response. This immune-mediated process becomes self-perpetuating even if the initiating factor is removed.[21] The end result of this imbalanced immune process is a systemic illness with immune cells localizing in synovial tissues, proliferating and producing soluble factors that are inflammatory and destructive to joint tissues.

RA causes inflammation that is centered in the synovial membrane. The joints that are affected by the inflammation associated with RA are lined by a thin tissue layer, the synovial membrane, which produces synovial fluid that nourishes the cartilage and lubricates the joint. Synovial membrane is not limited to joints alone but is found in many parts of the musculoskeletal system associated with motion, such as tendons, bursae, and ligaments. The inflammation associated with RA causes hypertrophy of this membrane along with the production of humoral factors that cause destruction of cartilage and bone cells. The end result of this inflammatory process, if left unchecked, is a destroyed joint with thinning cartilage, eroded bone, and disrupted supporting structures.

In the cervical spine, the structures lined with synovial membrane may be involved in RA. These structures include the atlantoaxial joint. This joint connects the atlas (C1) with the axis (C2) and is responsible for rotation of the skull on the cervical spine. Synovial tissue is located between the atlas and axis and between the ligaments and atlas (see Fig. 1–9 in Chapter 1). Other synovial joints include the zygapophyseal and uncovertebral. Bursae are also lined with synovial membrane and are found in the C1–C2 region and interspinous ligaments.[22]

RA causes disease in the cervical spine by causing chronic inflammatory changes to occur in the atlanto-occipital, atlantoaxial, zygapophyseal, and uncovertebral joints along with the discs and ligamentous and bursal structures. At the level of the atlantoaxial joint, synovial inflammation of the bursae and ligaments results in laxity of the transverse ligament that holds the atlas and axis together. Normally, the distance between the bones does not exceed 2.5 to 3 mm in adults.[23] The relaxation of supporting ligaments results in excess motion of the axis in relation to the atlas, atlantoaxial subluxation.[24] Luxation of the atlantoaxial joint may occur anteriorly, posteriorly, superiorly or vertically, or laterally.[25–28] Anterior subluxation is the most common form and results from insufficiency of the transverse ligament or fracture of the odontoid. Posterior subluxation occurs when C1 moves posteriorly on C2 and results from erosion or fracture of the odontoid. Vertical or superior subluxation results from destruction of the lateral atlantoaxial joints around the foramen magnum and is the rarest form. Lateral subluxation occurs with erosion of the lateral mass and odontoid.[29] Abnormal motion of this joint in any direction may result in compression of the cervical spinal cord or medulla oblongata, resulting in the development of neurologic symptoms and signs of myelopathy, including paresthesias, muscle weakness, reflex changes, spasticity, and incontinence.[30, 31] The vertebral arteries may be compressed during subluxation of the atlantoaxial joint by the odontoid process of the axis and the posterior arch of the atlas. The vertebral arteries are compressed as they travel through the foramina in the transverse processes of C1 and C2. Vertebral artery compression may cause tetraplegia, coma, or sudden death.[32, 33] Subluxation may occur in multiple directions in an individual.[34] Autopsy evaluation of RA patients with paralysis reveals spinal cords with mechanical neural compression with marked physical distortion, flattening, and destruction of the cord and vascular compression showing ischemic damage to the cord with necrosis of the lateral columns in the watershed regions supplied by anterior and posterior spinal arteries.[35]

Subluxation may occur between cervical vertebrae below the atlantoaxial joint. Common levels include C3–C4 and C4–C5. Inflammation in the zygapophyseal joints and surrounding bursae undermines the stability of these joints, resulting in excessive motion and angulation of the cervical spine.[36] The intervertebral discs may be invaded by growing synovial tissue, resulting in disc space narrowing.[6] The reported frequency of subaxial subluxation ranges from 7% to 29% of RA patients.[37]

Myelopathy may also occur in patients without atlantoaxial or cervical spine subluxation. In these patients, synovitis from the zygapophyseal joints along with intervertebral disc lesions may compromise the blood supply to the spinal cord through stenosis of vertebral vessels that feed the anterior spinal artery. Ischemic myelopathy is the result.[33] Sudden death may also be a consequence of thrombosis of vertebral vessels.[38]

The neurologic impairments from C1–C2 disease tend to be more severe than subluxations in other portions of the cervical spine. Cerebrospinal fluid flow may be impaired with the development of hydrocephalus or syringomyelia.[32] The kinds of neurologic deficits may vary depending on the specific tracts affected in the spinal cord. For example, cruciate paralysis occurs with compression of the upper corticospinal tract decussation in the center of the spinal cord without affecting the uncrossed tract supplying the lower extremities. The clinical result is bilateral weakness in the upper extremities and normal strength in the lower extremities.[39] Compression of the lateral aspect of the pyramidal decussation results in paresis of the ipsilateral arm and contralateral leg.[32]

Clinical History

Patients with RA develop joint pain, heat, swelling, and tenderness. The joint involvement is additive and symmetrical. The joints at greatest risk of being affected by the disease process include the proximal interphalangeal, metacarpal-carpal, wrist, elbow, hip, knee, ankle, and metatarsophalangeal joints. In the axial skeleton, the cervical spine is most frequently affected. Patients have joint pain and stiffness, which are most severe in the morning. Activity improves symptoms. This phenomenon, stiffness of a joint with rest, occurs frequently with active disease. As a component of systemic inflammation, afternoon fatigue, anorexia, and weight loss are common complaints.

The cervical spine is the most commonly affected component of the axial skeleton. Neck movement frequently precipitates or aggravates neck pain that is aching and deep in quality. Atlantoaxial disease is experienced in the upper part of the cervical spine, and pain radiates over the occiput into the temporal and frontal regions with increasing disease of the C1–C2 joint. Occipital headaches are frequently associated with active rheumatoid involvement of the cervical spine. Other symptoms of C1–C2 subluxation include a sensation of the head falling forward with flexion of the neck, loss of consciousness or syncope, incontinence, dysphagia, vertigo, convulsions, hemiplegia, dysarthria, nystagmus, or peripheral paresthesias.[40] Peripheral joint erosion is a harbinger of C1–C2 subluxation. Development of cervical subluxation occurs in patients who have joint erosions of hands and feet, serum rheumatoid factor, and subcutaneous nodules.[41, 42]

Pain associated with RA in the subaxial segments of the cervical spine is located in the lateral aspects of the neck and clavicles (C3–C4) and over the shoulders (C5–C6). Neurologic symptoms include paresthesias and numbness. The paresthesias have a burning quality that may be attributed to an entrapment neuropathy (carpal tunnel syndrome) but is sufficiently different, not to be confused with joint pain. Patients with sensory symptoms alone may have their symptoms ascribed to arthritis, delaying the diagnosis of cervical myelopathy.[31]

The appearance of spasticity, gait disturbance, muscular weakness, and incontinence (urinary or rectal) indicates significant compression of the spinal cord. Symptoms suggesting vertebrobasilar artery insufficiency include visual disturbances, dizziness, paresthesias of the face, ataxia, and dysarthria.[43, 44]

Patients with severe, generalized RA develop neck symptoms with cervical subluxation. However, patients may develop marked subluxation with little peripheral arthritis.[6] Similarly, the extent of cervical subluxation may not be closely correlated with the extent of neck pain or neurologic dysfunction. This may occur since there is adequate room at the C1–C2 level (the most capacious portion of the spinal canal) to allow the spinal cord to slip laterally around the odontoid, escaping compression.[5]

Physical Examination

Physical examination of an RA patient with cervical spine disease reveals diffuse peripheral joint involvement characterized by heat, swelling, bogginess, tenderness, and loss of motion. Nodules over the extensor surfaces are noted in 20% of RA patients. Examination of the cervical spine may show tenderness with palpation over the bony skeleton and limitation of all spinal movements. Pseudoaneurysm of the vertebral artery may be manifested as a pulsatile mass.[45] Inspection may show fixation of the head tilted down and to one side. This lateral tilt is caused by the asymmetrical destruction of the lateral atlantoaxial joints. The normal cervical lordosis may also be absent. With the neck flexed, the spinous process of the axis may be prominent in the midline of the neck of the patient with atlantoaxial subluxation. Palpation of the posterior pharynx during flexion may reveal abnormal separation of the anterior arch of the atlas from the body of the axis. Anteroposterior laxity may also be detected by applying pressure on the forehead while palpating the spinous process of the axis. In a patient with subluxation, the flexed head glides backward as the subluxation is reduced. This test is not frequently used, however, for fear of causing neurologic symptoms. Patients with subaxial subluxation may demonstrate abnormalities in the upper extremities. For example, compression of C6–C8 segments causes distinctive numb, clumsy hands and tactile agnosia.[46]

Neurologic abnormalities may include loss of sensation and weakness of muscles of the upper or lower extremities. Abnormal Babinski's signs may occur but are uncommon. Vertigo, nystagmus, dysphagia, or coma are present in the occasional patient with vertebral artery compression. Vertical subluxation may affect the medulla oblongata and cranial nerves. Abnormal neurologic signs in these patients may include internuclear ophthalmoplegia, facial diplegia, downbeat nystagmus, spastic quadriparesis, sleep apnea, loss of pinprick and light touch in the trigeminal nerve distribution, and dysfunction of cranial nerves IX, X, and XII.[32] In general, neurologic abnormalities are seen in approximately 7% of RA patients.[2]

Laboratory Data

Abnormal laboratory findings include anemia, elevated erythrocyte sedimentation rate, and increases in serum globulin levels. Thrombocytosis is found in patients with active RA. Rheumatoid factors (antibodies directed against host antibodies) are present in 80% of patients with RA. Antinuclear antibodies are present in 30% of RA patients. C-reactive protein, an acute-phase reactant, may be helpful when obtained in a serial manner to predict those individuals who are at increased risk for

joint deterioration and as a measure of response to therapy.[47] Synovial fluid analysis demonstrates an inflammatory fluid characterized by poor viscosity, increased numbers of white blood cells, decreased glucose level, and increased protein level.

Histologic examination of the synovium from affected joints demonstrates an inflammatory, hyperplastic tissue characterized by mononuclear cell infiltration, synovial cell proliferation, fibrin deposition, and necrosis. Examination of cervical spine apophyseal joints from autopsied RA patients has shown similar hyperplastic changes consistent with those synovial alterations associated with the inflammatory disease in peripheral joints.[6]

Somatosensory-evoked potentials are useful in detecting spinal cord impingement in patients with subluxation and severe arthritis. Neurologic signs may be difficult to elicit in patients with joint destruction. Somatosensory potentials may localize an area of cord impingement that may not be conclusively documented by physical examination or radiographs.[48]

Radiographic Evaluation

Characteristic roentgenographic changes of RA in peripheral joints include soft tissue swelling, bony erosion without reactive sclerotic bone, joint space narrowing, and periarticular osteopenia. Roentgenographic evaluation of the cervical spine includes anteroposterior, lateral with flexion and extension, oblique, and open-mouth frontal projection.

The roentgenographic criteria for the diagnosis of RA cervical spine disease as proposed by Bland and colleagues are the following: (1) atlantoaxial subluxation of 2.5 mm or more; (2) multiple subluxation of C2–C3, C3–C4, C4–C5, and C5–C6; (3) narrow disc spaces with little or no osteophytosis; (4) erosion of vertebrae, especially vertebral plates; (5) odontoid, small, pointed, eroded loss of cortex; (6) basilar impression; (7) apophyseal joint erosion, blurred facets; (8) cervical spine osteoporosis; (9) wide space (more than 5 mm) between posterior arch of the atlas and the spinous process of the axis (flexion to extension); and (10) secondary osteosclerosis, atlantoaxial occipital complex, which may indicate local degenerative change.[49]

Anterior subluxation is the most common form of cervical spine derangement. A variability exists in the frequency of anterior subluxation in RA patients. The variability may be related to the absence of all the roentgeno-graphic views (flexion) necessary to observe subluxation or to the difficulty in observing the anterior edge of the odontoid process. Anterior subluxation is present in 25% of all RA patients and in 70% of RA patients with neck pain.[50, 51] In postmortem studies, anterior subluxation is noted in 46% of RA patients.[52] The normal distance between the odontoid and atlas is 2.5 mm and 3.0 mm in women and men, respectively, as measured from the posteroinferior aspect of the tubercle of C1 to the nearest point on the odontoid[53] (Fig. 11–1). The posterior atlanto-odontoid interval is the remaining distance between the posterior surface of the odontoid process and the anterior edge of the posterior ring of the atlas. The mechanism of spinal cord compression with anterior subluxation has been studied by cineradiography.[54] During flexion, the atlas slowly separates anteriorly from the axis. With increasing displacement, the spinal canal is narrowed by the posterior arch of the atlas. In extension, subluxation persists as long as the head is below the horizontal. The atlas slides backwards and rests against the dens (producing a clicking sensation when motion is abrupt) when the horizontal plane is reached.

Posterior subluxation occurs in 6.7% of RA patients.[55] The atlas must be partially destroyed or malformed or the odontoid eroded, fractured, or congenitally absent for posterior subluxation to occur. Posterior subluxation may also occur if the atlas "jumps" over the axis, resting in a dorsal position resulting in posterior subluxation.[56, 57] Vertebrobasilar artery insufficiency associated with neurologic dysfunction is a manifestation of this form of subluxation.

Vertical subluxation of the dens through the foramen magnum into the posterior fossa occurs in 5% to 35% of RA patients.[55, 58, 59] Upward translocation occurs when the bony and ligamentous integrity of the atlanto-occipital

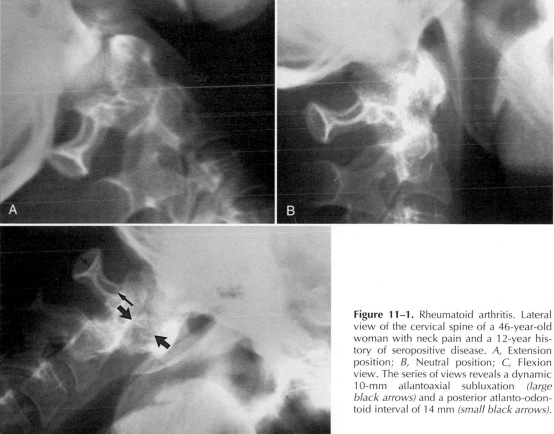

Figure 11–1. Rheumatoid arthritis. Lateral view of the cervical spine of a 46-year-old woman with neck pain and a 12-year history of seropositive disease. *A,* Extension position; *B,* Neutral position; *C,* Flexion view. The series of views reveals a dynamic 10-mm atlantoaxial subluxation *(large black arrows)* and a posterior atlanto-odontoid interval of 14 mm *(small black arrows).*

articulations is disrupted. Disease of the occipital condyles, lateral masses of the atlas, and lateral articulations of the axis results in bony erosions or collapse.[60] The extent of vertical migration may be measured by a number of methods[61] (Fig. 11–2). McRae's line defines the true foramen magnum with a line drawn between its anterior margin (basion) and its posterior margin (opisthion). The tip of the dens is below this line. Other lines have been described because the basion may be difficult to observe on lateral roentgenograms of the cervical spine. Chamberlain's line is drawn from the hard palate to the opisthion. The odontoid tip should not be more than 3 mm above this line. McGregor's line extends from the posterior margin of the hard palate to the most caudal point of the occiput. The dens should not project more than 4.5 mm above this line. These methods are based on the position of the tip of the odontoid. Because the location of the odontoid tip may be difficult to determine because of bony erosion, two alternative methods for vertical subluxation were devised. Ranawat's line is constructed by determining the coronal axis of C1 by connecting the center of the anterior arch of C1 with its posterior ring. The sclerotic ring in the center of C2 identifies the pedicle. The vertical distance along the dens axis is measured. In men, the distance is 17 +/− 2 mm, and in women the distance is 15 +/− 2 mm. Any distance less than 13 mm is indicative of superior migration.[53] The Redlund-Johnell line is determined by the vertical distance between the inferior border of the axis and McGregor's line.[62]

Rotatory-lateral subluxation occurs in up to 30% of RA patients.[37] Erosion of the lateral apophyseal joints allows for a rotational head tilt.[63] The open-mouth view may demonstrate narrowing of the atlanto-occipital and atlantoaxial joints as well as erosion of the odontoid. Subluxation occurs when the lateral masses of the atlas are displaced more than 2 mm with respect to those of the axis. Bony erosion is the most important factor in the development of severe lateral subluxation.[64]

In addition to changes in the upper cervical spine, radiographic abnormalities, including subaxial subluxation, apophyseal joint narrowing, and disc space narrowing, occur in the lower cervical spine. Subaxial subluxation occurs in up to 29% of RA patients.[61] Subaxial subluxation is present in instances of more than 3.5 mm malalignment. The stability of flexion and extension of the lower cervical spine depend on the integrity of the anterior and posterior longitudinal ligaments. Greater than 3.5 mm of malalignment is indicative of a mechanically unstable spine.[65] Multiple subluxations may occur, producing a "staircase" appearance on lateral radiographs.[61] Anterior subluxation is more frequent than posterior subluxation. Subaxial subluxation is most notable on a lateral flexion view of the cervical spine. Apophyseal joint disease includes narrowing, erosions, and sclerosis. Disc destruction in the cervical spine is associated with disc space narrowing and is caused by extension of erosive disease from uncovertebral joints or by ongoing trauma to vertebral end plates secondary to instability. The final stage of apophyseal disease is fibrous ankylosis of one or more levels, which may rarely simulate the appearance of ankylosing spondylitis.[66]

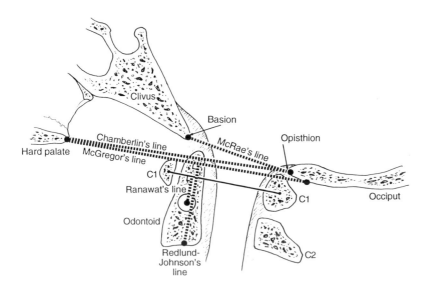

Figure 11–2. Vertical subluxation. Lines drawn at the base of the skull to determine subluxation of the dens into the foramen magnum.

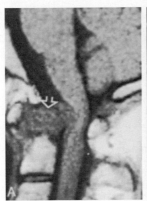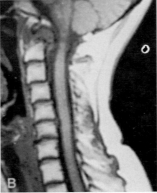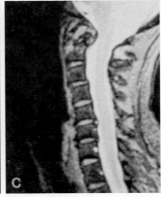

Figure 11–3. Magnetic resonance (MR) imaging in rheumatoid arthritis: evaluation of spinal involvement. Periodontoid disease. *A,* Sagittal T₁-weighted spin echo MR image (TR/TE 450/30) of the upper cervical spine reveals a mass of intermediate signal intensity *(arrow)* that is eroding the odontoid process and causing cord compression. (From Neuhold A, et al.: Medicamundi 32:38, 1987.) *B,* Sagittal T₁-weighted spin echo (TR/TE 600/11) and multiplanar gradient recalled. (From Resnick D: Rheumatoid arthritis. In: Resnick D [ed]: Diagnosis of Bone and Joint Disorders, 3rd ed. Philadelphia: WB Saunders Co, 1995, p 952.) *C,* Sagittal T₁-weighted spin echo (TR/TE 600/11). MR images show similar involvement in a different patient. Note the high signal intensity around the odontoid process. (Courtesy of C. Gundry, M.D., Minneapolis, Minnesota.)

Computerized tomography (CT) is a useful radiographic technique for detecting the extent of bony destruction of structures that may not be easily visualized with plain roentgenograms. CT scan detects the position of an eroded odontoid process that may not be seen on open-mouth view roentgenograms.[67] CT also demonstrates the posterior obliteration of subarachnoid space that marks those individuals at risk for progressive myelopathy.[68] In a comparison of plain roentgenograms and CT, Braunstein and colleagues reported on the usefulness of plain roentgenograms as the initial examination of choice.[69] CT visualized the transverse ligament but did not provide significant additional information. Others believe that CT images offer views of the spinal canal, spinal cord, and neural foramina that are useful in detecting the extent and severity of disease.[70]

Magnetic resonance (MR) imaging is a noninvasive method that is useful in detecting soft tissue abnormalities in the cervical spine of RA patients. MR imaging allows direct visualization of the spinal cord at sites of bony or soft tissue compression[71–73] (Fig. 11–3). MR imaging is able to detect pannus around the odontoid and alterations in the substance of the spinal cord.[74, 75] MR imaging may also be useful in documenting the response of pannus to therapy or the status of the spinal cord in the postoperative state.[76]

Differential Diagnosis

RA is a clinical diagnosis based on history of joint pain, distribution of joint involvement, and characteristic laboratory abnormalities (rheumatoid factor). Criteria for the classification of RA were published by the American College of Rheumatology[77] (Table 11–1). In the setting of generalized, active disease, the finding of neck pain associated with multiple abnormalities, including atlantoaxial subluxation, apophyseal joint erosion without sclerosis, disc space narrowing without osteophytes, and multiple subluxations, is most appropriately attributed to RA. The cervical spine abnormalities of ankylosing spondylitis, psoriatic arthritis, Reiter's syndrome, enteropathic arthritis, osteoarthritis, and diffuse idiopathic skeletal hyperostosis are associated with new bone formation or ligamentous calcification that differentiate them from RA. Occasionally, atlantoaxial subluxation may occur alone in the setting of little peripheral disease. In those circumstances, other disease processes that may cause subluxation include ankylosing spondylitis, psoriatic arthritis, Reiter's syndrome, trauma, or local infection.

Treatment

The treatment for control of generalized RA includes a regimen of patient education, physical therapy, nonsteroidal anti-inflammatory drugs (NSAIDs), remittive agents (gold, salts, penicillamine, or hydroxychloroquine), corticosteroids, and immunosuppressive agents (methotrexate).[21] The therapy has been organized into a therapeutic pyramid based on the use of less toxic therapies for all patients.

TABLE 11–1.   THE AMERICAN RHEUMATISM ASSOCIATION 1987 REVISED CRITERIA FOR THE CLASSIFICATION OF RHEUMATOID ARTHRITIS

1. Morning stiffness	Morning stiffness in and around the joints, lasting at least 1 hour before maximal improvement
2. Arthritis of three or more joint areas	At least three joint areas simultaneously have soft tissue swelling or fluid (not bony overgrowth)
3. Arthritis of hand joints	At least one area swollen (as defined above) in a wrist, metacarpophalangeal (MCP), or proximal interphalangeal (PIP) joint.
4. Symmetric arthritis	Simultaneous involvement of PIPs, MCPs, or metatarsophalangeals is acceptable without absolute symmetry
5. Rheumatoid nodules	Subcutaneous nodules, over bony prominences, extensor surfaces, or juxta-articular regions, observed by a physician
6. Serum rheumatoid factor	Demonstration of abnormal amounts of serum rheumatoid factor by any method for which the result has been positive in less than 5% of normal control subjects
7. Radiographic changes	Radiographic change typical of rheumatoid arthritis on posteroanterior hand and wrist radiographs, which must include erosions or unequivocal bony decalcification localized in or most marked adjacent to the involved joints (osteoarthritis changes alone do not qualify)

For classification purposes, a patient is said to have rheumatoid arthritis if the patient has satisfied at least four of seven criteria. Criteria 1 through 4 must have been present for at least 6 weeks. Patients with two clinical diagnoses are not excluded. Designation as classic, definite, or probable rheumatoid arthritis is not to be made.

Arnett FC, Edworthy SM, Block DA, et al.: The American Rheumatism Association 1987 revised criteria for the classification of rheumatoid arthritis. Arthritis Rheum 31:315, 1988.

Drugs of greater toxicity are added with increasing clinical activity of disease. A reassessment of the treatment regimen has been proposed.[78] This regimen initiates therapy with a multitude of drugs of increased toxicity compared with NSAIDs, with the proposition that the increased morbidity and mortality rates of RA require aggressive initial therapy.

Therapy is directed at the control of pain and stiffness, reduction of inflammation, maintenance of function, and prevention of deformity. Patients are educated about their disease so they may be an active participant in their care. They are encouraged to continue with as normal a lifestyle as possible. Physical therapy provides temperature modalities (heat or cold) that relieve pain, exercises that maintain muscle strength, and assistive devices (canes, crutches, and splints) that promote normal function and ambulation.

Medications to control pain and inflammation are useful in the patient with RA. Aspirin is a very effective agent for RA if given in adequate doses to reach a serum concentration of 20 to 25 mg/dL. For patients who are unable to take the number of tablets necessary to reach that serum level, who are intolerant of the drug, or on whom it has no effect, other NSAIDs are useful in controlling symptoms. These agents include ibuprofen, tolmetin, fenoprofen, naproxen, indomethacin, piroxicam, sulindac, mefenamic acid, ketoprofen, etodolac, diclofenac, nabumetone, and oxaprozin. The choice of agent is dependent on a number of factors, including drug half-life, formulation, dose range, and tolerability.[79]

Patients who continue with joint inflammation or who demonstrate joint damage (joint space narrowing, bony erosions, or cysts), despite adequate nonsteroidal therapy, are candidates for remittive therapy. Remittive agents, such as hydroxychloroquine, gold salts, and penicillamine, have a delayed onset of action compared with NSAIDs. Hydroxychloroquine has a moderate, disease-suppressive action with few adverse reactions at doses of 400 mg/day or less.[80] Injectable gold salts (50 mg/week) alter the natural history of RA.[81] The combination of D-penicillamine (125 to 750 mg/day) and sulfasalazine (2 gm/day) has been reported to have a beneficial effect on the inflammation of RA.[82] Methotrexate at doses from 7.5 to 15 mg/week is effective in decreasing the inflammation of RA and may also slow disease progression.[83] Methotrexate may be given all at once during the week. It is effective over a long duration of therapy.[84] In a study using methotrexate, 587 RA patients were followed for 70 months; 76% of patients remained on methotrexate for that period.[85] The drug remained effective in a majority of patients for the duration of the study. Patients who have a stable course may be able to take methotrexate every second week and maintain control of joint inflammation.[86]

Systemic corticosteroids are effective controlling the inflammatory components of RA. Corticosteroids are the most powerful and predictable remedy inducing immediate relief of joint inflammation in RA.[87] Corticosteroids at low doses may have a modest effect on reducing the rate of radiologically detected joint destruction.[88] Corticosteroids are also associated with a wide range of toxicities, from hypertension and diabetes to cataracts and osteonecrosis of bone. Glucocorticoid-induced osteoporosis is a significant complication of this therapy.[89] Intra-articular corticosteroid injections are used when a single joint remains active in the face of general control of the arthritic process.

Immunosuppressives are associated with severe toxicities (aplastic anemia and cancer), which limits their benefit to the severely affected patient. Only a small number of patients with RA require this therapy. Some of the immunosuppressives used in RA include azathioprine, chlorambucil, cyclophosphamide, and cyclosporin A.[90–93] A combination of cyclosporine and methotrexate may be an effective combination for therapy of patients with severe disease.[94]

Experimental therapy of RA includes the use of total lymph node irradiation, monoclonal antibodies, and antibiotics (minocycline). The studies of these agents are not conclusive to demonstrate their long-term beneficial effect on the course of RA.[95–97]

Major controversy remains concerning the role of surgery in the treatment of RA patients with cervical spine disease, particularly those who are asymptomatic. Myelopathic signs occur in up to 33% of patients.[61] Balanced against the potential for neurologic dysfunction is the mortality rate of 15% and a successful fusion rate of only 50%.[59] If neurologic function progresses to paralysis, the success of surgery to improve function is significantly compromised and surgical mortality increases.[98] Boden and colleagues reviewed the course of 20 years of 73 RA patients with cervical spine disease.[99] Forty-two of these patients developed paralysis. The posterior atlanto-odontoid interval and the diameter of the subaxial sagittal spinal canal were the measurements most closely associated with progression to paralysis. Patients with less than 10 mm of posterior atlanto-odontoid interval had no recovery after correction of atlantoaxial subluxation. Patients with vertical and atlantoaxial subluxation had neurologic recovery if the atlanto-odontoid interval was 13 mm. Good results with repair of subaxial subluxation required a diameter of 14 mm.

When surgical therapy is required for atlantoaxial subluxation, reducible atlantoaxial subluxations are managed with posterior arthrodesis.[100] Irreducible subluxation may require a transoral approach for decompression and posterior fusion.[101] Vertical subluxation with any evidence of cord compression requires surgical correction because of the high mortality associated with this lesion. These patients require tong traction to reduce subluxation, transoral anterior decompression, and occipitocervical fusion to prevent recurrent cranial settling.[61, 102] Patients with subaxial subluxation and compression should undergo reduction of the subluxation because granulation tissue may result in increased neural compression. One approach is that of posterior stabilization of the subluxed segment.[103] Other approaches are anterior decompression and fusion.[104] Common complications of RA cervical spine surgery include death (5% to 10%), infection, wound dehiscence, nonunion (5% to 20%), wire breakage and loss of reduction, and subluxation at the level below the fused segment.[105] Good outcomes occur when surgical intervention is undertaken before severe myelopathy is present.

Prognosis

The course of RA cannot be predicted at time of onset. Some patients develop sustained disease that is associated with joint destruction and resistance to therapy. Patients who are older with seropositive generalized disease with nodules are at greater risk of developing cervical spine disease. Not all patients develop subluxation. In a 5- to 14-year follow-up study, 25% of patients had an increase in subluxation, 50% had no change, and 25% had improvement.[3] In a 5-year study of 106 RA patients, the prevalence of cervical spine subluxation increased from 43% to 70%.[106] In subaxial disease, myelopathy was associated with narrowing of the canal, destruction of spinous processes, axial shortening, younger age of patient, longer duration of disease, higher dose of corticosteroids, and higher stage of disease.[36] Sudden death remains a complication of RA cervical spine disease, particularly in those with vertical subluxation.[107]

A practical consideration in the preoperative care of RA patients is the need for cervical spine roentgenograms. In 128 RA patients with no symptoms of cervical cord compression who underwent elective orthopedic surgery, unsuspected C1–C2 disease was detected in 5.5%. The results of the roentgenograms had little effect on the type of anesthesia given at the time of surgery. Alternative methods of anesthesia without the need for hyperextension of the neck were used without complication. Communication between the physician and anesthesiologist may negate the need for cervical spine roentgenograms in RA patients who are asymptomatic in regard to the cervical spine.[108]

References

RHEUMATOID ARTHRITIS

1. O'Sullivan JB, Cathcart ES: The prevalence of rheumatoid arthritis: follow-up evaluation of the effect of criteria on rates in Sudbury, Massachusetts. Ann Intern Med 76:573, 1972.
2. Colon PW, Isdale IC, Rose BS: Rheumatoid arthritis of the cervical spine: an analysis of 333 cases. Ann Rheum Dis 25:120, 1966.
3. Sharp J, Purser DW, Lawrence JS: Rheumatoid arthritis of the cervical spine in the adult. Ann Rheum Dis 17:303, 1958.
4. Bernhard G: Extra-articular rheumatoid arthritis: Clinical features and treatment overview. In: Utsinger PD, Zvaifler NJ, Ehrlich GE (eds): Rheumatoid Arthritis: Etiology, Diagnosis, Management. Philadelphia: JB Lippincott Co, 1985, p 337.
5. Bland JH, Davis PH, London MG, et al.: Rheumatoid arthritis of the cervical spine. Arch Intern Med 112:892, 1963.
6. Bland JH: Rheumatoid arthritis of the cervical spine. Bull Rheum Dis 18:471, 1967.
7. Bland JH: Rheumatoid arthritis of the cervical spine. J Rheumatol 1:319, 1974.
8. Stastny P: Immunogenetic factors in rheumatoid arthritis. Clin Rheum Dis 3:315, 1977.
9. Panayi GS: The immunopathogenesis of rheumatoid arthritis. Br J Rheumatol 32(suppl 1):4, 1993.
10. Simpson RW, McGinty L, Simon L, et al.: Association of parvoviruses with rheumatoid arthritis of humans. Science 223:1425, 1984.
11. Decker JL: Rheumatoid arthritis: evolving concept of pathogenesis and treatment. Ann Intern Med 101:810, 1984.
12. Baboonian C, Venables PJW, Williams DG, et al.: Cross-reaction of antibodies to a glycine-alanine repeat sequence of Epstein-Barr virus nuclear antigen-1 with collagen, cytokeratin, and actin. Ann Rheum Dis 50:772, 1991.
13. Van Boxel JA, Paget SA: Predominantly T-cell infiltrate in rheumatoid synovial membranes. N Engl J Med 293:517, 1975.
14. Janossy G, Panayi G, Duke O, et al.: Rheumatoid arthritis: a disease of lymphocytes, macrophage immunoregulation. Lancet 2:839, 1981.
15. Trentham DE, Dynesius RA, Rocklin RE, David JR: Cellular sensitivity to collagen in rheumatoid arthritis. N Engl J Med 299:327, 1978.
16. Alasalameh S, Mollenhauer J, Hain N, et al.: Cellular immune response toward human articular chondrocytes. Arthritis Rheum 33:1477, 1990.
17. Klimiuk PS, Clague RB, Grennan DM, et al: Autoimmunity to native type II collagen: a distinct genetic subset of rheumatoid arthritis. J Rheumatol 12:865, 1985.
18. Nepom GT, Byers P, Seyfried C, et al.: HLA genes associated with rheumatoid arthritis: identification of susceptibility alleles using specific oligonucleotide probes. Arthritis Rheum 32:15, 1989.
19. Harris ED Jr: Excitement in synovium: the rapid evolution of understanding of rheumatoid arthritis

and expectations for therapy. J Rheumatol 19(suppl 32):3, 1992.
20. Walport MJ, Ollier WER, Silman AJ: Immunogenetics of rheumatoid arthritis and the Arthritis and Rheumatism Council's national repository. Br J Rheumatol 31:701, 1992.
21. Harris ED Jr: Rheumatoid arthritis: pathophysiology and implications for therapy. N Engl J Med 322:1277, 1990.
22. Bywaters EGL: Rheumatoid and other disease of the cervical interspinous bursae, and changes in the spinous processes. Ann Rheum Dis 41:360, 1982.
23. Jackson H: Diagnosis of minimal atlanto-axial subluxation. Br J Radiol 23:672, 1950.
24. Mathews JA: Atlanto-axial subluxation in rheumatoid arthritis: a five-year follow-up study. Ann Rheum Dis 33:526, 1974.
25. Frigaard E: Posterior atlanto-axial subluxation in rheumatoid arthritis. Scand J Rheumatol 7:65, 1978.
26. Rana NA, Hancock DO, Taylor AR, Hill AGS: Upward translocation of the dens in rheumatoid arthritis. J Bone Joint Surg 55B:471, 1973.
27. Swinson DR, Hamilton EBD, Mathews JA, Yatres DAH: Vertical subluxation of the axis in rheumatoid arthritis. Ann Rheum Dis 31:359, 1972.
28. Burry HC, Tweed JM, Robinson RG, Howes R: Lateral subluxation of the atlanto-axial joint in rheumatoid arthritis. Ann Rheum Dis 37:525, 1978.
29. Nakano KK: Neurologic complications of rheumatoid arthritis. Orthop Clin North Am 6:861, 1975.
30. Meijers KAE, van Beusekom GT, Luyendijk W, et al.: Dislocation of the cervical spine with cord compression in rheumatoid arthritis. J Bone Joint Surg 56B:668, 1974.
31. Marks JS, Sharp J: Rheumatoid cervical myelopathy. Q J Med 199:307, 1981.
32. Zeidman SM, Ducker TB: Rheumatoid arthritis: neuroanatomy, compression, and grading of deficits. Spine 19:2259, 1994.
33. Editorial: Rheumatoid atlantoaxial subluxation. Br Med J 2:200, 1951.
34. Weiner S, Bassett L, Spiegel T: Superior, posterior, and lateral displacement of C1 in rheumatoid arthritis. Arthritis Rheum 25:1378, 1982.
35. Delamarter RB, Bohlman HH: Postmortem osseous and neuropathologic analysis of the rheumatoid cervical spine. Spine 19:2267, 1994.
36. Yonezawa T, Tsuji H, Matsui H, Hirano N: Subaxial lesions in rheumatoid arthritis: radiographic factors suggestive of lower cervical myelopathy. Spine 20:208, 1995.
37. Halla JT, Hardin JG, Vitek J, et al.: Involvement of the cervical spine in rheumatoid arthritis. Arthritis Rheum 32:652, 1989.
38. Webb F, Hickman J, Brew D: Death from vertebral artery thrombosis in rheumatoid arthritis. Br Med J 2:537, 1968.
39. Bell HS: Paralysis of both arms from injury of the upper portion of the pyramidal decussation: "cruciate paralysis." J Neurosurg 33:376, 1970.
40. Harris ED Jr: Clinical features of rheumatoid arthritis. In: Kelley WN, Harris ED Jr, Ruddy S, Sledge CB (eds): Textbook of Rheumatology, 4th ed. Philadelphia: WB Saunders Co, 1995, pp 874–911.
41. Winfield J, Young A, Williams P, et al.: Prospective study of the radiological changes in hands, feet, and cervical spine in adult rheumatoid disease. Ann Rheum Dis 42:613, 1983.
42. Wolfe BK, O'Keefe D, Mitchell DM, et al.: Rheumatoid arthritis of the cervical spine: early and progressive radiographic features. Radiology 165:145, 1987.

43. Jones MW, Kaufmann JCE: Vertebrobasilar artery insufficiency in rheumatoid atlantoaxial subluxation. J Neuro Neurosurg Psychiatry 39:122, 1976.

44. Mayer JW, Messner RP, Kaplan RJ: Brain stem compression in rheumatoid arthritis. JAMA 236:2094, 1976.

45. Fedele FA, Ho G Jr, Dorman BA: Pseudoaneurysm of the vertebral artery: a complication of rheumatoid cervical spine disease. Arthritis Rheum 29:136, 1986.

46. Chang MH, Liao KK, Cheung SC, et al.: "Numb, clumsy hands" and tactile agnosia secondary to high cervical spondylotic myelopathy: a clinical and electrophysiological correlation. Acta Neurol Scand 86:622, 1992.

47. Otterness IG: The value of C-reactive protein measurement in rheumatoid arthritis. Semin Arthritis Rheum 24:91, 1994.

48. Katz LM, Emsellem HA, Borenstein DG: Evaluation of cervical spine inflammatory arthritis with somatosensory evoked potentials. J Rheumatol 17:508, 1990.

49. Bland JH, Van Buskirk FW, Tampas JP, et al.: A study of roentgenologic criteria for rheumatoid arthritis of the cervical spine. AJR 95:949, 1965.

50. Matthews JA: Atlanto-axial subluxation in rheumatoid arthritis. Ann Rheum Dis 28:260, 1969.

51. Martel W: The occipito-atlanto-axial joints in rheumatoid arthritis and ankylosing spondylitis. AJR 86:223, 1961.

52. Bland JH: Rheumatoid subluxation of the cervical spine. J Rheumatol 17:134, 1990.

53. Komusi T, Munro T, Harth M: Radiologic review: the rheumatoid cervical spine. Semin Arthritis Rheum 14:187, 1985.

54. Park W, O'Neill M, McCall IW: The radiology of rheumatoid involvement of the cervical spine. Skeletal Radiol 4:1, 1979.

55. Weissman BNW, Aliabadi P, Weinfield MS, et al.: Prognostic features of atlanto-axial subluxation in rheumatoid arthritis patients. Radiology 144:745, 1982.

56. Teigland J, Magnaes B: Rheumatoid backward dislocation of the atlas with compression of the spinal cord. Scand J Rheumatol 9:253, 1980.

57. Lipson SJ: Cervical myelopathy and posterior atlanto-axial subluxation in patients with rheumatoid arthritis. J Bone Joint Surg 67A:593, 1985.

58. El-Khoury GY, Wener MH, Menezes AH, et al.: Cranial settling in rheumatoid arthritis. Radiology 137:637, 1980.

59. Morizono Y, Sakou T, Kawaida H: Upper cervical involvement in rheumatoid arthritis. Spine 12:721, 1987.

60. Martel W, Page JW: Cervical vertebral erosions and subluxation in rheumatoid arthritis and ankylosing spondylitis. Arthritis Rheum 3:546, 1960.

61. More J, Sen C: Neurological management of the rheumatoid cervical spine. Mt Sinai J Med 61:257, 1994.

62. Redlund-Johnell I, Pettersson H: Radiographic measurements of the cranio-vertebral region. Acta Radiol 25:23, 1984.

63. Halla JT, Fallahi S, Hardin JG: Nonreducible rotational head tilt and lateral mass collapse. Arthritis Rheum 25:1316, 1982.

64. Bogduk N, Major GAC, Carter J: Lateral subluxation of the atlas in rheumatoid arthritis: a case report and post-mortem study. Ann Rheum Dis 43:341, 1984.

65. White AA III, Johnson RM, Panjabi MM, et al.: Biomechanical analysis of clinical stability in the cervical spine. Clin Orthop 109:737, 1978.

66. Wong RL, Wilson AJ, Ingenito FS, et al: Apophyseal joint ankylosis of the cervical spine in adult-onset rheumatoid arthritis. Arthritis Rheum 28:958, 1985.

67. Westmark KD, Weissman BN: Complications of axial arthropathies. Orthop Clin North Am 21:423, 1990.

68. Raskin RJ, Schnapf DJ, Wolf CR, et al.: Computerized tomography in evaluation of atlantoaxial subluxation in rheumatoid arthritis. Arthritis Rheum 10:33, 1983.

69. Braunstein EM, Weissman BN, Seltzer SE, et al.: Computed tomography and conventional radiographs of the craniocervical region in rheumatoid arthritis: a comparison. Arthritis Rheum 27:26, 1984.

70. Kaufman RL, Glenn WV Jr: Rheumatoid cervical myelopathy: evaluation by computerized tomography with multiplanar reconstruction. J Rheumatol 10:33, 1983.

71. Pettersson H, Larsson EM, Holtos A, et al.: Magnetic resonance imaging of the cervical spine in rheumatoid arthritis. AJNR 9:573, 1988.

72. Aisen AM, Martel W, Ellis JH, McCune WJ: Cervical spine involvement in rheumatoid arthritis: magnetic resonance imaging. Radiology 165:159, 1987.

73. Breedveld FC, Algra PR, Veilvoye CJ, Cats A: Magnetic resonance imaging in the evaluation of patients with rheumatoid arthritis and subluxations of the cervical spine. Arthritis Rheum 30:624, 1987.

74. Kawaida H, Sakou T, Morizono Y, et al.: Magnetic resonance imaging of upper cervical disorders in rheumatoid arthritis. Spine 14:1144, 1989.

75. Dvorak J, Grob D, Baumgartner H, et al: Functional evaluation of the spinal cord by magnetic resonance imaging in patients with rheumatoid arthritis and instability of upper cervical spine. Spine 14:1057, 1989.

76. Larsson EM, Holtas S, Zygmunt S: Pre- and postoperative MR imaging of the craniocervical junction in rheumatoid arthritis. AJR 152:561, 1989.

77. Arnett FC, Edworthy SM, Block DA, et al.: The American Rheumatism Association 1987 revised criteria for the classification of rheumatoid arthritis. Arthritis Rheum 31:315, 1988.

78. Wilske KR, Healey LA: Remodeling the pyramid, a concept whose time has come. J Rheumatol 16:565, 1989.

79. Brooks PM, Day RO: Nonsteroidal anti-inflammatory drugs—differences and similarities. N Engl J Med 324:1716, 1991.

80. Tett SE, Cutler D, Day RO: Antimalarials in rheumatic diseases. Clin Rheumatol 4:467, 1990.

81. Capell HA, Lewis D, Carey J: A three-year follow-up of patients allocated to placebo, or oral or injectable gold therapy for rheumatoid arthritis. Ann Rheum Dis 45:705, 1986.

82. Taggart AJ, Hill J, Asbury C, et al.: Sulphasalazine alone or in combination with D-penicillamine in rheumatoid arthritis. Br J Rheumatol 26:32, 1987.

83. Scully CJ, Anderson CJ, Cannon GW: Long-term methotrexate therapy for rheumatoid arthritis. Semin Arthritis Rheum 20:317, 1991.

84. Sany J, Anaya JM, Lussiez V, et al.: Treatment of rheumatoid arthritis with methotrexate: a prospective open long-term study of 191 cases. J Rheumatol 18:1323, 1991.

85. Buchbinder R, Hall S, Sambrook PN, et al.: Methotrexate therapy in rheumatoid arthritis: a life table review of 587 patients treated in community practice. J Rheumatol 20:639, 1993.

86. Kremer JM, Davies JMS, Rynes RI, et al.: Every-other-week methotrexate in patients with rheumatoid arthritis: a double-blind, placebo-controlled prospective study. Arthritis Rheum 38:601, 1995.

87. Harris ED Jr, Emkey RD, Nichols JE, et al.: Low

dose prednisone therapy in rheumatoid arthritis: a double-blind study. J Rheumatol 10:713, 1983.

88. Kirwan JR: The effect of glucocorticoids on joint destruction in rheumatoid arthritis. N Engl J Med 333:142, 1995.

89. Lukert BP, Raisz LG: Glucocorticoid-induced osteoporosis: pathogenesis and management. Ann Intern Med 112:352, 1990.

90. Luqmani RA, Palmer RG, Bacon PA: Azathioprine, cyclophosphamide and chlorambucil. Clin Rheumatol 4:595, 1990.

91. van Rijthoven AW, Dijkmans BA, Thè HS, et al.: Comparison of cyclosporine and D-penicillamine for rheumatoid arthritis: a randomized, double-blind, multicentre study. J Rheumatol 18:815, 1991.

92. Dougados M, Duchesne L, Awada H, et al.: Assessment of efficacy and acceptability of low dose cyclosporine in patients with rheumatoid arthritis. Ann Rheum Dis 48:550, 1989.

93. Cash JM, Klippel JH: Second-line drug therapy for rheumatoid arthritis. N Engl J Med 330:1368, 1994.

94. Tugwell P, Pincus T, Yocum D, et al.: Combination therapy with cyclosporine and methotrexate in severe rheumatoid arthritis. N Engl J Med 333:137, 1995.

95. Soden M, Hassan J, Scott DL, et al.: Lymphoid irradiation in intractable rheumatoid arthritis. Arthritis Rheum 32:523, 1989.

96. Horneff G, Burmester GR, Emrich F, et al.: Treatment of rheumatoid arthritis with an anti-CD4 monoclonal antibody. Arthritis Rheum 32:523, 1989.

97. Tilley BC, Alarcon GS, Heyse SP, et al.: Minocycline in rheumatoid arthritis: a 48-week, double-blind, placebo-controlled trial. Ann Intern Med 122:81, 1995.

98. Zoma A, Sturrock RD, Fisher WD, et al.: Surgical stabilization of the rheumatoid cervical spine: a review of indications and results. J Bone Joint Surg 69B:8, 1987.

99. Boden SD, Dodge LD, Bohlman HH, Rechtine GR: Rheumatoid arthritis of the cervical spine: a long-term analysis with predictors of paralysis and recovery. J Bone Joint Surg 75A:1282, 1993.

100. Clark CR, Goetz DD, Menezes AH: Arthrodesis of the cervical spine in rheumatoid arthritis. J Bone Joint Surg 71A:381, 1989.

101. Crockard HA, Pozo JL, Ransford HO, et al.: One-stage transoral anterior decompression and posterior stabilization in cervical myelopathy complicating rheumatoid arthritis. J Bone Joint Surg 67B:498, 1985.

102. Boden SD: Rheumatoid arthritis of the cervical spine: surgical decision making based on predictors of paralysis and recovery. Spine 19:2275, 1994.

103. Lipson SJ: Rheumatoid arthritis in the cervical spine. Clin Orthop 239:121, 1989.

104. Santavirta S, Konittinen YT, Sandelin J, et al.: Operations for the unstable cervical spine in rheumatoid arthritis: sixteen cases of subaxial subluxation. Acta Orthop Scand 61:106, 1990.

105. Conaty JP, Mongan ES: Cervical fusion in rheumatoid arthritis. J Bone Joint Surg 63A:1218, 1991.

106. Pellicci PM, Ranawat CS, Tsairis P, Bryan WJ: A prospective study of the progression of rheumatoid arthritis of the cervical spine. J Bone Joint Surg 63A:342, 1981.

107. Mikulowski P, Wollheim FA, Rotmil P, Olsen I: Sudden death in rheumatoid arthritis with atlanto-axial dislocation. Acta Med Scand 198:445, 1975.

108. Campbell RSD, Wou P, Watt I: A continuing role for preoperative cervical spine radiography in rheumatoid arthritis? Clin Radiol 50:157, 1995.

ANKYLOSING SPONDYLITIS

Capsule Summary

Frequency of neck pain—common
Location of neck pain—cervical spine
Quality of neck pain—ache
Symptoms and signs—morning stiffness, decreased neck motion
Laboratory and x-ray tests—increased erythocyte sedimentation rate, squaring vertebral bodies on plain roentgenogram
Treatment—range-of-motion exercises, nonsteroidal anti-inflammatory drugs, muscle relaxants

Prevalence and Pathogenesis

Ankylosing spondylitis (AS) (Greek *ankylos*, bent; *spondylos*, vertebra) is a chronic inflammatory disease characterized by a variable symptomatic course and progressive involvement of the sacroiliac and axial skeletal joints. It is the prototype of the seronegative spondyloarthropathies. This disease complex is characterized by axial skeletal arthritis, the absence of rheumatoid factor in serum (seronegative), the lack of rheumatoid nodules, and the presence of a tissue factor on host cells, human leukocyte antigen (HLA)-B27. AS is a disease of antiquity, having been found in the remains of mummies from Egypt and having been known to Hippocrates.[1] A reappraisal of skeletal remains from a period from Egyptian dynasties to the 19th century suggests that AS may not have been as common as once suspected. Forestier's disease (diffuse idiopathic skeletal hyperostosis), Reiter's syndrome, or psoriatic spondylitis may have occurred more commonly.[2] During that period and to the present, AS has had many names, including rheumatoid spondylitis, Marie-Strümpell disease, von Bechterew's disease, and rheumatoid variant.

AS affects about 1% to 2% of whites, a number equal to the prevalence for rheumatoid arthritis.[3, 4] Some studies have suggested that 6.7% of white adults in certain populations may have AS.[5] Initially, the male-to-female ratio was thought to be 10:1. More recent studies have demonstrated the ratio to be in the range of 3:1.[6] Women tend to be less symptomatic and develop less severe disease, and this may explain their small representation in earlier studies. Women may also present more often with cervical spine disease with minimal lumbar spine symptoms. In addition, the specific-

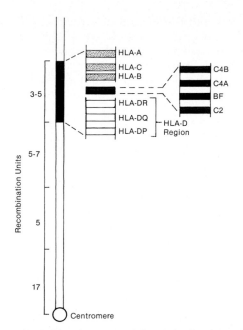

Figure 11–4. The short arm of the sixth chromosome of humans containing the histocompatibility locus (human leukocyte antigen). Included in this area are the A, B, C, and D loci. The D locus includes three alleles (DR, DQ, and DP). Interposed between the B and D loci is the genetic material that codes for some of the complement components (C4B, C4A, BF, C2).

ity of criteria necessary for diagnosis of AS also has an effect on the number of people who have the disease.

The pathogenesis of AS is unknown. In the past, infections, trauma, and heredity were thought to be involved. A genetic predisposition to AS and to the seronegative spondyloarthropathies in general does exist. HLAs are cell surface markers that are present on all nucleated mammalian cells. The portion of the short arm of the sixth chromosome of humans that determines the expression of the HLA antigen is the major histocompatibility complex (MHC), which is associated with control of the immune response of the host (Fig. 11–4). In the MHC region are loci that code for the A, B, C, and D HLA antigens. A, B, and C loci are class I antigens, which are serologically (antibody) defined. The antigen consists of two polypeptide chains: a large glycosylated chain that carries antigenic specificity and a small chain (B_2-microglobulin) (Fig. 11–5). MHC class I genes are expressed on all nucleated cells. The heavy chain is divided into five distinct regions: three extracellular domains, a transmembrane region, and a cytoplasmic domain. There are many alleles for each locus (HLA-A: 20 alleles, HLA-B: 40 alleles, HLA-C: 12 alleles).[7] The D locus or class II antigens are determined by interaction with specific lymphocytes (mixed lymphocyte reaction). The class II antigen consists of two membrane-inserted glycosylated polypeptides that are noncovalently bound (Fig. 11–5). Humans have at least three sets of genes for class II molecules: HLA-DR, HLA-DP, and HLA-DQ. Different alleles exist for each class II molecule. MHC class II antigens are expressed on cells that present antigens to CD4+ T lymphocytes. The class II molecules have an alpha and beta chain. Each chain has two domains: a transmembrane segment and an intracytoplasmic tail. Investigators have identified specific antigens associated with each locus.

A strikingly high association between HLA-B27 and AS has been demonstrated. HLA-B27 is present in more than 90% of white patients with AS compared with a frequency of 8% in a normal white population.[8] Approximately 2% of white patients with HLA-B27 have AS.[9] HLA-B27 is present in 50% of American blacks with AS, with a prevalence of 4% in the normal black population.[10] African blacks do not have the HLA-B27 antigen and rarely develop AS. Other ethnic groups, such as the Haida and Pima Indians, have a large proportion of peo-

Figure 11–5. Major histocompatibility complex (MHC) class I molecules consist of a single alpha chain forming three domains along with beta-microglobulin that acts as a stabilizer for the alpha chain. MHC class II molecules consist of two separate alpha and beta chains that form four extracellular domains.

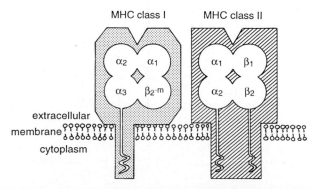

ple affected by AS associated with an increased prevalence of HLA-B27. Approximately 20% of the people who have HLA-B27 have evidence of spondylitis.[6] However, genetic factors alone do not result in the expression of the disease. Many individuals who have HLA-B27 have no evidence of a spondyloarthropathy. Identical twins who have HLA-B27 may be discordant for AS. One twin may have AS, and the other may be normal or develop symptoms and signs of a form of spondyloarthropathy other than AS.[11]

Part of this discordance may be related to the fact that there are at least three different epitopes (antigenic specificities) carried by B27 (M_1, M_2+, M_2-). These HLA-B27 epitopes were defined by murine monoclonal antibodies. The antibody reacting with M_1 was an immunoglobulin G (IgG), and the antibody reacting with M_2 was an IgM. Studies of these B27 epitopes show the following: (1) B27 M_1 is shared by all B27 individuals; (2) M_2 is on most B27 molecules and cross-reacts with Bw47; (3) B27 antigens are M_2-positive or M_2-negative; (4) M_2 variant is more commonly found in Asians than in white populations; (5) B27 M_2-negative molecule is more strongly related to AS than other B27 variants; and (6) B27 M_2-positive molecule may be associated with Reiter's syndrome.[12–15]

Additional evidence for certain subclasses of B27 individuals being at increased risk of developing AS arises from the observation that spondylitis is more common among B27-positive relatives of spondylitics than in B27-positive relatives of healthy B27 control subjects. Susceptibility may be related to the B27 epitope or to the presence of additional or linked genes that increase susceptibility.[16–18] Because genetic information in the MHC region other than class I antigen (complement components—class III antigens) does not increase susceptibility to spondylitis, additional genetic information that predisposes to spondylitis is probably distant from the B27 locus.[19]

Since the report by Calin and colleagues,[18] significant progress has been made in regard to understanding the heterogeneity of HLA-B27. HLA-B27 has been subdivided into nine subtypes.[20, 21] B*2705 is the major subtype of B27. This subtype is present in 90% of B27-positive whites. B*2703 is found only in American blacks.[22] The heterogeneity of HLA-B27 is apparent when its physical structure is examined.[23] The structure of the molecule forms an antigen-binding pocket. The floor of the antigen-binding site is formed by the beta strands and the margins are formed by alpha helices. Certain residues are highly variable and are associated with the subtypes of HLA-B27 (Fig. 11–6).[24] This binding site is the location for the attachment of antigen that is presented to the T cell receptor for processing as an antigen.[25] The various B27 alleles differ from each other by one to six amino acids scattered throughout the peptide-binding groove of the class I molecule. The subtypes associated with AS and the related spondyloarthropathies include B*2701, B*2702, B*2704, B*2705, and B*2707.[26] Additional studies are being reported in regard to identification of HLA-B27 subtypes associated with the various spondyloarthropathies.[27] Currently, the HLA-B27 subtypes are similar between groups.

The mechanism by which HLA-B27 antigen results in spondylitis is not known. The proposed hypotheses to explain this occurrence have included B27 as a receptor site for infectious agents; B27 as a marker for an immune response gene that determines susceptibility to an environmental trigger; and B27 as a factor that induces tolerance to cross-reactive foreign antigens.[28, 29]

A genetically determined host response to an environmental factor in genetically susceptible individuals seems to be the most likely basis for the pathogenesis of the spondyloarthropathies. B27 is not sufficient to develop AS and is supported by the fact that not all individuals with B27 develop disease, that B27 even in a homogeneous form does not cause disease, and that a small number of AS patients do not have B27. Recent studies in animals suggest that the HLA-B27 molecule

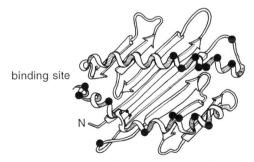

Figure 11–6. Structure of the major histocompatibility complex class I peptide-binding groove. The alpha 1 and 2 domains of the polypeptide chain form a beta-pleated sheet platform and two alpha helices that form the walls of groove into which the antigen peptides can bind. The filled circles correspond to residues critical in defining serologic epitopes on the alpha 1 and 2 domains.

plays a role in the pathogenesis of spondylitis. In transgenic rats made to express high levels of B27, an illness similar to AS develops.[30] The environmental component that may play a role in disease pathogenesis may be intestinal flora. Transgenic rats that are bacteria-free do not develop AS manifestations, whereas those exposed to bacteria subsequently develop the disease. This model provides direct evidence for the participation of the HLA-B27 molecule and environmental factors in disease pathogenesis.[31]

Although not frequently mentioned in the context of spondylitis, DR antigens may play a role in the appearance of certain disease manifestations. Miehle and colleagues reported an increased prevalence of peripheral joint arthritis in HLA-DR4–positive patients with AS.[32]

The role of incidental trauma to the cervical spine in the initiation of the inflammatory process of AS is unknown. Patients with AS may present with radicular arm pain that is thought to be secondary to a herniated cervical disc. Some of these patients have had laminectomies, then later developed classic changes of AS in the axial skeleton. One of the potential complications of total hip joint replacement in a patient with AS is myositis ossificans, or the calcification of soft tissues surrounding a joint. It may be possible that in the patients predisposed to this disease, significant tissue injury to the cervical spine or peripheral joints can result in an inflammatory process that promotes tissue calcification and joint ankylosis.[33]

The difficulty substantiating the role of spine trauma and the development of AS is illustrated by two histories. In the case of fraternal twin brothers, one was asymptomatic with no evidence of AS. The other brother, who was asymptomatic before a fall at work, developed low back pain. He had a decompression procedure (laminectomy) for a suspected herniated lumbar disc. Subsequently, he developed progressive fusion of the lumbar, thoracic, and cervical spine and peripheral arthritis of the hip. In another case, an Egyptian soldier who had symptoms of low back pain compatible with AS was wounded with shrapnel in the lumbar spine and thighs. He was immobilized for an extended period and experienced marked limitation of axial skeleton motion, including the cervical spine. Radiographic evaluation demonstrated increased spondylitic changes in his entire axial skeleton. Did significant tissue damage to the axial skeleton or peripheral joints in those patients with

active AS result in an exacerbation of symptoms and progression of disease in the injured area? Would AS have developed to the same extent in the absence of spinal surgery or tissue injury? Jacoby and colleagues have reported on their experience with five patients who developed spondylitic symptoms after trauma. Radiograph evaluation of these patients revealed disease already present at the time of the injury.[34] They suggest that trauma does not cause spondylitis but brings the patient to medical attention.

Infective agents have also been proposed as initiators of the inflammatory process that causes AS. *Klebsiella* pneumonia has been singled out as the most likely pathogen.[35] Immunologic abnormalities specific to individuals with HLA-B27 antigen have been described.[36] Certain bacteria (*Klebsiella, Shigella, Yersinia*) cause alterations in lymphocyte responses in patients who are B27 M_1- or M_2-positive.[37, 38] However, findings demonstrating the increased colonization of the gut and heightened lymphocyte sensitivity to Klebsiella organisms in AS patients have not been borne out in other investigations.[39, 40] Increased sensitivity of lymphocytes from B27 patients has also not been found with exposure to outer membrane proteins from *Klebsiella,* pneumoniae nitrogenase, or *Yersinia.*[41]

The complete role of the HLA-B27 molecule in the pathogenesis of AS and related spondyloarthropathies remains to be determined. HLA-B27 has the potential to affect the pathogenesis of the illness in multiple ways. Infection with arthrogenic micro-organisms produces proteins that bind to HLA-B27 that triggers an immune response by CD8 + T cells. Bacterial products may also be disseminated to distant tissues like synovium, resulting in persistent inflammation. Alternatively, HLA-B27 receptor sites may recognize bacterial proteins with induction of autoreactivity to host tissues that share identical epitopes. HLA-B27 may select a clone of T cells that specifically react with microbial antigens.[42, 43]

AS is a disease of the synovial and cartilaginous joints of the axial skeleton, including sacroiliac joints, spinal apophyseal joints, and symphysis pubis. The large appendicular joints, hips, shoulders, knees, elbows, and ankles are also affected in 30% of patients. The inflammatory process is characterized by chondritis (inflammation of cartilage) or osteitis (inflammation of bone) at the junction of the cartilage and bone in the spine. An inflammatory granulation tissue forms and erodes the vertebral body margins. As opposed to rheumatoid arthritis, which is associated with osteoporosis as an early manifestation of disease, the inflammation of AS is characterized by ankylosis of joints and ossification of ligaments surrounding the vertebrae (syndesmophytes) and other musculotendinous structures, such as the heels and pelvis.

Clinical History

The classic AS patient is a man from 15 to 40 years of age with intermittent dull low back pain and stiffness slowly progressing for months.[44] Back pain, which occurs throughout the disease in 90% to 95% of patients, is greatest in the morning and is increased by periods of inactivity. Patients may have difficulty sleeping because of pain and stiffness; they may awaken at night and find it necessary to leave bed and move about for a few minutes before returning to sleep.[45] The back pain improves with exercise. The mode of onset is variable, with a majority of the patients developing pain in the lumbosacral region. In a small number, peripheral joints (hips, knees, and shoulders) are initially involved, but occasionally acute iridocyclitis (eye inflammation) or heel pain may be the first manifestation of disease. Rarely, patients may develop ankylosis of the spine without any back pain.[46] Conversely, back pain may be severe, with radiation into the lower extremities, mimicking acute lumbar disc herniation. The patients have symptoms related to the piriformis syndrome.[47] The belly of the piriformis muscle crosses over the sciatic nerve. Inflammation in the sacroiliac joint, where the muscle attaches, results in muscle spasm and nerve compression. There are no abnormal, persistent neurologic signs associated with the sciatic pain. The symptoms are reversible with medical therapy that relieves joint inflammation. This symptom complex of radicular pain is referred to as pseudosciatica.

The usual patient has a moderate degree of intermittent aching pain localized to the lumbosacral area. Paraspinal musculoskeletal spasm may also contribute to the discomfort. With progression of the disease, pain develops in the dorsal and cervical spine and rib joints.

Cervical spine disease in AS occurs less frequently than lumbosacral involvement and at a later time in the course of the illness. Studies of large groups of AS patients report cervical spine involvement to range from 0% to 53.9%.[48–50] Cervical involvement occurs about 5 to 8 years after the onset of the illness in the lumbosacral spine.[51] Studies of different populations have demonstrated increased frequency of cervical spine disease in both women and men when the sexes are compared.[52, 53] A number of reasons may explain the underestimation of AS in women.[54] Women do not have radiographs taken as often as men. They have a more benign course. Peripheral arthritis occurs more commonly in women, suggesting an alternative diagnosis (rheumatoid arthritis). The disease has a slower progression in women. Women have cervical spine disease characteristic of AS with little lumbar spine involvement.[55] The primary symptom of cervical spine disease is neck stiffness and pain. Patients may develop intermittent episodes of torticollis. Involvement of the cervical spine causes the head to protrude forward, making it difficult to look straight ahead.

Spinal involvement is manifested by flattening of the lumbar spine and loss of normal lordosis. Thoracic spine disease causes decreased motion at the costovertebral joints, reduced chest expansion, and impaired pulmonary function. Back pain; back stiffness; thigh, hip, or groin pain; and sciatica are the initial symptoms in 81% of patients. Pain in peripheral joints is the initial complaint of 13%; pain in the chest of 2%, and generalized aches of 1%.[48]

Peripheral joint arthritis (hips, knees, ankles, shoulders, and elbows) occurs in 30% of patients within the first 10 years of disease.[56] Joint disease first appears as pain and stiffness. The inflammatory process may proceed to joint space narrowing and contractures. Fixed flexion contractures of the hips give rise to difficulty with walking and cause a rigid gait. Hip disease is the most frequent limiting factor in mobility rather than spinal stiffness. In fact, peripheral joint disease, particularly of the hips, which appears in the first 10 years of disease, is associated with greater disease activity and more extensive restriction of spinal motion.

Ankylosis may also occur in cartilaginous joints, such as the symphysis pubic, sternomanubrial, and costosternal joints. Erosions of the plantar surface of the calcaneus at the attachment of the plantar fascia result in an enthesopathy (inflammation of an enthesis—attachment of tendon to bone).[57] This inflammation causes a fasciitis and periosteal reaction, which causes heel pain and the formation of heel spurs. Achilles tendinitis is another enthesopathy associated with heel pain and AS.

AS is also associated with many nonarticular abnormalities. Constitutional manifestations of disease, such as fever, fatigue, and weight loss, are seen in a small number of patients with active disease, particularly in those with peripheral joint manifestations. Iritis, inflammation of the anterior uveal tract of the eye, may be the presenting complaint of 25% of the patients with AS and is present in up to 40% of patients over the course of the disease. It is usually unilateral and recurrent and is most often independent of the severity of the joint disease. Iritis is normally treated with topical corticosteroids along with the occasional use of systemic corticosteroids. Mild visual loss may be associated with iritis, but blindness is rare.

Neurologic complications of AS are secondary to nerve impingement or trauma to the spinal cord. In a study of 33 patients with AS and neurologic complications, cervical abnormalities were the most common cause of neurologic compromise.[58] Atlantoaxial subluxation occurs in the setting of AS but less often than in rheumatoid arthritis.[59–61] In rare instances, symptoms of atlantoaxial subluxation may be the presenting manifestation of AS.[62] Significant instability may occur without symptoms in rheumatoid arthritis because of generalized ligamentous laxity and erosion of bone. AS patients have symptoms and signs of nerve impingement more frequently in the setting of instability secondary to the immobilized state of the calcified structures surrounding the spine. Patients with peripheral joint disease are at greater risk of C1–C2 subluxation (6 of 17 AS patients in one study), implying a generalized synovitis affecting a wide field of joints, including those at the atlantoaxial junction.[63] Symptoms of subluxation with impingement of the upper nerve roots include severe neck pain radiating into the occipital and mastoid areas. Spinal cord compression is associated with myelopathic symptoms, including sensory deficits, spasticity, paresis, and incontinence.

AS causes two significant changes to occur in the spine over time. Although the disease is associated with calcification of ligaments and joints, the loss of motion in the spine causes the vertebrae to become osteoporotic. Osteoporosis is a process in which there is a loss of bone calcium. Osteoporotic bones are weaker and are at greater risk of fracture.[64] The other change is the loss of normal flexibility because of ankylosis of the spinal joints and ligaments. The spine in this ankylosed state is much more brittle and is prone to fracture, even with minimal trauma. The most common location for fracture is the cervical spine, although dorsal and lumbar spine fractures have also been described.[65, 66] The occurrence of traumatic cervical spine injury is 3.5 times greater in AS patients than in the normal population.[67] The frequency of AS as the cause of spinal cord injury is 0.3% to 0.5%.[68–71] The lower cervical spine (C6–C7) is the most frequent location for fracture, which is often associated with a fall. Patients who develop fractures may complain of nothing more than localized pain and decreased or increased spinal motion, but severe sensory and motor functional loss corresponding to the location of the lesion may develop. The onset of neurologic dysfunction may be delayed for weeks after initial trauma.[65] In AS patients, an unexpected increase of neck pain, neck motion, or appearance of neurologic symptoms with or without the history of recent trauma is an indication for radiographic evaluation of the axial spine, because multiple fractures may occur.[72] The diagnosis of fracture may be delayed because of the difficulty of detecting fractures in osteoporotic bone with plain roentgenograms. Magnetic resonance (MR) imaging evaluation of these patients may identify the location of the fracture.[66] Radiographic evaluation, including MR imaging, is helpful in detecting the rare disc herniation or epidural hematoma in association with a fracture. An MR image may be difficult to obtain in AS patients because the shape of their spine does not allow entry into the gantry to obtain an optimum scan. Therapy usually consists of external fixation with a brace when neurologic symptoms are minimal, but surgical decompression and fusion for severe neurologic abnormalities such as paraplegia are required.[73] Fractures that mend with external bracing or with surgical fusion heal with normal bone formation. Neurologic deficits may persist despite surgical intervention in as many as 85.7% of patients.[73, 74] A mortality rate from 35% to 50% may be found particularly in AS patients who are elderly, who have complete cord lesions, or who develop pulmonary complications after fracture.[64, 69, 71, 75]

Another complication of long-standing AS is spondylodiscitis, a destructive lesion of the disc and its surrounding vertebral bodies.[76–79] This lesion is associated with a new onset of localized pain in the spine, which uncharacteristically for the AS patient is improved with bed rest. The cause of these lesions may be localized inflammation or minor trauma. In one study, AS patients who did heavy manual labor were at greater risk of developing this abnormality than those who had sedentary occupations.[77] In most cases, external immobilization was effective in controlling symptoms, and surgical fusion was reserved for the more severely affected patients.

Cardiac involvement occurs in 10% of patients with disease durations of 30 years or longer. Mild features include tachycardia, conduction defects, and pericarditis. The most serious cardiac abnormality is proximal aortitis, which results in aortic valve insufficiency, heart failure, and death.[80] Aortic disease may be more common in patients with peripheral arthritis.[81] Prosthetic valve replacement may forestall cardiac deterioration. AS may also be a cause of cardiac conduction disturbances. In a study of patients with pacemakers, 8.5% of 223 men had evidence of sacroiliitis and spondylitis.[82]

Pulmonary involvement is manifested by decreased chest expansion, which limits lung capacity. In addition, a fibrotic process affects the apical segments of the lung as a late and rare complication.[83, 84]

Amyloid, a deposition of a protein-like material in a number of visceral organs, is a very rare complication of AS.[85] Another form of proteinuria associated with AS patients is IgA nephropathy. Patients have increased IgA levels, proteinuria, and renal impairment.[86]

Physical Examination

A careful musculoskeletal examination is necessary, particularly of the lumbosacral spine, to discover the early findings of limitation of motion of the axial skeleton, which is especially noticeable with lateral bending or hyperextension. Percussion over the sacroiliac joints elicits pain in most circumstances.

Measurements of spinal motion, including Schober's test (lumbar spine motion), lateral bending of the lumbosacral spine, occiput to wall (cervical spine motion), and chest expansion are important in ascertaining limitations of motion and following the progression of the disease (Fig. 11–7). Paraspinous muscles may be tender on palpation and in spasm, resulting in limitation of back motion. Finger-to-floor measurements should be done but are more to determine flexibility, which is more closely associated with hip motion than with back mobility. Rotation may be checked with the patient seated. This fixes the pelvis, limiting pelvic rotation. Chest expansion is measured at the fourth intercostal space in men and below the breasts in women. Patients raise their hands over their head and are asked to

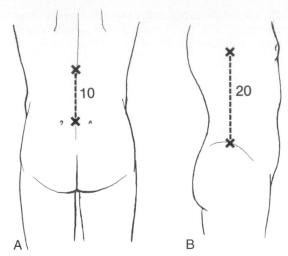

Figure 11–7. Measurement of anterior spinal flexion *(A)* and right and left lateral flexion *(B)*.

take a deep inspiration. Normal expansion is 2.5 cm or greater. Cervical spine evaluation includes measurement of all planes of motion. Peripheral joint examination is also indicated. Careful hip examination is necessary to determine the potential loss of function involved with simultaneous arthritis of the back and hip.[48] Examination of the eyes, heart, lungs, and nervous system may uncover unsuspected extra-articular disease.

Laboratory Data

Laboratory results are nonspecific and add little to the diagnosis of AS. Only 15% of patients have mild anemia. Erythrocyte sedimentation rate is increased in 80% of patients with active disease.[87] Patients with normal sedimentation rates with active arthritis may have elevated levels of C-reactive protein.[88] The rheumatoid factor and antinuclear antibody are characteristically absent.

Histocompatibility testing (for HLA) is positive in 90% of AS patients but is also present in an increased percentage of patients with other spondyloarthropathies (Reiter's syndrome, psoriatic spondylitis, and spondylitis with inflammatory bowel disease). It is not a diagnostic test for AS. HLA testing may be useful in the young patient with early disease for whom the differential diagnosis may be narrowed by the presence of HLA-B27.[89] The presence of HLA-B27 homozygosity was evaluated in 100 patients with AS.[90] Homozygosity was associated with more severe disease but did not impart a greater risk for spondylitis in families of patients with AS.

Radiographic Evaluation

Characteristic changes of AS in the sacroiliac joints and lumbosacral spine are helpful in making a diagnosis but may be difficult to determine in the early stages of the disease.[91] The disease affects synovial and cartilaginous joints as well as sites of tendon and ligament attachment to bone (enthesis). The areas of the skeleton most frequently affected include the sacroiliac, apophyseal, discovertebral, and costovertebral joints.

The disease affects the sacroiliac joints initially and then appears in the upper lumbar and thoracolumbar areas.[92, 93] Subsequently, in ascending order, the lower lumbar, thoracic, and cervical spine are involved. The radiographic progression of disease may be halted at any stage, although sacroiliitis alone is a rare finding except in some women with spondylitis or in men in the early stage of disease.[45, 52] The combination of roentgenographic findings of sacroiliitis and cervical spondylitis without lumbar or thoracic involvement occurs more commonly in women than men.[52] In the peripheral skeleton, the hips and shoulders (glenohumeral) joints are most commonly affected, followed by knees, hands, wrists, and feet, including the heels.[94–96]

Evaluation of the sacroiliac joints is difficult on conventional anteroposterior supine view of the pelvis because of bony overlap and the oblique orientation of the joint. A Ferguson's view of the pelvis (x-ray tube tilted 15° to 30° in a cephalad direction) provides a useful view of the anterior portion of the joint, the initial area of inflammation in sacroiliitis. Radiographic evaluation of the sacroiliac joints is based on five observations: (1) distribution, (2) subchondral mineralization, (3) cystic or erosive bony change, (4) joint width, and (5) osteophyte formation.[97] The symmetry of involvement must be compared with the same areas of the joint (superior—fibrous, inferior—synovial) and to the iliac (thinner cartilage) and sacral (thicker cartilage) sides of the joint.

Sacroiliitis in AS is a bilateral, symmetrical process. Early sacroiliitis appears in the inferior portion of the joint on the iliac side of the articulation. Patchy periarticular osteopenia appears along with areas of subchondral bony sclerosis. During the next stage, the artic-

ular space becomes "pseudowidened" secondary to joint surface erosions. With continued inflammation, the area of sclerosis widens and is joined by proliferative bony changes that cross the joint space. In the final stages of sacroiliitis, complete ankylosis with total obliteration of the joint space occurs. Ligamentous structures surrounding the sacroiliac joint may also calcify. The radiographic changes associated with sacroiliitis may be graded from 0 (normal) to 5 (complete ankylosis) (Table 11–2).[98]

Abnormalities also occur in the lumbar, thoracic, and cervical spine. Classic AS causes vertebral column disease in association with sacroiliac disease. The occurrence of spondylitis without sacroiliitis in AS is an extremely rare finding.[99] This pattern of involvement is much more common in Reiter's syndrome or psoriatic spondylitis.

While osteopenia of the bony structures appears, calcification of disc and ligamentous structures emerges. Thin, vertically oriented calcifications of the annulus fibrosus and anterior and posterior longitudinal ligaments are termed syndesmophytes. Bamboo spine is the term used to describe the spine of a patient with AS with extensive syndesmophytes encasing the axial skeleton.[100]

The discovertebral junction may be affected centrally, peripherally, or in combination.[78] Central erosions cause irregularity of the superior and inferior vertebral margins with surrounding sclerosis. Peripheral lesions cause erosions in the noncartilaginous portion of the junction. The radiographic findings include anterior or posterior bony erosion. Combined lesions affecting the central and peripheral portion of the discovertebral junction may cause ballooning of the disc space ("fish vertebrae") or narrowing of the disc space

TABLE 11–2. RADIOGRAPHIC GRADING OF SACROILIITIS

Grade 0: Normal—normal width, sharp joint margins

Grade 1: Suspicious changes—radiologist is uncertain whether Grade 2 changes are present

Grade 2: Definite early changes—pseudowidening with erosion or sclerosis on both sides of the joint

Grade 3: Unequivocal abnormality—erosions; sclerosis; widening, narrowing, or partial ankylosis

Grade 4: Severe abnormalities—with narrowed joint space, ankylosis

Grade 5: Ankylosis of body joints with regression of surrounding sclerosis

Adapted from Dale K: Radiographic grading of sacroiliitis in Bechterew's syndrome and allied disorders. Scand J Rheumatol Suppl 32:92, 1979.

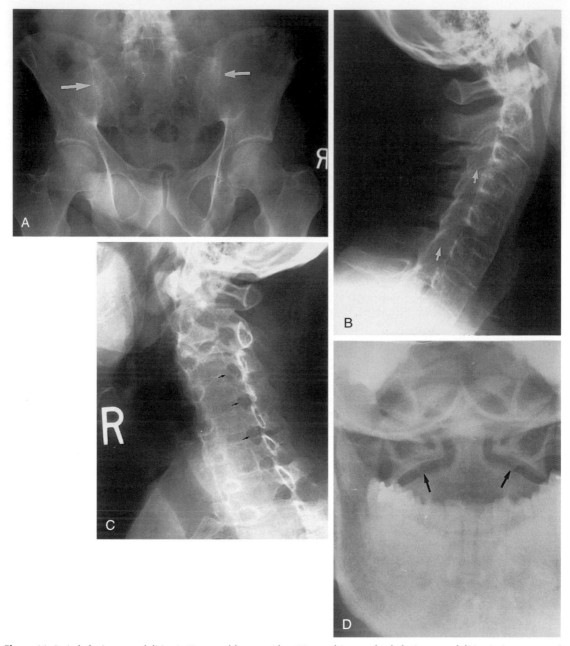

Figure 11–8. Ankylosing spondylitis. A 42-year-old man with a 20-year history of ankylosing spondylitis. *A,* Anteroposterior view of pelvis reveals bilateral sacroiliitis with fusion of these joints *(arrows). B,* Lateral view of cervical spine. There are anterior and posterior syndesmophytes from C3 to C7. Apophyseal joint fusion is noted from C3 to C7 *(arrows). C,* Oblique view of cervical spine. Maintenance of the space for the neural foramina is noted *(arrows). D,* Open-mouth view of the C1–C2 articulation. Despite severe disease in other portions of the cervical spine, the atlantoaxial articulations are intact *(arrows).*

(spinal pseudoarthrosis).[101, 102] This latter finding occurs most commonly in patients with AS of long duration who sustain trauma to the spine. In the cervical spine discovertebral erosion may occur without apophyseal joint disease and before the appearance of syndesmophytes.[103] Intervertebral disc narrowing and

bony sclerosis in vertebral bodies may be accompanying findings.

The apophyseal joints are also affected in the illness. As the disease progresses, fusion of the apophyseal joints occurs. Radiographs of the spine may demonstrate the loss of joint space and complete fusion of the joints. Cervical spine ankylosis may be particularly severe. Complete obliteration of articular spaces between the posterior elements of C2 through C7 results in a column of solid bone[103] (Fig. 11–8). Patients with complete ankylosis of the apophyseal joints and syndesmophytes may develop extensive bony resorption of the anterior surface of the lower cervical vertebrae late in the course of the illness. Bone under the ligaments connecting the spinous processes may also be eroded in the setting of apophyseal joint ankylosis.

The C1–C2 joints may become eroded and subluxed. Synovial tissue around the dens may cause erosion of the odontoid process.[60] Further damage of the surrounding ligaments results in instability that is measured by the movement of the odontoid process from the posterior aspect of the atlas with flexion and extension views of the cervical spine. Widening of the space is indicative of a dynamic subluxation. No movement of the distance between the atlas and axis suggests a fixed subluxation. In addition to atlantoaxial subluxation, migration of the odontoid into the foramen magnum and rotary subluxation may occur.[104–106] Subaxial subluxation is more characteristic of rheumatoid arthritis than AS.

The use of other radiographic techniques in the diagnosis of AS is of marginal additional benefit. They have been used primarily for the evaluation of sacroiliitis. Scintigraphy, computerized tomography, or MR imaging evaluation of the cervical spine would be useful in the setting of spinal fracture or subluxation to determine the location of fracture and the status of the spinal cord (Fig. 11–9). From a diagnostic and clinical perspective, plain roentgenograms provide adequate information at a reasonable cost. Plain roentgenograms remain the usual radiographic technique for the diagnosis of AS.

Differential Diagnosis

Two sets of diagnostic criteria exist for AS. The Rome clinical criteria, used in studies of AS, include bilateral sacroiliitis on radiologic examination and low back pain for more than 3 months that is not relieved by rest, pain in the thoracic spine, limited motion in the lumbar spine, and limited chest expansion or iritis.[107] When these criteria proved to lack sensitivity in identifying patients with spondylitis, the Rome criteria were modified at a New York symposium in 1966 (Table 11–3). These criteria included a grading system for radiographs of the sacroiliac joints in addition to limited spine motion, chest expansion, and back pain.[108] Although these criteria are used mostly for studies of patient populations, they are helpful in the office setting. The criteria are not ideal for population surveys because radiographic sacroiliitis may not be to the ex-

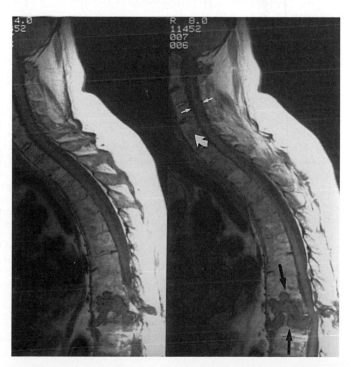

Figure 11–9. Ankylosing spondylitis. Magnetic resonance scan of the cervical spine. T₁-weighted sagittal image reveals pseudoarthrosis in the thoracic spine with compression of the thoracic spinal cord *(black arrows)*. The cervical spine is ankylosed, with calcification of the anterior and posterior longitudinal ligaments and fusion of intervertebral disc spaces *(curved white arrow)*. The spinal canal has adequate room for the cervical spinal cord with cerebrospinal fluid anterior and posterior to the cord *(small white arrows)*.

TABLE 11–3. CLINICAL CRITERIA FOR ANKYLOSING SPONDYLITIS

ROME CRITERIA[107]

A. Clinical Criteria

1. Low back pain and stiffness >3 months not relieved by rest
2. Pain and stiffness in the thoracic region
3. Limited motion in the lumbar spine
4. Limited chest expansion
5. History of evidence of iritis or its sequelae

B. Radiologic Criterion

1. X-ray showing bilateral sacroiliac changes characteristic of ankylosing spondylitis
   Diagnosis: Criterion B + one clinical criterion
           or
   four clinical criteria in absence of radiologic sacroiliitis

NEW YORK CRITERIA[108]

A. Clinical Criteria

1. Limitation of motion of the lumbar spine in anterior flexion, lateral flexion, and extension
2. History of or presence of pain at the dorsolumbar junction or in the lumbar spine
3. Limitation of chest expansion to ≤1 inch

B. Radiologic Criteria

Sacroiliitis
Grade 3—unequivocal abnormality; moderate or advanced sacroiliitis with one or more erosions; sclerosis; widening, narrowing, or partial ankylosis.
Grade 4—severe abnormality, total ankylosis
Diagnosis: Definite—Grade 3–4 bilateral sacroiliitis + one clinical criterion
        or
Grade 3–4 unilateral or Grade 2 bilateral sacroiliitis with clinical criteria 1 or 2 and 3
Probable—Grade 3–4 bilateral sacroiliitis alone

---

tent to satisfy criteria, thereby missing early disease.[109] Some of the measures of decreased mobility and chest expansion are imprecise. In the office setting, a physician makes the diagnosis of AS when the patient is a young male with bilateral sacroiliac pain, lumbar spine stiffness improves with activity, recurring radicular pain alternates side to side, there is a history of iritis and radiologic changes of spondylitis, and HLA-B27 status is determined. However, in the early stages of the disease, clinical symptoms may be mild or atypical and radiologic changes nonexistent, preventing early diagnosis. Suggestions have been made offering a weighing to individual characteristics of the illness to allow better codification of the diagnosis.[110] Others have also pointed out that the diagnostic criteria are too restrictive for certain patients with early disease or an undifferentiated spondyloarthropathy. The European Spondyloarthropathy Study Group has developed a preliminary classification system for spondyloarthropathy in general (Table 11–4).[111]

Although spondyloarthropathies are a common inflammatory musculoskeletal disorder, this group of illnesses is frequently overlooked by nonrheumatologists.[112] A delay in diagnosis from the onset of symptoms and referral to a rheumatologist ranged from 6 to 264 months.

The differential diagnosis of neck pain in a young patient includes other spondyloarthropathies, herniated cervical disc, rheumatoid arthritis, osteoarthritis, fibromyalgia, infection, and tumors. Characteristics of these specific diseases are listed in Table 11–5. The course

TABLE 11–4. EUROPEAN SPONDYLOARTHROPATHY STUDY GROUP CLASSIFICATION CRITERIA FOR SPONDYLOARTHROPATHY

Inflammatory spinal pain or synovitis		
Asymmetrical		
Predominantly in the lower extremities		
And one of the following:		
Positive family history		
Psoriasis		
Inflammatory bowel disease	sensitivity	77%
Alternate buttock pain	specificity	89%
Enthesopathy		
Adding		
Sacroiliitis	sensitivity	86%
	specificity	87%

TABLE 11–5. DIFFERENTIAL DIAGNOSIS OF ANKYLOSING SPONDYLITIS

	ANKYLOSING SPONDYLITIS	REITER'S SYNDROME	PSORIATIC ARTHRITIS	ENTEROPATHIC ARTHRITIS	REACTIVE ARTHROPATHY	HERNIATED NUCLEUS PULPOSUS	OSTEOARTHRITIS OF THE SPINE	RHEUMATOID ARTHRITIS	FIBROMYALGIA	INFECTION	TUMORS
Sex	Male	Male	=	=	=	=	=	Female	Female		=
Age at onset (yr)	15–40	20–30	30–40	15–45	Any age	20–40	40–50	20–60	30–50	Any age	Young—benign Older—malignant
Presentation	Neck pain	Arthritis Urethritis Conjunctivitis	Extremity arthritis Psoriasis Back pain	Abdominal pain	Gastrointestinal, genitourinary infection	Radicular pain	Neck pain	Peripheral arthritis	Generalized fatigue Sleeplessness Tender points	Acute, severe neck pain	Slowly progressive insidious pain
Axial skeleton	+	+/−	+/−	+	+/−	−	+	(Cervical spine)	−	−	−
Peripheral joints	Lower	Lower	Upper	Lower	Lower	−	Lower	Upper and lower	−	−	−
Enthesopathy	+	+	+	−	+/−	−	−	−	−	−	−
Erythrocyte sedimentation rate	Elevated	Elevated	Elevated	Elevated	Elevated	Normal	Normal	Elevated	Normal	Elevated	Elevated (malignant)
Rheumatoid factor (%)	−	−	−	−	−	−	−	80	−	−	−
HLA-B27 (%)	90	80	60 (Spondylitis)	50 (Spondylitis)	90	8	8	8	8	8	8
Course	Continuous	Relapsing	Continuous	Continuous	Self-limited or continuous	Episodic	Relapsing	Continuous	Continuous	Episodic	Continuous
Therapy	Nonsteroidals Exercise	Nonsteroidals Gold Methotrexate	Nonsteroidals Gold Methotrexate	Nonsteroidals Corticosteroids Antibiotics	Nonsteroidals Antibiotics	Nonsteroidals Epidural corticosteroids Surgery	Nonsteroidals	Nonsteroidals Gold Methotrexate	Tricyclic antidepressants Nonsteroidals	Antibiotics Bracing	En bloc excision Chemotherapy Radiotherapy
Disability	Hip	Lower extremity	Lower extremity	Hip	—	Neurologic dysfunction	Neurologic dysfunction	Generalized joint deformities (cervical subluxation anterior, posterior vertical, lateral)	Muscle pain	Neurologic dysfunction	Local invasion—benign Metastases—malignant
Miscellaneous	Neck pain early in women	Neck pain rare		Similar to ankylosing spondylitis in spine involvement							

of AS may be complicated by other common arthritic diseases. AS and rheumatoid arthritis have developed in the same patient. The hosts (AS in men, RA in women) and disease pattern are different, suggesting that the diseases are unassociated.[113] Another disease that may occur in the setting of spondylitis is diffuse idiopathic skeletal hyperostosis (DISH). The convergence of two common diseases in the same host, a middle-aged man, is likely. The occurrence of AS and DISH of the cervical spine has been reported.[114] Reactive arthritis secondary to *Yersinia enterocolitica* has been reported to cause atlantoaxial arthritis in a patient with AS.[115]

Treatment

The goals of therapy, as with other forms of inflammatory arthritis, are to control pain and stiffness, reduce inflammation, maintain function, and prevent deformity with avoidance of undue toxicity. Patients require a comprehensive program of education, physiotherapy, medications, and other measures. Patients are educated about their disease. They are told what they can reasonably expect from treatment and are encouraged to continue with as normal a lifestyle as possible. Patients are taught proper posture and mobilizing and breathing exercises to prevent the tendency to stoop forward and lose chest motion. The importance of a firm upright chair for sitting and a hard mattress with no pillows for sleeping is stressed. Physical therapy with range-of-motion exercises may improve neck movement.[116] The physician gives encouragement and support to patients to adopt their lives to their disease. When the physician cannot give patients adequate time to quell their concern, the physician should arrange additional support for the patients in the form of a social worker, psychiatrist, or vocational counselor. The genetic implications of the disease are placed in perspective. Offspring are at 10% risk of developing AS if a parent is HLA-B27–positive. Also, the importance of self-help groups, such as the Spondylitis Association of America in Sherman Oaks, California, cannot be underestimated. These organizations offer medical literature, exercises, and other resources that are useful to AS patients. Medications to control pain and inflammation are useful to the patient with AS.[117] In the patient with mild spinal or peripheral joint disease, aspirin may be somewhat effective. However, in the patient with more severe disease, aspirin is usually ineffective. If salicylates are used, anti-inflammatory salicylate serum concentrations (20 to 25 mg/dL) should be maintained. Other nonsteroidal anti-inflammatory drugs (NSAIDs) that have been demonstrated to be effective in AS are indomethacin and phenylbutazone. These drugs are effective in controlling spinal and peripheral joint disease but are associated with potentially serious side effects.[118] In a retrospective radiographic study, phenylbutazone decreased the rate of progression of axial skeletal disease in AS.[119] Phenylbutazone is not readily available from pharmaceutical manufacturers and is not used for therapy for the usual AS patient. A follow-up study of 14 patients with AS who took indomethacin for 18 years reported a beneficial effect for the majority, including remission in 28% of patients.[120] NSAIDs such as ibuprofen, tolmetin, fenoprofen, piroxicam, diclofenac, etodolac, flurbiprofen, ketoprofen, sulindac, and mefenamic acid may also be effective in AS.[121, 122] Sulindac has been compared to indomethacin and has comparable efficacy and a tolerance advantage of a twice-a-day dose regimen.[123] This drug has Food and Drug Administration (FDA) approval for use in AS. Naproxen also has FDA approval, and studies have shown efficacy of the drug in the treatment of AS patients.[124] As mentioned, other NSAIDs may be useful for control of joint symptoms but are not approved by the FDA for use in patients with spondylitis.

Patients with acute AS may develop severe muscle spasm with associated limited motion that may hinder their return to normal, daily activities. In these patients, the addition of a muscle relaxant to an NSAID helps decrease muscle pain and muscle spasm and improve back motion. Muscle relaxants, such as cyclobenzaprine, at low-dosage levels (10 mg/day) are helpful while limiting possible drug toxicity. The sleepiness associated with muscle relaxants with long half-lives can be limited by giving the medication 2 hours before bedtime.

Systemic corticosteroids are rarely needed and are ineffective for the articular disease of AS. For the occasional patient with continued joint symptoms, while receiving maximum doses of NSAIDs, adding small doses of corticosteroids (5 mg of prednisone/day) may prove to be useful. Larger doses of corticosteroids cause appreciably more toxicity without an increased benefit. Occasionally, systemic corticosteroids are needed to control persistent iritis. Intra-articular injection of a long-acting steroid preparation is indicated if a patient has peripheral joint disease with persistent effusions.

Pulse intravenous methylprednisolone has caused improvement in patients who failed to respond to nonsteroidal drugs. The use of intravenous pulses yielded dramatic responses lasting 14 months.[125] In another study, pulse methylprednisolone was helpful, but improvement in spinal motions lasted only 2 months.[126]

Intramuscular gold salt injections are not indicated for the axial skeletal disease of AS, but they may be helpful in the rare patient with peripheral joint disease who demonstrates persistent synovitis and joint destruction. Antimalarials have not been used on a regular basis in AS patients. Immunosuppressive medications, primarily methotrexate, have been used for AS in only a small number of patients with some success.[127, 128] A double-blind, placebo-controlled trial of penicillamine in AS detected no significant difference between the test drug and placebo in clinical and laboratory indices.[129]

Orthopedic appliances, such as a heel cup for plantar fasciitis, or a temporary spinal brace to prevent forward flexion, are useful in appropriate patients. Transcutaneous nerve stimulators, in addition to non-narcotic analgesics, are useful in reducing pain in patients with partial response to nonsteroidal drugs. In the patients with fixed flexion deformities of the hip, total joint replacement relieves pain and increases mobility.[130] Surgical procedures on the spine, such as a lumbar spine osteotomy, are limited to patients who have such a degree of forward flexion as to prevent them from looking up from the ground.[131] This operation has multiple potential complications and is viewed as a procedure of last resort. Bradford and colleagues have reported good outcome of spinal osteotomy in 20 of 21 patients, including two with progressive paraplegia.[132]

Radiation therapy was used frequently in patients with AS up to the 1960s, and it was effective at controlling pain and stiffness in the lumbosacral spine.[133] The effects of this therapy, however, were transient and did not prevent progression of the disease. In addition, long-term follow-up studies on these patients demonstrated an increased mortality secondary to leukemia. A Canadian study has shown decreased survival of men who received radiation therapy to the spine after a 27-year follow-up period.[134] The therapy has been abandoned except for the rarest of patients who are intolerant of all other treatment. Lo-cal radiation therapy may be considered for the patient with spondylodiscitis who fails all other therapies.[135]

Prognosis

The general course of AS is benign and is characterized by exacerbations and remissions. Many patients with AS may have sacroiliitis with mild involvement of the lumbosacral spine. Limitation of lumbosacral motion may be mild. The disease can become quiescent at any time. Patients who go on to develop total fusion of the spine may feel better because ankylosis of the spinal joints is associated with decreased pain. In a study of 1,492 patients for 2 years, the frequency of patients with a total remission of disease was less than 2%.[136]

The role of HLA-B27 homozygosity on the course and severity of AS has been controversial. It has been suggested that homozygosity for HLA-B27 increases both the risk and the severity of AS and may be associated with severe peripheral arthritis along with axial disease.[137, 138] Other investigators have been unable to confirm this finding.[139, 140] Suarez-Almazor and Russell reported their experience of the effects of homozygosity on the severity of disease and familial penetrance of spondylitis in association with HLA-B27.[90] HLA-B27 was associated with statistically significant more severe disease in homozygous patients but was not associated with earlier onset of disease or increased risk of family members to develop spondylitis.

The prognosis of men and women with AS has been reported to be different.[141, 142] Women were reported to have a milder course, more peripheral disease, and less radiographic change in the axial skeleton. Gran and colleagues compared 44 women and 82 men with AS and found no difference between the sexes in respect to age at onset, initial symptoms, work performance, restriction of spinal motion, or peripheral joint involvement.[53]

Most studies report that the majority of patients remain functional and employed over the course of the disease.[56] The prime predictor of more severe dysfunction is the presence of peripheral joint involvement, particularly in the hips, and this usually appears within the first 10 years of disease. A majority of these patients developed severe spinal restriction. Patients with fixed flexion contractures of the hips and ankylosis of the spine are severely limited in their functional capacity; however, total hip joint replacement may improve their mobility. Patients with spinal rigidity but normal hip function have minimal disability. However, they should avoid heavy labor, such as lifting objects heavier than 40 pounds.

References

ANKYLOSING SPONDYLITIS

1. Ruffer A: Arthritis deformans and spondylitis in ancient Egypt. J Pathol 22:159, 1918.
2. Rogers J, Watt I, Dieppe P: Paleopathology of spinal osteophytosis, vertebral ankylosis, ankylosing spondylitis and vertebral hyperostosis. Ann Rheum Dis 44:113, 1985.
3. Gran JT, Husby F, Hordvik M: Prevalence of ankylosing spondylitis in males and females in a young middle-aged population of Tromso, Northern Norway. Ann Rheum Dis 44:359, 1985.
4. Hochberg MC: Epidemiology. In: Calin A (ed): Spondyloarthropathies. Orlando: Grune & Stratton, 1984, pp 21–42.
5. Khan MA: An overview of clinical spectrum and heterogeneity of spondyloarthropathies. Rheum Dis Clin North Am 18:1, 1992.
6. Calin A, Fries JF: Striking prevalence of ankylosing spondylitis in "healthy" W27 positive males and females: a controlled study. N Engl J Med 293:835, 1975.
7. Engleman EG, Rosenbaum JT: HLA and disease: An overview. In: Calin A (ed): Spondyloarthropathies. Orlando: Grune & Stratton, 1984, pp 279–296.
8. Schlosstein L, Terasaki PI, Bluestone R, Pearson CM: High association of an HL antigen, W27, with ankylosing spondylitis. N Engl J Med 288:704, 1973.
9. Khan MA, van der Linden SM: Ankylosing spondylitis and other spondyloarthropathies. Rheum Dis Clin North Am 16:551, 1990.
10. Good AE, Kawaniski H, Schultz JS: HLA-B27 in blacks with ankylosing spondylitis or Reiter's disease. N Engl J Med 294:166, 1976.
11. Hochberg MC, Bias WB, Arnett FC Jr: Family studies in HLA-B27 associated arthritis. Medicine 57:463, 1978.
12. Grumet FC, Calin A, Engleman EG, et al.: Studies of HLA-B27 using monoclonal antibodies: Ethnic and disease associated variants. In: Ziff M, Cohen SB (eds): The Spondyloarthropathies: Advances in Inflammation Research, vol 9. New York: Raven Press, 1985, p 41.
13. Grumet FC, Fendly BM, Fish L, et al.: Monoclonal antibody (B27 M$_2$) subdividing HLA-B27. Hum Immunol 5:61, 1982.
14. Karr RW, Hahn Y, Schwartz BD: Structural identity of human histocompatibility leukocyte antigen-B27 molecules from patients with ankylosing spondylitis and normal individuals. J Clin Invest 69:443, 1982.
15. Kaneoka H, Engleman EG, Grumet FC: Immunochemical variants of HLA-B27. J Immunol 130:1288, 1983.
16. Ebringer A, Shipley M (eds): Pathogenesis of HLA-B27–associated disease. Br J Rheumatol 2(suppl):1, 1983.
17. Engleman EG, Calin A, Grumet FC: Analysis of HLA-B27 antigen with monoclonal antibodies. J Rheumatol Suppl 10:59, 1983.
18. Calin A, Marder A, Becks E, Burns T: Genetic differences between B27 positive patients with ankylosing spondylitis and B27 positive healthy controls. Arthritis Rheum 26:1460, 1983.
19. Gran JT, Teiberg P, Olaissen B, et al.: HLA-B27 and allotypes of complement components in ankylosing spondylitis. J Rheumatol 11:324, 1984.
20. Lopez de Castro JA, Bragado R, Lauzurica P, et al.: Structure and immune recognition of HLA-B27 antigens: implications for disease association. Scand J Rheumatol Suppl 87:21, 1990.
21. Del Porto P, D'Amato M, Fiorillo MT, et al.: Identification of a novel HLA-B27 subtype by restriction analysis of a cytotoxic gamma delta T cell clone. J Immunol 153:3093, 1994.
22. Hill AVS, Kwiatkowski D, Greenwood BM, et al.: HLA class I typing by PCR: HLA-B27 and an African B27 subtype. Lancet 337:640, 1991.
23. Matsumura M, Fremont DH, Peterson PA, et al.: Emerging principles for the recognition of peptide antigens by MHC class I molecules. Science 257:927, 1992.
24. Bjorkman PJ, Saper MA, Samraoui B, et al.: Structure of the human class I histocompatibility antigen, HLA-A2. Nature 329:506, 1987.
25. Breur-Vriesendorp BS, Vingerhoed J, Kuijpers KC, et al.: Effect of a Tyr-to-His point-mutation at position 59 in the alpha-1 helix of the HLA-B27 class-I molecule on allospecific and virus-specific cytotoxic T-lymphocyte recognition. Scand J Rheumatol Suppl 87:36, 1990.
26. Khan MA: HLA-B27 and its subtypes in world populations. Curr Opin Rheumatol 7:263, 1995.
27. Maclean IL, Iqball S, Woo P, et al.: HLA-B27 subtypes in the spondyloarthropathies. Clin Exp Immunol 91:214, 1993.
28. Calin A: The relationship between genetics and environment in the pathogenesis of rheumatic diseases. West J Med 131:205, 1979.
29. Geczy AF, Prendergast JK, Sullivan JS, et al.: HLA-B27, molecular mimicry and ankylosing spondylitis: popular misconceptions. Ann Rheum Dis 46:171, 1987.
30. Hammer RE, Maika SD, Richardson JA, et al.: Spontaneous inflammatory disease in transgenic rats expressing HLA-B27 and human beta 2m: an animal model of HLA-B27 associated human disorders. Cell 63:1099, 1990.
31. Taurog JD, Richardson JA, Croft JT, et al.: The germ-free state prevents development of gut and joint inflammatory disease in HLA-B27 transgenic rats. J Exp Med 180:2359, 1994.
32. Miehle W, Schattenkirchner M, Albert D, Bunge M: HLA-DR4 in ankylosing spondylitis with different patterns of joint involvement. Ann Rheum Dis 44:39, 1985.
33. Resnick D, Dwosh IL, Goergen TG, et al.: Clinical and radiographic "reankylosis" following hip surgery in ankylosing spondylitis. AJR 126:1181, 1976.
34. Jacoby RK, Newell RLM, Hickling P: Ankylosing spondylitis and trauma: the medicolegal implications. A comparative study of patients with nonspecific back pain. Ann Rheum Dis 44:307, 1985.
35. Geczy AF, Alexander K, Bashir HV, et al.: HLA-B27, *Klebsiella,* and ankylosing spondylitis: bacteriologic and chemical studies. Immunol Rev 70:23, 1983.
36. Sullivan JS, Geczy AF: The modification of HLA-B27-positive lymphocytes by the culture filtrate of *Klebsiella* K43 BTS 1 is a metabolically active process. Clin Exp Immunol 62:672, 1985.
37. Van Bohemen GG, Grumet FC, Zanen HC: Identifi-

cation of HLA-B27 M_1 and M_2 cross-reactive antigens in *Klebsiella, Shigella,* and *Yersinia.* Immunology 52:607, 1984.

38. Sheldon PJ, Pell PA: Lymphocyte proliferative responses to bacterial antigens in B-27 associated arthropathies. J Rheumatol 24:11, 1985.
39. Warren RE, Brewerton DA: Faecal carriage of *Klebsiella* by patients with ankylosing spondylitis and rheumatoid arthritis. Ann Rheum Dis 39:37, 1980.
40. Edmonds J, Macauley D, Tyndall A, et al.: Lymphocytotoxicity of anti-*Klebsiella* antisera in ankylosing spondylitis and related arthropathies: patient and family studies. Arthritis Rheum 24:1, 1981.
41. Lahesmaa R, Skurnik M, Gransfors K, et al.: Molecular mimicry in the pathogenesis of spondyloarthropathies: a critical appraisal of cross-reactivity between microbial antigens and HLA-B27. Br J Rheumatol 31:221, 1992.
42. Lopez de Castro JA: Structural polymorphism and function of HLA-B27. Curr Opin Rheumatol 7:270, 1995.
43. Careless DJ, Inman RD: Etiopathogenesis of reactive arthritis and ankylosing spondylitis. Curr Opin Rheumatol 7:290, 1995.
44. Neustadt DH: Ankylosing spondylitis. Postgrad Med 61:124, 1977.
45. Wilkinson M, Bywaters EGL: Clinical features and course of ankylosing spondylitis as seen in a follow-up of 222 hospital referred cases. Ann Rheum Dis 17:209, 1958.
46. Hochberg MC, Borenstein DG, Arnett FC: The absence of back pain in classical ankylosing spondylitis. Johns Hopkins Med J 143:181, 1978.
47. Pace JB, Nagle D: Piriformis syndrome. West J Med 124:435, 1976.
48. Hart FD, MacLagen NF: Ankylosing spondylitis: a review of 184 cases. Ann Rheum Dis 34:87, 1975.
49. Lehtinen K: 76 patients with ankylosing spondylitis seen after 30 years of disease. Scand J Rheumatol 12:5, 1983.
50. Hart FD, Robinson KC: Ankylosing spondylitis in women. Ann Rheum Dis 18:15, 1959.
51. Moller P, Vinje O, Kass E: How does Bechterew's syndrome (ankylosing spondylitis) start? Scand J Rheumatol 12:289, 1983.
52. Resnick D, Dwosh IL, Goergen TG, et al.: Clinical and radiographic abnormalities in ankylosing spondylitis: a comparison of men and women. Radiology 119:293, 1978.
53. Gran JT, Ostensen M, Husby G: A clinical comparison between males and females with ankylosing spondylitis. J Rheumatol 12:126, 1985.
54. Gran JT, Husby G: Ankylosing spondylitis in women. Semin Arthritis Rheum 19:303, 1990.
55. Calin A, Elswood J: The relationship between pelvic, spinal and hip involvement in ankylosing spondylitis: one disease process or several? Br J Rheumatol 27:393, 1988.
56. Carette S, Graham D, Little H, et al.: The natural disease course of ankylosing spondylitis. Arthritis Rheum 26:186, 1983.
57. Ball J: Enthesopathy of rheumatoid and ankylosing spondylitis. Ann Rheum Dis 30:213, 1971.
58. Fox MW, Onofrio BM, Kilgore JE: Neurological complications of ankylosing spondylitis. J Neurosurg 78:781, 1993.
59. Sharp J, Purser DW: Spontaneous atlanto-axial dislocation in ankylosing spondylitis and rheumatoid arthritis. Ann Rheum Dis 20:47, 1961.
60. Martel W: The occipito-atlanto-axial joints in rheu-

matoid arthritis and ankylosing spondylitis. AJR 86:223, 1961.
61. Sorin S, Askari A, Moskowitz RW: Atlantoaxial subluxation as a complication of early ankylosing spondylitis. Arthritis Rheum 22:273, 1979.
62. Hamilton MG, MacRae ME: Atlantoaxial dislocation as the presenting symptom of ankylosing spondylitis. Spine 18:2344, 1993.
63. Suarez-Almazor ME, Russell AS: Anterior atlantoaxial subluxation in patients with spondyloarthropathies: association with peripheral disease. J Rheumatol 15:973, 1988.
64. Hunter T, Dubo H: Spinal fractures complicating ankylosing spondylitis. Ann Intern Med 88:546, 1978.
65. Broom MJ, Raycroft JF: Complications of fractures of the cervical spine in ankylosing spondylitis. Spine 13:763, 1988.
66. Iplikcioglu AC, Bayar MA, Kokes F, et al.: Magnetic resonance imaging in cervical trauma associated with ankylosing spondylitis: report of two cases. J Trauma 36:412, 1994.
67. Detwiler KN, Loftus CM, Godersky JC, et al.: Management of cervical spine injuries in patients with ankylosing spondylitis. J Neurosurg 72:210, 1990.
68. Bohlman HH: Acute fractures and dislocations of the cervical spine: an analysis of three hundred hospitalized patients and review of the literature. J Bone Joint Surg 61A:1119–1142, 1979.
69. Foo D, Sarkarati M, Marcelino V: Cervical spinal cord injury complicating ankylosing spondylitis. Paraplegia 23:358, 1985.
70. Guttmann L: Traumatic paraplegia and tetraplegia in ankylosing spondylitis. Paraplegia 4:188, 1966.
71. Young JS, Cheshire DJE, Pierce JA, et al.: Cervical ankylosis with acute spinal cord injury. Paraplegia 15:133, 1977.
72. Osgood CP, Abbasy M, Mathews T: Multiple spine fractures in ankylosing spondylitis. J Trauma 15:163, 1975.
73. Rowed DW: Management of cervical spinal cord injury in ankylosing spondylitis: the intervertebral disc as a cause of cord compression. J Neurosurg 77:241, 1992.
74. Foo D, Rossier AB: Post-traumatic spinal epidural hematoma. Neurosurgery 11:25, 1982.
75. Weinstein PR, Karpman RR, Gall EP, et al.: Spinal cord injury, spinal fracture, and spinal stenosis in ankylosing spondylitis. J Neurosurg 57:609, 1982.
76. Wholey MH, Pugh DG, Bickel WH: Localized destructive lesions in rheumatoid spondylitis. Radiology 74:54, 1960.
77. Dihlmann W, Delling G: Discovertebral destructive lesions (so-called Andersson lesions) associated with ankylosing spondylitis. Skeletal Radiol 3:10, 1978.
78. Cawley MID, Chalmers TM, Kellgren JH, Ball J: Destructive lesions of vertebral bodies in ankylosing spondylitis. Ann Rheum Dis 31:345, 1972.
79. Dunn N, Preston B, Jones KL: Unexplained acute backache in longstanding ankylosing spondylitis. Br Med J 291:1632, 1985.
80. Bulkey BH, Roberts WC: Ankylosing spondylitis and aortic regurgitation: description of the characteristic cardiovascular lesion from study of eight necropsy patients. Circulation 48:1014, 1973.
81. Graham DC, Smythe HA: The carditis and aortitis of ankylosing spondylitis. Bull Rheum Dis 9:171, 1958.
82. Bergfeldt L, Edhag O, Vedin H, Vallin H: Ankylosing spondylitis: an important cause of severe disturbances of the cardiac conduction system. Prevalence among 223 pacemaker-treated men. Am J Med 73:187, 1982.

83. Rosenow EC III, Strimlan CV, Muhm JR, Ferguson RH: Pleuropulmonary manifestations of ankylosing spondylitis. Mayo Clin Proc 52:641, 1977.

84. Applerouth D, Gottlieb NL: Pulmonary manifestations of ankylosing spondylitis. J Rheumatol 2:446, 1975.

85. Cruickshank B: Pathology of ankylosing spondylitis. Clin Orthop 74:43, 1971.

86. Lai KN, Li PKT, Hawkins B, et al.: IgA nephropathy associated with ankylosing spondylitis: occurrence in women as well as in men. Ann Rheum Dis 48:435, 1989.

87. Kendal MJ, Lawrence DS, Shuttleworth GR, Whitefield AGW: Hematology and biochemistry of ankylosing spondylitis. Br Med J 2:235, 1973.

88. Nashel DJ, Petrone DL, Ulmer CC, Sliwinsi AJ: C-reactive protein: a marker for disease activity in ankylosing spondylitis and Reiter's syndrome. J Rheumatol 13:364, 1986.

89. Khan MA, Khan MK: Diagnostic value of HLA-B27 testing in ankylosing spondylitis and Reiter's syndrome. Ann Intern Med 906:70, 1982.

90. Suarez-Almazor ME, Russell AS: B27 homozygosity and ankylosing spondylitis. J Rheumatol 14:302, 1987.

91. McEwen C, DiTata D, Ling GC, Porini A, et al.: Ankylosing spondylitis and spondylitis accompanying ulcerative colitis, regional enteritis, psoriasis, and Reiter's disease: a comparative study. Arthritis Rheum 14:291, 1971.

92. Kinsella TD, MacDonald FR, Johnson LG: Ankylosing spondylitis: a late re-evaluation of 92 cases. Can Med Assoc J 95:1, 1966.

93. Rosen PS, Graham DC: Ankylosing (Strümpell-Marie) spondylitis (a clinical review of 128 cases). AIR 5:158, 1962.

94. Resnick D: Patterns of peripheral joint disease in ankylosing spondylitis. Radiology 110:523, 1974.

95. Ginsburg WW, Cohen MD: Peripheral arthritis in ankylosing spondylitis: a review of 209 patients followed up for more than 20 years. Mayo Clin Proc 58:593, 1983.

96. Dwosh IL, Resnick D, Becker MA: Hip involvement in ankylosing spondylitis. Arthritis Rheum 19:683, 1976.

97. Cone RD, Resnick D: Roentgenographic evaluation of the sacroiliac joints. Orthop Rev 12:95, 1983.

98. Dale K: Radiographic grading of sacroiliitis in Bechterew's syndrome and allied disorders. Scand J Rheumatol Suppl 32:92, 1979.

99. Cheatum DE: "Ankylosing spondylitis" without sacroiliitis in a woman without the HLA-B27 antigen. J Rheumatol 3:420, 1976.

100. Dale K: Radiographic changes of the spine in Bechterew's syndrome and allied disorders. Scand J Rheumatol Suppl 32:103, 1979.

101. Spencer DG, Park WM, Dick HM, et al.: Radiological manifestations in 200 patients with ankylosing spondylitis: correlation with clinical features and HLA-B27. J Rheumatol 6:305, 1979.

102. Martel W: Spinal pseudoarthrosis: a complication of ankylosing spondylitis. Arthritis Rheum 21:485, 1978.

103. Resnick D, Niwayama G: Ankylosing spondylitis. In: Resnick D (ed): Diagnosis of Bone and Joint Disorders, 3rd ed. Philadelphia: WB Saunders Co, 1995, pp 1008–1074.

104. Little H, Swinson DR, Cruickshank B: Upward subluxation of the axis in ankylosing spondylitis. Am J Med 60:279, 1976.

105. Baron M, Tator CH, Little H: Hangman's fracture in ankylosing spondylitis preceded by vertical subluxation of the axis. Arthritis Rheum 23:850, 1980.

106. Leventhal MR, Maguire JK Jr, Christian CA: Atlantoaxial rotary subluxation in ankylosing spondylitis: a case report. Spine 15:1374, 1990.

107. Kellgren JH: Diagnostic criteria for population studies. Bull Rheum Dis 13:291, 1962.

108. Bennett PH, Wood PHN: Population studies of the rheumatic diseases: proceedings of the 3rd International Symposium, New York, 1966. Amsterdam: Excerpta Medica, 1968, p 456.

109. Moll JMH, Wright V: New York clinical criteria for ankylosing spondylitis. Ann Rheum Dis 32:354, 1973.

110. Moll JM: Criteria for ankylosing spondylitis: facts and fallacies. Br J Rheumatol 27(suppl):34, 1988.

111. Khan MA, van der Linden SM: A wider spectrum of spondyloarthropathies. Semin Arthritis Rheum 20:107, 1990.

112. Kidd BL, Cawley MID: Delay in diagnosis of spondylarthritis. Br J Rheumatol 27:230, 1988.

113. Clayman MD, Reinertsen JL: Ankylosing spondylitis with subsequent development of rheumatoid arthritis, Sjögren's syndrome, and rheumatoid vasculitis. Arthritis Rheum 21:383, 1978.

114. Williamson PK, Reginato AJ: Diffuse idiopathic skeletal hyperostosis of the cervical spine in a patient with ankylosing spondylitis. Arthritis Rheum 27:570, 1984.

115. Gran JT, Paulsen AQ, Gaskjenn H, Schulz T: Reactive arthritis of the cervical spine due to *Yersinia enterocolitica* in patients with preexisting ankylosing spondylitis. Scand J Rheumatol 21:95, 1992.

116. O'Driscoll SL, Jayson MIV, Baddeley H: Neck movements in ankylosing spondylitis and their responses to physiotherapy. Ann Rheum Dis 37:64, 1978.

117. Godfrey RG, Calabro JJ, Mills D, Matty BA: A double blind crossover trial of aspirin, indomethacin and phenylbutazone in ankylosing spondylitis. (Abstract) Arthritis Rheum 15:110, 1972.

118. Fowler P: Phenylbutazone and indomethacin. Clin Rheum Dis 1:267, 1975.

119. Boersma JW: Retardation of ossification of the lumbar vertebral column in ankylosing spondylitis by means of phenylbutazone. Scand J Rheumatol 5:60, 1976.

120. Calabro JJ: Appraisal of efficacy and tolerability of Indocin (indomethacin, MSD) in acute gout and moderate to severe ankylosing spondylitis. Semin Arthritis Rheum 12(suppl 1):112, 1982.

121. Simon LS, Mills JA: Nonsteroidal anti-inflammatory drugs. N Engl J Med 302:1179, 1237, 1980.

122. Gran JT, Husby G: Ankylosing spondylitis: current drug treatment. Drugs 44:585, 1992.

123. Calin A, Britton M: Sulindac in ankylosing spondylitis: double-blind evaluation of sulindac and indomethacin. JAMA 242:1885, 1979.

124. Ansell BM, Major G, Liyanage G, et al.: A comparative study of butacote and Naprosyn in ankylosing spondylitis. Ann Rheum Dis 37:436, 1978.

125. Mintz G, Enriquez RD, Mercado U, et al.: Intravenous methylprednisolone pulse therapy in severe ankylosing spondylitis. Arthritis Rheum 24:734, 1981.

126. Richter MB: Management of the seronegative spondyloarthropathies. Clin Rheum Dis 11:147, 1985.

127. Handler RP: Favorable results using methotrexate in the treatment of patients with ankylosing spondylitis. Arthritis Rheum 32:234, 1989.

128. Ferraz MB, da Silva HC, Altra E: Low dose methotrexate with leucovorin rescue in ankylosing spondylitis. J Rheumatol 18:146, 1991.

129. Steven MM, Morrison M, Sturrock RD: Penicillamine

in ankylosing spondylitis: a double blind placebo controlled trial. J Rheumatol 12:735, 1985.

130. William F, Taylor AR, Arden GP, Edwards DH: Arthroplasty of the hip in ankylosing spondylitis. J Bone Joint Surg 59B:393, 1977.

131. Scudese VA, Calabro JJ: Vertebral wedge osteotomy: correction of rheumatoid (ankylosing) spondylitis. JAMA 186:627, 1963.

132. Bradford DS, Schumacher WL, Lonstein JE, Winter RB: Ankylosing spondylitis: experience in surgical management of 21 patients. Spine 12:238, 1987.

133. Brown WMC, Doll R: Mortality from cancer and other causes after radiotherapy for ankylosing spondylitis. Br Med J 2:1327, 1965.

134. Kaprove RE, Little AH, Graham DC, Rosen PS: Ankylosing spondylitis: survival in men with and without radiotherapy. Arthritis Rheum 23:57, 1980.

135. Creemers MCW, van Riel PLCM, Franssen MJAM, et al.: Second-line treatment in seronegative spondyloarthropathies. Semin Arthritis Rheum 24:71, 1994.

136. Kennedy LG, Edmunds L, Calin A: The natural history of ankylosing spondylitis: does it burn out? J Rheumatol 20:688, 1993.

137. Kahn MA, Kushner I, Braun WE, et al.: HLA-B27 homozygosity in ankylosing spondylitis: relationship to risk and severity. Tissue Antigens 11:434, 1978.

138. Arnett FC, Schacter BZ, Hochberg M, et al.: Homozygosity for HLA-B27: impact on rheumatic disease expression in two families. Arthritis Rheum 20:797, 1977.

139. Spencer DG, Dick HM, Dick WC: Ankylosing spondylitis: the role of HLA-B27 homozygosity. Tissue Antigens 14:379, 1979.

140. Moller P, Berg K: Family studies in Bechterew's syndrome (ankylosing spondylitis). III: genetics. Clin Genet 24:73, 1983.

141. Hill HFH, Hill AGS, Bodmer JG: Clinical diagnosis of ankylosing spondylitis in women and relation to presence of HLA-B27. Ann Rheum Dis 35:267, 1976.

142. Jeannet M, Saudan Y, Bitter T: HLA-27 in female patients with ankylosing spondylitis. Tissue Antigens 6:262, 1975.

PSORIATIC ARTHRITIS

Capsule Summary

Frequency of neck pain—uncommon

Location of neck pain—cervical spine

Quality of neck pain—ache

Symptoms and signs—morning stiffness, skin rash with plaques, neck tenderness, decreased motion

Laboratory and x-ray tests—increased erythrocyte sedimentation rate; nonmarginal syndesmophytes on plain roentgenogram, with or without sacroiliitis

Treatment—topical drugs, nonsteroidal anti-inflammatory drugs, methotrexate

Prevalence and Pathogenesis

Patients with psoriasis who develop a characteristic pattern of joint disease have psoriatic arthritis. French physicians Bazin and Bourdillon in the last century were the first to name the disease and describe it in detail.[1, 2] In the United States, there was hesitancy in ascribing joint disease to psoriasis. Many physicians thought that two common diseases—psoriasis and rheumatoid arthritis—were occurring in patients simultaneously. More recent studies, however, have clearly demonstrated the association of psoriasis and arthritis.[3] Moll has suggested a working definition of the disease to include three components: psoriasis (skin or nail), inflammatory arthritis (peripheral or axial), and negative test for rheumatoid factor.[4] However, the disease should be considered as a range with patients developing components gradually. Some patients have inflammatory arthritis compatible with psoriatic disease before the appearance of skin lesions. Like Reiter's syndrome, incomplete forms of the disease are relevant to the clinical disease.

Precise data concerning the prevalence of psoriasis are not available. Many patients with mild disease may never be seen by physicians. Therefore, only estimates of prevalence have been made; they suggest that 1% to 3% of the population is affected by psoriasis. Psoriasis does, however, occur more commonly in people from temperate climate zones. Prevalence of psoriasis in the United States and Japan is similar. People from eastern and northern Africa are also similarly affected. Psoriasis is rare in southern and western Africa, and this is reflected in the low percentage of American blacks affected, most of whom originated from western Africa. Psoriatic arthritis occurs in 5% to 7% of individuals with psoriasis, and in 0.1% of the general population.[5, 6] Others have suggested a higher prevalence of arthritis of 20% to 34% in patients with psoriasis.[7–9] Psoriasis and psoriatic arthritis occur with equal frequency in both sexes. In a study of 220 patients with psoriatic arthritis, 47% were men and 53% were women.[10]

The basic abnormality, which results in the increased metabolic activity of the skin, is unknown. Some investigators believe this abnormality resides in the most superficial layers of the skin (epidermis), and others believe that the inner layers of the skin (dermis) are the source of the increased metabolic activity. A psoriatic diathesis exists in patients who are at risk for disease. Abnormalities in protein synthesis, blood flow, and metabolism are present in normal-appearing skin, hair, and nails in these individuals. Recent experiments have shown a hyperproliferative effect on normal keratinocytes by psoriatic skin fibroblasts. These cells undergo unrestrained growth, which reflects the condition of the skin in vivo.[11]

A genetic predisposition for the development of psoriasis and psoriatic arthritis does exist. Although a positive family history is obtained in about one third of patients with psoriasis, a definite pattern of inheritance has not been established. Psoriatic arthritis occurs more frequently in family members.[12] The skin disease of psoriasis has been associated with human leukocyte antigen B13, (HLA)-Bw17, HLA-Cw6, and HLA-DRw6 antigens.[13] More recent population studies have identified HLA-B13, HLA-B17, HLA-B37, HLA-Cw6, and HLA-DR7 as haplotypes associated with psoriasis.[14] Genetic factors also play a role in psoriatic arthritis. Patients with peripheral psoriatic arthritis have an increased frequency of HLA-Bw38, HLA-DR4 and HLA-DR7 antigens.[15] Others have reported HLA-Bw57, HLA-Bw39, HLA-Bw6, and HLA-Bw7 associated with peripheral arthropathy.[16] Other reported haplotypes associated with psoriatic arthritis include HLA-B13, HLA-B17, HLA-B38, HLA-B39, HLA-DR4, and HLA-DR7.[17] Psoriatic spondylitis is associated with increased frequency of HLA-B27.[18]

Like ankylosing spondylitis and Reiter's syndrome, psoriatic arthritis may develop after exposure to a number of environmental factors. Trauma has been reported by a number of investigators as the initiator of arthritis or osteolysis (bone loss) in psoriasis.[19–22] Chronic arthritis has developed after trauma to normal joints in patients with psoriasis uncomplicated by arthritis. In a comparison of environmental events immediately preceding the onset of arthritis, 12 patients (9%) with psoriatic arthritis versus 2 patients (1%) with rheumatoid arthritis had an acute traumatic event, including operation, articular trauma, abortion, myocardial infarction, thrombophlebitis, or drug exposure.[23]

Synovial joints in psoriasis patients may be more liable to damage owing to an enzyme deficiency of synovial fluid.[24] Psoriatic synovium has fewer macrophages, greater number of blood vessels, and less expression of the endothelial adhesion molecule-1 compared with rheumatoid synovium.[25] Genetic control of cell growth may be impaired in psoriasis patients. The oncogene c-*myc* is expressed to a greater degree in skin and synovium of psoriasis patients compared to normal cells. The greater turnover of skin and synovial cells may be directly related to the role of the oncogenes

of cell proliferation.[14] The decline in the number of CD4+ cells may also play a role in the development of arthritis in light of the expression of more severe disease in individuals infected with the human immunodeficiency virus.[26] Other immunologic abnormalities associated with psoriasis include increased levels of complement activation fragments, decreased T cell subpopulations, lipoxygenase products, and local release of cytokines, including interferon gamma.[27–30] Other environmental factors including infections with *Staphylococcus aureus* and *Clostridium perfringens* and delayed hypersensitivity have also been suggested as important in the development of psoriatic arthritis.[31, 32]

Clinical History

Psoriatic arthritis has more than one clinical form, and this initially caused confusion in the description of the illness (Table 11–6).[33–35] Classic psoriatic arthritis is described as involving distal interphalangeal (DIP) joints and associated nail disease alone. This pattern occurs in 5% of patients. The most common form of the disease, affecting 70% of patients with psoriatic arthritis, is an asymmetrical oligoarthritis; a few large or small joints are involved. Dactylitis, diffuse swelling of a digit, is most closely associated with this form of the disease. Skin activity and joint symptoms do not correlate—patients with little skin activity may experience continued joint pain and stiffness. As opposed to rheumatoid arthritis, the clinical appearance of an involved joint does not necessarily correlate with patient symptoms. Patients with severely affected joints may be asymptomatic. Symmetrical polyarthritis, which affects the small joints of the hands and feet and resembles rheumatoid arthritis, occurs in 15% of patients. Arthritis mutilans,

TABLE 11–6. CLASSIFICATION OF PSORIATIC ARTHRITIS

FORM	INCIDENCE			
	Moll[33]	*Kammer*[34]	*Alonso*[35]	*Veale*[36]
Asymmetrical oligoarthritis	70	54	37	43
Symmetrical "rheumatoid arthritis-like"	15	25	36	33
Psoriatic spondylitis	5	21	23	14
Distal interphalangeal predominant	5		8	
Arthritis mutilans	5		4	2

characterized by extensive destruction of bone in hands, is found in 5% of patients. Spondylitis with or without peripheral joint disease occurs in 5% of patients.

In one report, clinical forms of psoriatic arthritis were simplified to three major types—asymmetrical, oligoarticular arthritis (54%); symmetrical arthritis (25%); and spondyloarthritis (21%).[34] DIP involvement occurred most commonly in the asymmetrical oligoarthritis group and rarely in the spondyloarthropathy group. Arthritis mutilans occurred rarely in all groups.

Other large studies have reported on the subsets of psoriatic arthritis patients. These groups of patients are listed in Table 11–6.[35, 36] The largest subset in all the studies is the group with asymmetrical oligoarthritis. Spondyloarthropathy is found in a minority of patients, ranging from 5% to 23% of patients with psoriatic arthritis.

Patients who develop axial skeletal disease, sacroiliitis or spondylitis, are usually men who have the onset of psoriasis later in life.[37] The number of psoriatic patients with involvement of the cervical spine varies from 45% to 70% of individuals.[38, 39] The variation depends on the definition of involvement, characterized as clinical symptoms or radiographic abnormalities. In one study 40% and in another 45% of psoriatic arthritis patients had symptoms of inflammatory cervical spine disease, including neck pain or prolonged stiffness.[38, 39]

Patients who first develop psoriatic arthritis before the age of 20 years may be more likely to develop arthritis mutilans. Low back pain, which is indistinguishable from the pain associated with the other spondyloarthropathies, is present in the majority of patients with axial skeletal disease. These patients may have back pain or peripheral joint symptoms as their initial complaint. Asymmetrical or symmetrical peripheral joint involvement may antedate the development of axial skeletal disease.

The typical patient with the symmetrical or asymmetrical form of psoriatic arthritis is a man or woman from 35 to 45 years of age. Patients with more severe disease have an onset of symptoms at an earlier age, manifested by inflammation in a few joints or by diffuse swelling of an entire digit (dactylitis). Psoriasis antedates the arthritis in a majority of patients (Table 11–7).[40] From 10% to 20% of patients have characteristic arthritis before the appearance of psoriatic lesions. Patients with severe skin involvement are more likely to develop arthritis.[41] However, even patients with minimal skin involvement still have some risk of developing joint disease. Nail involvement, characterized by pitting, horizontal ridging, onycholysis (opacification of the nail bed), and discoloration, occurs in 80% of patients with psoriatic arthritis in contrast with a 30% incidence in patients with uncomplicated psoriasis. The activity of skin and nail disease does not necessarily correlate with joint symptoms because any of the forms of psoriatic skin disease, whether guttate, pustular, seborrheic, or others, may be associated with joint involvement.[42, 43]

TABLE 11–7. ONSET OF PSORIATIC ARTHRITIS

	%
Psoriasis before arthritis	70
Psoriasis simultaneous with arthritis	20
Arthritis before psoriasis	10

Although constitutional symptoms of fever, anorexia, and weight loss are rare in patients with psoriatic arthritis, fatigue and morning stiffness are common. Ocular involvement includes conjunctivitis in 20%, iritis in 10%, and scleritis in 2% of patients with psoriatic arthritis.[44] Iritis is more commonly seen in patients with axial skeletal disease. Cardiac complications, such as aortic insufficiency as seen in ankylosing spondylitis, are rare and are usually associated with spondylitis.[45]

Physical Examination

An extensive examination of the skin is an essential part of the investigation of a patient with suspected psoriatic arthritis. The diagnosis of psoriasis is not difficult to make when the patient has the characteristic erythematous, raised, circumscribed, dry, scaling lesions over the elbows, knees, and scalp and pitting of the nails. Skin lesions may be hidden in the scalp, gluteal folds, perineum, rectum, or umbilicus, and may remain undetected unless a complete skin examination is done. Nails are examined for the presence of pitting, ridges, opacification, and hyperkeratosis.[46]

A complete musculoskeletal examination is essential in determining the extent of joint involvement. Patients may be asymptomatic in a specific joint, although physical examination demonstrates decreased function. They may have dactylitis of a toe and may be unaware of the change until pointed out by the physician. Examination of the axial skeleton should be completed even in the asymptomatic patient. A loss of spinal motion may be a manifestation of axial skeleton disease. Sacroiliac involvement may be unilateral or bilateral. Percussion over the sacroiliac joints can elicit symptoms over the affected side. Patients may develop spondylitis in the absence of sacroiliitis, and this has maximal tenderness with percussion over the spine above the sacrum. In the cervical spine, limitation of motion is a primary manifestation of neck involvement. Patients may have radiographic evidence of cervical spine arthritis with normal movement of the neck.[39]

Laboratory Data

The findings of anemia, mild leukocytosis, and elevated erythrocyte sedimentation rate occur in a minority of patients.[47] C-reactive protein (CRP), an acute phase reactant, may be elevated. CRP is a marker of clinical disease activity and may be persistently elevated in those with extensive joint destruction.[48] An elevated uric acid level, hyperuricemia, is detected in 20% of patients. This may be secondary to an increased metabolic rate and protein breakdown in patients with extensive skin involvement. These patients may develop secondary gout. Psoriatic synovial fluid is inflammatory but has no diagnostic features. Rheumatoid factor and antinuclear antibody (ANA) are usually absent. If they are present, the rheumatoid factor and ANA occur in the same frequency as found in age-matched controls. HLA-B27 is detected in approximately 35% to 60% of patients with axial skeleton disease.[49] In one study, patients with sacroiliitis and spondylitis were 90% positive for HLA-B27, and in another study patients with spondylitis and normal sacroiliac joints were 43% positive.[18, 37] In a study of 180 patients, 85% of patients with bilateral sacroiliitis were B27-positive, and 22% of those with asymmetric sacroiliitis were B27-positive.[35] Peripheral joint disease is associated with HLA-B38 and HLA-B39, and psoriasis alone is associated with HLA-B13, HLA-B17, and HLA-Cw6.[50, 51]

Radiographic Evaluation

Whereas radiologic features of psoriatic arthritis and rheumatoid arthritis may be similar, certain features of DIP and proximal interpha-langeal (PIP) joints in psoriatic arthritis are distinctive.[52, 53] The joint involvement is oligoarticular with erosive changes in the DIP joint and terminal phalanx, especially the big toe. The "pencil-in-cup" deformity, osteolysis of the proximal phalanx and widening of the distal phalanx, is characteristic of psoriatic arthritis. Periosteal reaction occurs along the shafts of the long bones, as opposed to the periosteal changes in Reiter's syndrome that are localized to the metatarsal and phalanges of the feet and hands.

Axial skeleton involvement was first emphasized by Dixon and Lience.[54] Up to 25% of patients have sacroiliac involvement manifested by sacroiliitis, which can be unilateral or bilateral.[55–57] Symmetrical involvement, from side to side and severity of disease, predominate over asymmetrical disease. Sacroiliitis may occur without spondylitis. Radiographic characteristics of sacroiliitis include erosions and sclerosis predominantly on the ilium, along with joint widening. Joint ankylosis occurs less commonly than in ankylosing spondylitis. Sacroiliitis with psoriasis has no radiographic changes that can be considered specific for the disease.[58] Spondylitis is characterized by asymmetric involvement of the vertebral bodies and nonmarginal syndesmophytes. Spondylitis with normal sacroiliac joints may show up radiographically. Rare patients have been described with axial skeletal disease that mirrors the involvement characteristic of ankylosing spondylitis. Paravertebral ossification separated from the vertebral body may occur in the thoracolumbar region.[59] Squaring of vertebral bodies, osteitis of bone, and facet joint ankylosis occur less frequently in psoriatic spondylitis than in ankylosing spondylitis.[60] Spinal disease progression occurs in a random rather than orderly fashion, ascending the spine as commonly noted in ankylosing spondylitis.

In psoriatic spondylitis, the cervical spine is affected less frequently than the lumbar spine.[61] Cervical spine disease may occur in the absence of sacroiliitis or lumbar spondylitis.[39] Alterations in the cervical spine include joint space sclerosis and narrowing and anterior ligamentous calcification.[62] This form of involvement follows the pattern of the spondyloarthropathies characterized by ankylosis and calcification (Fig. 11–10). These patients may have nonmarginal or marginal syndesmophytes. Another group of patients has disease characterized by erosions and subluxations in the absence of ligamentous calcifications, more reminiscent of the alterations associated

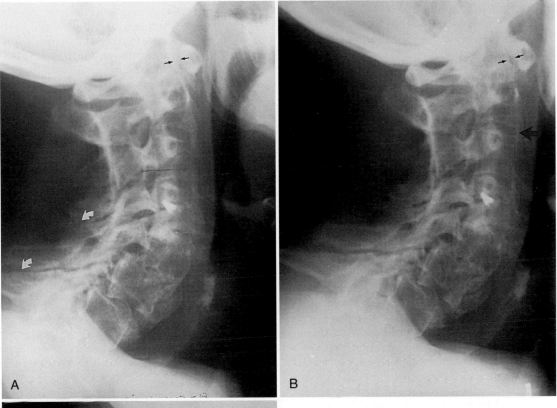

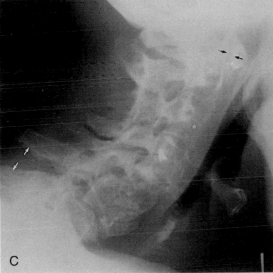

Figure 11–10. Psoriatic arthritis. A 57-year-old woman with arthritis mutilans, neck pain, and no neurologic deficits. She had seronegative polyarthritis for 20 years before a psoriatic skin rash appeared. *A*, Lateral view of cervical spine, extension; *B*, Neutral; *C*, Flexion. Anterior syndesmophytes are present in *B* from C2 to C5 *(large black arrow)*. Fusion is present between spinous process of C3–C4. Pseudoarticulation and erosion of the spinous processes of C4–C5 and C6–C7 are present in *A (curved white arrows)*. Atlantoaxial subluxation of 4 mm remains the same in all views *(small black arrows)*. Anterior subluxation with total loss of intervertebral disc space is noted at the C5–C6 interspace. The C6–C7 interspace is subluxed and mobile. With flexion of the neck, C6 moves forward on C7 and the distance between the spinous processes widens in *C (small white arrows)*. The triangular metal item is the tip of a knife, resulting from a physical assault.

with rheumatoid arthritis (Fig. 11–10).[38] The "rheumatoid-like" group has subaxial subluxations and/or instability at the atlantoaxial joint.[63] Subluxations may occur without spinal cord compression.[39]

As with the other spondyloarthropathies, a scintiscan may demonstrate increased activity over the sacroiliac joints or axial skeleton before radiographic changes are detectable.[64] Other radiographic techniques, computerized tomography (CT) or magnetic resonance (MR) imaging, do not offer specific abnormalities that help identify psoriatic arthritis patients from others. CT or MR imaging may be of value in the patient with cervical spine arthritis and neurologic symptoms compatible with myelopathy or radiculopathy. These radiographic techniques can identify the occasional patient with psoriatic spondylitis and neural compression.

Differential Diagnosis

The diagnosis of psoriatic arthritis is easily made when the patient has characteristic skin lesions and joint changes. The diagnosis is more difficult in the patient who presents with joint symptoms before the appearance of skin lesions. The differential diagnosis for such a patient should include Reiter's syndrome, gout, erosive osteoarthritis, and rheumatoid arthritis. Reiter's syndrome may be differentiated by urethritis, predominantly lower extremity involvement, and periosteal changes. Acute gout is confirmed by the detection of monosodium urate crystals in synovial fluid. Erosive osteoarthritis occurs in postmenopausal women and is characterized by inflammation in the DIP and PIP joints and radiographic findings of osteophytes, sclerosis, and cysts in these joints. The erythrocyte sedimentation rate remains normal. The clinical appearance of symmetrical polyarthritis in psoriatic arthritis and rheumatoid arthritis is similar. The absence of rheumatoid nodules, rheumatoid factor, and the presence of DIP involvement and periostitis helps differentiate the patient with psoriatic arthritis from the one with rheumatoid arthritis (Table 11–5).

Treatment

The goals of therapy are the maintenance and improvement of function through the reduction of inflammation. Therapy includes patient education, nonsteroidal anti-inflammatory drugs (NSAIDs), immunosuppressives, and physical therapy. The importance of appropriate skin care must be stressed. Whereas in the past no correlation between improvement in skin and joint symptoms could be demonstrated, a recent study reported the improvement of nonspondylitic psoriatic arthritis in patients who responded to photochemotherapy for their skin disease.[65] NSAIDs, particularly indomethacin and phenylbutazone, are useful in controlling pain and stiffness in the peripheral and axial joints. Phenylbutazone has limited availability and is not an initial agent for the therapy of this illness. Mefenamic acid has also been suggested as a useful drug for the control of joint symptoms. The NSAIDs are given in maximum doses tolerated by patients to better control the inflammation associated with their joint disease (indomethacin 150 mg/day, naproxen 1,500 mg/day, and sulindac 400 mg/day). The drugs should be given for 4 to 6 weeks before deciding on the efficacy of the agent. A series of NSAIDs should be tried before deciding on the inefficacy of this group of drugs in an individual patient. The primary toxicity of the NSAID is gastrointestinal. These agents do not increase the severity of psoriatic skin disease.[66] NSAIDs do not alter the progression of axial skeletal joint disease. However, they are helpful in decreasing joint stiffness and pain, allowing for greater neck motion. This benefit of joint motion should not be overlooked in the treatment of spondylitis patients. NSAIDs may allow for greater ease with activities of daily living that improve patient comfort on a recurring basis.

Drugs with skin rash as a potential toxicity have been contraindicated in the past; however, recent studies have demonstrated the efficacy and lack of skin toxicity for hydroxychloroquine and gold salts.[34, 67, 68] These drugs are given in the same doses and frequency as those used with rheumatoid arthritis patients. These drugs are most helpful for the patient with refractory peripheral arthritis. Sulfasalazine has been studied for the treatment of psoriatic arthritis. Patients receiving the drug have had a modest improvement but with gastrointestinal and cutaneous toxicities. In general, sulfasalazine has not been recommended for psoriatic arthritis patients.[69]

In patients with severe and extensive skin disease and destructive arthritis, immunosuppressive therapy with methotrexate, 6-mercaptopurine, and azathioprine is indicated.[70–72] The drug 6-mercaptopurine is associated with excessive toxicity and has been supplanted by methotrexate for the treatment of psoriatic arthritis. Methotrexate is usually given orally (2.5 mg every 12 hours or as a single dose) for a total dose of 7.5 mg. This is given once a week to limit toxicity. Liver fibrosis is the most common serious toxicity of methotrexate. Liver biopsy has been recommended in the past when the patient received 2 gm of medicine.[73] However, the complications associated with liver biopsy outweigh the benefits associated with identifying the rare individual with liver fibrosis associated with methotrexate. A cost analysis of liver biopsy did not demonstrate a definite benefit unless the risk of cirrhosis was high.[74] Only a few rheumatologists in Canada obtain liver biopsies before or after a cumulative dose of methotrexate.[75] Liver biopsy should be reserved for individuals with elevated liver function tests or complications such as hepatitis and ethanolism who are at increased risk for cirrhosis.[74]

Methotrexate has been shown to be a safe,

effective agent for the therapy of psoriatic arthritis. A multicenter study demonstrated methotrexate to be helpful in patients with psoriasis, compared with control subjects, for skin lesion improvement and subjective physician assessment.[76] A study of 40 patients documented the control of peripheral arthritis, skin, and nail disease in a majority of psoriatic arthritis patients.[77] These drugs have the potential for liver toxicity and leukopenia. Patients receiving this drug were monitored closely on a monthly basis.

Systemic corticosteroids are rarely used for skin or joint disease because a rebound phenomenon appears when the drug is discontinued.[78] Intra-articular corticosteroids are useful in the patient with psoriatic monarthritis and persistent effusion, usually of the knee. The immunosuppressive and corticosteroids are more effective for control of peripheral arthritis than for axial skeletal disease.

Retinoids (vitamin A) have recently been associated with improvement in psoriatic arthritis.[79] Maintenance therapy was required to prevent relapse. Of interest is the observation that less psoralen treatment was needed to achieve a clinical response when it was used in conjunction with retinoids. The need for less psoralen for control of psoriasis may decrease the incidence of squamous cell cancer of the skin, which is noted in patients on psoralens for an average of 5.7 years.[80]

Cyclosporin A has been used in the therapy of psoriatic arthritis patients. The response to joint and skin disease was modest, but the renal toxicity was persistent. In addition, this drug is expensive compared with other agents. The drug should be limited to only the most severely affected and drug-resistant psoriatic patient.[81]

Prognosis

The course of psoriatic arthritis is unpredictable.[40] A small percentage of patients develop destructive, disabling disease, whereas a majority have less pain and disability than seen in rheumatoid arthritis. In one large study, 97% of psoriatic patients were able to work at their jobs, missing less than 12 months of work during a minimum 10-year follow-up period.[40] Another survey found that women who developed symmetrical large- and small-joint disease had more destructive arthritis.[34]

Patients who develop psoriatic spondylitis develop varying degrees of restriction of spinal motion. There is no consistent correlation between the severity of peripheral joint disease and axial skeletal disease. A study of patients with ankylosing spondylitis, psoriatic spondylitis, and enteropathic spondylitis found the psoriatic patients to be the most severely affected.[82] Another study found the ankylosing spondylitis patients to be more severely affected.[83] Other studies have demonstrated radiographic progression of spondylitis without an increase in symptoms or decreased spinal mobility.[84] The results of these studies leave the physician to follow each patient to identify an individual course. Psoriatic arthritis may not be as benign a disease as previously thought. Patients with longer duration disease, or those with HLA-B39 and HLA-DR4 and radiocarpal erosions, may be at increased risk for psoriatic spondyloarthropathy involving the cervical spine.[38, 39] Patients with psoriatic arthritis may develop atlantoaxial subluxation with evidence of cervical myelopathy on rare occasions.[85] Greater respect should be given to the destructive potential of psoriatic arthritis. Patients with this disease should be treated earlier and more aggressively.[86]

References

PSORIATIC ARTHRITIS

1. Bazin P: Lecons Theoriques et Cliniques sur les Affections Cutanees de Nature Arthritique et Darteux. Paris: Delahaye, 1860, pp 154–161.
2. Bourdillon C: Psoriasis et Arthropathies. Paris: These, 1888.
3. Wright V: Rheumatism and psoriasis: a re-evaluation. Am J Med 27:454, 1959.
4. Moll JMH: The place of psoriatic arthritis in the spondarthritides. Baillieres Clin Rheumatol 8:465, 1994.
5. Baker H: Epidemiological aspects of psoriasis and arthritis. Br J Dermatol 78:249, 1966.
6. Hellgren L: Association between rheumatoid arthritis and psoriasis in total populations. Acta Rheum Scand 15:316, 1969.
7. Scarpa R, Oriente P, Pulino A, et al.: Psoriatic arthritis in psoriatic patients. Br J Rheumatol 23:246, 1984.
8. Stern RS: The epidemiology of joint complaints in patients with psoriasis. J Rheumatol 12:315, 1985.
9. Smiley JD: Psoriatic arthritis. Bull Rheum Dis 44:1, 1995.
10. Gladman DD, Shuckett R, Russell ML, et al.: Psoriatic arthritis (PSA): an analysis of 220 patients. Q J Med 238:127, 1987.
11. Saiag P, Coulomb B, Lebreton C, et al.: Psoriatic fibroblasts induce hyperproliferation of normal keratinocytes in a skin equivalent model in vitro. Science 230:669, 1985.
12. Moll JMH, Wright V: Familial occurrence of psoriatic arthritis. Ann Rheum Dis 32:181, 1973.
13. McKendry RJR, Sengar DPS, DesGroseilliers JP, Dunne JV: Frequency of HLA antigens in patients with psoriasis or psoriatic arthritis. Can Med Assoc J 130:411, 1984.

14. Gladman DD: Psoriatic arthritis: recent advances in pathogenesis and treatment. Rheum Dis Clin North Am 18:247, 1992.
15. Espinoza LR, Vasey FB, Gaylord SW, et al.: Histocompatibility typing in the seronegative spondyloarthropathies: a survey. Semin Arthritis Rheum 11:375, 1982.
16. Beaulieu AD, Roy R, Mathon G, et al.: Psoriatic arthritis: risk factors for patients with psoriasis—a study based on histocompatibility antigen frequencies. J Rheumatol 10:633, 1983.
17. Metzger AL, Morris RI, Bluestone R, Teraski PI: HLA-W27 in psoriatic arthropathy. Arthritis Rheum 18:111, 1975.
18. Buckley WR, Raleigh RL: Psoriasis with acro-osteolysis. N Engl J Med 261:539, 1959.
19. Williams KA, Scott JT: Influence of trauma on the development of chronic inflammatory polyarthritis. Ann Rheum Dis 26:532, 1967.
20. Langevitz P, Buskila D, Gladman DD: Arthritis precipitated by physical trauma. J Rheumatol 17:695, 1990.
21. Pages M, Lassoued S, Fournile B, et al.: Psoriatic arthritis precipitated by physical trauma: destructive arthritis or associated with reflex sympathetic dystrophy? J Rheumatol 19:185, 1992.
22. Scarpa R, Del Puente A, di Girolamo C, et al.: Interplay between environmental factors, articular involvement, and HLA-B27 in patients with psoriatic arthritis. Ann Rheum Dis 51:78, 1992.
23. Cotton DWK, Mier PD: An hypothesis on the aetiology of psoriasis. Br J Dermatol 76:519, 1969.
24. Veale D, Yanni G, Rogers S, et al.: Reduced synovial membrane macrophage numbers, ELAM-1 expression, and lining layer hyperplasia in psoriatic arthritis as compared with RA. Arthritis Rheum 36:893, 1993.
25. Reveille JD: The interplay of nature versus nurture in predisposition to the rheumatic diseases. Rheum Dis Clin North Am 19:15, 1993.
26. Arnett FC, Reveille JD, Duvic M: Psoriasis and psoriatic arthritis associated with human immunodeficiency virus infection. Rheum Dis Clin North Am 17:59, 1991.
27. Rosenberg EW, Noah PW, Wyatt RJ, et al.: Complement activation in psoriasis. Clin Exp Dermatol 15:16, 1990.
28. Rubins AY, Merson AG: Subpopulations of T lymphocytes on psoriasis patients and their changes during immunotherapy. J Am Acad Dermatol 17:972, 1987.
29. Voorhees JJ: Leukotrienes and other lipoxygenase products in the pathogenesis and therapy of psoriasis and other dermatoses. Arch Dermatol 119:541, 1983.
30. O'Connell PG, Gerber LH, Digiovanna JJ, Peck GL: Arthritis in patients with psoriasis treated with gamma-interferon. J Rheumatol 19:80, 1992.
31. Landau JW, Gross BG, Newcomer VD, Wright ET: Immunologic response of patients with psoriasis. Arch Dermatol 91:607, 1965.
32. Mansson I, Olhagen B: Intestinal *Clostridium perfringens* in rheumatoid arthritis and other connective tissue disorders: studies of fecal flora, serum antitoxin levels, and skin hypersensitivity. Acta Rheum Scand 12:167, 1966.
33. Moll JMH, Wright V: Psoriatic arthritis. Semin Arthritis Rheum 3:55, 1973.
34. Kammer GM, Soter WA, Gibson DJ, Schur PH: Psoriatic arthritis: a clinical, immunologic and HLA study of 100 patients. Semin Arthritis Rheum 9:75, 1979.
35. Alonso JCT, Perez AR, Castrillo AMA, et al.: Psoriatic arthritis (PA): A clinical, immunological and radiological study of 180 patients. Br J Rheumatol 30:245, 1991.
36. Veale D, Rogers S, Fitzgerald O: Classification of clinical subsets in psoriatic arthritis. Br J Rheumatol 33:133, 1994.
37. Lambert JR, Wright V: Psoriatic spondylitis: a clinical radiological description of the spine in psoriatic arthritis. Q J Med 46:411, 1977.
38. Jenkinson T, Armas J, Evison G, et al.: The cervical spine in psoriatic arthritis: a clinical and radiological study. Br J Rheumatol 33:255, 1994.
39. Salvarani C, Macchioni P, Cremonesi W, et al.: The cervical spine in patients with psoriatic arthritis: a clinical, radiological and immunogenetic study. Ann Rheum Dis 51:73, 1992.
40. Roberts MET, Wright V, Hill AGS, Mehra AC: Psoriatic arthritis: follow-up study. Ann Rheum Dis 35:206, 1976.
41. Leczinsky CG: The incidence of arthropathy in a ten-year series of psoriasis cases. Acta Derm Venereol 28:483, 1948.
42. Wright V, Roberts MD, Hill AGS: Dermatologic manifestations in psoriatic arthritis: a follow-up study. Acta Derm Venereol 59:235, 1979.
43. Eastmoral CJ, Wright V: Nail dystrophy of psoriatic arthritis. Ann Rheum Dis 38:226, 1979.
44. Lambert JR, Wright V: Eye inflammation in psoriatic arthritis. Ann Rheum Dis 35:354, 1976.
45. Roller DH, Muna WF, Ross AM: Psoriasis, sacroiliitis and aortitis. Chest 75:641, 1979.
46. Goodfield M: Skin lesions in psoriasis. Baillieres Clin Rheumatol 8:295, 1994.
47. Baker H, Golding DH, Thompson M: Psoriasis and arthritis. Ann Intern Med 58:909, 1963.
48. Troughton PR, Morgan AW: Laboratory findings and pathology of psoriatic arthritis. Baillieres Clin Rheumatol 8:439, 1994.
49. Brewerton DA, Coffrey M, Nicholls A, et al.: HLA-B27 and arthropathies associated with ulcerative colitis and psoriasis. Lancet 1:956, 1974.
50. Espinoza LR, Vasey FB, Oh JH, et al.: Association between HLA-Bw38 and peripheral psoriatic arthritis. Arthritis Rheum 21:72, 1978.
51. Eastmond CJ: Genetics and HLA antigens. Baillieres Clin Rheumatol 8:263, 1994.
52. Avila R, Pugh DG, Slocumb CH, Winkelman RK: Psoriatic arthritis: a roentgenographic study. Radiology 75:691, 1960.
53. Wright V: Psoriatic arthritis: a comparative study of rheumatoid arthritis and arthritis associated with psoriasis. Ann Rheum Dis 20:123, 1961.
54. Dixon AS, Lience E: Sacroiliac joint in adult rheumatoid arthritis and psoriatic arthropathy. Ann Rheum Dis 20:247, 1961.
55. Harvie JN, Lester RS, Little AH: Sacroiliitis in severe psoriasis. AJR 127:579, 1976.
56. Maldonado-Cocco JA, Porrini A, Garcia-Morteo O: Prevalence of sacroiliitis and ankylosing spondylitis in psoriasis patients. J Rheumatol 5:311, 1978.
57. McEwen C, DiTata D, Lingg C, et al.: Ankylosing spondylitis and spondylitis accompanying ulcerative colitis, regional enteritis, psoriasis and Reiter's disease: a comparative study. Arthritis Rheum 14:291, 1971.
58. Molin L: Sacroiliitis in psoriasis. Scand J Rheumatol Suppl 32:133, 1979.
59. Bywaters EGL, Dixon ASJ: Paravertebral ossification in psoriatic arthritis. Ann Rheum Dis 24:313, 1965.
60. Oriente P, Biondi-Oreinte C, Scarpa R: Clinical manifestations. Baillieres Clin Rheumatol 8:277, 1994.
61. Porter GG: Plain radiology and other imaging techniques. Baillieres Clin Rheumatol 8:465, 1994.
62. Kaplan D, Plotz CM, Nathanson L, Frank L: Cervical

spine in psoriasis and in psoriatic arthritis. Ann Rheum Dis 23:50, 1964.

63. Blau R, Kaufman RL: Erosive and subluxing cervical spine disease in patients with psoriatic arthritis. J Rheumatol 14:111, 1987.

64. Barraclough D, Russell AS, Percy JS: Psoriatic spondylitis: a clinical radiological and scintiscan survey. J Rheumatol 4:282, 1977.

65. Perlman SG, Gerber LH, Roberts RM, et al.: Photochemotherapy and psoriatic arthritis: a prospective study. Ann Intern Med 91:717, 1979.

66. Scarpa R, Pucino A, Iocco M et al.: The management of 138 psoriatic arthritis patients. Acta Derm Venereol 146:199, 1989.

67. Dorwart BB, Gall EP, Schumacher HR, Krauser RE: Chrysotherapy in psoriatic arthritis: efficacy and toxicity compared to rheumatoid arthritis. Arthritis Rheum 21:513, 1978.

68. Sayers ME, Mazanec DJ: Use of antimalarial drugs for the treatment of psoriatic arthritis. Am J Med 93:474, 1992.

69. Cuellar ML, Citera G, Espinoza LR: Treatment of psoriatic arthritis. Baillieres Clin Rheumatol 8:483, 1994.

70. Black RL, O'Brien WM, Van Scott EJ, et al.: Methotrexate therapy in psoriatic arthritis: double-blind study in 21 patients. JAMA 189:743, 1964.

71. Baum J, Hurd E, Lewis D, et al.: Treatment of psoriatic arthritis with 6-mercaptopurine. Arthritis Rheum 16:139, 1973.

72. DuVivier A, Munro DD, Verbov J: Treatment of psoriasis with azathioprine. Br Med J 1:49, 1974.

73. Roenigk HH, Auerbach RM, Mailbach HI, Weinstein GD: Methotrexate guidelines revised. J Am Acad Dermatol 6:145, 1982.

74. Bergquist SR, Felson DT, Prashker MJ, Freedberg KA: The cost-effectiveness of liver biopsy in rheumatoid arthritis patients treated with methotrexate. Arthritis Rheum 38:326, 1995.

75. Collins D, Bellamy N, Campbell J: A Canadian survey of current methotrexate prescribing practices in rheumatoid arthritis. J Rheumatol 21:1220, 1994.

76. Willkens RF, Williams JH, Ward JR, et al.: Randomized, double-blind, placebo-controlled trial of low-dose pulse methotrexate in psoriatic arthritis. Arthritis Rheum 27:376, 1984.

77. Espinoza LR, Zaraoui L, Espinoza CG, et al.: Psoriatic arthritis: clinical response and side effects to methotrexate therapy. J Rheumatol 19:872, 1992.

78. Hollander JL, Brown EM, Jessar RA, et al.: The effect of triamcinolone on psoriatic arthritis: a two-year study. Arthritis Rheum 2:513, 1959.

79. Farber EM, Abel EA, Charuworn A: Recent advances in the treatment of psoriasis. J Am Acad Dermatol 8:311, 1983.

80. Skern RS, Laud N, Melski J, et al.: Cutaneous squamous cell carcinoma in patients treated with PUVA. N Engl J Med 310:1156, 1984.

81. Donnelly S, Doyle DV: Cyclosporin A (CyA)—long-term assessment of tolerability in psoriatic arthritis. Br J Dermatol Suppl 3:25, 1992.

82. Edmunds L, Elswood J, Kennedy LG, et al.: Primary ankylosing spondylitis, psoriatic and enteropathic spondyloarthropathy: a controlled analysis. J Rheumatol 118:696, 1991.

83. Scarpa R, Oriente P, Pucino A, et al.: The clinical spectrum of psoriatic spondylitis. Br J Rheumatol 27:133, 1988.

84. Hanly JG, Russell ML, Gladman DD: Psoriatic spondyloarthropathy: a long-term prospective study. Ann Rheum Dis 47:386, 1988.

85. Lee S, Lui T: Psoriatic arthritis with C1–C2 subluxation as a neurosurgical complication. Surg Neurol 26:428, 1986.

86. Gladman DD: Natural history of psoriatic arthritis. Baillieres Clin Rheumatol 8:379, 1994.

REITER'S SYNDROME

Capsule Summary

Frequency of neck pain—rare

Location of neck pain—cervical spine

Quality of neck pain—ache

Symptoms and signs—morning stiffness, conjunctivitis, urethritis, decreased spinal motion

Laboratory and x-ray tests—increased erythrocyte sedimentation rate, spondylitis on plain roentgenogram

Treatment—exercises, nonsteroidal anti-inflammatory drugs

Prevalence and Pathogenesis

Reiter's syndrome is a disease associated with the triad of urethritis (inflammation of the lower urinary tract), arthritis, and conjunctivitis. Reiter's syndrome is the most common cause of arthritis in young men and primarily affects the lower extremity joints and the low back. Involvement of the cervical spine is rare. The disease results from the interaction of an environmental factor, usually a specific infection, and a genetically predisposed host. The course of the disease, although usually benign, may be chronic and remitting, resulting in significant disability.

Many physicians, including Hippocrates, have written about the apparent relation between venereal and gastrointestinal infections and the development of arthritis. In 1916 Reiter as well as Fiessinger and Leroy described young soldiers with an acute febrile illness that included conjunctivitis, urethritis, and polyarthritis appearing after dysenteric illness.[1, 2] However, the triad and the term Reiter's syndrome were not associated until Bauer and Engleman in 1942 referred to the findings of urethritis, conjunctivitis, and arthritis in World War II soldiers as Reiter's disease.[3]

Reiter's syndrome occurs throughout the world in patients who have no racial or ethnic predisposition. Approximately 1% of patients with the common infection, nongonococcal urethritis, develop the syndrome.[4] A more recent study suggests that 3% of individuals with nonspecific urethritis develop Reiter's syndrome.[5] The syndrome develops in 0.2% to 3% of all patients with enteric infections secondary to *Shigella, Salmonella, Campylobacter,* and *Yersinia.*[6] The male to female ratio in venereal infection is in the range of 10:1, and the ratio is 1:1 in large outbreaks secondary to enteric infection. The ratio may also be 1:1 in patients with no antecedent infection or where urogenital symptoms may be a manifestation of the disease instead of a primary infection.[7, 8] In one study, the incidence was 3.5/100,000 men younger than 50 years of age.[9]

The etiology of Reiter's syndrome is unknown. However, the relationship of the environment to genetics is crucial in the pathogenesis of illness.[10] The initiation of the disease is thought to be related to dysenteric (epidemic) or venereal (endemic) infections. The postdysenteric form of Reiter's syndrome follows infections by *Shigella dysenteriae* and *Shigella flexneri, Salmonella enteritidis, Yersinia enterocolitica,* and *Campylobacter jejuni.*[11–16] In a recent epidemic of *Salmonella* infection in Finland, Reiter's syndrome was diagnosed in 6.9% of exposed individuals.[17] In another example, 19 of 260 (7.6%) individuals infected with *Salmonella typhimurium* developed Reiter's syndrome.[18] The relationship of sexually acquired genital infections with *Chlamydia trachomatis* and *Ureaplasma urealyticum* and the precipitation of joint disease is not clearly established. Although the evidence for *Ureaplasma* is weak, there is increasing evidence in the medical literature connecting the pathogenesis of reactive arthritis with *Chlamydia* infection.[19] The distinction of urethritis as an initiating event and as an integral manifestation of the syndrome is a difficult one to make. Patients with enteric infections develop urethritis without urethral infection.[11] *C. trachomatis* is cultured in 50% to 69% of patients with Reiter's syndrome at the onset of joint disease.[20, 21] Patients with Reiter's syndrome may also have higher prevalences and titers of antichlamydial antibodies than control subjects and demonstrate higher lymphocyte transformation stimulation indices than control subjects.[22] No correlation was found between Reiter's syndrome and *Mycoplasma hominis* or *U. urealyticum* by the same authors.[22] The role of *Neisseria gonorrhoeae* in Reiter's syndrome is not clear because 40% of patients with gonococcal infection also have chlamydial infection simultaneously.[23]

Reiter's syndrome may develop in patients who deny enteric or venereal infection. Some of these patients associate the onset of their disease with an episode of joint trauma.[24] The trauma is associated with swelling, stiffness, and pain in the traumatized joint, and this is followed by the emergence of additional joint symptoms, urethritis, conjunctivitis, or cutaneous lesions. Another possible manifestation of a response to trauma in these patients is the presence of bony bridging or nonmarginal syndesmophytes in the spine in the absence of sacroiliitis or axial symptoms.[25, 26] However, there is no scientific evidence to substantiate the role of trauma as an initiator of Reiter's syndrome.

Characteristic of the spondyloarthropathies in general, Reiter's syndrome is associated with the human leukocyte antigen (HLA)-B27. From 60% to 80% of whites are positive for HLA-B27. In blacks the prevalence of HLA-B27 has varied from 15% to 75%.[27–29] A majority of those who are negative for this antigen have HLA-B antigens that cross-react with B27, including B7, Bw22, B40, and Bw42.[27] HLA-B27 and related antigens may be linked to genes controlling the cellular immune response to certain infectious agents, and these genes cause an abnormal immune response. Alternately, the HLA-B27 antigen may cross-react immunologically with certain infectious agents (molecular mimicry).[30]

Despite its association with Reiter's syndrome, the HLA-B27 haplotype is not the only determinant for disease expression; only a minority of HLA-B27 individuals develop Reiter's syndrome after exposure to infectious agents. In addition, HLA-B27 is associated with a wide range of diseases that cause spondyloarthropathy. There may be genetic material closely linked to HLA-B27 that actually determines the expression of Reiter's syndrome or other spondyloarthropathies.[31]

Evaluation of the HLA molecule reveals an antigen-binding groove that appears to serve the function of capturing appropriate corresponding antigen and presenting it to T cell receptors of the CD8+ cytotoxic cell. An explanation for the variability of HLA-B27 being associated with a variety of arthritides might be explained by the variability of key amino acid residues that affect the form of the binding site. HLA-B27 has been divided into six subtypes. These include B*2701 through B*2706. Different subtypes are associated with particular ethnic groups and susceptibility for spondyloarthropathy.[32]

Clinical History

The classic Reiter's syndrome patient is a young man about 25 years old who develops urethritis and a mild conjunctivitis, followed by the onset of a predominantly lower extremity oligoarthritis. The symptoms of urethritis are usually mild with a mucopurulent discharge and dysuria. Men may also develop acute or chronic prostatitis. Women may have vaginitis or cervicitis, although many with these manifestations of genitourinary tract involvement in Reiter's syndrome may be asymptomatic. This paucity of symptoms from the genitourinary tract may in part explain the infrequency of the diagnosis of Reiter's syndrome in women.[7] Urethritis occurs in both epidemic and endemic forms of the disease. Up to 93% of patients with Reiter's syndrome have genitourinary symptoms during the course of their illness.[33]

The conjunctivitis is usually mild and is manifested by an erythema (redness) and crusting of the lids. Conjunctival inflammation is usually bilateral and gradually resolves in a few days, but it may recur spontaneously. Acute iritis occurs in 20% of Reiter's syndrome patients and is marked by severe pain, photophobia, and scleral injection.

Arthritis may occur 1 to 3 weeks after the initial infection. In many patients, arthritis is the only manifestation of disease.[34] The term reactive arthritis is used for patients who develop only the arthritis of Reiter's syndrome after an enteric or genitourinary infection. The weight-bearing joints—knees, ankles, and feet—are most frequently affected in an asymmetrical manner. A minority of patients have a persistent monarthritis as their only articular abnormality. The involved joints are acutely inflamed, with some joints developing large effusions.

Neck pain is a rare symptom of patients with Reiter's syndrome. Most studies of Reiter's syndrome do not include patients with neck symptoms. Cervical spine disease in Reiter's syndrome occurs in 2.2% to 2.4% of patients.[6, 35, 36] In a study of 153 men and 119 women, cervical spine disease occurred in Reiter's syndrome patients in 2.5% and 5.0%, respectively.[8] On occasion, patients with Reiter's syndrome may develop torticollis, indicative of cervical spine involvement.[37]

Low back pain occurs more frequently as part of the symptoms associated with Reiter's syndrome. During the acute course, 31% to 92% of the patients may develop pain in the lumbosacral region.[33, 38, 39] The pain is of an aching quality and is improved with activity. Occasionally the pain radiates into the posterior thighs but rarely below the knees; it may be unilateral. This finding corresponds to the asymmetrical involvement of the sacroiliac joints, and it contrasts with the symmetrical involvement of ankylosing spondylitis.[40] Sacroiliitis is the cause of back pain in a majority of patients in the acute phase of the disease, as measured by increased activity over the sacroiliac joints on scintiscan.[41] Radiographic evidence of sacroiliitis is usually restricted to those patients with severe disease. In retrospective studies, sacroiliitis can be detected radiographically in 9% of patients in the acute phase of disease and in up to 71% of patients who have had disease activity longer than 5 years.[4] Spondylitis affecting the lumbar, thoracic, and cervical spine occurs less commonly than sacroiliitis—up to 23% of patients with severe disease show such involvement.[42]

Another musculoskeletal manifestation of Reiter's syndrome is inflammation of the insertion of tendons and fascia. This anatomic structure is called an enthesis, and a process that results in its inflammation is an enthesopathy. Heel pain, "lover's heel," secondary to plantar fascia inflammation, is a common finding.[43] Other manifestations of enthesopathy in Reiter's syndrome patients are Achilles tendinitis, chest wall pain, dactylitis or "sausage digit," and low back pain with no evidence of active sacroiliitis.

Although not part of the classic triad of the disease, mucocutaneous lesions are characteristic of Reiter's syndrome. Keratoderma blennorrhagicum is a skin rash characterized by waxy, macular lesions that become vesicular and scaly. They are found predominantly on the palms and soles. Histologically, they are indistinguishable from pustular psoriasis. Keratoderma, which appears on the glans penis, is referred to as circinate balanitis. It occurs in up to 31% of patients. Oral ulcers occur on the palate, tongue, buccal mucosa, and lips. These lesions are shallow and painless and occur in 33% of patients. Nail involvement is characterized by opacification and hyperkeratosis, but not pitting.

Constitutional symptoms occur in about one third of patients and are characterized by fever, anorexia, weight loss, and fatigue. Cardiac complications, including heart block and aortic regurgitation, occur as a late manifestation of disease and in 2% of patients.[44] Neurologic disease occurs in 1% of patients and is associated with peripheral neuropathy, hemiplegia, and cranial nerve abnormalities.[45] Amyloidosis is also a rare and late complication of Reiter's syndrome.[46]

Physical Examination

Physical examination should include all organ systems that may be involved in the disease process. Many of the manifestations of Reiter's syndrome may be overlooked by patients. Important findings, such as oral ulcers, circinate balanitis, and limitation of axial motion, may be missed if not sought by the physician. Conjunctivitis is manifested by erythema of the conjunctivae and crusting of the lids. Urethritis may be detected only by "milking" the urethra before urination for the presence of a mucopurulent discharge.

A complete musculoskeletal examination should include both upper and lower extremities as well as the axial skeleton. Men tend to have involvement in the knees, ankles, and feet, and women have more upper extremity disease.[7] The usual patient has six or fewer joints affected. Percussion tenderness over the sacroiliac joints may be unilateral, correlating with asymmetrical involvement in Reiter's syndrome. The mobility of the lumbosacral and cervical spine should be measured in all planes of motion. Patients with cervical spine involvement may have straightening of the neck. Paracervical muscles should be palpated for increased tension. A search for evidence of enthesopathy, heel pain, or Achilles tendon tenderness is also required.

An examination of the oropharynx, genitals, palms, soles, and nails covers the areas that are associated with the mucocutaneous lesions of Reiter's syndrome.

Laboratory Data

Laboratory results are nonspecific and not helpful in making the diagnosis of Reiter's syndrome. A mild anemia of chronic disease, an elevated white blood cell count (leukocytosis), and an elevated platelet count (thrombocytosis) are demonstrated in about one third of patients.[24] The erythrocyte sedimentation rate is increased in 70% to 80% of patients, but it does not follow the course of the disease. The C-reactive protein level is elevated, particularly in patients with reactive arthritis.[47] Rheumatoid factor and antinuclear antibodies are not present in this illness. HLA-B27 or one of the cross-reactive antigens is present in 80% of patients. HLA-B27–positivity is helpful in differentiating Reiter's syndrome from rheumatoid arthritis (this is more easily done by clinical examination). The test, however, is not helpful in differentiating Reiter's syndrome from the other spondyloarthropathies. Histocompatibility testing should not be regarded as a routine diagnostic test. Testing may be most helpful early in the course of an arthropathy in which no typical extra-articular features are present.[48] Synovial fluid analysis demonstrates an inflammatory fluid with no specific abnormalities. Synovial lymphocyte proliferation to a variety of organisms associated with Reiter's syndrome has been documented in patients with cultures of body fluids without growth.[49, 50] These proliferation assays are research tests and should not be used for therapeutic decisions.

Radiographic Evaluation

In patients who do not manifest the complete triad of Reiter's syndrome, radiographic changes are helpful in confirming the diagnosis.[36] Joint destruction is most severe in the feet. The hips and shoulders are usually spared. The radiologic correlate of the enthesopathy of Reiter's syndrome is periosteal new-bone formation at the attachments of the plantar fascia and Achilles tendon into the calcaneus. The incidence of sacroiliac disease increases with disease chronicity and may be more common in postvenereal HLA-B27 patients.[41] Sacroiliac involvement may mimic ankylosing spondylitis (symmetric disease) or may be asymmetrical in severity of joint changes. Unilateral sacroiliac disease occurs early in the disease process.[38] Bone erosion is more common on the iliac than sacral side of the joint. Variable amounts of sclerosis are associated with erosions. Widening of the joint (erosion), then narrowing (fusion), is the progression of radiographic changes. Fusion of the joints occurs less frequently than in ankylosing spondylitis.

Spondylitis is discontinuous in its involvement of the axial skeleton (skip lesions) and is characterized by nonmarginal bony bridging of vertebral bodies. These vertebral hyperostoses are markedly thickened compared with the thin syndesmophytes of ankylosing spondylitis. Cervical spine disease is associated with hyperostoses at the anteroinferior corners of one or more cervical vertebrae.[36] Extensive syndesmophytes may be present in the cervical spine, without similar lesions in the thoracic or lumbar spine.[35] Atlantoaxial subluxation is a rare complication of Reiter's syndrome[51, 52] (Fig. 11–11). In rare circumstances, Reiter's syndrome may have an initial presentation with atlantoaxial subluxation.[53] Patients who develop nonreducible rotational head tilt may have involvement of the craniocervical junction.[54]

Paravertebral ossification may appear about

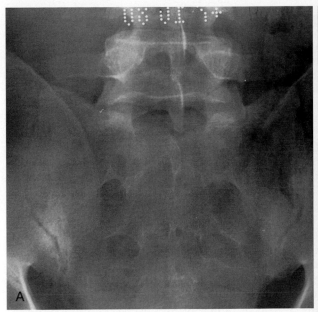

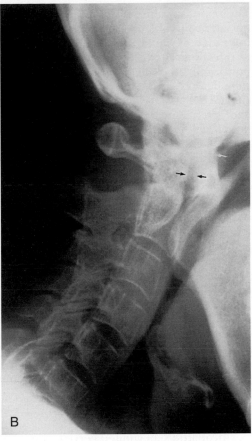

Figure 11–11. Reiter's syndrome. A 26-year-old man with neck pain. *A,* Spot view of the pelvis reveals greater involvement of the right sacroiliac joint characterized by joint sclerosis and erosion. *B,* Lateral view of the cervical spine reveals atlantoaxial subluxation of 10 mm *(arrows).* (Courtesy of Anne Brower, M.D.)

the lower three thoracic and upper three lumbar vertebrae.[55] This roentgenographic finding may antedate the appearance of sacroiliac or peripheral joint alterations.[56] Paravertebral ossification may be the source of nonmarginal syndesmophytes. Ossification may skip areas of the spine as opposed to the continuous vertebral involvement of ankylosing spondylitis. Reiter's syndrome patients may also develop typical thin syndesmophytes similar to those of ankylosing spondylitis. The apophyseal joints may fuse, but the frequency of this finding is less than in classic ankylosing spondylitis.[57]

Whether spinal disease should be considered a complication of Reiter's syndrome or a manifestation of HLA-B27 disease is unclear. The difference in the appearance of spondylitis in Reiter's syndrome and ankylosing spondylitis suggests that the spondylitic process is dissimilar in the two conditions. The fact that spinal disease is often asymmetrical and has skip areas and little squaring of vertebral bodies, along with the finding of increased spinal involvement with severe, long-standing Reiter's syndrome, suggests that the process is related to Reiter's syndrome itself rather than HLA-B27. Spondylitis in Reiter's syndrome occurs in an older age group than ankylosing spondylitis.

Differential Diagnosis

Preliminary criteria for the diagnosis of acute Reiter's syndrome have recently been reported by the American Rheumatism Association.[58] Patients with Reiter's syndrome were distinguished from patients with other spondyloarthropathies and gonococcal arthritis by an episode of peripheral arthritis of more than 1 month's duration, occurring in association with urethritis or cervicitis or both.

Reactive arthritis may be considered a subset of Reiter's syndrome or a separate disease entity. Reactive arthritis refers to an inflammatory joint disease that follows an infection elsewhere in the body without microbial invasion of the synovial space.[59] Ahvonen and colleagues introduced the term reactive arthritis to describe the nonpurulent joint inflammation associated with a *Yersenia enterocolitica* and *Yersinia pseudotuberculosis* enteric infection.[60]

The reasons for the development of arthropathy alone in reactive arthritis instead of the full range of Reiter's syndrome after exposure to infectious agents are unknown.[61] The infectious agents include *Salmonella*,[12] *Shigella*,[11] *Yersinia*,[13] and *Campylobacter*[15]; parasites, including *Giardia*,[62, 63] *Chlamydia*,[20] *Neisseria gonorrhoeae*,[64] and streptococci[65]; and nonspecific chronic urogenital infections.[66, 67] About 80% of patients with reactive arthritis are HLA-B27–positive.[68, 69] Like epidemic Reiter's syndrome, young men and women are affected equally. The onset and pattern of disease of reactive arthritis is similar to that of Reiter's syndrome. Approximately 30% of patients with reactive arthritis develop back pain.[69] These patients are HLA-B27–positive. These patients also are at greater risk of developing radiographic evidence of sacroiliitis. Patients with reactive arthritis respond to the same therapy that is effective for Reiter's syndrome. At the time of a 5-year follow-up, one third of patients with reactive arthritis may continue to have back pain and show evidence of sacroiliitis.[69, 70]

The differential diagnosis of the patient who presents with neck pain and no other manifestation of Reiter's syndrome is the same as that presented for ankylosing spondylitis. This differential diagnosis includes the other spondyloarthropathies, herniated cervical disc, diffuse idiopathic skeletal hyperostosis, and tumors (Table 11–5). In the patient who presents with acute monarticular disease after sexual intercourse, the diagnosis of infectious arthritis secondary to *N. gonnorhoeae* must not be overlooked.[71] Bacterial cultures of the urethra, rectum, pharynx, and synovial fluid are necessary to detect the presence of the bacterium. Examination of synovial fluid for bacterial fatty acids, particularly succinic acid, helps differentiate those individuals with septic arthritis from those with effusions secondary to Reiter's syndrome.[72]

Human Immunodeficiency Virus (HIV). HIV infection was first recognized during the early 1980s.[73] The disease is characterized by fever, weight loss, anorexia, lymphadenopathy, multiple infections, and Kaposi's sarcoma. The cause of HIV infection is a ribonucleic acid retrovirus that has a high affinity for the CD4 receptor that is expressed preferentially on T helper/inducer lymphocytes. These cells are killed by the virus, resulting in dysfunction in the surveillance function of the immune system. The absence of this function results in opportunistic infections and malignancies. Many organ systems are affected by the immune dysfunction and the persistent infections.[74] Compared with other organ systems, the musculoskeletal system is spared. In a study of 556 patients with HIV infection, only 11% had musculoskeletal disorders and 0.5% had Reiter's syndrome.[75] Reiter's syndrome was the first distinct rheumatologic disorder described in association with HIV infection.[76] Reiter's syndrome may precede or follow the onset of acquired immunodeficiency syndrome (AIDS). The usual articular symptoms are asymmetric oligoarthritis of large joints, enthesopathy, and skin lesions.[77] Interestingly, patients with axial skeleton disease have involvement of the cervical spine to a greater degree in Reiter's patients with HIV infection than Reiter's unassociated with HIV.[75, 78] Cervical spine disease includes straightening of the neck, with evidence of sclerosis and apophyseal joint narrowing on roentgenograms. The thoracic and lumbar spine may be affected in the presence or absence of sacroiliitis. Radiographic alterations of the spine occur, and 66% of patients are HLA-B27–positive. Therapy directed at controlling arthritis has the potential to exacerbate the underlying immunodeficiency.[78] Patients who develop Reiter's syndrome are severely ill. Debate remains regarding the association of AIDS with Reiter's syndrome. Reports have suggested a clear association.[79] Other studies have suggested that the increased risk is from risk behaviors associated with AIDS (bowel infections) and not to the virus itself.[80]

Treatment

The therapeutic regimen includes patient education, medications, and physical therapy. Patients are confused by the association of Reiter's syndrome and sexual relations. Many develop guilt or anxiety over sexual intercourse. The fact that urethritis may recur without any obvious cause must be made clear to the patient.

Acute joint symptoms are treated symptomatically with nonsteroidal anti-inflammatory drugs (NSAIDs) and the modalities of physical therapy. The drugs that are most effective for Reiter's syndrome are reviewed in Section IV. The joint and enthesopathic manifestations of Reiter's syndrome appear to respond better to indomethacin, phenylbutazone, or the other newer NSAIDs than to aspirin. The drugs are continued as long as the patient remains symptomatic. The effect of these agents on the long-term course of the disease is unknown. In patients with decreased range of motion of the spine associated with Reiter's syndrome,

NSAIDs are useful to decrease pain. The addition of muscle relaxants in these patients can also be helpful in improving that component of immobility secondary to muscle tightness and spasm that are associated with arthritis or enthesopathy.

The role of antibiotic therapy in the acute phase of Reiter's syndrome remains controversial. A study demonstrated that antibiotic therapy did not influence the appearance of Reiter's syndrome in patients with nonspecific urethritis.[20] A recent double-blind, placebo-controlled study of 3 months' duration evaluating the treatment with a lysine conjugate of tetracycline showed that those with *Chlamydia*-associated reactive arthritis recovered more rapidly than those with post-*Yersinia* arthritis.[81]

A recent review studied the role of second-line agents (gold, sulfasalazine, methotrexate, and azathioprine) for the treatment of spondyloarthropathies, including Reiter's syndrome.[82] Gold salt therapy may be helpful in the patient with progressive, destructive, peripheral joint disease. Sulfasalazine has been reported to improve spine pain and swollen joints in patients with Reiter's syndrome and reactive arthritis. The usual dose of sulfasalazine is 2 gm/day in divided doses. The immunosuppressive, methotrexate, is reserved for the patient with uncontrolled progression of joint disease and unresponsive, extensive skin involvement.[83] The dose of methotrexate used ranges from 7.5 to 50 mg weekly. Most individuals have a beneficial response in regard to improved joint symptoms without toxicity. Azathioprine has been shown to be effective in controlling activity of intractable Reiter's syndrome in a placebo-controlled, crossover study.[84] Corticosteroids are used as drops for iritis and as long-acting preparations for intra-articular injection. Systemic corticosteroids have less of an effect in Reiter's syndrome than they do in rheumatoid arthritis and are rarely used.

Prognosis

Reiter's syndrome has no cure. The course of the illness is unpredictable. About 30% to 40% of patients have a self-limited illness, lasting 3 months to 1 year. Another 30% to 50% develop a relapsing pattern of illness with periods of complete remission. The final 10% to 25% develop chronic, unremitting disease associated with significant disability.[33, 85] Measuring C-reactive protein level may be a better method for following activity of disease than erythrocyte sedimentation rate in Reiter's syndrome in addition to looking for clinical parameters (such as morning stiffness and joint swelling).[86] Patients who develop significant disability from Reiter's syndrome typically have painful or deformed feet or visual loss from iritis. A 5-year follow-up study of 131 consecutive patients with Reiter's syndrome revealed that 83% of the patients had some disease activity.[33] Fifty-one percent of patients had continued low back pain, and 45% had persistent foot or heel pain. Thirty-four percent of patients had disease activity that interfered with their job; 26% had to changes jobs or were unemployed. Heel involvement at the time of diagnosis was the finding most closely associated with a poor functional outcome. The presence of HLA-B27 did not correlate with functional outcome; however, a report from Finland suggested that the HLA-B27 status of the patient was associated with disease severity.[69] Patients who were HLA-B27–positive had more frequent back pain and mucocutaneous and genitourinary symptoms. They also had a longer duration of disease and more frequent chronic low back pain and sacroiliitis. Chronic joint symptoms continued in 68% of 140 Reiter's syndrome patients studied, and 41% had chronic back pain. Most patients were able to lead normal lives, although 16% of the group had chronic destructive peripheral arthritis. Another report suggested that homozygosity for HLA-B27 may also be associated with more severe disease.[87]

In contrast, a study of 55 Reiter's patients followed for 9.3 years showed a 40% incidence of sacroiliitis. Sacroiliitis was rarely associated with spondylitis, 33 patients had mild limitation of back motion, and only 1 patient was functionally impaired by back disease.[88] The patients with sacroiliitis had more iritis, prolonged disease duration, and HLA-B27–positivity.

Reiter's syndrome is no longer considered a benign disease. Most patients do not have significant impairment secondary to cervical spine disease. Impairment is more closely associated with disease in other locations in the skeleton and in other organ systems. Early therapy with NSAIDs, physical therapy, and appropriate shoes may have beneficial effects on patient function. Unfortunately, even aggressive therapy is unable to prevent disease activity and progressive disability in many of Reiter's syndrome patients.

References

REITER'S SYNDROME

1. Reiter H: Über eine bisher unerkannte Spirochaeteninfektion (Spirochaetosis arthritica). Dtsch Med Wochenschr 42:1535, 1916.

2. Fiessinger N, Leroy E: Contribution a l'etude d'une epidemie de dysenterie dans le somme. Bull Soc Med Hop Paris, 40:2030, 1916.

3. Bauer W, Engleman EP: A syndrome of unknown etiology characterized by urethritis, conjunctivitis, and arthritis (so-called Reiter's disease). Trans Assoc Am Physicians 57:307, 1942.

4. Csonka GW: The course of Reiter's syndrome. Br Med J 1:1088, 1958.

5. Keat AC, Maini RN, Nkwazi GC, et al.: Role of *Chlamydia trachomatis* and HLA-B27 in sexually acquired reactive arthritis. Br Med J 1:605, 1978.

6. Noer HR: An "experimental" epidemic of Reiter's syndrome. JAMA 198:693, 1966.

7. Neuwelt CM, Borenstein DG, Jacobs RP: Reiter's syndrome: a male and female disease. J Rheumatol 9:268, 1982.

8. Yli-Kerttua UI: Clinical characteristics in male and female uro-arthritis or Reiter's syndrome. Clin Rheumatol 3:351, 1984.

9. Michet CJ, Machado EBV, Ballard DJ, et al.: Epidemiology of Reiter's syndrome in Rochester, Minnesota: 1950–1980. Arthritis Rheum 31:428, 1988.

10. Calin A: The relationship between genetics and environment in the pathogenesis of rheumatic diseases (medical progress). West J Med 131:205, 1979.

11. Paronen I: Reiter's disease: a study of 344 cases observed in Finland. Acta Med Scand Suppl 212:1, 1948.

12. Good AE, Schultz JS: Reiter's syndrome following *Shigella flexneri* 2a. Arthritis Rheum 20:100, 1977.

13. Jones RAK: Reiter's disease after *Salmonella typhimurium* enteritis. Br Med J 1:1391, 1977.

14. Solem JH, Lassen J: Reiter's disease following *Yersinia enterocolitica* infection. Scand J Infect Dis 8:83, 1971.

15. Laitenen O, Leirisalo M, Skylv G: Relation between HLA-B27 and clinical features in patients with *Yersinia* arthritis. Arthritis Rheum 20:121, 1977.

16. Van de Putte LBA, Berden JHM, Boerbooms AM, et al.: Reactive arthritis after *Campylobacter jejuni* enteritis. J Rheumatol 7:531, 1980.

17. Mattila L, Leirisalo-Repo M, Koskimies S, et al.: Reactive arthritis following an outbreak of *Salmonella* infection in Finland. Br J Rheumatol 33:1136, 1994.

18. Inman RD, Johnston MEA, Hodge M, et al.: Postdysenteric reactive arthritis: a clinical and immunogenetic study following an outbreak of salmonellosis. Arthritis Rheum 31:1377, 1988.

19. Rahman MU, Hudson AP, Schumacher HR Jr: *Chlamydia* and Reiter's syndrome (reactive arthritis). Rheum Dis Clin North Am 18:67, 1992.

20. Keat AC, Thomas BJ, Taylor-Robinson D, et al.: Evidence of *Chlamydia trachomatis* infection in sexually acquired reactive arthritis. Ann Rheum Dis 39:431, 1980.

21. Kousa M, Saikku P, Richmond S, Lassus A: Frequent association of chlamydial infection with Reiter's syndrome. Sex Transm Dis 5:57, 1978.

22. Martin DH, Pollock S, Kuo C, et al.: *Chlamydia trachomatis* infections in men with Reiter's Syndrome. Ann Intern Med 100:207, 1984.

23. Holmes KK, Handsfield HH, Wang SP, et al.: Etiology of nongonococcal arthritis. N Engl J Med 292:1199, 1975.

24. Arnett FC Jr: Reiter's syndrome. Johns Hopkins Med J 150:39, 1982.

25. Calin A, Fries JF: Striking prevalence of ankylosing spondylitis in "healthy" W27-positive males and females: a controlled study. N Engl J Med 293:835, 1975.

26. Cohen LM, Mittal KK, Schmid FR, et al.: Increased risk for spondylitis stigmata in apparently healthy HLA-W27 men. Ann Intern Med 84:1, 1976.

27. Arnett FC, Hochberg MD, Bias WB: Cross-reactive HLA antigens in B27-negative Reiter's syndrome and sacroiliitis. John Hopkins Med J 141:193, 1977.

28. Khan MA, Askari AD, Braun WE, Aponte CJ: Low association of HLA-B27 with Reiter's syndrome in blacks. Ann Intern Med 90:202, 1979.

29. Good AE, Kawaniski H, Schultz JS: HLA-B27 in blacks with ankylosing spondylitis or Reiter's disease. N Engl J Med 294:166, 1976.

30. McDevitt HO, Bodmer WF: HLA, immune response genes and disease. Lancet 1:1269, 1974.

31. Reveille JD, McDaniel DO, Barger BO, et al.: Restriction fragment length polymorphism (RFLP) analysis in familial ankylosing spondylitis: independent segregation of a 9.2 Kb PVU II RFLP from B27 haplotypes (Abstract). Arthritis Rheum 30:S36, 1987.

32. Khan MA: An overview of clinical spectrum and heterogeneity of spondyloarthropathies. Rheum Dis Clin North Am 18:1, 1992.

33. Fox R, Calin A, Gerber RC, Gibson D: The chronicity of symptoms and disability in Reiter's syndrome: an analysis of 131 consecutive patients. Ann Intern Med 91:190, 1979.

34. Arnett FC, McClusky E, Schacter BZ, Lordon RE: Incomplete Reiter's syndrome: discriminating features and HLA-W27 in diagnosis. Ann Intern Med 84:8, 1976.

35. Sholkoff SD, Glickman MG, Steinbach HL: Roentgenology of Reiter's syndrome. Radiology 97:497, 1970.

36. Martel W, Braunstein EM, Borlaza G, et al.: Radiologic features of Reiter's disease. Radiology 132:1, 1979.

37. Oates JK, Hancock JAH: Neurological symptoms and lesions occurring in the course of Reiter's disease. Am J Med Sci 238:79, 1959.

38. Oates JK, Young AC: Sacroiliitis in Reiter's disease. Br Med J 1:1013, 1959.

39. Popert AJ, Gill AJ, Laird SM: A prospective study of Reiter's syndrome: an interim report on the first 82 cases. Br J Vener Dis 40:160, 1964.

40. Russell AS, Davis P, Percy JS, Lentle GC: The sacroiliitis of acute Reiter's syndrome. J Rheumatol 4:293, 1977.

41. Russell AS, Lentle BC, Percy JS: Investigation of sacroiliac disease: comparative evaluation of radiological and radionuclide techniques. J Rheumatol 2:45, 1975.

42. Good AE: Reiter's syndrome: long-term follow-up in relation to development of ankylosing spondylitis. Ann Rheum Dis 38:39, 1979.

43. Ball J: Enthesopathy of rheumatoid and ankylosing spondylitis. Ann Rheum Dis 30:213, 1971.

44. Ruppert GB, Lindsay J, Barth WF: Cardiac conduction abnormalities in Reiter's syndrome. Am J Med 73:335, 1982.

45. Good AE: Reiter's disease: a review with special attention to cardiovascular and neurologic sequelae. Semin Arthritis Rheum 3:253, 1974.

46. Miller LD, Brown EC, Arnett FC: Amyloidosis in Reiter's syndrome. J Rheumatol 6:225, 1979.

47. Kvien TK, Glennas A, Melby K, et al.: Reactive arthritis: incidence, triggering agents, and clinical presentation. J Rheumatol 21:115, 1994.

48. Calin A: HLA-B27: to type or not to type? Ann Intern Med 92:208, 1980.

49. Sieper J, Kingsley G, Palacios-Boix A, et al.: Synovial T lymphocyte specific immune response to *Chlamydia trachomatis* in Reiter's disease. Arthritis Rheum 34:588, 1991.

50. Sieper J, Braun J, Wu P, et al.: The possible role of *Shigella* in sporadic enteric reactive arthritis. Br J Rheumatol 32:582, 1993.

51. Latchaw RE, Meyer GW: Reiter disease with atlanto-axial subluxation. Radiology 126:303, 1978.
52. Kransdorf MJ, Wehrle PA, Moser RP Jr: Atlantoaxial subluxation in Reiter's syndrome: a report of three cases and review of the literature. Spine 13:12, 1988.
53. Melsom RD, Benjamin JC, Barnes CG: Spontaneous atlantoaxial subluxation: an unusual presenting manifestation of Reiter's syndrome. Ann Rheum Dis 48:170, 1989.
54. Halla JT, Bliznak J, Hardin JG: Involvement of the craniocervical junction in Reiter's syndrome. J Rheumatol 15:1722, 1988.
55. Cliff JM: Spinal bony bridging and carditis in Reiter's disease. Ann Rheum Dis 30:171, 1971.
56. Sundaram M, Patton JT: Paravertebral ossification in psoriasis and Reiter's disease. Br J Radiol 48:628, 1975.
57. Ford DK: Natural history of arthritis following venereal urethritis. Ann Rheum Dis 12:177, 1953.
58. Willkens RF, Arnett FC, Bitter T, et al.: Reiter's syndrome: evaluation of preliminary criteria for definite disease. Bull Rheum Dis 32:31, 1982.
59. Reactive arthritis (editorial). Br Med J 281:311, 1980.
60. Ahvonen P, Sievers K, Aho K: Arthritis associated with *Yersinia enterocolitica* infection. Acta Rheum Scand 15:232, 1969.
61. Amor B: Reiter's syndrome and reactive arthritis. Clin Rheumatol 2:315, 1983.
62. Goobar JP: Joint symptoms in giardiasis. Lancet 1:1010, 1977.
63. Bocanegra TS, Espinoza LR, Bridgeford PH, et al.: Reactive arthritis induced by parasitic infestation. Ann Intern Med 94:207, 1981.
64. Rosenthal L, Olhagen B, Ek S: Aseptic arthritis after gonorrhea. Ann Rheum Dis 39:141, 1980.
65. Hubbard WN, Hughes GRV: Streptococci and reactive arthritis. Ann Rheum Dis 41:435, 1982.
66. Olhagen B: Postinfective or reactive arthritis. Scand J Rheumatol 9:193, 1980.
67. Szanto E, Hagenfeldt K: Sacro-iliitis and salpingitis. Scand J Rheumatol 8:129, 1979.
68. Aho K, Ahvonen P, Lassus A, et al.: HLA-27 in reactive arthritis: a study of Yersinia arthritis and Reiter's disease. Arthritis Rheum 17:521, 1974.
69. Leirisalo M, Skylv G, Kousa M, et al.: Follow-up study on patients with Reiter's disease and reactive arthritis, with special reference to HLA-B27. Arthritis Rheum 25:249, 1982.
70. Marsal L, Winblad S, Wollheim FA: *Yersinia enterocolitica* arthritis in southern Sweden: a four-year follow-up study. Br Med J 283:101, 1981.
71. McCord WC, Nies KM, Louie JS: Acute venereal arthritis: comparative study of acute Reiter's syndrome and acute gonococcal arthritis. Arch Intern Med 137:858, 1977.
72. Borenstein DG, Gibbs CA, Jacobs RP: Gas-liquid chromatographic analysis of synovial fluid. Arthritis Rheum 25:947, 1982.
73. Siegal FP, Lopez C, Hammer GS, et al.: Severe acquired immunodeficiency in male homosexuals, manifested by chronic perianal ulcerative herpes simplex lesions. N Engl J Med 305:1439, 1981.
74. Sande MA, Volberding PA: The Medical Management of AIDS, 3rd ed. Philadelphia: WB Saunders Co, 1992, p 525.
75. Fernandez SM, Cardenal A, Balsa A, et al.: Rheumatic manifestations in 556 patients with human immunodeficiency virus infection. Semin Arthritis Rheum 21:30, 1991.
76. Winchster R, Bernstein DH, Fischer HD, et al.: The co-occurrence of Reiter's syndrome and acquired immunodeficiency. Ann Intern Med 106:19, 1987.
77. Keat A, Rowe I: Reiter's syndrome and associated arthritides. Rheum Dis Clin North Am 17:25, 1991.
78. Rowe IF, Forster SM, Seifert MH, et al.: Rheumatological lesion in individuals with human immunodeficiency virus infection. Q J Med 73:1167, 1989.
79. Espinoza LR, Jara LJ, Espinoza CG, et al.: There is an association between human immunodeficiency virus infection and spondyloarthropathies. Rheum Dis Clin North Am 18:257, 1992.
80. Clark MR, Solinger AM, Hochberg MC: Human immunodeficiency virus is not associated with Reiter's syndrome: data from three large cohort studies. Rheum Dis Clin North Am 18:267, 1992.
81. Lauhio A, Leirisalo-Repo M, Lahdevirta J, et al.: Double-blind, placebo-controlled study of three-month treatment with lymecycline in reactive arthritis, with special reference to *Chlamydia* arthritis. Arthritis Rheum 34:6, 1991.
82. Creemers MCW, van Riel PLCM, Franssen MJAM, et al.: Second-line treatment in seronegative spondyloarthropathies. Semin Arthritis Rheum 24:71, 1994.
83. Farber GA, Forshner JG, O'Quinn SE: Reiter's syndrome: treatment with methotrexate. JAMA 200:171, 1967.
84. Calin A: A placebo-controlled, crossover study of azathioprine in Reiter's syndrome. Ann Rheum Dis 45:653, 1986.
85. Good AE: Involvement of the back in Reiter's syndrome: follow-up study of thirty-four cases. Ann Intern Med 57:44, 1962.
86. Nashel DJ, Petrone DL, Ulmer CC, Sliwinski AJ: C-reactive protein: a marker for disease activity in ankylosing spondylitis and Reiter's syndrome. J Rheumatol 13:364, 1986.
87. Arnett FC, Schacter BZ, Hochberg MC, et al.: Homozygosity for HLA-B27: impact on rheumatic disease expression in two families. Arthritis Rheum 20:797, 1977.
88. McGuigan LE, Hart HH, Gow PJ, et al.: The functional significance of sacroiliitis and ankylosing spondylitis in Reiter's Syndrome. Clin Exp Rheumatol 3:311, 1985.

ENTEROPATHIC ARTHRITIS

Capsule Summary

Frequency of neck pain—rare
Location of neck pain—cervical spine
Quality of neck pain—ache
Symptoms and signs—morning stiffness, abdominal pain or cramps
Laboratory and x-ray tests—increased erythrocyte sedimentation rate, blood in stool, syndesmophytes on plain roentgenogram
Treatment—exercises, nonsteroidal anti-inflammatory drugs

Prevalence and Pathogenesis

Ulcerative colitis and Crohn's disease are inflammatory bowel diseases. Ulcerative colitis is limited to the colon; Crohn's disease, or regional enteritis, may involve any part of the gastrointestinal tract. Inflammation of the gut results in numerous gastrointestinal symptoms, including abdominal pain, fever, and weight loss. These inflammatory diseases are also associated with extraintestinal manifestations, including arthritis. Articular involvement in these inflammatory bowel diseases includes both peripheral and axial skeleton joints. Peripheral arthritis is generally nondeforming and follows the activity of the underlying bowel disease. Axial skeleton disease is similar to ankylosing spondylitis and follows a course independent of activity of bowel inflammation.

The association of arthritis and ulcerative colitis was first elucidated by Bargen in the 1920s.[1] Crohn's disease was described by Crohn and colleagues in 1932.[2] The association of arthritis and Crohn's disease was commented on by Van Patter and colleagues and by Steinberg and colleagues in the 1950s.[3, 4]

Ulcerative colitis occurs four times more commonly in whites than nonwhites and more commonly among Jews than non-Jews. In a white population, the annual incidence of disease is up to 10 per 100,000 people.[5, 6] Symptomatic ulcerative colitis usually occurs from 25 to 45 years of age, and the disease is more common among women than among men.

Crohn's disease occurs in all races and is distributed worldwide. In the United States, the annual incidence of the disease is 4 per 100,000 people.[5] The disease appears most often from 15 to 35 years of age. Men and women are equally affected. Patients from urban backgrounds and with high levels of education are at greater risk.

The frequency of peripheral arthritis is 11% in ulcerative colitis and 20% in Crohn's disease, and the occurrence of axial arthritis is equal in both sexes.[7, 8] Spondylitis occurs in 3% to 4% of both diseases, and radiographic sacroiliitis occurs in 10%.[9, 10] Women and men are equally affected by Crohn's disease; women are affected half as often as men in ulcerative colitis with spondylitis.

The etiology of both these inflammatory bowel diseases is unknown.[6] Specific infections with bacteria, overproduction of enzymes, vascular disorders, and hypersensitivity to foods are a few of the unproven theories suggested as possible causes. No specific genetic predisposition for these illnesses has been discovered, although there may be a familial predilection.[11, 12]

The pathogenesis of peripheral and axial arthritis may be different. Peripheral arthritis may evolve as a complication of active bowel disease. Hypothetically, endogenous or exogenous antigens may be absorbed through the bowel wall, initiating an immune response (antigen-antibody complexes) that would collect in peripheral joints and cause synovitis. This scheme has clinical correlations in the close association of activity of bowel disease and peripheral arthritis and the association of peripheral arthritis and other extraintestinal manifestations of disease, including erythema nodosum and iritis.[13] A similar immune complex mechanism may also explain the arthritis associated with another bowel abnormality, intestinal bypass arthritis.[14, 15] Polyarthritis, including peripheral arthritis, and spondylitis have been associated with ileal pouch surgery after proctocolectomy. The development of arthritis after bowel surgery suggests the role of exposure to bowel antigens in the development of joint disease.[16]

Axial arthritis of inflammatory bowel disease may be a hereditary accompaniment of the disease and not a manifestation of activity of bowel disease itself. Familial aggregation of spondylitis and sacroiliitis in relatives of inflammatory bowel disease patients has been reported.[17, 18] Both non–human leukocyte antigen (HLA)-related factors and HLA-B27 may play a role. Enlow and colleagues reported an incidence of HLA-B27 in 30% of patients with axial arthritis and inflammatory bowel disease.[19] In the same study, when relatives of the HLA-B27–negative spondylitis patients were studied, four were found to have axial arthritis without inflammatory bowel disease. No specific HLA haplotype was associated with axial arthropathy. This study suggests that both HLA-B27 and non-HLA genetic determinants predispose to axial arthropathy in patients with inflammatory bowel disease. In patients with enteropathic spondylitis, HLA-B27 is positive in 50% to 75% of patients.[20] Although no association is reported between the activity of bowel disease and axial arthritis, Mielants and Veys have described silent inflammatory gut disease identified by colonoscopy.[21] Patients with chronic spondyloarthropathy in association with peripheral arthritis have a higher frequency of inflammatory bowel disease than patients with axial skeletal disease alone. Crohn's disease in an early stage is the cause of bowel lesions in 26% of these patients with chronic axial and peripheral arthritis.[22]

Clinical History

The early symptoms of ulcerative colitis are frequent bowel movements with blood or mucous. Mild disease is associated with some abdominal pain and a few bowel movements per day. Severe disease is characterized by fatigue, weight loss, fever, and extracolonic involvement. Crohn's disease is frequently an indolent illness characterized by generalized fatigue, mild nonbloody diarrhea, anorexia, weight loss, and cramping lower abdominal pain. Patients may have symptoms for years before the diagnosis is made.

Articular involvement in these inflammatory bowel diseases is divided into two forms: peripheral and spondylitic. In ulcerative colitis, peripheral arthritis starts as an acute monarticular or oligoarticular arthritis affecting the knee, ankle, elbow, proximal phalangeal, wrist, or shoulder joints in patients with active bowel disease.[23] The attacks are painful and sometimes associated with effusions. They subside after 6 to 8 weeks and are nondeforming.[24] Joint symptoms follow the activity of the bowel disease. Patients with arthritis frequently demonstrate other extracolonic manifestations of ulcerative colitis, such as erythema nodosum, pyoderma gangrenosum, and uveitis, as well as extensive and chronic bowel disease with pseudopolyps and perianal disease.[25]

The peripheral joint involvement in Crohn's disease is similar in onset and distribution to those of ulcerative colitis.[26] However, the correlation of bowel inflammation and joint symptoms may continue while gastrointestinal complaints subside. The lack of association is probably secondary to the more scattered nature of Crohn's disease throughout the gut compared with the colonic involvement of ulcerative colitis and the difficulty in ascertaining complete remission of the illness.[18] Patients with colonic involvement with Crohn's disease may be at greater risk of developing peripheral arthritis.[27] On rare occasions, the peripheral arthritis may mimic the distribution of rheumatoid arthritis in the absence of rheumatoid factor.[28]

Axial skeleton involvement in ulcerative colitis and Crohn's disease is similar. Three groups of patients with inflammatory bowel disease and spondylitis have been described by Dekher-Saeys and colleagues.[29] In about one third of patients, spondylitis antedates bowel disease. This interval may be as long as 10 to 20 years.[10] Seventy percent were HLA-B27–positive, 68% had radiographic changes of spondylitis, and 25% had iritis. An association between sacroiliitis and iritis in ulcerative colitis was also reported by Wright and colleagues.[30] One fourth of patients developed bowel symptoms before the onset of spondylitis. Thirteen percent were HLA-B27–positive, 36% had radiographic changes of spondylitis, and none had iritis. These patients had severe disease of the gut. The remaining patients had simultaneous onset of gut and spine disease. The spondylitis of inflammatory bowel disease has a course totally independent of that of the bowel disease. The clinical and radiographic findings are similar to those of ankylosing spondylitis, including involvement of shoulders and hips, although some have suggested that it is a milder disease and has an increased proportion of women with spondylitis.[31] Patients with spondylitis complain of aching low back pain with stiffness that is maximal in the early morning, similar to ankylosing spondylitis.[32] As in uncomplicated ankylosing spondylitis, the development of cervical spine stiffness and pain is a manifestation of disease progression to generalized spondylitis. In a study of classic ankylosing spondylitis, only 7.6% of patients had an initial complaint of neck pain.[33] Neck pain occurs in patients after the disease has been present for a number of years. In a study lasting 15 years, 33% of enteropathic arthritis patients developed cervical spine disease.[31] Occasional patients with Crohn's disease have been reported with severe back pain, limitation of lumbar motion, and decreased chest expansion, even though they have no radiographic changes of spondylitis. In these patients, improvement in bowel disease was associated with improved musculoskeletal function.[29] This form of arthritis is a secondary phenomenon of the activity of Crohn's disease. Other musculoskeletal complications of inflammatory bowel disease include clubbing and periostitis, avascular necrosis of bone, septic arthritis of the hips, and granulomatous inflammation of synovium, bone, and muscle.[34, 35]

Physical Examination

The general physical examination concentrates on the abdomen and gastrointestinal tract, including inspection of the oropharynx, perineum, and rectum. Examination for extraintestinal disease, such as aphthous ulcers, iritis, erythema nodosum, and pyoderma gangrenosum, is indicated. The musculoskeletal examination must include both peripheral joints and axial skeleton. Patients with spondyloarthropathy may have decreased motion of the spine in all planes and percussion tenderness over the sacroiliac joints. In rare circumstances, chest expansion is diminished. Patients with more extensive disease have limitation of motion of the cervical spine. Straightening is the main postural abnormality.[31] Occiput-to-wall measurements document the immobility of the entire axial skeleton, including the cervical spine. In a small number of patients, peripheral and axial skeleton disease may coexist.

Laboratory Data

Usual laboratory test results, such as decreased hematocrit level, increased white blood cell (WBC) count, increased platelet count, hypoalbuminemia, and hypokalemia, are abnormal but are nonspecific. The inflammatory findings of increased WBC count with poor mucin clot in the synovial fluid is also nondiagnostic. Rheumatoid factor and antinuclear antibodies are absent. No specific HLA antigen has been associated with ulcerative colitis, Crohn's disease, or peripheral joint disease. Approximately 50% of patients with symptomatic spondylitis and inflammatory bowel disease are HLA-B27–positive.[36]

Radiographic Evaluation

Radiographs of peripheral joints demonstrate soft tissue swelling and occasionally joint effusions.[25, 37, 38] Findings of joint destruction, joint space narrowing, erosions, and periosteal proliferation are rare.[39] The radiographic changes of spondylitis in inflammatory bowel disease are indistinguishable from those with classic ankylosing spondylitis.[40] They include squaring of vertebral bodies, erosions, widening and fusion of the sacroiliac joints, symmetrical involvement of sacroiliac joints, and marginal syndesmophytes involving the lumbar, thoracic, or cervical spine[31] (Fig. 11–12). No correlation between colonic disease and spondylitis could be ascertained in a study of patients with Crohn's disease.[41] Asymptomatic radiographic sacroiliitis is demonstrated in up to 15% of patients with inflammatory bowel disease. In contrast to classic ankylosing spondylitis, these patients have no association with HLA-B27, and women and men have equal involvement.[42] Scintigraphic evaluation of sacroiliac joints in inflammatory bowel disease patients has detected increased uptake of radiotracer in 52%.[43] The clinical significance of these findings remains to be determined.

The clinical diagnosis of inflammatory bowel disease is suspected in an individual with diarrhea, rectal bleeding, abdominal cramps, abdominal pain, perianal fistula or abscess, and an abdominal mass along with erythema nodosum, iritis, or arthritis. Radiographic evaluation of ulcerative colitis reveals mucosa ulceration, edema, and varying lengths of bowel.

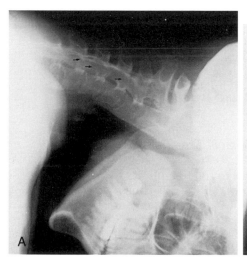
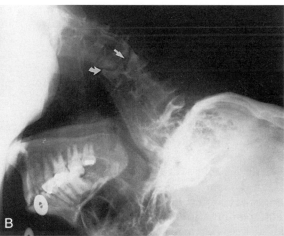

Figure 11–12. Crohn's disease. A 30-year-old woman with a 14-year history of Crohn's disease had a 9-year history of spine pain and stiffness. The patient had a chest expansion of 2 cm and no movement of the lumbar spine with flexion. Fusion of sacroiliac joints and the apophyseal joint were prominent. Cervical spine disease resulted in neck pain and gradual neck flexion, with her chin coming to rest on her chest wall. She was to undergo vertebral osteotomy when she sustained a spontaneous fracture of the cervical spine without any neurologic deficits. She was placed in a halo cast and healed in a more functional position. *A*, 7/3/90—Lateral view of the cervical spine reveals fusion of all facet joints *(arrows)* and space between the mandible and chest wall. *B*, 2/26/91—Lateral view of the cervical spine shows fracture through C4–C5 interspace *(straight arrow)* and anterior subluxation *(curved arrow)*.

Crohn's disease causes deep ulcerations with strictures, fistulization, loop separation, and mass effect in a discontinuous pattern that may involve the small intestine as well as the colon.

Differential Diagnosis

A specific diagnosis of ulcerative colitis or Crohn's disease is made from the histologic examination of biopsy material from the gut. The inflammatory abnormalities of ulcerative colitis are limited to the superficial layers of the gut, mucosa, and submucosa. The most characteristic findings in ulcerative colitis are atrophy of mucosal glands and inflammatory cells in the crypts of the colon, causing crypt abscesses with no skip areas. Crohn's disease is characterized by a transluminal granulomatous inflammation. Whereas biopsy material yields supportive evidence for one or the other illness, the final differentiation rests heavily on the history, clinical course, and barium contrast studies of the gut. The differential diagnosis for the bowel disease includes infectious colitis, diverticulitis, pseudomembranous colitis, and ischemic colitis. Infectious agents associated with colitis include *Shigella, Salmonella, Campylobacter fetus, Yersinia enterocolitica,* cytomegalovirus, amebiasis, and histoplasmosis.

Culture of an early-morning stool specimen is an important part of the evaluation of a patient with chronic diarrhea. Special stains of biopsy material may discover an unsuspected organism. Diverticulitis causes localized pain, fever, and diarrhea. Radiographic studies help identify the localized nature of the disorder caused by an infection of a colonic diverticulum. Patients who receive oral or parenteral antibiotics may develop, up to 4 weeks later, a nonbloody, watery diarrhea that on endoscopic examination is associated with a yellowish-white pseudomembrane on the colonic surfaces. Stool cultures that grow *Clostridium difficile* or reveal *C. difficile* toxin virtually ensure the diagnosis of pseudomembranous colitis. The abrupt onset of abdominal cramps with bleeding in a patient 60 years of age or older with preexisting atherosclerotic cardiovascular disease suggests an ischemic insult to the bowel. An abdominal flat plate film may demonstrate scalloping ("thumb printing") of the wall. This finding is consistent with ischemic colitis. Of the various entities included in the preceding differential diagnosis of inflammatory bowel disease, bacterial infection of the gut is the only entity associated with spondyloarthropathy (reactive arthritis).[44] See the preceding section on Reiter's syndrome.

The diagnosis of enteropathic arthritis is not difficult to make in the patient with ulcerative colitis or Crohn's disease with nondeforming peripheral arthritis. As most patients develop peripheral arthritis after the onset of gastrointestinal symptoms, the possibilities for the cause of their arthritis are limited. The real difficulty arises in the patient with back symptoms before the onset of bowel disease; their differential diagnosis includes the other spondyloarthropathies, including ankylosing spondylitis and Reiter's syndrome. The lower frequency of HLA-B27 may help differentiate enteropathic arthritis from ankylosing spondylitis. The absence of conjunctivitis, urethritis, and periostitis, particularly in the heels, may help to distinguish it from Reiter's syndrome.

The patient with enteropathic spondyloarthropathy commonly presents with back pain in the absence of gastrointestinal symptoms. The finding of morning stiffness should raise the suspicion of a spondyloarthropathy. The factors that help make the diagnosis of enteropathic spondyloarthropathy are the pattern of peripheral arthritis if present (upper extremity disease uncommon in ankylosing spondylitis and Reiter's syndrome; bilateral ankle arthritis uncommon in psoriatic disease), erythema nodosum, and iritis.

Patients who have undergone intestinal bypass surgery for morbid obesity may develop polyarthritis as a complication of this procedure. Most patients are women who develop a polyarthritis most commonly after jejunocolostomy probably secondary to a systemic reaction to bacterial products.[15, 45] The arthritis affects the knees, hands, feet, wrists, elbows, and hips. Involvement of the axial skeleton, particularly the sacroiliac joints, has been only rarely reported.[46] Radiographs of these patients reveal erosions, sclerosis, and articular space narrowing at the sacroiliac joint and syndesmophytes of the spine. HLA-B27 antigen may be detected in patients with axial joint involvement. Nonsteroidal anti-inflammatory drugs (NSAIDs) may be somewhat helpful in controlling joint pain. Patients with severe symptoms unresponsive to drugs may obtain improvement with revision of the bypass.[47]

Treatment

Treatment for peripheral arthritis must be directed toward control of the underlying bowel disease. Therapy might include sulfasalazine (Azulfidine, 4 to 6 gm/day), metronidazole, corticosteroid enemas, oral corticosteroids, and colectomy for the severe patient with ulcerative colitis.[48–50] A variety of therapies has been developed for the treatment of Crohn's disease. There are newer forms of sulfasalazine that contain only the active moiety, 5-aminosalicylic acid such as olsalazine and mesalamine, which have fewer side effects and may be given orally or as a suppository.[51] These drugs may be used for the treatment of mild, initial attacks or for prophylaxis of recurrent attacks of ulcerative colitis.[52, 53] In active, severe disease, the combination of sulfasalazine and corticosteroids is effective in 90% of patients.[54] Corticosteroids are effective when given orally or rectally.[55] Occasionally immunosuppressive drugs in the form of azathioprine or mercaptopurine are needed to control severe Crohn's disease. Mercaptopurine is given in doses of 50 mg/day. Clinical effect may take months to appear as a result of the slow-acting nature of the drug.[56, 57] Colectomized patients with ulcerative colitis do not have recurrences of peripheral joint disease.[23] Surgery is not nearly as effective in Crohn's disease because the disease may have more extensive distribution through the gastrointestinal tract.

The therapeutic program for peripheral joint disease may also include NSAIDs, intra-articular injections of corticosteroids, and physical therapy. There is no evidence of increased gastrointestinal adverse effects with NSAIDs in these patients with inflammatory bowel disease. Initially, lower therapeutic doses of the NSAIDs may be tried to test drug tolerability. Increased dosage can be used if the patient tolerates the medicine but experiences inadequate relief of symptoms. If a patient has a good response to an NSAID but develops gastrointestinal symptoms, the addition of medications to control those symptoms may be added to the patient's therapeutic program. In rare circumstances, NSAIDs have been implicated as factors causing an exacerbation of inflammatory bowel disease.[58, 59]

Therapy for enteropathic spondylitis is similar to that for classic ankylosing spondylitis. This program includes patient education, NSAIDs, and physical therapy. Control of bowel disease does not necessarily correlate with improvement in axial skeleton symptoms. In ulcerative colitis, colectomy should not be done with the expectation of resolution of spondylitic symptoms.

Prognosis

The ultimate course and outcome of these patients depend on the severity of their bowel disease. Patients with severe ulcerative colitis have a mortality rate of 10% to 20% over 5 years. Patients with a severe initial attack, continuous clinical activity, involvement of the entire colon, and disease for 10 years or longer have a higher risk of developing cancer of the colon.[60] These patients may require colectomy. Although Crohn's disease is associated with frequent recurrences, the overall mortality rate of 5% for the first 5 years of disease is much less than in ulcerative colitis.[61]

Patients with peripheral enteropathic arthritis have nondeforming disease of short duration. These patients experience little disability from the arthritis and are able to work. The disability associated with enteropathic spondylitis is similar to that of ankylosing spondylitis in severely affected patients. The association of hip disease and spondylitis results in a marked decrease in mobility. Patients with spinal rigidity are at risk for fracture. These patients should not perform heavy labor associated with lifting.

References

ENTEROPATHIC ARTHRITIS

1. Bargen JA: Complications and sequelae of chronic ulcerative colitis. Ann Intern Med 3:335, 1929.
2. Crohn BB, Ginzburg L, Oppenheimer GD: Regional ileitis: a pathologic and clinical entity. JAMA 99:1323, 1932.
3. Van Patter WN, Bargen JA, Dockerty MB, et al.: Regional enteritis. Gastroenterology 26:347, 1954.
4. Steinberg VL, Storey G: Ankylosing spondylitis and chronic inflammatory lesions of the intestines. Br Med J 2:1157, 1957.
5. Monk M, Mendeloff AI, Siegel CI, Lilienfeld A: An epidemiological study of ulcerative colitis and regional enteritis among adults in Baltimore: hospital incidence and prevalence, 1960 to 1963. Gastroenterology 53:198, 1967.
6. Kirsner JB, Shorter RG: Recent developments in nonspecific inflammatory bowel disease. N Engl J Med 306:837, 1982.
7. Greenstein AJ, Janowitz HD, Sachar DB: The extraintestinal complications of Crohn's disease and ulcerative colitis: a study of 700 patients. Medicine 55:401, 1976.
8. Haslock F, Wright V: The musculoskeletal complications of Crohn's disease. Medicine 52:217, 1973.
9. Dekher-Saeys BJ, Meuwissen SGM, van den Berg-Loonen EM, et al.: Prevalence of peripheral arthritis, sacroiliitis and ankylosing spondylitis in patients suffering from inflammatory bowel disease. Ann Rheum Dis 37:33, 1978.
10. Acheson ED: An association between ulcerative colitis, regional enteritis and ankylosing spondylitis. Q J Med 29:489, 1960.
11. Almy TP, Sherlock P: Genetic aspects of ulcerative colitis and regional enteritis. Gastroenterology 51:757, 1966.
12. Paulley JW: Ulcerative colitis: a study of 173 cases. Gastroenterology 16:566, 1950.

13. Hochberg MC, Feinstein RS, Moser RL, Ryan MJ: Colitic arthritis. Johns Hopkins Med J 151:173, 1982.

14. Stein HB, Schlappner OLA, Boyko W, et al.: The intestinal bypass arthritis-dermatitis syndrome. Arthritis Rheum 24:684, 1981.

15. Wands JR, Lamont JT, Mann E, Isselbacher KJ: Arthritis associated with intestinal-bypass procedure for morbid obesity: complement activation and characterization of circulating cryoproteins. N Engl J Med 294:121, 1976.

16. Axon JMC, Hawley PR, Huskisson EC: Ileal pouch arthritis. Br J Rheumatol 32:586, 1993.

17. Macrae I, Wright V: A family study of ulcerative colitis. Ann Rheum Dis 32:16, 1973.

18. Haslock I: Arthritis and Crohn's disease: a family study. Ann Rheum Dis 32:479, 1973.

19. Enlow RW, Bias WB, Arnett FC: The spondylitis of inflammatory bowel disease: evidence for a non–HLA-linked axial arthropathy. Arthritis Rheum 23:1359, 1980.

20. Weiner SR, Clarke J, Taggart NA, et al.: Rheumatic manifestations of bowel disease. Semin Arthritis Rheum 20:353, 1991.

21. Mielants H, Veys EM: The gut in the spondyloarthropathies. J Rheumatol 17:7, 1990.

22. Leirisalo-Repo M, Turunen U, Stenman S, et al.: High frequency of silent inflammatory bowel disease in spondyloarthropathy. Arthritis Rheum 37:23, 1994.

23. Wright V, Watkinson G: The arthritis of ulcerative colitis. Br Med J 2:670, 1965.

24. Palumbo PJ, Ward LE, Sauer WG, Scudamore HH: Musculoskeletal manifestations of inflammatory bowel disease: ulcerative and granulomatous colitis and ulcerative proctitis. Mayo Clin Proc 48:411, 1973.

25. McEwen C, Lingg C, Kirsner JB, Spencer JA: Arthritis accompanying ulcerative colitis. Am J Med 33:923, 1962.

26. Ansell BM, Wigley RAD: Arthritic manifestations in regional enteritis. Ann Rheum Dis 23:64, 1964.

27. Norton KI, Eichenfield AH, Rosh JR, et al.: Atypical arthropathy associated with Crohn's disease. Am J Gastroenterol 88:948, 1993.

28. Cornes JS, Stecher M: Primary Crohn's disease of the colon and rectum. Gut 2:189, 1961.

29. Dekher-Saeys BJ, Meuwissen SGM, van den Berg-Loonen EM, et al.: Clinical characteristics and results of histocompatibility typing (HLA-B27) in 50 patients with both ankylosing spondylitis and inflammatory bowel disease. Ann Rheum Dis 37:36, 1978.

30. Wright R, Lumsden K, Luntz MH, et al.: Abnormalities of the sacro-iliac joints and uveitis in ulcerative colitis. Q J Med 134:229, 1965.

31. McEwen C, DiTata D, Lingg C, et al.: Ankylosing spondylitis and spondylitis accompanying ulcerative colitis, regional enteritis, psoriasis and Reiter's disease: a comparative study. Arthritis Rheum 14:291, 1971.

32. Bowen GE, Kirsner JB: The arthritis of ulcerative colitis and regional enteritis ("intestinal arthritis"). Med Clin North Am 49:17, 1965.

33. Gran JT, Ostensen M, Husby G: A clinical comparison between males and females with ankylosing spondylitis. J Rheumatol 12:126, 1985.

34. Neale G, Kelsall AR, Doyle FH: Crohn's disease and diffuse symmetrical periostitis. Gut 9:383, 1968.

35. London D, Fitton JM: Acute septic arthritis complicating Crohn's disease. Br J Surg 57:536, 1970.

36. Morris RI, Metzger AL, Bluestone R, Terasaki PI: HLA-w27—a useful discriminator in the arthropathies of inflammatory bowel disease. N Engl J Med 290:1117, 1974.

37. Clark RL, Muhletaler CA, Margulies SI: Colitic arthritis: clinical and radiographic manifestations. Radiology 101:585, 1971.

38. Bywaters EGL, Ansell BM: Arthritis associated with ulcerative colitis: a clinical and pathological study. Ann Rheum Dis 17:169, 1958.

39. Frayha R, Stevens MB, Bayless TM: Destructive monoarthritis and granulomatous synovitis as the presenting manifestations of Crohn's disease. Johns Hopkins Med J 137:151, 1975.

40. Zvaifler NJ, Martel W: Spondylitis in chronic ulcerative colitis. Arthritis Rheum 3:76, 1960.

41. Mueller CE, Seeger JF, Martel W: Ankylosing spondylitis and regional enteritis. Radiology 112:579, 1974.

42. Hyla JF, Franck WA, Davis JS: Lack of association of HLA-B27 with radiographic sacroiliitis in inflammatory bowel disease. J Rheumatol 3:196, 1976.

43. Davis P, Thomson ABR, Lentle B: Quantitative sacroiliac scintigraphy in patients with Crohn's disease. Arthritis Rheum 21:234, 1978.

44. Olhagen B: Postinfective or reactive arthritis. Scand J Rheumatol 9:193, 1980.

45. Shagrin JW, Frame B, Duncan H: Polyarthritis in obese patients with intestinal bypass. Ann Intern Med 75:377, 1971.

46. Rose E, Espinoza LR, Osterland CK: Intestinal bypass arthritis: association with circulating immune complexes. J Rheumatol 4:129, 1977.

47. Leff RD, Aldo-Benson MA, Madura JA: The effect of revision of the intestinal bypass on post-intestinal bypass arthritis. Arthritis Rheum 26:678, 1983.

48. Peppercorn MA: Sulfasalazine: pharmacology, clinical use, toxicity, and related new-drug development. Ann Intern Med 101:377, 1984.

49. Present DW, Korelitz BI, Wise HN, et al.: Treatment of Crohn's disease with 6-mercaptopurine: a long-term randomized double-blind study. N Engl J Med 302:981, 1980.

50. Summers RW, Switz DM, Session JT, et al.: National Cooperative Crohn's disease study: results of drug treatment. Gastroenterology 77:847, 1979.

51. Jarnerot G: Newer 5-aminosalicylic acid-based drugs in chronic inflammatory bowel disease. Drugs 37:76, 1989.

52. Rao SS, Dundas SA, Hildsworth CD, et al.: Olsalazine or sulfasalazine in first attacks of ulcerative colitis: a double-blind study. Gut 30:675, 1989.

53. Ireland A, Mason CH, Jewell DP: Controlled trial comparing olsalazine and sulfasalazine for the maintenance treatment of ulcerative colitis. Gut 29:835, 1988.

54. Rijk MC, Hogezand RA, van Lier HJ, et al.: Sulphasalazine and prednisone compared with sulfasalazine for treating active Crohn's disease: a double-blind, randomized multicenter trial. Ann Intern Med 114:445, 1991.

55. Linn FV, Peppercorn MA: Drug therapy for inflammatory bowel disease: part I. Am J Surg 164:85, 1992.

56. Marsh JW, Vehe KL, White HM: Immunosuppressants. Gastroenterol Clin North Am 21:679, 1992.

57. Linn FV, Peppercorn MA: Drug therapy for inflammatory bowel disease: part II. Am J Surg 164:178, 1992.

58. Kaufmann HJ, Taubin HL: Nonsteroidal anti-inflammatory drugs activate quiescent inflammatory bowel disease. Ann Intern Med 107:513, 1988.

59. Gran JT, Husby G: Ankylosing spondylitis: current drug treatment. Drugs 44:585, 1992.

60. Farmer RG, Hawk WA, Turnbull RB Jr: Carcinoma associated with mucosal ulcerative colitis, and with

transmural colitis and enteritis (Crohn's disease). Cancer 28:289, 1971.

61. Lock MR, Farmer RG, Fazio VW, et al.: Recurrence and reoperation for Crohn's disease: the role of disease in prognosis. N Engl J Med 304:1586, 1981.

DIFFUSE IDIOPATHIC SKELETAL HYPEROSTOSIS

Capsule Summary

Frequency of neck pain—common

Location of neck pain—cervical spine

Quality of neck pain—ache

Symptoms and signs—dysphagia, decreased neck motion

Laboratory and x-ray tests—flowing calcification of the anterolateral aspect of four contiguous vertebral bodies on plain roentgenogram

Treatment—nonsteroidal anti-inflammatory drugs, range-of-motion exercises

Prevalence and Pathogenesis

Diffuse idiopathic skeletal hyperostosis (DISH) is a disease characterized clinically by spinal stiffness and pain and radiographically by exuberant calcification of spinal and extraspinal structures. Despite impressive radiographic abnormalities, patients rarely have significant loss of function or disability from the illness except for the rare individual who develops difficulty swallowing (dysphagia) secondary to cervical spine involvement. This disease has been known by many different names, including spondylitis ossificans ligamentosa, vertebral osteophytosis, ankylosing hyperostosis of Forestier and Rotes-Querol, and Forestier's disease. DISH was suggested in 1975 by Resnick and Niwayama as a more appropriate name in light of the diffuse bone growth that develops in both spinal and extraspinal locations.[1]

DISH is a common entity found in 6% to 28% of autopsy populations.[2–4] The usual patient is a man from the ages of 48 to 85 years.[5] The ratio of men to women is 2:1.[6] The prevalence rate increases in both sexes with weight and age.[7, 8] The disease occurs most commonly in whites and rarely in blacks. The disease has been described in populations from all the continents, except Antarctica.

The etiology of DISH is unknown. In one study, occupational stress or spinal trauma was reported in 57% of patients with this condition.[1] The patients usually had occupations that included construction, ranching, and roofing and required a moderate degree of physical activity. Other people in the same study had no history of occupational or accidental trauma. Endocrinologic abnormalities associated with bony hyperostosis, acromegaly, and hypoparathyroidism have been suggested as causes of DISH. No abnormalities in growth hormone (acromegaly) or parathormone (hypoparathyroidism) have been found.[5] Diabetes mellitus occurs in 30% of patients with the disease; however, this frequency of diabetes mellitus may be related to the age of the population rather than being a true association of the two disorders.[1] Impaired glucose tolerance occurs in DISH patients to a greater degree than in control subjects.[9] The level of glucose intolerance does not correlate with the extent of bony overgrowth. In addition, elevated concentrations of insulin have been measured in DISH patients compared with control subjects.[10] Insulin may be acting as a growth-like factor for new bone formation. The systemic exposure from insulin would be compatible with distribution of DISH lesions throughout the skeleton. Elevated levels of endogenous retinoic acids are present in DISH patients compared with control subjects.[11] The elevation in 13-*cis* and all *trans*retinoic acid and associated bone growth may be similar to the increased concentration of retinoids found in patients with hyperostosis who use these agents in the treatment of psoriasis and acne.

A specific genetic predisposition to the development of the problem has not been identified. Human leukocyte antigen (HLA)-B27–positivity was found in 34% of DISH patients in one study,[12] but a subsequent study found no significant association with HLA antigens.[13] Until further data are obtained to the contrary, DISH should not be classified with the HLA-B27–positive, seronegative spondyloarthropathies (ankylosing spondylitis and Reiter's syndrome).

Clinical History

The principal musculoskeletal complaint in 80% of patients is spinal stiffness.[1] The duration of spinal stiffness before diagnosis may be 10 to 20 years, with onset when the patient is 40 to 50 years of age. Morning stiffness dissipates within an hour, only to recur in the late evening.[6] Symptoms may increase with inclement weather. Immobility increases symptoms as well. Back pain in the thoracolumbar spine occurs in 57% of patients as their initial complaint.[1] Back pain is usually mild, intermittent, and rarely radiating. A minority of patients have cervical spine pain as the initial complaint. Neck pain is a complaint of more than 50% of patients with DISH during the course of the illness.[14] Subsequently, cervical stiffness may become the prominent symptom.[15] Dysphagia is seen in 17% to 28% of patients.[5] Dysphagia may be an initial complaint of patients with cervical anterior osteophytes.[16] Dysphagia occurs secondary to constriction of the esophagus by anteriorly located cervical osteophytes. Osteophytes located adjacent to the location of esophageal fixation near the cricoid cartilage (C5–C6) are those most closely associated with esophageal compression and dysphagia.[17] Patients with DISH and anterior osteophytes may also be at risk for aspiration and pneumonia.[18] Intubation may be difficult in patients with DISH of the cervical spine.[19]

Extraspinal manifestations of DISH occur in 37% of patients. In 20%, extraspinal pain was the initial or predominant complaint. The most common extraspinal skeletal areas that are symptomatic secondary to an enthesopathy include the shoulders, knees, elbows, and heels.

Physical Examination

Physical examination usually reveals little limitation of motion in the cervical and lumbar spine.[20] Occasionally a slight decrease in cervical lordosis may be present.[1] A minority of patients are tender to percussion over the cervical spine. On palpation of the neck, bilateral fullness may be appreciated lateral to the trachea.[21] A rare patient may develop neurologic signs from spinal cord compression secondary to DISH.[22] Patients with extraspinal disease may have diminished range of motion and pain on palpation over affected areas. Areas that may show abnormalities include the hips, subtalar joints, shoulders, knees, elbows, heels, and ankle joints.

Laboratory Data

Laboratory parameters are essentially normal in patients with DISH.[13] Occasionally a mildly elevated erythrocyte sedimentation rate (ESR) is noted. Because patients who develop the disease are elderly, laboratory abnormalities may be secondary to another illness affecting the patient. Therefore, elevations of fasting and 2-hour postprandial glucose are probably secondary to impending diabetes rather than to DISH.

Pathologic evaluation of the axial skeleton is not necessary for diagnosis of DISH. However, pathologic findings do correlate with the radiographic characteristics of DISH. These findings include fibrous tissue separating anterior calcification and the annulus fibrosus of the intervertebral disc, normal disc height, and close proximity of anterior calcifications without fusion in most circumstances.[3]

The location for the initiation of the process that results in DISH is the enthesis, the attachment of tendon to bone. The earliest changes are connective tissue proliferation followed by fibrocartilaginous metaplasia. Chondrocytes develop, producing proteoglycans, with subsequent ossification. Preferential ossification occurs close to an enthesis.[8] The source of pain in patients with DISH is not clear. Pain may result from the enthesopathy or secondary to the abnormal biomechanical stresses placed across a skeletal structure. Of the two, the latter is more likely as many DISH lesions are asymptomatic.

Radiographic Evaluation

The diagnosis of DISH is a radiographic one. It is made, not uncommonly, in asymptomatic people who happen to have characteristic bony changes in the thoracic spine on a chest radiograph. The three criteria for spinal involvement include flowing calcification along the anterolateral aspect of four contiguous vertebral bodies; preservation of intervertebral disc height; and absence of apophyseal joint bony ankylosis and sacroiliac joint sclerosis, erosion, or fusion.[2] These criteria help differentiate DISH from spondylosis deformans, intervertebral disc degeneration, and ankylosing spondylitis. The fact that the posterior spinal elements are not affected permits almost normal range of motion on physical examination. Radiographic abnormalities are seen most frequently in the thoracic and lumbar spine.[1] A majority of patients also develop cervical spine lesions.

In the cervical spine, the lower vertebrae (C4–C7) are most commonly affected[23] (Fig. 11–13). Calcification occurs initially along the anterior aspect of the vertebral body. Bony excrescences are in an anterosuperior position near the disc margin and extend upward across the intervertebral disc space (Fig. 11–14). A flowing pattern, like candle wax, may

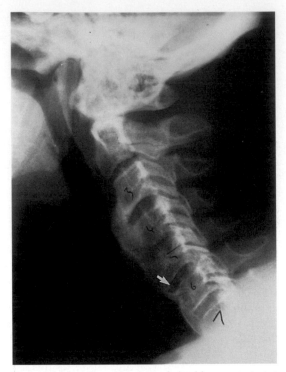

Figure 11–13. Diffuse idiopathic skeletal hyperostosis. Lateral view of the cervical spine reveals "flowing" anterior ligament calcification involving C3–C7. Notice radiolucent extension at the level of the intervertebral disc *(arrow)*.

result with interruption of the column with radiolucent disc extensions at the intervertebral discs. An ossicle, a small triangular bony fragment, may form anterior to the intervertebral disc. The excrescences are thick in comparison with syndesmophytes. Anterior calcifications may reach the size to impinge on anterior soft tissue structures of the throat, including the esophagus (Fig. 11–15). A thin radiolucent line that separates the vertebral body proper and the anterior calcification occurs less commonly in the cervical spine than the thoracic or lumbar spine. In contrast to other locations in the axial skeleton, posterior vertebral abnormalities, including osteophytes of the posterior vertebral bodies, and ligament calcification occur in the cervical spine.[24] Hyperostosis may also affect midline structures, including the atlantoaxial joint and the base of the occiput.[17] The stylohyoid ligament may become ossified in patients with DISH. These patients with Eagle's syndrome may complain of throat pain, dysphagia, otalgia, and foreign body sensation.[25]

Extraspinal radiographic changes include bony proliferation or "whiskering," ligamentous calcification, and para-articular osteophytes.[6] Common locations for these changes

are in the pelvis, heels, feet, patellae, elbows, shoulders, and wrists.

Differential Diagnosis

The diagnosis of DISH is based on the presence of characteristic radiographic changes and an absence of clinical abnormalities suggestive of another illness. Resnick and Niwayama have proposed the following criteria for the diagnosis of DISH:[1]

1. Flowing calcification and ossification along the anterolateral aspect of four contiguous vertebral bodies with or without associated localized pointed excrescences at the intervening vertebral body–intervertebral disc junctions.

2. Relative preservation of intervertebral disc height in the involved vertebral segment and the absence of radiographic evidence of degenerative disc disease.

3. Absence of apophyseal joint bony ankylosis and sacroiliac joint erosion, sclerosis, or intra-articular osseous fusion.

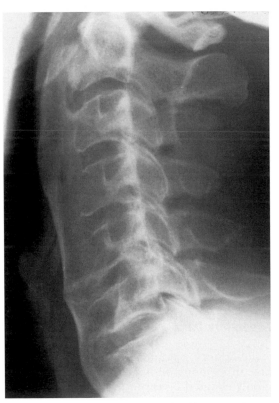

Figure 11–14. Diffuse idiopathic skeletal hyperostosis. Lateral view of the cervical spine reveals "flowing" anterior calcification extending from C2 to C7. (Courtesy of Anne Brower, M.D.)

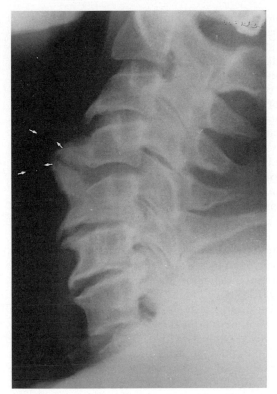

Figure 11–15. Diffuse idiopathic skeletal hyperostosis. A 65-year-old woman with dysphagia. Lateral view of the cervical spine shows large anterior bony projection at the C4–C5 level. The soft tissues and hollow viscus anterior to this bony projection are constricted (arrows). (Courtesy of Anne Brower, M.D.)

There are a number of causes of bony outgrowths of the spine, including spondyloarthropathies, acromegaly, hypoparathyroidism, fluorosis, ochronosis, neuropathic arthropathy, and trauma. Specific abnormalities associated with each of these entities, which are reviewed in other sections of this chapter, help differentiate these diseases from DISH.

Spondyloarthropathies are frequently associated with cervical spine disease. The syndesmophytes associated with ankylosing spondylitis are thin and vertically oriented. These patients with ankylosing spondylitis are young and have prolonged morning stiffness that improves with activity during the day. The simultaneous occurrence of DISH with other diseases does occur. For example, a patient with a diagnosis of DISH and ankylosing spondylitis has been reported.[26] Patients may have DISH of the cervical spine and spondylitis of the lumbosacral spine. Currently, eight patients have been reported in the medical literature with coexistent DISH and ankylosing spondylitis. Only four of these patients are HLA-B27–positive.[27]

Acromegaly is associated with posterior scalloping of the vertebral body and increased intervertebral disc space height in the thoracic and lumbar spine. In the cervical spine, elongation and widening of the vertebral bodies are observed. These alterations of vertebral bodies and disc spaces are similar to those associated with spondylosis deformans. Osteophytes may bridge the intervertebral disc space. Patients with DISH do not have soft tissue hypertrophy or joint space enlargement.[28] Patients with hypoparathyroidism develop osteophytes with preservation of intervertebral disc spaces. Hypoparathyroidism is associated with hypocalcemia and tetany, which are not associated with DISH. Fluorosis causes generalized bone sclerosis to a greater extent than with DISH.[29] Ochronotic involvement of the vertebral column is manifested by disc height loss and calcifications.[30] Neuropathic arthropathy causes disorganization and destruction of bone in combination with bone formation. Trauma causes callus formation in localized areas of the spine.

Sternocostoclavicular Hyperostosis (SCCH). SCCH is one of the illnesses associated with the SAPHO syndromes (*s*ynovitis, *a*cne, *p*ustules, *h*yperostosis, *o*steitis). SCCH is a rare syndrome, is found most commonly in Japan, and is characterized by hyperostosis and soft tissue ossification between the clavicle and anterior part of the upper ribs.[31] Men who are 30 to 50 years of age are at greatest risk for this illness. Swelling, tenderness, erythema, and pain are prominent over the anterior chest wall. Patients with cervical spine disease have pain in the neck with radiation to the shoulders.[32] Physical examination of the cervical spine reveals varying degrees of limited motion, depending on the extent of spine involvement. Swelling over the clavicles or sternum may be prominent. Pustulosis palmaris et plantaris, a cutaneous disorder affecting palms and soles, is associated with SCCH in up to 50% of patients.[33] Laboratory abnormalities are nonspecific, compatible with an inflammatory state. The ESR remains increased during the course of the illness. The radiographic abnormalities associated with SCCH may occur without disease in other portions of the axial skeleton. In contrast to the frequent occurrences of clinical symptoms, the radiologic signs of disease progression take several years to become detectable. SCCH has characteristics that resemble ankylosing spondylitis, DISH, and psoriatic spondylitis. New bone formation in the cervical spine is occasionally exuberant, predominating in the anterior aspect of the vertebral bodies and intervertebral discs and leading to obliteration of the anterior vertebral surface[34] (Fig. 11–16). Other roentgenographic findings of the cervical spine include ossification of the anterior and posterior longitudinal ligaments, apophyseal joint ankylosis, atlantoaxial subluxation, endplate erosions, and sclerosis of vertebral bodies.[35–37] In addition, hyperostosis of the sternum, manubriosternal junction, clavicle, or upper ribs is encountered. Bone scintigraphy is helpful in documenting increased activity in joints that may be difficult to visualize with plain roentgenograms.[38] Arthro-osteitis is the term used to describe this illness if spinal and extraspinal abnormalities are present in the absence of anterior chest involvement.[34] The use of computerized tomography (CT) to identify retrosternal proliferation of soft tissue is valuable because the finding helps differentiate SCCH from other benign hyperostotic processes.[39] Alteration in intervertebral discs and vertebral end plates may resemble infec-

tious processes. Biopsy of these discal lesions usually reveals nonspecific chronic inflammation with scar formation.[39] Treatment for the disease includes nonsteroidal anti-inflammatory drugs (NSAIDs) and antibiotics.[37] The course of the disease is protracted with periods of remissions and exacerbations. The disease starts as an enthesopathy that ends decades later with total ankylosis of affected structures.

Ossification of the Posterior Longitudinal Ligament (OPLL). OPLL is a disease of unknown etiology that results in the calcification of the posterior longitudinal ligament, particularly in the cervical spine. Terayama and colleagues are credited with naming the disease.[40] The disease is found most frequently in Japanese.[41] The incidence of OPLL in the Japanese has been reported to be 1% to 2% of the population with cervical spine symptoms.[42, 43] OPLL may affect people of other Asian or non-Asian nationalities.[44, 45] OPLL occurs in a male-to-female ratio of 2:1.[46]

Most patients with the disease are from 50 to 60 years of age. The onset of disease is insidious. Twenty percent of patients may have an acute onset associated with minor trauma caused by slipping or a fall.[42] Ono and colleagues divided 166 symptomatic OPLL patients with musculoskeletal and neurologic abnormalities into three groups: myelopathy with motor and sensory signs in the lower extremities (56%); segmental signs with motor and sensory signs in the upper extremities (16%); and cervicobranchialgia manifested by pain in the neck, shoulder, and arm (28%).[47] A combination of sensory and motor signs in the upper extremity may be so severe as to affect daily living habits. Gait disturbances occur in 25% and inability to ambulate occurs in 10%.[42] Myelopathic findings occurred when the thickness of the calcification exceeded 30% to 60% of the sagittal diameter of the cervical spinal canal. This may also be affected by the rapidity of compression.[48] Acute quadriparesis has been reported in OPLL patients.[49] Physical examination may reveal decreased neck motion and stiffness along with neurologic signs corresponding to areas of nerve compression. Laboratory findings include an elevated ESR but are nonspecific. Pathologic findings include cortical bone with Haversian canals and immature bone marrow. Proposed mechanisms of ligamentous calcification have included proliferation of cartilage cells in the ligament, mucoid degeneration of the ligament, and coalescence of hydroxyapatite crystals to form calcifying masses.[46] Ossification starts on the dural side of the ligament and

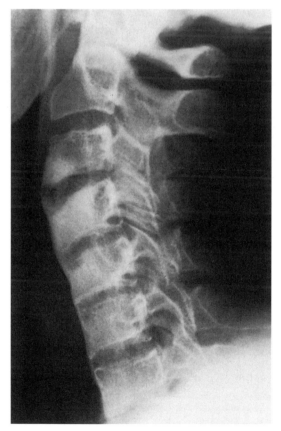

Figure 11–16. Sternocostoclavicular hyperostosis. Observe hyperostotic changes involving the anterior portion of the third and seventh cervical vertebral bodies and the development of syndesmophytes. (Courtesy of C. Resnick, M.D., Baltimore, Maryland.)

progresses in a posteroanterior direction to involve the deep layers of the ligament. In the final stage, the ligament becomes fused with the vertebral body and dura. OPLL is a radiologic diagnosis.[41] On lateral roentgenograms, a dense, ossified strip 1 to 5 mm long is evident along the posterior margin of the vertebral bodies and intervertebral discs. The ossification may be continuous or segmental. A thin radiolucent zone separates the vertebral body and the layer of ossification. The intervertebral discs and apophyseal joints are spared, although anterior osteophytes are common. The midcervical region (C3–C5) is the most frequently affected spinal level. Thoracic and lumbar ligaments are affected in 10% of OPLL patients.[42] Thoracic and lumbar lesions may be identified in people who do not have cervical spine disease.[50] Anterior calcifications may be indicative of DISH. Resnick and colleagues have reported OPLL in 50% of DISH patients.[51] Other investigators have also reported the simultaneous occurrence of these two illnesses[44, 52] (Fig. 11–17). DISH may be present in 40% of OPLL patients.[53] CT scan is able to detect the size and location of the ossified ligament to a greater extent than can plain roentgenograms. Nose and colleagues reported that midline lesions were associated with myelopathy, and lateral lesions were associated with radiculopathy when viewed with CT myelography.[54] Magnetic resonance evaluation allows for the detection of marrow in the ossified ligament and the status of the spinal cord in regard to compression.[55] Conservative treatment for OPLL consists of rest, traction, and bracing and is effective in 70% of patients.[56] Indications for surgical intervention include persistent neurologic impairment, intractable pain, and risk of additional cord damage. Surgical techniques may approach the calcification from an anterior or posterior direction, but they may not stop postoperative progression of calcification.[57] Japanese and non-Japanese patients have similar clinical characteristics and respond to therapy in the same manner.[58]

Treatment

Treatment is directed to relieving pain and maximizing function. In patients with neck pain and stiffness, NSAIDs may be helpful. Exercise programs are designed to encourage maximum ranges of motion throughout the axial skeleton. Local injections of lidocaine

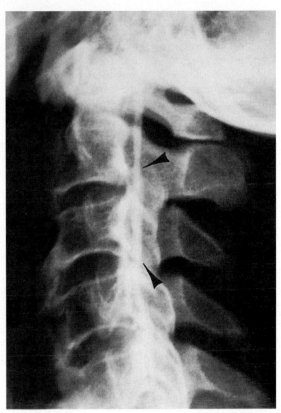

Figure 11–17. Coexistent ossification of the posterior longitudinal ligament and diffuse idiopathic skeletal hyperostosis (DISH). Extensive posterior ligamentous ossification *(arrows)* is combined with anterior vertebral changes typical of DISH. (From Resnick D: Calcification and ossification of the posterior spinal ligaments and tissues. In: Resnick D [ed]: Diagnosis of Bone and Joint Disorders, 3rd ed. Philadelphia: WB Saunders Co, 1995, p 1503.)

and corticosteroid are used in areas of bony overgrowth, such as the heel, for pain relief.

Patients with severe dysphagia may require removal of the offending hyperostosis.[21] A possible complication of surgical excision of exostoses is recurrence of bony overgrowth. Some patients with DISH who have had hip joint replacements have developed postoperative heterotopic ossification.[59] Procedures for removal of osteophytes are successful in most circumstances. In a series of 19 patients, only 2, one with unrecognized esophageal cancer and another with postoperative apnea, had a poor outcome.[60]

Prognosis

The course of DISH is usually benign. Confusion in diagnosis may occur in patients who present in their 40s with neck pain with no physical findings or early radiographic changes. The differential diagnosis for such a patient requires investigation for a number of illnesses that affect the axial skeleton. Patients with DISH have a slow, progressive course. They may have aching neck pain and stiffness for an extended period but rarely develop any limitations in their activities or morbidity from their disease. Patients with DISH are at risk of developing fracture through ankylosed segments. Fracture occurs most commonly in the cervical spine.[61] Patients with fractures develop neurologic dysfunction immediately or on a delayed basis.[62] Most fractures occur through vertebral bodies in the midportion of the ankylosed segment. Less commonly, fractures may occur through discs at levels above or below the ankylosed segment. This is in contrast to ankylosing spondylitis fractures that occur through discs, the weakest part of the ankylosed spine. The trauma that causes a fracture may be minimal.[61] Spinal fractures may result in quadriplegia in 7 of 15 DISH patients. Only 3 of 15 patients had no neurologic damage after a fracture. Fractures heal with early stabilization. Death is a potential result of fracture if the fracture is not recognized.

References

DIFFUSE IDIOPATHIC SKELETAL HYPEROSTOSIS

1. Resnick D, Niwayama G: Radiographic and pathologic features of spinal involvement in diffuse idiopathic skeletal hyperostosis (DISH). Radiology 119:559, 1976.
2. Resnick D, Shaul SR, Robins JM: Diffuse idiopathic skeletal hyperostosis (DISH): Forestier's disease with extraspinal manifestations. Radiology 115:513, 1975.
3. Vernon-Roberts B, Pirie CJ, Trenwith V: Pathology of the dorsal spine in ankylosing hyperostosis. Ann Rheum Dis 33:281, 1974.
4. Boachie-Adjei O, Bullough PG: Incidence of ankylosing hyperostosis of the spine (Forestier's disease) at autopsy. Spine 12:739, 1987.
5. Utsinger PD, Resnick D, Shapiro R: Diffuse skeletal abnormalities in Forestier disease. Arch Intern Med 136:763, 1976.
6. Forestier J, Lagier R: Ankylosing hyperostosis of the spine. Clin Orthop 74:65, 1971.
7. Utsinger PD: Diffuse idiopathic skeletal hyperostosis. Clin Rheum Dis 11:325, 1985.
8. Fornasier VL, Littlejohn GO, Urowitz MB, et al.: Spinal entheseal new bone formation: the early changes of diffuse idiopathic skeletal hyperostosis. J Rheumatol 10:939, 1983.
9. Forgacs SS: Diabetes mellitus and rheumatic disease. Clin Rheum Dis 12:729, 1986.
10. Littlejohn GO, Smythe HA: Marked hyperinsulinemia after glucose challenge in patients with diffuse idiopathic skeletal hyperostosis. J Rheumatol 8:965, 1981.
11. Periquet B, Lambert W, Garcia J, et al.: Increased concentrations of endogenous 13-*cis*- and all-*trans*-reti-

noic acids in diffuse idiopathic skeletal hyperostosis as demonstrated by HPLC. Clin Chim Acta 203:57, 1991.
12. Shapiro RF, Utsinger PD, Wiesner KB, et al.: The association of HLA-B27 with Forestier's disease (vertebral ankylosing hyperostosis). J Rheumatol 3:4, 1976.
13. Spagnola AM, Bennet PH, Terasaki PI: Vertebral ankylosing hyperostosis (Forestier's disease) and HLA antigens in Pima Indians. Arthritis Rheum 21:467, 1978.
14. Harris J, Carter AR, Glick EN, Storey GO: Ankylosing hyperostosis: I. Clinical and radiological features. Ann Rheum Dis 33:210, 1974.
15. Spilberg I, Lieberman DM: Ankylosing hyperostosis of the cervical spine. Arthritis Rheum 15:208, 1972.
16. Meeks LW, Renshaw TS: Vertebral osteophytosis and dysphagia. J Bone Joint Surg 55A:197, 1973.
17. Resnick D, Niwayama G: Diffuse idiopathic skeletal hyperostosis (DISH): Ankylosing hyperostosis of Forrestier and Rotes-Querol. In: Resnick D (ed): Diagnosis of Bone and Joint Disorders, 3rd ed. Philadelphia: WB Saunders Co, 1995, pp 1463–1495.
18. Warnick C, Sherman MS, Lesser RW: Aspiration pneumonia due to diffuse cervical hyperostosis. Chest 98:763, 1990.
19. Crosby ET, Grahovac S: Diffuse idiopathic skeletal hyperostosis: a unique cause of difficult intubation. Can J Anaesth 40:54, 1993.
20. Julkunen H, Heinonen OP, Pyorala K: Hyperostoses of the spine in an adult population: its relationship to hyperglycemia and obesity. Ann Rheum Dis 30:605, 1971.
21. Kritzer RO, Parker WD: DISH: a cause of anterior cervical osteophyte-induced dysphagia. Spine 13:130, 1988.
22. Algenhat JP, Hallet M, Kido DK: Spinal cord compression in diffuse idiopathic skeletal hyperostosis. Radiology 142:119, 1982.
23. Suzuki K, Ishida Y, Ohmori K: Long term follow-up of diffuse idiopathic skeletal hyperostosis in the cervical spine: analysis of progression of ossification. Neuroradiology 33:427, 1991.
24. Ono K, Ota H, Tada K, et al.: Ossified posterior longitudinal ligament: a clinicopathologic study. Spine 2:126, 1977.
25. Eagle W: Elongated styloid process: further observations and a new syndrome. Arch Otolaryngol 47:630, 1948.
26. Williamson PK, Reginato AJ: Diffuse idiopathic skeletal hyperostosis of the cervical spine in a patient with ankylosing spondylitis. Arthritis Rheum 27:570, 1984.
27. Maertens M, Mielants H, Verstraete K, et al.: Simultaneous occurrence of diffuse idiopathic skeletal hyperostosis and ankylosing spondylitis in the same patient. J Rheumatol 19:1978, 1992.
28. Lang EK, Bessler WT: Roentgenologic features of acromegaly. AJR 86:321, 1961.
29. Soriano M, Manchon F: Radiological aspects of a new type of bone fluorosis, periostitis deformans. Radiology 87:1089, 1966.
30. O'Brien WM, Banfield WG, Sokoloff L: Studies on the pathogenesis of ochronotic arthropathy. Arthritis Rheum 4:137, 1961.
31. Resnick D: Hyperostosis and ossification in the cervical spine. Arthritis Rheum 27:564, 1984.
32. Resnick CS, Ammann AM: Cervical spine involvement in sternocostoclavicular hyperostosis. Spine 10:846, 1985.
33. Sonozaki H, Kawashima M, Hongo O, et al.: Incidence of arthro-osteitis in patients with pustulosis palmaris. Ann Rheum Dis 40:554, 1981.
34. Resnick D, Niwayama G: Enostosis, hyperostosis, and periostitis. In: Resnick D (ed): Diagnosis of Bone and

Joint Disorders, 3rd ed. Philadelphia: WB Saunders Co, 1995, pp 4396–4466.

35. Fallet GH, Arroyo J, Vischer TL: Sternocostoclavicular hyperostosis: case report with a 31-year follow-up. Arthritis Rheum 26:784, 1983.

36. Resnick D: Sternocostoclavicular hyperostosis. AJR: 135:1278, 1980.

37. Chigira M, Maehara S, Nagase M, et al.: Sternocostoclavicular hyperostosis: a report of nineteen cases with special reference to etiology and treatment. J Bone Joint Surg 68A:103, 1986.

38. Prevo RL, Rasker JJ, Kruijsen MWM: Sternocostoclavicular hyperostosis or pustulotic arthro-osteitis. J Rheumatol 16:1602, 1989.

39. Fritz P, Baldauf G, Wilke H, Reitter I: Sternocostoclavicular hyperostosis: its progression and radiological features: a study of 12 cases. Ann Rheum Dis 51:658, 1992.

40. Terayama K, Maruyama S, Miyashita R, et al.: Ossification of the posterior longitudinal ligament of the cervical spine (Jpn). Jpn Orthop Surg (Tokyo) 15:1083, 1964.

41. Jones MD, Pais MJ, Omiya B: Bony overgrowths and abnormal calcification about the spine. Radiol Clin North Am 26:1213, 1988.

42. Tsuyama N: Ossification of the posterior longitudinal ligament of the spine. Clin Orthop 184:71, 1984.

43. Nahanshi T, Mannen T, Toyokura Y: Asymptomatic ossification of the posterior longitudinal ligament of the cervical spine: incidence and roentgenographic findings. J Neurol Sci 19:375, 1973.

44. McAfee PC, Regan JJ, Bohlman HH: Cervical cord compression from ossification of the posterior longitudinal ligament in non-Orientals. J Bone Joint Surg 69B:569, 1987.

45. Harsh GR IV, Sypert GW, Weinstein PR, et al.: Cervical spine stenosis secondary to ossification of the posterior longitudinal ligament in non-Orientals. J Neurosurg 67:349, 1987.

46. Resnick D: Calcification and ossification of the posterior spinal ligaments and tissues. In: Resnick D (ed): Diagnosis of Bone and Joint Disorders, 3rd ed. Philadelphia: WB Saunders Co, 1995, pp 1496–1507.

47. Ono K, Ota H, Tada K, et al.: Ossified posterior longitudinal ligament: a clinicopathologic study. Spine 2:126, 1977.

48. Firooznia H, Rafii M, Golimbu C, et al.: Computed tomography of calcification and ossification of posterior longitudinal ligament of the spine. J Comput Assist Tomogr 8:317, 1984.

49. Pouchot J, Watts CS, Esdaile JM, Hill RO: Sudden quadriplegia complicating ossification of the posterior longitudinal ligament and diffuse idiopathic skeletal hyperostosis. Arthritis Rheum 30:1069, 1987.

50. Ono M, Russell WJ, Kudo S, et al.: Ossification of the thoracic posterior longitudinal ligament in a fixed population: radiological and neurological manifestations. Radiology 143:469, 1982.

51. Resnick D, Guerra J Jr, Robinson CA, et al.: Association of DISH and calcification and ossification of the PLL. AJR 131:1049, 1978.

52. Griffiths ID, Fitzjohn TP: Cervical myelopathy, ossification of the posterior longitudinal ligament, and diffuse idiopathic skeletal hyperostosis: problems in investigation. Ann Rheum Dis 46:166, 1987.

53. Arlet PJ, Pujol M, Buc A, et al.: Role de l'hyperostose vertebrale dans les myelopathies cervicales. Rev Rhum Mal Osteoartic 43:167, 1976.

54. Nose T, Egashira T, Enomoto T, et al.: Ossification of the posterior longitudinal ligament: a clinico-radiolog-

ical study of 74 cases. J Neurol Neurosurg Psychiatry 50:321, 1987.

55. Otake S, Matusi M, Nishizawa S, et al.: Ossification of the posterior longitudinal ligament: MR evaluation. AJNR 13:1059, 1992.

56. Klara PM, McDonnell DE: Ossification of the posterior longitudinal ligament in Caucasians: diagnosis and surgical intervention. Neurosurgery 19:212, 1986.

57. Hirabayashi K, Miyakawa J, Satomi K, et al.: Operative results and postoperative progression of ossification among patients with ossification of cervical posterior longitudinal ligament. Spine 6:354, 1981.

58. Trojan DA, Pouchot J, Pokrupa R, et al.: Diagnosis and treatment of ossification of the posterior longitudinal ligament: report of eight cases and literature review. Am J Med 92:296, 1992.

59. Resnick D, Linovitz RJ, Feingold ML: Postoperative heterotopic ossification in patients with ankylosing hyperostosis of the spine (Forestier's disease). J Rheumatol 3:313, 1976.

60. Sobol S, Rigual N: Anterolateral extrapharyngeal approach for cervical osteophyte-induced dysphagia. Ann Otol Rhinol Laryngol 93:498, 1984.

61. Hendrix RW, Melany M, Miller F, Rogers LF: Fracture of the spine in patients with ankylosis due to diffuse idiopathic skeletal hyperostosis: clinical and imaging findings. AJR 162:899, 1994.

62. Paley D, Schwartz M, Cooper P, et al.: Fractures of the spine in diffuse idiopathic skeletal hyperostosis. Clin Orthop 267:22, 1991.

POLYMYALGIA RHEUMATICA

Capsule Summary

Frequency of neck pain—very common

Location of neck pain—paracervical muscles, shoulders

Quality of neck pain—diffuse ache with stiffness

Symptoms and signs—morning stiffness, normal strength, diffuse muscle pain in proximal musculature

Laboratory and x-ray tests—increased erythrocyte sedimentation rate, anemia

Treatment—corticosteroids 15 to 25 mg daily initially, decreasing doses with improvement

Prevalence and Pathogenesis

Polymyalgia rheumatica (PMR) is a clinical syndrome characterized by severe stiffness, tenderness, and aching of the proximal musculature of the upper and lower extremities. Patients who are 50 years of age or older are most commonly affected by this syndrome, and they have an elevated erythrocyte sedimentation rate (ESR) as the primary abnormal laboratory finding. There is no pathognomonic pathologic abnormality that helps physicians diagnose this disease; therefore, other diseases that may be associated with proximal muscle pain must be eliminated as possible causes of pain before a diagnosis of PMR is made.

The incidence of PMR depends to a great extent on the patient population studied. In one population study of whites older than 50 years of age, the incidence of PMR was 19.8 per 100,000 population of people 50 to 59 years of age up to 112.2 per 100,000 in people 70 to 79 years of age. In the total population, the incidence rate was 11 per 100,000 population.[1] A follow-up study completed in Olmstead County, Minnesota, from 1970 to 1991 found a prevalence of PMR in people older than 50 years of age to be 6 per 1,000 and an incidence of 52.5 per 100,000.[2] The prevalence of the disease increases in older age groups, with a majority of patients being 60 years of age or older.[3] The male-to-female ratio is 1:4. The Olmstead County study found a ratio of 39.9% men and 61.7% women.[2] Blacks rarely develop the illness.[4] However, reports of temporal arteritis occurring in blacks have appeared in the literature.[5]

The pathogenesis of PMR is unknown.[6] No familial or genetic predisposition has been shown. Efforts to prove a viral etiology have not been successful.[7] A report of a married couple developing PMR simultaneously is supportive for an environmental pathogenesis.[8] Also, seasonal clustering associated with the onset of the disease during the summer months (May to August) suggests a temporal or environmental mechanism for initiation.[9]

Some have suggested that PMR is an arthritic condition affecting the axial joints.[10, 11] The joints primarily affected include the sternoclavicular and humeroscapular. Synovitis has been demonstrated in these joints on bone scan. However, the relatively small proportion of patients with PMR and synovitis and the distribution of involved joints (relative absence in hip joints) make this mechanism unlikely. Additional studies have reported supporting the presence or absence of joint disease in PMR patients. Investigations of PMR patients, including radiographic studies and necropsy, have been unable to demonstrate synovitis in PMR patients.[10, 11] However, clinical reports have presented data describing patients with synovitis that may be confused with rheumatoid arthritis (RA) who develop classic PMR. Studies supporting increased presence of haplotype DR4 in PMR patients provide additional evidence for a relationship between PMR and RA. Human leukocyte antigen-DR4 is found to be increased in PMR patients compared with control subjects.[12, 13]

Immunologic mechanisms including circulating immune complexes, cell-mediated immunity, and shifts in lymphocyte population have been studied in patients with PMR. No consistent correlation in immune complex amount or composition or the status of lymphocyte numbers or function has been clearly associated with disease pathogenesis.[14–16] Additional studies have demonstrated alteration in lymphocyte distribution and the elevation in a variety of cytokines, including interleukin-6, interleukin-2 receptors, and intercellular adhesion molecule 1.[17–19] However, no consistent correlation has been reported demonstrating normalization of these abnormalities with patient clinical improvement during an extended period.

A new area of study has been the investigation of muscle from PMR patients by the electron microscope. The mitochondria in affected muscle are abnormal. In one study 71% contained crystals that may impair their metabolic activity.[20]

Barber in 1957 was the first to propose the name of polymyalgia rheumatica for the clinical syndrome.[21] PMR has had numerous names, including senile rheumatic gout, polymyalgia arteritica, and anarthritic rheumatoid disease.

Clinical History

The classic PMR patient is a woman older than 50 years of age who develops pain and stiffness symmetrically in the muscles of the neck and shoulder girdle.[22] Discomfort in the low back, pelvic girdle, and thighs is also commonly experienced. Pain starts initially in the shoulders and neck more commonly than in the low back or pelvis. The pain is worse in the morning, such that getting out of bed is difficult. Activity decreases the pain. Symptoms reappear when the patient becomes inactive. The onset of symptoms may be abrupt or gradual. There may also be constitutional symptoms, including fever, malaise, fatigue, anorexia, weight loss, and depression. In about one third of patients, a history of a prodromal viral illness may be elicited.

Physical Examination

Physical examination demonstrates muscle tenderness on palpation and muscle pain with motion, but atrophy and weakness are not present. Although active range of motion of joints may be limited by pain, passive motion is normal. Neck motion is not limited. Occasionally joint swelling, particularly in the sternoclavicular area, may be seen.[23]

Laboratory Data

The characteristic laboratory finding is an increased ESR, and it is present in almost every case of PMR.[24] ESR is more sensitive than C-reactive protein for assessment of disease in PMR patients.[25] Patients with active disease may also develop a hypochromic anemia.[26] Increases in leukocytes and platelets may be more closely related to giant cell arteritis (GCA), which may accompany PMR, than to PMR itself.[27] Chemical studies are usually normal except for about one third of patients with abnormal liver function tests, particularly alkaline phosphatase.[28] Tests for rheumatoid factor and antinuclear antibody are usually negative or these elements are present in the same proportion as found in normal age-matched control subjects. Antimitochondrial antibodies have been reported in a minority of patients with PMR.[29] Their clinical significance remains in doubt. Muscle enzyme levels are normal. Anticardiolipin antibodies, immunoglobulin IgG or IgM, are elevated in only 27% of PMR patients, whereas 80% of GCA patients have antibodies. GCA patients with both antibodies may be at risk for more severe vascular complications.[30]

Pathologic examinations of muscle biopsy specimens from PMR patients are unremarkable.[31] Synovial biopsy demonstrates nonspecific inflammation of the synovium.[32, 33]

Radiographic Evaluation

Plain radiographs demonstrate typical changes in the skeleton that might be expected in patients of this age group. PMR is unassociated with any specific radiographic abnormality, but joint scans with technetium pertechnetate may demonstrate increased uptake in the shoulder joints.[34]

Differential Diagnosis

PMR is a diagnosis made after a number of other diseases with similar symptoms are excluded. Other diseases associated with proximal muscle pain include viral infections, subacute bacterial endocarditis, malignancy, osteoarthritis, rheumatoid arthritis, polymyositis, GCA, fibromyalgia, thyroid dysfunction, and parathyroid dysfunction. A complete history, physical examination, and laboratory evaluation can usually differentiate these diseases. In some instances in which clinical symptoms or laboratory abnormalities are not absolutely characteristic, a tentative diagnosis of PMR is made and therapy is initiated. These patients are then continuously observed to be sure that another illness is not causing their muscle symptoms. When other diseases have been excluded and a patient demonstrates shoulder pain of a month's duration, is 50 years of age or older, has an increased ESR, and responds to corticosteroid therapy, a diagnosis of PMR can be made.

The diagnosis of PMR should not be considered until at least 6 weeks after onset of symptoms. Viral syndromes frequently resolve in this time period. Subacute bacterial endocarditis causes cardiac abnormalities (murmur or change in heart size) that are not associated with PMR. Malignancy does not usually respond to the dose of corticosteroids that is effective for PMR. For example, patients with renal cell carcinoma and lymphoma have presented with PMR symptoms resistant to therapy.[35, 36] Osteoarthritis causes symptoms that are maximum at the end of the day and is associated with a normal ESR. Rheumatoid arthritis affects more joints in the peripheral skeleton than is usually noted in PMR. In the initial states of rheumatoid arthritis in the elderly patient, symptoms of arthritis and muscle pain may be difficult to differentiate from those associated with PMR. The presence of rheumatoid nodules may be helpful in these circumstances. In one study, PMR patients were differentiated from rheumatoid arthritis patients by the presence of upper arm tenderness, the lack of rheumatoid factor, and normal ceruloplasmin levels.[37] Fibromyalgia causes muscle pain in specific locations and has a normal ESR. Signs of thyroid disease (tachycardia and hyperreflexia) and parathyroid disease (polyuria and ulcer disease), for example, should help differentiate these endocrine abnormalities from PMR.

Patients with GCA, an inflammation of blood vessels, frequently have symptoms of PMR.[38] However, in addition to the symptoms of PMR, these patients also have symptoms of headache, pain in the jaw with chewing (jaw claudication), and visual changes, including scotoma, or blindness. The major complication of GCA is blindness caused by the occlusion of the artery that supplies the retina. The diagnosis of GCA is suspected in a patient with PMR who has headache, visual symptoms, or jaw claudication and has the diagnosis confirmed by biopsy of the temporal artery. Almost all GCA patients have an ESR that is markedly increased. In rare circumstances, the ESR may be normal or minimally increased. This unusual presentation may occur when patients have received low-dose corticosteroids that may suppress the ESR without controlling the disease.[39]

Polymyositis is an inflammatory disease of muscle associated with muscle weakness. Muscle pain occurs in polymyositis in 50% of patients. Muscle weakness and pain occur in the shoulder and pelvic girdle, but low back pain can rarely be an associated symptom. A muscle biopsy showing inflammatory changes helps differentiate polymyositis from PMR.[40] The presence of increased serum creatine kinase concentrations also should raise the suspicion for a diagnosis of polymyositis. Polymyositis may be associated with tumors, such as gastric or ovarian cancers. PMR may be associated with tumors, particularly myelodysplastic syndromes.[41]

Bird and colleagues suggested seven criteria for the diagnosis of PMR.[42] They are: (1) bilateral shoulder pain and stiffness, (2) onset of illness of less than 2 weeks' duration, (3) initial ESR greater than 40 mm/h, (4) duration of morning stiffness exceeding 1 hour, (5) age 65 years or older, (6) depression or weight loss, and (7) bilateral tenderness of the upper arm. The diagnosis of PMR is probable if three or more criteria are met.

Treatment

The generally accepted treatment for PMR is daily corticosteroids. Patients with PMR respond rapidly to corticosteroids with dramatic relief of symptoms. The prompt response is regarded as additional confirmation of the diagnosis. The use of steroids may also help the vasculitis that may be associated with GCA. However, the doses needed to control GCA are higher, and patients have been reported to develop GCA while on corticosteroids for PMR.[43–45]

The dose of corticosteroids is usually 15 mg of prednisone every morning. Many patients have a remarkable diminution of symptoms within 24 to 48 hours.[46] If the patient remains symptomatic, an increase to 25 mg is in order. Doses of 10 mg or less per day of prednisolone are inadequate to control symptoms.[47] If patients remain symptomatic at this dosage, splitting the dose in the morning and evening may be helpful while limiting any further increase in prednisone dosage. Alternate-day therapy is usually not effective.[47] Intramuscular injections of depot methylprednisolone also have been used to control PMR disease activity. An injection of 120 mg every 3 weeks followed by monthly injections resulted in disease control without suppression of the adrenal gland.[48, 49]

The patient's response to therapy is monitored by a normalization of the ESR. The C-reactive protein (CRP) level may fall more rapidly with therapy and may be a better test acutely if it is available from a convenient clinical laboratory.[49] CRP is a most helpful monitoring response to therapy during the early stages of the illness. Subsequently, ESR is a more sensitive measure of disease activity. As the ESR or CRP normalizes, the prednisone dose may be tapered slowly. Initially the decrements may be made by 2.5 mg until 7.5 mg is reached. The usual time between reductions is 1 month. Once 7.5 mg is reached, the reductions are 1 mg in magnitude. The goal is to have the patient off corticosteroids by the end of a year, if possible.

Approximately 30% of patients who discontinue steroids before a 2-year period of therapy has concluded are at risk of a relapse.[50] A patient with an exacerbation of symptoms has an associated rise in ESR. The prednisone should be raised to that patient's initial dosage level. The level can be tapered quickly once symptoms are controlled. After an exacerbation of symptoms, the maintenance dose of prednisone should be kept at a higher level (10 mg) and the pace of tapering slowed to 1 mg every 2 to 3 months. In a study of 210 patients with PMR and GCA, the mean duration of treatment was 27.5 months for PMR and 30.9 months for GCA.[51] Return of hypothalamic-pituitary-adrenal axis function does not require alternate-day corticosteroid therapy. Patients who are controlled with the equivalent of 5 mg of prednisone have return of function despite daily doses of medicine. The cumulative dose does not effect return of function.[52]

Corticosteroids have many toxicities, including osteopenia, that may be particularly troublesome in elderly women. These same women are the individuals at greatest risk of developing PMR. Nonsteroidal anti-inflammatory drugs may be useful at diminishing symptoms in PMR patients. They may act as steroid-sparing agents. However, in general, they are useful only in patients with mild disease whose diagnosis may be called into question. Deflazacort, another form of corticosteroid, is effective for controlling disease activity of PMR without the toxicities associated with prednisone. Cortisol secretion is not suppressed and calcium excretion is increased by deflazacort.[53] A very rare but potentially serious manifestation of corticosteroid toxicity is epidural lipomatosis.[54] A patient with epidural lipomatosis is at risk of developing neurologic deficits from neural compression. Immunosuppressive drugs, particularly azathioprine, have been used to decrease steroid dependence of patients with PMR.[55] This is particularly so in patients with compression fractures secondary to chronic corticosteroid use. The immunosuppressives are not benign drugs and increase a patient's risk of developing an infection or a malignancy. Immunosuppressives should be used only after other alternative therapies have been tried.

Patients with GCA require high-dose (60 mg or more) corticosteroids to control disease. These higher doses are necessary to diminish the risk of developing blindness.[43] The frequency of steroid toxicities may be as high as 66% of patients, if weight gain is included as a side effect, with doses of prednisolone of 30 mg/day or greater.[56]

Prognosis

The course of PMR is usually benign. Most patients are able to have their disease controlled at a mean prednisone dosage of 22.8 mg/day, in one study of 76 patients.[57] Ayoub and colleagues suggest PMR may be divided into two patient groups.[57] The first group has limited disease that lasts about 2 years. The second group has disease that is active for 3 to 4 years. These patients require higher doses for a longer period.[57] No specific characteristic could be ascertained that helped predict the classification of individual patients.

References

POLYMYALGIA RHEUMATICA

1. Chuang TY, Hunder GG, Ilbtrup DM, Kurland LT: Polymyalgia rheumatica: a 10-year epidemiologic and clinical study. Ann Intern Med 97:672, 1982.
2. Salvarani C, Gabriel SE, O'Fallon WM, Hunder GG: Epidemiology of polymyalgia rheumatica in Olmstead County, Minnesota, 1970–1991. Arthritis Rheum 38:369, 1995.
3. Mowat AG, Hazelman BL: Polymyalgia rheumatica: a clinical study with particular reference to arterial disease. J Rheumatol 1:190, 1974.
4. Bell W, Klinefelter HF: Polymyalgia rheumatica. Johns Hopkins Med J 121:175, 1967.
5. Bielroy L, Ogunkoya A, Frohman LP: Temporal arthritis in blacks. Am J Med 86:707, 1989.
6. Hunder GG: Giant cell arteritis and polymyalgia rheumatism. In: Kelley WN, Harris ED, Ruddy S Jr, Sledge CB (eds): Textbook of Rheumatology, 4th ed. Philadelphia: WB Saunders Co, 1993, pp 1103–1112.
7. Liang M, Greenberg H, Pincus T, Robinson WS: Hepatitis B antibodies in polymyalgia rheumatica. Lancet 1:43, 1976.
8. Faerk KK: Simultaneous occurrence of polymyalgia rheumatica in a married couple. J Intern Med 231:621, 1992.
9. Cimmino MA, Caporali R, Montecucco CM, et al.: A seasonal pattern in the onset of polymyalgia rheumatica. Ann Rheum Dis 49:521, 1990.
10. Coomes EN, Sharp J: Polymyalgia rheumatica—a misnomer? Lancet 2:1328, 1961.
11. Bruk MI: Articular and vascular manifestations of polymyalgia rheumatica. Ann Rheum Dis 26:103, 1967.
12. Cid MC, Ercilla G, Vilaseca J, et al.: Polymylagia rheumatica: a syndrome associated with HLA-DR4 antigen. Arthritis Rheum 31:678, 1988.
13. Sakhas LI, Loqueman N, Panayi GS, et al.: Immunogenetics of polymyalgia rheumatica. Br J Rheumatol 29:331, 1990.
14. Park JR, Jones JG, Harkiss GD, Hazelman BL: Circulating immune complexes in polymyalgia and giant cell arteritis. Ann Rheum Dis 40:360, 1981.
15. Papaioannou CC, Hunder CG, McDuffie FC: Cellular immunity in polymyalgia rheumatica and giant cell arteritis: lack of response to muscles or artery homogenates. Arthritis Rheum 22:740, 1979.
16. Chelazzi G, Broggini M: Abnormalities of peripheral blood T lymphocyte subsets in polymyalgia rheumatica. Clin Exp Rheumatol 2:333, 1984.
17. Dasgupta D, Panayi GS: Interleukin-6 in serum of patients with polymyalgia rheumatica and giant cell arteritis. Br J Rheumatol 29:456, 1990.
18. Salvarini C, Macchioni P, Boiardi L, et al.: Soluble interleukin-2 receptors in polymyalgia rheumatica/giant cell arteritis: clinical and laboratory correlations. J Rheumatol 19:1100, 1992.
19. Macchioni P, Boiardi L, Meliconi R, et al.: Elevated soluble intercellular adhesion molecule 1 in the serum of patients with polymyalgia rheumatica: influence of steroid treatment. J Rheumatol 21:1860, 1994.
20. Fassbender R, Simmling-Annefeld M: Ultrastructural examination of the skeletal muscles in polymyalgia rheumatica. J Pathol 137:181, 1982.
21. Barber HS: Myalgic syndrome with constitutional effects: polymyalgia rheumatica. Ann Rheum Dis 16:230, 1957.
22. Fernandez-Herlihy L: Polymyalgia rheumatica. Semin Arthritis Rheum 1:236, 1971.
23. Miller LD, Stevens MB: Skeletal manifestations of polymyalgia rheumatica. JAMA 240:27, 1978.
24. Kyle V, Cawston TE, Hazelman BL: Erythrocyte sedimentation rate and C-reactive protein in the assessment of polymyalgia rheumatica/giant cell arteritis on presentation and during followup. Ann Rheum Dis 48:667, 1989.
25. Healy LA, Parker F, Wilske KR: Polymyalgia rheumatica and giant cell arteritis. Arthritis Rheum 14:138, 1971.
26. Gordon I: Polymyalgia rheumatica: a clinical study of 21 cases. Q J Med 29:473, 1960.

27. Bengtsson BA, Malmvall BE: Giant cell arteritis. Acta Med Scand 658(S):1, 1982.

28. Von Knorring, Wasastjerna C: Liver involvement in polymyalgia rheumatica. Scand J Rheumatol 8:197, 1976.

29. Sattar MA, Cawley MID, Hamblin TJ, Robertson JC: Polymyalgia rheumatica and antimitochondrial antibodies. Ann Rheum Dis 43:264, 1984.

30. Espinoza LR, Jara LJ, Silveira LH, et al.: Anticardiolipin antibodies in polymyalgia rheumatica–giant cell arteritis: association with severe vascular complications. Am J Med 90:474, 1991.

31. Brooke MH, Kaplan H: Muscle pathology in rheumatoid arthritis, polymyalgia rheumatica and polymyositis: a histochemical study. Arch Pathol 94:101, 1972.

32. Gordon I, Rennie AM, Branwood AW: Polymyalgia rheumatica: biopsy studies. Ann Rheum Dis 23:447, 1964.

33. Chou C, Schumacher HR Jr: Clinical and pathologic studies of synovitis in polymyalgia rheumatica. Arthritis Rheum 27:1107, 1984.

34. O'Duffy JD, Wahner HW, Hunder GG: Joint imaging in polymyalgia rheumatica. Mayo Clin Proc 51:519, 1976.

35. Sidhom DA, Basalaev M, Sigal LH: Renal cell carcinoma presenting as polymyalgia rheumatica: resolution after nephrectomy. Arch Intern Med 153:2043, 1993.

36. Montanaro M, Bizarri F: Non-Hodgkin's lymphoma and subsequent acute lymphoblastic leukemia in a patient with polymyalgia rheumatica. Br J Rheumatol 31:277, 1992.

37. Hantzschel H, Bird HA, Seidel W, et al.: Polymyalgia rheumatica and rheumatoid arthritis of the elderly: a clinical, laboratory, and scintigraphic comparison. Ann Rheum Dis 50:619, 1991.

38. Hamilton CR, Shelley WM, Tumulty PA: Giant cell arteritis including temporal arteritis and polymyalgia rheumatica. Medicine 50:1, 1971.

39. Wise CM, Agudelo CA, Shelley WM, Tumulty PA: Giant cell arteritis with low erythrocyte sedimentation rate: a review of five cases. Arthritis Rheum 34:1571, 1991.

40. Bohan A, Peter JB, Bowman RL, Pearson CM: A computer-assisted analysis of 153 patients with polymyositis and dermatomyositis. Medicine 56:255, 1977.

41. Kohli M, Bennett RM: An association of polymyalgia rheumatica with myelodysplastic syndromes. J Rheumatol 21:1357, 1994.

42. Bird HA, Esselinck W, Dixon A, et al.: An evaluation of criteria for polymyalgia rheumatica. Ann Rheum Dis 38:434, 1979.

43. Hunder GG, Allen GL: Giant cell arteritis: a review. Bull Rheum Dis 29:980, 1978.

44. Hunder GG, Sheps SG, Allen GI, Joyce JW: Daily and alternate-day corticosteroid regimens in treatment of giant cell arteritis: comparison in prospective study. Ann Intern Med 82:613, 1975.

45. Papadakis MA, Schwartz ND: Temporal arteritis after normalization of erythrocyte sedimentation rate in polymyalgia rheumatica. Arch Intern Med 146:2283, 1986.

46. Davison S, Spiera H: Concepts and treatment in polymyalgia rheumatica. J Mt Sinai Hosp NY 35:473, 1968.

47. Kyle V, Hazelman BL: Treatment of polymyalgia rheumatica and giant cell arteritis: I. steroid regimens in the first two months. Ann Rheum Dis 48:658, 1991.

48. Dasgupta B, Gray J, Fernandes I, et al.: Treatment of polymyalgia rheumatica with intramuscular injection of depot methylprednisolone. Ann Rheum Dis 50:942, 1991.

49. Mallya RK, Hind CR, Berry H, Pepys MB: Serum C-reactive protein in polymyalgia rheumatica: a prospective serial study. Arthritis Rheum 28:383, 1985.

50. Fauchald P, Rygvold O, Ystsese B: Temporal arteritis and polymyalgia rheumatica: clinical and biopsy findings. Ann Intern Med 77:845, 1972.

51. Delecoueillerie G, Joly P, Cohen de Lara A, et al.: Polymyalgia rheumatica and temporal arteritis: a retrospective analysis of prognostic features and different corticosteroid regimens (1-year survey of 210 patients). Ann Rheum Dis 47:733, 1989.

52. LaRochelle GE, LaRochelle AG, Ratner RE, et al.: Recovery of the hypothalamic-pituitary-adrenal (HPA) axis in patients with rheumatic disease receiving low-dose prednisone. Am J Med 95:258, 1993.

53. Gray RE, Doherty GM, Galloway J, et al.: A double-blind study of deflazacort and prednisone in patients with chronic inflammatory disorders. Arthritis Rheum 34:287, 1991.

54. Tabron J: Epidural lipomatosis as a cause of spinal cord compression in polymyalgia rheumatica. J Rheumatol 18:286, 1991.

55. De Silva M, Hazelman BL: Azathioprine in giant cell arteritis–polymyalgia rheumatica: a double-blind study. Ann Rheum Dis 45:136, 1986.

56. Kyle V, Hazelman BL: Treatment of polymyalgia rheumatica and giant cell arteritis: II. relation between steroid dose and steroid-associated side effects. Ann Rheum Dis 48:662, 1989.

57. Ayoub WT, Franklin CM, Torretti D: Polymyalgia rheumatica: duration of therapy and long-term outcome. Am J Med 79:309, 1985.

FIBROMYALGIA

Capsule Summary

Frequency of neck pain—very common

Location of neck pain—paracervical muscles, occiput

Quality of neck pain—general ache, sharp pain with pressure over tender points

Symptoms and signs—generalized fatigue, muscle soreness, multiple tender points

Laboratory and x-ray tests—normal

Treatment—rest, aerobic exercise, antidepressants, nonsteroidal anti-inflammatory drugs

Prevalence and Pathogenesis

Fibromyalgia (FM) is a soft tissue, pain amplification syndrome. It is characterized by chronic pain in discrete tender point areas and specific sleep disturbance that occurs in a perfectionist, compulsive individual. FM is unassociated with any structural abnormalities of muscle, bone, or cartilage. However, the persistent pain and chronic fatigue associated with the syndrome prevent patients from achieving their full potential.

The prevalence and incidence of FM are unknown; however, many primary care physicians believe FM to be a common disease, with more than 10 million Americans affected.[1] In the family practice setting 2.1% of patients have FM.[2] In rheumatology practices, the syndrome is present in 12% to 20% of new patients.[3, 4] The syndrome occurs most commonly in white women with a mean age of 29 years, or 34 years if all patients with other rheumatic conditions are excluded.[4] The prevalence in a general community population was reported at 2%, with 3.4% women and 0.5% men, with a mean age of 59 years.[5] The syndrome has also been found in other populations in Europe, Africa, and Asia.[6, 7]

The exact etiology of the disease is unknown. The hypothesis that best explains the clinical symptoms is that of a disorder of central pain signalling, with the central nervous system (CNS) functioning in an overly sensitive manner to nociceptive and non-nociceptive stimuli. Moldofsky and colleagues have suggested that specific disturbances in sleep may result in patients developing FM.[8] The abnormality in sleep is the superimposition of light stages of sleep, characterized by alpha waves on electroencephalogram, on deep stages of sleep, characterized by delta waves (non–rapid eye movement sleep). In a second study, Moldofsky produced FM symptoms in healthy volunteers when their deep sleep was interrupted by loud noises for 3 days.[9] Sleep disturbances are frequent complaints of patients with FM.[10, 11] FM may be a disorder of nonrestorative sleep in which a disorder of serotonin metabolism results in musculoskeletal pain. Chlorpromazine, a drug that increases delta sleep, decreased patients' pain and tender points in one study.[11] However, the role of sleep in the pathogenesis of FM remains in question because other studies have not been able to reproduce the findings of Moldofsky, and other groups of patients (those with depression) have similar sleep disturbances without pain.[12–14]

Abnormalities with sleep are thought to disorder the processing of painful stimuli by the CNS.[15] The CNS is capable of modifying the way it processes a variety of impulses (neuronal plasticity).[16] These abnormalities can lower pain thresholds. Substance P levels in the CNS (not in serum) are higher in FM patients than in control subjects.[17, 18] Other measures of CNS dysfunction include abnormal cortisol response, decreased somatomedin C levels, and decreased serotonin levels.[19–21] The sensitivity of tender points and secondary manifestations of FM are related to autonomic system activity and may be modified by sympathetic inhibition.[22] These abnormalities are not exclusive to FM and may be of secondary importance and not the mechanism causing the disease.

Fowler and Kraft have suggested that patients with fibrositis have increased muscle tone.[23] When performing a standardized task, they have 50% more electrical activity on electromyogram than normal control subjects. In a study of fatigue characteristics as measured by surface integrated electromyogram activity, FM patients had findings similar to those of control subjects.[24] Individuals with increased muscle tension and abnormal sleep patterns may be at risk of developing FM. Muscle metabolism may be disordered in patients with FM. A decrease in levels of adenosine triphosphate, adenosine diphosphate, and phosphoryl creatine and an increase in the levels of adenosine monophosphate and creatine were found in the trapezius muscle of patients with FM. These findings suggest that the source of pain in patients with FM may be local tissue hypoxia.[25]

Smythe has suggested that trauma in a single incident or repeated episodes may be a cause of FM.[26] In the anxious, perfectionist-type person, trauma in areas of increased sensitivity may result in perpetuation of pain long after the injury and associated pain should have subsided. For example, cab drivers may develop cervical FM, and bus drivers may develop FM of the back. The association of trauma and FM remains a conjecture because no prospective study has been completed that demonstrates this association. A 10-year follow-up study of patients who were traumatized in motor vehicle accidents, work injuries, surgery, or sports injuries revealed that 56 of 67 (83%) had 11 or more tender points. Other symptoms were similar to those of primary FM patients.[27] The relationship between trauma in the workplace and FM remains to be determined.[28]

FM was also thought to be a psychogenic disorder and was classified with psychogenic rheumatism.[29] Most recent studies have shown no increased prevalence of psychological disorders in patients with FM compared with normal control subjects.[30] The majority of patients with FM do not have any psychiatric disorder.[31] Some of the psychiatric difficulties associated with these patients may be related to chronic pain and dysfunction.[32]

The concept of fibrositis has evolved over many years. The central theme of the disease has been the tender point or fibrositic nodule, which was first described in 1824 by Balfour.[33] These areas were only tender with pressure. This was in contrast with trigger points, which were soft tissue regions that spontaneously caused radiating pain.[34] Myofascial pain syndromes were defined as muscle disorders with symptoms that were amplified by abnormalities in the CNS.[35] Subsequently, Gowers introduced the term fibrositis, although no inflammatory alterations could be identified in muscle.[36] More recently, a specific set of symptoms and signs have become associated with FM.[37] Although some authors do not believe that FM is a distinct entity, this disease has been reported by other rheumatologists to have a prevalence in the United States of 3 to 6 million.[38, 39]

Clinical History

Patients with FM complain of generalized aching pain associated with profound stiffness and fatigue. Areas of pain are confined to articular and periarticular structures, including ligaments, tendons, muscles, and bony prominences. The pain may be unremitting, with durations of 20 years or longer. Generalized stiffness is most notable in the morning, usually lasting up to an hour. A smaller percentage of patients have evening stiffness, and some patients have day-long stiffness. Fatigue is also a prominent feature of patients with FM. Characteristically, these patients arise in the morning after a restless sleep, feeling exhausted. Some patients complain of unrelenting fatigue. Other clinical features include polyarthralgias, occasionally associated with hand swelling, numbness, headaches, and anxiety.

Cold or humid weather, overactivity, total inactivity, and poor sleep exacerbate FM. Patients with FM have increased symptoms with changes in barometric pressure.[40] Factors that improve symptoms include moderate activity; warm, dry weather; and massage.

FM also occurs in older patients who have clinical findings similar to these of younger patients. In a study of 31 older patients with FM, only 17% had the disease diagnosed before referral to a rheumatologist. A significant number of these patients were treated inappropriately with corticosteroids.[41] In a spine center setting, 12% of 125 referred patients had FM. The diagnosis was not recognized by the majority of physicians who referred these patients. These patients had clinical symptoms and signs of FM when examined for the disease.[42]

Physical Examination

Physical examination demonstrates specific areas that are tender on palpation. These areas are referred to as tender points and are localized to certain anatomic sites. The most commonly affected areas include the upper border of the trapezius, medial part of the knees, lateral border of the elbows, posterior iliac crest, and the lumbar spine. Pressure over the area results in a pattern of local pain (Fig. 11–18). There is no tenderness outside the local area. In one study, patients had 4 to 33 tender points.[4] Usually, patients with primary FM have 12 or more discrete areas. The exact location that differentiates patients with FM from control subjects continues to be evaluated. Some areas that may be useful include the anterior shoulder, anterior chest, posterior scapula, and medial knee.[43]

Patients with FM may have fibrositic nodules located about the sacrum and posterior iliac crest. The nodules are mobile, firm, and tender on palpation. Results of biopsy of these nodules demonstrate fibrofatty tissue without inflammation. Other than the findings of tender points and nodules, the physical examination is normal, with full range of motion of the cervical and lumbosacral spine.

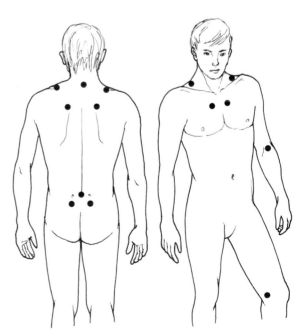

Figure 11–18. Diagram of common sites of tenderness on palpation in fibromyalgia patients.

TABLE 11–8. DIAGNOSTIC CRITERIA FOR FIBROMYALGIA

MAJOR CRITERIA

Chronic, generalized aches, pains, or stiffness (involving ≥3 anatomic sites for ≥3 months)
Absence of other systemic condition to account for these symptoms
Multiple tender points at characteristic locations

MINOR CRITERIA

Disturbed sleep
Generalized fatigue or tiredness
Subjective swelling, numbness
Pain in neck, shoulders
Chronic headaches
Irritable bowel symptoms

Modified from Goldenberg DL: Fibromyalgia syndrome: an emerging but controversial condition. JAMA 257:2782, 1987. Copyright 1987, American Medical Association.

Laboratory Data

Laboratory parameters are normal. Blood chemistries, hematologic parameters, the erythrocyte sedimentation rate (ESR), rheumatoid factor, and antinuclear antibody are all normal in primary FM. Among the findings that are normal are serum tryptophan levels, absence of autoantibodies, and distribution of human leukocyte antigens.[44–46] Assessment of the hypothalamic-pituitary-adrenal axis reveals low 24-hour urinary-free cortisol, hyporesponsiveness of the adrenal gland to stimulation, and decreased levels of neuropeptide Y.[47] The clinical importance of these laboratory tests has not been determined.

Pathologic evaluation of muscle biopsies is unrevealing on histoimmunochemical and ultrastructural studies. The biopsy may be important only to eliminate other disorders as the cause of muscle pain.[48]

Radiographic Evaluation

Radiographic findings are normal in patients with FM. The results of bone scintiscans are no different in FM patients than in control subjects.[49]

Differential Diagnosis

The diagnosis of primary FM is based on the presence of characteristic musculoskeletal abnormalities in the absence of stigmata of other diseases. Patients who have diffuse aching and fatigue of at least 3 months' duration, at least 12 tender points, and disturbed sleep

patterns probably have FM. There are no specific physical or laboratory findings that are pathognomonic for this disease. Therefore, the diagnosis of FM is one of exclusion, and these patients require constant reevaluation. A variety of diagnostic criteria have been proposed for fibrositis.[4, 37] Goldenberg has divided the clinical characteristics of the disease into major and minor criteria[50] (Table 11–8). The presence of three major criteria and four of six minor criteria was necessary for the diagnosis of FM by Goldenberg's approach. In 1990, a committee of the American College of Rheumatology presented classification criteria for FM (Table 11–9).[51]

Repeat evaluation is necessary to detect early physical or laboratory findings that are indicative of an underlying disease process, such as rheumatoid arthritis or a malignancy. Patients with an underlying disease and muscle pain have secondary FM. Other diseases associated with secondary FM include rheumatoid arthritis, osteoarthritis, spondyloarthropathies, connective tissue diseases, malignancies, hypothyroidism, hyperparathyroidism, chronic infections, and sarcoidosis.[52] Patients with human immunodeficiency virus infection also develop FM.[53] Characteristic physical findings, inflammatory joint signs, laboratory abnormalities, increased ESR, and positive rheumatoid factor help differentiate these diseases from primary FM.

FM must also be differentiated from psychogenic rheumatism, which is characterized by significant anxiety, depression, or neurosis.[54] Patients with psychogenic rheumatism have severe pain of a burning or cutting quality. The pain is excruciating in intensity and without any recognizable anatomic boundaries. The patients usually deny stiffness. On examination, they have a marked response to

TABLE 11–9. AMERICAN COLLEGE OF RHEUMATOLOGY CLASSIFICATION CRITERIA FOR FIBROMYALGIA

1. History of widespread pain. Pain is on both sides of the body and above and below the waist. Low back pain is considered lower segment pain.
2. Pain in 11 of 18 tender points on digital palpation—4 kg of force should be applied with digital pressure. The site must be painful, not tender.

Widespread pain should be present for ≥3 months. A second clinical disorder does not exclude the diagnosis of fibromyalgia.

Modified from Wolfe F, Smythe HA, Yunus MB, et al.: The American College of Rheumatology 1990 criteria for the classification of fibromyalgia: report of the multicenter criteria committee. Arthritis Rheum 33:160, 1990, Karger, Basel.

minimal pressure on palpation. Their areas of tenderness do not correspond to the tender points of FM. The laboratory evaluation of these patients is normal, and their complaints are resistant to all forms of therapy.

Chronic fatigue syndrome is another disorder that has a clinical spectrum that overlaps with FM. This syndrome is associated with chronic fatigue that does not resolve with bed rest, no other complicating illness, mild fever, sore throat, painful lymph nodes, muscle weakness, headaches, arthralgias, and insomnia.[55] The severity of fatigue is greater in patients with chronic fatigue syndrome. In a review of patients with FM, only 20% fulfilled the criterion of fatigue.[56]

Myofascial Pain Syndrome (MPS). MPS is a regional pain syndrome characterized by two major components: the first is a localized area of deep muscle tenderness (trigger point) that is accompanied by a palpable abnormality in muscle consistency (fibrositic nodule), and the second is a specific area of referral pain distant from the trigger point.[57] The muscles in MPS have extreme tenderness on palpation, decreased flexibility, abnormal consistency, pain on contraction, and localized "twitch response" to rapid snapping of the trigger point or fibrositic nodules. Pressure over a trigger point results in a dull, aching pain in a referral pattern that does not follow any characteristic myotomal structure. A trigger point may be a muscle region of increased energy consumption with an inadequate oxygen supply.[58] Neck pain is a common symptom associated with MPS.[59] Neck muscles associated with MPS and their associated pain radiations are listed in Table 11–10. MPS and FM are not the same disease, although superficially they seem quite similar. MPS is a localized pain syndrome with sudden onset and trigger points with distant referred pain. FM is a diffuse pain syndrome with gradual onset, multiple tender points, and disturbed sleep. Controversy remains whether MPS exists as a separate clinical entity. The characteristic clinical findings of MPS, including trigger points, may not be differentiated in patients with MPS from patients with FM or normal control subjects.[60] Therapy for MPS consists of injection with local anesthetics of trigger points along with the use of superficial cooling in association with muscle stretching. In patients with chronic MPS symptoms, local injection of botulinum toxin (which blocks release of acetylcholine) has decreased pain for a small number.[61] Several clinical, psychological, and sociological factors are associated with poor response to trigger point injections. These factors (unemployment, constant pain, and poor coping ability) suggest that factors affecting pain associated with MPS go beyond abnormal muscle physiology.[62]

Treatment

Treatment of FM requires a multifactorial approach.[63] In many circumstances, educating patients about their illness is reassuring and relieves some symptoms. Many patients are encouraged by having a specific diagnosis for their ailments. Their symptoms are no longer "in their head." They are told that their condition is not life-threatening, deforming, or degenerating, but that it causes chronic pain.

Rest and relaxation are important for patients who are overworked. Patients are encouraged to remain at work, but they should not become excessively fatigued.[4] Some pa-

TABLE 11–10. PAIN LOCATION AND MUSCLES ASSOCIATED WITH MYOFASCIAL PAIN SYNDROME OF THE NECK

MUSCLE WITH TRIGGER POINT	PHYSICAL ABNORMALITY WITH PAIN	REFERRED PAIN DISTRIBUTION
Trapezius	Active rotation head toward opposite side, side bending	Upper posterolateral neck, scapulae
Levator scapulae	Decreased neck rotation	Base of neck, medial scapulae
Splenius capitis	Decreased neck flexion, rotation same side	Vertex of head
Splenius cervicis	Decreased neck flexion, rotation same side	Occiput, back of orbit, angle of neck
Semispinalis capitis/ cervicis/multifidis	Decreased neck flexion, extension, rotation	Occiput, above orbit, angle of neck
Suboccipital	Decreased head flexion, rotation, side bending	Occiput, back of orbit

Travell JG, Simons DG: Myofascial Pain and Dysfunction: The Trigger Point Manual: The Upper Extremities. Baltimore: Williams & Wilkins, 1983, p 713.

tients require a change in their job status to lighter duty. Simple interventions in the environment, including chairs with cervical supports, cervical pillows, firm mattress, and comfortable work position, may have a beneficial effect on pain. Range-of-motion and stretching exercises encourage improved muscle function. Patients are also encouraged to participate in an aerobic exercise program. Studies have demonstrated the benefit of cardiovascular training in reducing pain in FM patients.[64] The exercise program should also contain a home component so that patients become an active participant in their own care.[65] Heat treatments are also useful. Drug therapy in the form of aspirin or other nonsteroidal anti-inflammatory drugs (NSAIDs) is helpful in reducing the pain associated with FM.[52] Injection of tender points with a combination of anesthetic agent and a long-acting corticosteroid is helpful in controlling localized pain.[66] Systemic corticosteroids are not used in patients with primary FM.[67] Narcotics are also not indicated for this disease.

With the thought that abnormal serotonin metabolism plays a role in the pathogenesis of FM, antidepressants and muscle relaxants that increase serotonin levels have been studied in controlled short-term, placebo-based drug trials. Cyclobenzaprine hydrochloride (Flexeril), a tricyclic muscle relaxant, at dosages of 10 to 40 mg/day caused significant improvement in pain, sleep, and tender points compared with placebo.[68] Improvement was also seen in another study with another tricyclic drug, amitriptyline hydrochloride (Elavil), at a dose of 50 mg at bedtime.[69] Amitriptyline, when effective, results in decreased symptoms within 2 weeks of starting therapy.[70] A report of a controlled study of 208 patients on a 6-month trial of cyclobenzaprine, amitriptyline, and placebo demonstrated no benefit of active drugs versus placebo after the first few weeks of therapy.[71] Imipramine hydrochloride at 50 to 75 mg/day had no beneficial effect on the symptoms of FM.[72] Marginal benefit has been associated with aprazolam.[73] The antidepressant fluoxetine is not helpful in decreasing pain in FM patients.[74]

The basic program of therapy for a patient with FM is a tricyclic agent along with patient education and controlled activity in a physical therapy program. The addition of an NSAID is optional, depending on the patient's muscle pain. Injection of tender points is useful if they are few in number.

All these modes of therapy do have a beneficial effect on the symptoms of FM; however, FM is a chronic disease that may be exacerbated by a number of factors, including increased tension, cold exposure, or sleep disturbances. Compliance with a program is essential for long-term management. Appropriate rest, exercise, and stress management may control disease symptoms without the need to use medications or injections.

Men with FM may have sleep apnea as a cause of their chronic pain syndrome. These patients may benefit from therapy directed at improving their sleep apnea.[75]

Prognosis

The course of FM is one of exacerbations and remissions. Patients have neck, low back, knee, and chest pain that hinders their ability to perform up to their potential. Wood, in a study of English workers, reported that nonarticular rheumatism, which included patients with FM, accounted for 10.9% of absences from work and corresponded to 10.5% of days lost from work.[76] FM may go unrecognized for an extended period. In such circumstances, a person may be thought of as a malingerer who is unwilling to do a full day's work. FM is a chronic condition. In a 4-year follow-up study of FM patients, 97% continued to experience symptoms and 85% fulfilled diagnostic criteria for FM.[77] The disease is associated with functional disability and high levels of anxiety and depression despite therapy.[78]

Although FM is not disabling in the same sense as the spondyloarthropathies, it is associated with reduced productivity and absenteeism. Recognition of the disease and institution of appropriate therapy can have a beneficial effect on a patient's outlook and work performance.

References

FIBROMYALGIA

1. The American Rheumatism Association Committee on Rheumatologic Practice: A description of rheumatology practice. Arthritis Rheum 20:1278, 1977.
2. Hartz A, Kirchdoerfer E: Undetected fibrositis in primary care practice. J Fam Pract 25:365, 1987.
3. Wolfe F, Cathey MA: Prevalence of primary and secondary fibrositis. J Rheumatol 10:965, 1983.
4. Yunus M, Masi AT, Calabro JJ, et al.: Primary fibromyalgia (fibrositis): clinical study of 50 patients with matched normal controls. Semin Arthritis Rheum 11:151, 1981.
5. Wolfe F, Ross K, Anderson J, et al.: The prevalence and characteristics of fibromyalgia in the general population. Arthritis Rheum 38:19, 1995.

6. Forseth KO, Gran JT: The prevalence of fibromyalgia among women aged 20–49 years in Arendal, Norway. Scand J Rheumatol 21:74, 1992.

7. Buskila D, Press J, Gedalia A, et al.: Assessment of nonarticular tenderness and prevalence of fibromyalgia in children. J Rheumatol 20:368, 1993.

8. Moldofsky H, Scarisbrick P, England R, Smythe H: Musculoskeletal symptoms and non-REM sleep disturbance in patients with "fibrositis syndrome" and healthy subjects. Psychosom Med 37:341, 1975.

9. Moldofsky H, Scarisbrick P: Induction of neurasthenic musculoskeletal pain syndrome by selective sleep stage deprivation. Psychosom Med 38:35, 1976.

10. Campbell SM, Clark S, Tyndall EA, et al.: Clinical characteristics of fibrositis: I. a "blinded" controlled study of symptoms and tender points. Arthritis Rheum 26:817, 1983.

11. Moldofsky A, Lue FA: The relationship of alpha and delta EEG frequencies to pain and mood in fibrositis patients treated with chlorpromazine and L-tryptophan. Electroencephalogr Clin Neurophysiol 50:71, 1980.

12. Golden H, Weber SM, Bergen D: Sleep studies in patients with fibrositis syndrome. Arthritis Rheum 26:S32, 1983.

13. Moldofsky H: Workshop on sleep studies. Am J Med 81:(suppl 3A) 107, 1986.

14. Wittig R, Zorick FJ, Blumer D, et al.: Disturbed sleep in patients complaining of chronic pain. J Nerv Ment Dis 170:429, 1982.

15. Yunus MB: Toward a model of pathophysiology of fibromyalgia-aberrant central pain mechanism with peripheral modulation. J Rheumatol 19:846, 1992.

16. Dubner R: Hyperalgesia and expanded receptive fields. Pain 48:3, 1992.

17. Vaeroy H, Helle R, Forre O, et al.: Elevated CSF levels of substance P and high incidence of Raynaud's phenomenon in patients with fibromyalgia: new features for diagnosis. Pain 32:21, 1988.

18. Reynolds WJ, Chiu B, Inman RD: Plasma substance P levels in fibrositis. J Rheumatol 15:1802, 1988.

19. McCain GA, Tilbe KS: Diurnal hormone variation in fibromyalgia syndrome: a comparison with rheumatoid arthritis. J Rheumatol Suppl 19:154, 1989.

20. Bennett RM, Clark SR, Campbell SM, et al.: Low levels of somatomedin C in patients with fibromyalgia syndrome: a possible link between sleep and muscle pain. Arthritis Rheum 35:550, 1992.

21. Russell IJ, Vaeroy H, Javors M, et al.: Cerebrospinal fluid biogenic amine metabolites in fibromyalgia/fibrositis syndrome and rheumatoid arthritis. Arthritis Rheum 35:550, 1992.

22. Bengtsson M, Bengtsson A, Jorfeldt L: Diagnostic epidural opioid blockade in primary fibromyalgia at rest and during exercise. Pain 39:171, 1989.

23. Fowler RS Jr, Kraft GH: Tension perception in patients having pain associated with chronic muscle tension. Arch Phys Med Rehabil 55:28, 1974.

24. Stokes MJ, Colter C, Klevstov A, et al.: Normal paraspinal muscle electromyographic fatigue characteristics in patients with primary fibromyalgia. Br J Rheumatol 32:71, 1993.

25. Bengtsson A, Henriksson KG, Larsson J: Reduced high-energy phosphate levels in the painful muscle of patients with primary fibromyalgia. Arthritis Rheum 24:817, 1986.

26. Smythe HA: Non-articular rheumatism and psychogenic musculoskeletal syndromes. In: McCarty DJ Jr (ed): Arthritis and Allied Conditions, 10th ed. Philadelphia: Lea & Febiger, 1985, pp 1083–1094.

27. Waylonis GW, Perkins RH: Post-traumatic fibromyalgia: a long-term follow-up. Am J Phys Med Rehabil 73:403, 1994.

28. Littlejohn GO: Fibrositis/fibromyalgia syndrome in the workplace. Rheum Dis Clin North Am 15:45, 1989.

29. Savage O: Management of rheumatic diseases in the armed forces. Br Med J 2:336, 1942.

30. Clark S, Campbell SM, Forehand ME, et al.: Clinical characteristics of fibrositis. Arthritis Rheum 28:132, 1985.

31. Goldenberg DL: Psychiatric and psychologic aspects of fibromyalgia syndrome. Rheum Dis Clin North Am 15:105, 1989.

32. Merskey H: Physical and psychological considerations in the classification of fibromyalgia. J Rheumatol Suppl 16:72, 1989.

33. Balfour W: Observations with cases illustrative of a new, simple, and expeditious mode of curing rheumatism and sprains. Lond Med Phys J 51:446, 1824.

34. Kellgren JH: Observations on referred pain arising from muscle. Clin Sci 3:175, 1938.

35. Travell J, Ringler SH: The myofascial genesis of pain. Postgrad Med 11:425, 1952.

36. Gowers WR: Lumbago: its lessons and analogues. Br Med J 1:117, 1904.

37. Wolfe F, Cathey MA: The epidemiology of tender points: a prospective study of 1520 patients. J Rheumatol 12:1164, 1985.

38. Hadler WM: Medical Management of the Regional Musculoskeletal Disease. New York: Grune and Stratton, 1985.

39. Wallace DJ: Systemic lupus erythematosus, rheumatology, and medical literature: current trends. J Rheumatol 12:913, 1985.

40. Guedj D, Weinberger A: Effect of weather conditions on rheumatic patients. Ann Rheum Dis 49:158, 1990.

41. Yunus MB, Holt GS, Masi AT: Fibromyalgia syndrome among the elderly: comparison with younger patients. J Am Geriatr Soc 36:987, 1988.

42. Borenstein D: Prevalence and treatment outcome of primary and secondary fibromyalgia in patients with spinal pain. Spine 20:796, 1995.

43. Simms RW, Goldenberg DL, Felson DT, et al.: Tenderness in 75 anatomic sites: distinguishing fibromyalgia patients from controls. Arthritis Rheum 31:182, 1988.

44. Yunus MB, Dailey JW, Aldag JC, et al.: Plasma tryptophan and other amino acids in primary fibromyalgia: a controlled study. J Rheumatol 19:90, 1992.

45. Bengtsson A, Ernerudh J, Vrethem M, et al.: Absence of autoantibodies in primary fibromyalgia. J Rheumatol 17:1682, 1990.

46. Horven S, Stiles TC, Holst A, et al.: HLA antigens in primary fibromyalgia syndrome. J Rheumatol 19:1269, 1992.

47. Crofford LJ, Pillemer SR, Kalogera KT, et al.: Hypothalamic-pituitary-adrenal axis perturbations in patients with fibromyalgia. Arthritis Rheum 37:1583, 1994.

48. Drewes A, Andreasen A, Schnider HD, et al.: Pathology of skeletal muscle in fibromyalgia: a histo-immuno-chemical and ultrastructural study. Br J Rheumatol 32(suppl):479, 1993.

49. Yunus MB, Berg BC, Masi AT: Multiphase skeletal scintigraphy in primary fibromyalgia syndrome: a blinded study. J Rheumatol 16:1466, 1989.

50. Goldenberg DL: Fibromyalgia syndrome: an emerging but controversial condition. JAMA 257:2782, 1987.

51. Wolfe F, Smythe HA, Yunus MB, et al.: The American College of Rheumatology 1990 criteria for the classification of fibromyalgia: report of the multicenter criteria committee. Arthritis Rheum 33:160, 1990.

52. Beetham WP Jr: Diagnosis and management of fibro-

sitis syndrome and psychogenic rheumatism. Med Clin North Am 63:433, 1979.

53. Simms RW, Zerbini CA, Ferrante N, et al.: Fibromyalgia syndrome in patients infected with human immunodeficiency virus: the Boston City Hospital clinical AIDS team. Am J Med 92:368, 1992.

54. Rotes-Querol J: The syndromes of psychogenic rheumatism. Clin Rheum Dis 5:797, 1979.

55. Holmes GP, Kaplan JE, Gabtz NM, et al.: Chronic fatigue syndrome: a working case definition. Ann Intern Med 108:387, 1988.

56. Norregaard J, Bulow PM, Prescott E, et al.: A four-year follow-up study in fibromyalgia: relationship to chronic fatigue syndrome. Scand J Rheumatol 22:35, 1993.

57. Travell JG, Simons DG: Myofascial Pain and Dysfunction. The Trigger Point Manual: the Upper Extremities, vol 1. Baltimore: Williams & Wilkins, 1992.

58. Simons DG: Myofascial pain syndromes: where are we? where are we going? Arch Phys Med Rehabil 69:207, 1988.

59. Campbell SM: Regional myofascial pain syndromes. Rheum Dis Clin North Am 15:31, 1989.

60. Wolfe F, Simons DG, Fricton J, et al.: The fibromyalgia and myofascial pain syndromes: a preliminary study of tender points and trigger points in persons with fibromyalgia, myofascial pain syndrome, and no disease. J Rheumatol 19:944, 1992.

61. Cheshire WP, Abashian SW, Mann JD: Botulinum toxin in the treatment of myofascial pain syndrome. Pain 59:65, 1994.

62. Hopwood MB, Abram SE: Factors associated with failure of trigger point injections. Clin J Pain 10:227, 1994.

63. Goldenberg DL: Treatment of fibromyalgia syndrome. Rheum Dis Clin North Am 15:61, 1989.

64. McCain GA, Bell DA, Mai FM, et al.: A controlled study of the effects of supervised cardiovascular fitness training program on the manifestations of primary fibromyalgia. Arthritis Rheum 31:1135, 1988.

65. Rosen NB: Physical medicine and rehabilitation approaches to the management of myofascial pain and fibromyalgia syndromes. Baillieres Clin Rheumatol 8:881, 1994.

66. Kraus H: Triggerpoints. NY State J Med 73:1310, 1973.

67. Clark S, Tindall E, Bennett RM: A double-blind crossover trial of prednisone versus placebo in the treatment of fibrositis. J Rheumatol 12:980, 1985.

68. Bennett RM, Gatter RA, Campbell SM, et al.: A comparison of cyclobenzaprine and placebo in the management of fibrositis: a double-blind controlled study. Arthritis Rheum 31:1535, 1988.

69. Carette S, McCain GA, Bell DA, Fam AG: Evaluation of amitriptyline in primary fibrositis. Arthritis Rheum 29:655, 1986.

70. Jaechke R, Adachi J, Guyatt G, et al.: Clinical usefulness of amitriptyline in fibromyalgia: the results of 23 N-of-1 randomized controlled trials. J Rheumatol 18:447, 1991.

71. Carette S, Bell MJ, Reynolds WJ, et al.: Comparison of amitriptyline, cyclobenzaprine, and placebo in the treatment of fibromyalgia: a randomized, double-blind clinical trial. Arthritis Rheum 37:32, 1994.

72. Wysenbeek AJ, Mor F, Lurie Y, Weinberger A: Imipramine for the treatment of fibrositis: a therapeutic trial. Ann Rheum Dis 44:752, 1985.

73. Russell IJ, Fletcher EM, Michalek JE, et al.: Treatment of primary fibrositis/fibromyalgia syndrome with ibuprofen and alprazolam: a double-blind, placebo-controlled study. Arthritis Rheum 34:552, 1991.

74. Wolfe F, Cathey MA, Hawley DJ: A double-blind placebo-controlled trial of fluoxetine in fibromyalgia. Scand J Rheumatol 23:255, 1994.

75. May KP, West SG, Baker MR, et al.: Sleep apnea in male patients with the fibromyalgia syndrome. Am J Med 94:505, 1993.

76. Wood PHN: Rheumatic complaints. Br Med Bull 27:82, 1971.

77. Ledingham J, Doherty S, Doherty M: Primary fibromyalgia syndrome: an outcome study. Br J Rheumatol 32:139, 1993.

78. Hudson JI, Goldenberg DL, Pope HG, et al.: Comorbidity of fibromyalgia with medical and psychiatric disorders. Am J Med 92:363, 1992.

12

Infections of the Cervical Spine

Infections of the cervical spine are uncommon causes of neck pain; however, these disorders must be included in the differential diagnosis of the patient with systemic neck pain. This is particularly important because the outcome of these infections is excellent if the disease processes are recognized early and treated appropriately. When spinal infections are not promptly recognized, however, they can lead to catastrophic complications, including spinal deformity and spinal cord compression with associated paralysis, incontinence, and, ultimately, death.

The clinical symptoms and course of spinal infections depend on the organism involved. Bacterial infections cause acute, toxic symptoms, whereas tuberculous and fungal diseases are more indolent in onset and course. The primary symptom of patients with spinal infection is neck pain that tends to be localized over the anatomic structure involved. Physical examination demonstrates decreased motion, muscle spasm, and percussion tenderness over the involved area. Results of common laboratory tests are not always present, and they are nonspecific. Radiographic abnormalities including vertebral body subchondral bone loss, disc space narrowing, and erosions of contiguous bony structures are helpful when present but often lag behind clinical symptoms by weeks to months. Patients may present with nondescript neck pain ascribed to "degenerative disc disease" on plain roentgenograms, only to develop increasing neck pain, neurologic dysfunction, and marked bony destruction on radiographic evaluation over a short period.

The definitive diagnosis of spinal infection requires identification of the offending organism by culturing aspirated or biopsied material from the lesion. Treatment consists of antimicrobial drugs directed against the specific organism causing the infection, immobilization with bed rest to relieve pain, a cast if spinal instability is present, and surgical drainage of abscesses to relieve spinal cord compression. Patients who have a prompt diagnosis and appropriate antimicrobial therapy are able to combat the infection without residual disability. Significant disability from persistent pain, spinal instability, and spinal cord compression may occur when there has been a delay in diagnosing persistent osteomyelitis or epidural abscess. These patients require surgical decompression and stabilization.

Herpes zoster is a viral infection of dorsal root ganglia that causes severe neck pain in association with a rash. The diagnosis of this infection is easy in the presence of a dermatomal skin rash but quite difficult in the period before the rash appears. Postherpetic neuralgia, a complication of the infection, causes significant morbidity with persistent neck pain, particularly in the elderly population.

Lyme disease is a spirochetal infection caused by *Borrelia burgdorferi*. Neck pain is a manifestation associated with the early stage of the illness and the appearance of a characteristic skin rash, erythema migrans. In later stages of the illness, polyradiculitis affecting the upper extremities may develop. The diagnosis of Lyme disease is established by a history of tick exposure, characteristic symptoms and signs, and confirmatory laboratory tests. The illness is treated by the use of oral or intravenous antibiotics.

VERTEBRAL OSTEOMYELITIS

Capsule Summary

Frequency of neck pain—very common

Location of neck pain—cervical spine, involved bone

Quality of neck pain—sharp ache, radicular with nerve compression

Symptoms and signs—general malaise, percussion tenderness, fever

Laboratory and x-ray tests—leukocytosis, increased erythrocyte sedimentation rate; subchondral bone loss on plain roentgenogram, soft tissue mass on computerized tomography scan, abnormal signal on magnetic resonance imaging

Treatment—antibiotics, immobilization, fusion for instability

Prevalence and Pathogenesis

Vertebral osteomyelitis is a disease process caused by the growth of a potentially wide variety of organisms in the bones that comprise the axial skeleton. These organisms include the following bacteria: *Staphylococcus aureus, Escherichia coli,* and *Brucella abortus*; mycobacteria: *Mycobacterium tuberculosis*; fungi: *Coccidioides immitis*; spirochetes: *Treponema pallidum*; and parasites: *Echinococcus granulosus.* Vertebral osteomyelitis develops most commonly from hematogenous spread through the blood stream. The clinical symptoms and course depend on the infecting organism and the associated host inflammatory response. Bacterial infections are generally associated with an acute, toxic reaction, whereas granulomatous infections caused by tuberculous or fungal organisms are more indolent in onset and course. The diagnosis of vertebral osteomyelitis is frequently missed because patient symptoms are ascribed to more common causes of neck pain, such as muscle strain, and radiographic changes lag behind the evolution of the infection.

Over a 10-year period, 348 cases of vertebral osteomyelitis were reported in the medical literature.[1] Vertebral involvement has been found to account for 2% to 4% of all cases of osteomyelitis.[2] In one study, more than 52% of patients with vertebral osteomyelitis were 50 years of age or older.[3] Another article reviewed 397 vertebral osteomyelitis patients in the literature and reported the mean age of adults with the disease to be from 45 to 62 years of age.[4] Those in the seventh decade of life represented the single largest group. The male-to-female ratio is up to 3:1.

Vertebral body bone is most frequently infected by hematogenous spread through the blood stream. It is supplied by the paravertebral venous system and nutrient arteries.[5, 6] The venous Batson's plexus is a network of valveless veins that lines the vertebral column, and the flow in this venous system is modified by changes in intra-abdominal pressure. Increased pressure tends to force blood from infected areas into the veins of the vertebral column. The presence of cellular bone marrow and the sluggish venous blood flow have been suggested as predisposing factors for bone infection.[7] Although genitourinary infections are more frequent in women than men, the incidence of vertebral osteomyelitis is higher in men. A possible explanation is the highly vascularized tissue around the longer urethra, which may develop metastatic infection after urologic manipulation.[3] Other potential hematogenous sources of infection include soft tissue infection, infective endocarditis, dental extraction, furunculosis, and intravenous drug abuse.[3, 8]

On the other hand, the localization of early foci of osteomyelitis in vertebral bodies in the subchondral region corresponds to an area richly supplied by nutrient arteries.[6] The spread of infection from extraspinal foci is associated with the constitutional symptoms of septicemia. It is probable that both routes may be involved in individual patients.

Infection from contiguous sources, direct implantation by cisternal puncture or disc operations, is relatively rare compared with those caused by hematogenous spread. Occasional patients with vertebral osteomyelitis may have a history of prior trauma to the spine, but trauma usually does not play a role in the pathogenesis of hematogenous vertebral osteomyelitis.[9] Studies of patients with vertebral osteomyelitis and epidural abscess, however, report a significant percentage with a history of substantial trauma prior to the development of the infection.[10] Hematoma associated with trauma can become a culture medium for hematogenously spread organisms. The role of minor trauma, such as muscle strain, as a predisposing factor for vertebral osteomyelitis is uncertain. The importance of unrelated and coincident minor trauma may be overestimated in some patients with vertebral osteomyelitis, thus confusing the diagnosis and delaying the initiation of appropriate antibiotic therapy to the disadvantage of the patient. Injection into the jugular vein by heroin addicts is a form of trauma that is associated with the increased risk of cervical osteomyelitis.[11] Hematogenous or contiguous spread may be the mechanism of infection in patients who develop cervical osteomyelitis after endotracheal intubation, dental extraction, or esophagoscopy.[12–14]

Grisel's syndrome, spontaneous atlantoaxial subluxation in association with infection in neighboring soft tissue structures, may occur secondary to hematogenous spread from the pharyngovertebral veins to the periodontoidal venous plexus.[15] This syndrome occurs in children most often and is associated with infections in the throat, including pharyngitis, tonsillitis, alveolar periostitis, adenitis, and pharyngeal ulcers.[16] These people experience neck pain and torticollis.

Approximately 40% or more of patients with vertebral osteomyelitis have an unequivocal extraspinal primary source for infection.[17] The usual locations for these infections include the genitourinary tract, skin, and respiratory tract (Table 12–1).[4] Parenteral drug abusers also develop vertebral osteomyelitis, particularly with *Pseudomonas aeruginosa*.[18] Any person with a chronic disease that decreases host immunity, such as diabetes mellitus, chronic alcoholism, malignancy, and sickle cell anemia, is also at risk of developing vertebral osteomyelitis.[4] Cervical vertebral osteomyelitis may be a complication of older people with cervical spondylosis who undergo manipulation by a chiropractor.[19]

The organisms gain entrance into the verte-bral bodies in the subchondral area, which is richly supplied by nutrient arterioles on the anterior surface and by the main nutrient artery entering through the posterior vertebral nutrient foramen.[6] The infection may spread across the periphery of the disc to involve the adjacent vertebra or may rupture through the end plates into the disc. The posterior elements are affected less often and later in the course of the infection. The infection spreads through the disc material to reach the opposite end plate and vertebra. The disc material is quickly destroyed by bacterial enzymes. This is in contrast with tuberculous infection that causes bony destruction but little damage to the intervertebral disc.[20] Infection of three or more vertebral bodies is quite rare. Involvement of the posterior elements of the vertebrae is unusual.

An infection of a vertebral body may extend beyond the bone into the soft tissues. Infections in the cervical spine can produce a retropharyngeal abscess that can become very large.[21] Paravertebral masses may cause draining sinuses. Inferior dissection along fascial planes may cause a mediastinitis. The infection may also drain into the spinal canal, causing an epidural abscess, or penetrate the dura, causing a picture of meningitis.[10] In addition, bone destruction may cause instability of the spine, which may result in compression of the spinal cord or nerve roots.[22]

The most frequently encountered organism causing infection is *Staphylococcus aureus* in up to 60% of cases (Table 12–2).[4] In rare circumstances, *S. epidermidis* may cause vertebral osteomyelitis in immunocompetent people.[23] Other gram-positive organisms causing osteomyelitis include streptococci, including *Streptococcus pneumoniae*, and group B streptococci from the vaginal tract.[24] Group G streptococcal osteomyelitis of the spine has been reported in elderly individuals with malignancies.[25] Gram-negative organisms, including *E. coli, Pseudomonas, Klebsiella, Pasteurella,* and *Salmonella,* are relatively uncommon.[26] Other rare gram-negative organisms include *Proteus mirabilis* and polymicrobial infections, including *Bacteroides fragilis.*[27–31] Anaerobic organisms cause infection in 3% or less of patients.[4, 30] Even more infrequent as causes of infection are mycobacteria, fungi, spirochetes, and parasites.

The cervical spine is a rare location for osteomyelitis of the spine. Approximately 8% of patients with vertebral osteomyelitis have cervical involvement (Table 12–3).[4] In intravenous drug users, the cervical vertebrae are involved in 27% of patients with vertebral os-

TABLE 12–1. SOURCE OF INFECTION IN PYOGENIC VERTEBRAL OSTEOMYELITIS (n = 370 patients)

	NUMBER OF PATIENTS	PERCENT OF PATIENTS WITH SOURCE IDENTIFIED
Source identified	188	
Genitourinary tract	87	46
Skin	35	19
Respiratory tract	27	14
Spinal surgery	16	9
Bowel	7	4
Intravenous drug abuse	6	3
Intravenous catheter	5	3
Dental	4	2
Bacterial endocarditis	1	1
No source identified	182	

From Schwartz ST, Spiegel M, Ho G Jr: Bacterial vertebral osteomyelitis and epidural abscess. Semin Spine Surg 2:95, 1990.

TABLE 12–2. BACTERIOLOGY OF PYOGENIC VERTEBRAL OSTEOMYELITIS (n = 220 bacteria)

	NUMBER OF CASES	PERCENT OF BACTERIAL ISOLATES
Gram-positive aerobic cocci	159	72
Staphylococcus aureus	139	63
Staphylococcus coagulase-negative	5	2
Streptococcal species	15	7
Gram-negative aerobic bacilli	55	24
Escherichia coli	35	16
Proteus species	11	5
Pseudomonas species	3	1
Klebsiella species	3	1
Other*	3	1
Anaerobic bacteria†	6	3

Serratia species, *Enterobacter agglomerans, Eikenella corrodens.*
†*Corynebacterium diphtheriae, Bacteroides fragilis, Peptostreptococcus,* and *Propionibacterium.*
From Schwartz ST, Spiegel M, Ho G Jr: Bacterial vertebral osteomyelitis and epidural abscess. Semin Spine Surg 2:95, 1990.

teomyelitis.[31] In a study of 40 patients with vertebral osteomyelitis, 30% had cervical osteomyelitis, 27.5% had thoracic disease, and 42.5% had lumbar infection.[32]

Clinical History

The primary symptom of patients with cervical vertebral osteomyelitis is neck pain. Local spine pain is present in 98% of patients with vertebral osteomyelitis, with radicular symptoms in 30%.[32] Dysphagia and persistent sore throat may be seen in about 11% of patients with cervical spine involvement.[3] Patients may also complain of neck stiffness associated with occipital headache. Pain may develop over 8 to 12 weeks before the diagnosis is established.

TABLE 12–3. VERTEBRAL SITE OF PYOGENIC VERTEBRAL OSTEOMYELITIS (n = 396 patients)

VERTEBRAL SITE	NUMBER OF PATIENTS	PERCENT OF PATIENTS
Cervical	32	8.0
Cervical thoracic	1	0.3
Thoracic	137	35.0
Thoracolumbar	31	8.0
Lumbar	168	42.0
Lumbosacral	26	7.0
Sacral	1	0.3

From Schwartz ST, Spiegel M, Ho G Jr: Bacterial vertebral osteomyelitis and epidural abscess. Semin Spine Surg 2:95, 1990.

A history of a recent primary infection, or an invasive diagnostic procedure, is common. Pain may be intermittent or constant, may be present at rest, and is exacerbated by motion. Paralysis is an occasional complication of cervical vertebral osteomyelitis.[33]

Patients with certain underlying illnesses may develop vertebral osteomyelitis secondary to specific organisms. *S. aureus* is associated with soft tissue infection, endocarditis, or infected intravenous lines. Pneumococci are associated with respiratory infection. Those with diabetes mellitus or chronic urinary tract infections develop vertebral osteomyelitis secondary to gram-negative bacteria.[9] Parenteral drug abusers develop *Pseudomonas* and *Candida* osteomyelitis.[34] Patients with sickle-cell anemia may get *Salmonella* osteomyelitis. Fungal osteomyelitis secondary to *Candida* has been reported to complicate vertebral osteomyelitis previously infected with *Serratia marcescens.*[35]

Brucellosis, a disease caused by *Brucella,* affects patients who ingest unpasteurized milk products, or more commonly, since the advent of pasteurization, workers involved with meat processing.[36] The infection, passed from lower animals, cattle, or hogs to humans, occurs in government meat inspectors, veterinarians, farmers, stockworkers, rendering-plant workers, and laboratory personnel. The *Brucella* organism, *Brucella melitensis,* the most virulent, *Brucella suis, Brucella canis,* or *B. abortus,* penetrates the mucous membranes of the oropharynx or enters through breaks in the skin, traverses the lymph nodes, and enters the blood stream where it spreads to the reticuloendothelial system. The clinical manifestations of brucellosis vary and may be classified into asymptomatic or serologic, acute systemic or localized, and chronic or relapsing forms.[37] The most common complication is osseous, occurring in up to 70% of cases. Patients with brucella spondylitis are men, older than 50 years of age, with preexisting spine disease.[38] The lumbosacral spine is affected most often, with cervical spine disease a rare occurrence.[39–42] The range of involvement of the cervical spine is between 1% to 3% in large study populations from endemic areas.[43, 44] The disease has an insidious onset with intermittent fever, chills, weakness, weight loss, and headache. Patients commonly complain of tenderness of pain over the vertebral bodies, which is worse with activity and relieved by rest.[43, 44] Radiation of pain is associated with nerve root irritation of a mechanical or inflammatory nature.[44]

Elderly patients, alcoholics, and drug abusers are at greatest risk of developing vertebral osteomyelitis secondary to *M. tuberculosis*.[45] Prior to antibiotic therapy, children were most frequently affected, but more recent data from patients with skeletal tuberculosis in the United States show average ages of 40 to 51 years.[46, 47] Skeletal tuberculosis occurs as a result of hematogenous spread from another source, usually pulmonary, during an acute infection; or as a reactivation of a quiescent focus present in bone for many years after initial seeding.[48, 49] From 50% to 60% of patients with skeletal tuberculosis have axial skeletal disease.[48] This may be explained in part by the affinity of this organism to relatively high oxygen concentrations that exist in the cancellous bone of the vertebral bodies. Tuberculous spondylitis begins in the subchondral area of the vertebral body adjacent to the intervertebral disc, and the organism creates an inflammatory process characterized by the formation of granulomas and caseation necrosis of bone. Initially, only the vertebral body is affected; however, the infection can spread to involve contiguous structures, which include the intervertebral disc, other vertebral bodies, and soft tissues such as muscle and ligaments, to form a paravertebral abscess, or can spread to the spinal cord and meninges. The more extensive the destruction, the greater the potential for deformity of the axial skeleton with kyphoscoliosis and associated spinal cord compression.[50] Cervical involvement is a rare complication of tuberculous osteomyelitis. In a review of 1,000 people with skeletal tuberculosis, cervical involvement was identified in 3.5%.[51] In people with tuberculosis, the cervical spine is affected in 0.03%.[52]

The clinical presentation of a patient with tuberculous osteomyelitis consists of two primary forms. Younger children develop more diffuse and extensive involvement, the formation of the large abscesses, and a lower incidence of quadriplegia. The adult type is more localized and produces less pus but has a higher incidence of paraplegia.[53] In children, pain is found over the involved vertebrae associated with stiffness and with radiation into a shoulder or upper extremity. Low-grade fever and weight loss of varying duration may occur. Patients with more advanced disease may present with neurologic symptoms. Angular deformities of the neck with loss of height occurs less commonly than lesions in the thoracic spine unless three or more vertebral bodies are involved, because the weight of the head is borne through the articular processes rather than the vertebral body. However, when infec-

tion in the lower cervical spine spreads down to the upper dorsal region, forward subluxation or dislocation of the cervical spine may occur on the thoracic spine so that the undersurface of the lowest remaining cervical vertebra comes to rest on the anterior surface of the uppermost thoracic vertebra.[51] These lesions may heal with spontaneous fusion of the posterior apophyseal joints.

The second primary form affects adults. The disease is more localized and does not spread as extensively as it does in children. However, quadriplegia is a more common complication of the infection in adults. In a series of 40 patients, 13 of 16 older than 10 years of age with tuberculosis of the lower cervical spine had cord compression versus 4 of 24 younger than 10 years of age.[53] Possible explanations for the increased frequency of quadriplegia may include progressive narrowing of the spinal canal from degenerative disease, loss of flexibility, and inelasticity of the prevertebral fascia.[51] Tuberculous osteomyelitis in adults may spread over more than one intervertebral segment in the cervical spine.[54] This occurs as the infection lifts the supporting longitudinal ligaments and spreads to contiguous structures. The disease may also present as a lesion of a single intervertebral segment or a vertebral body. Solitary lesions are not uncommon in the upper and lower portions of the cervical spine, including the atlantoaxial area.[55–57]

The onset of symptoms is gradual and the time before presentation to a physician may be as long as 3 years.[58] Paraplegia may be the first manifestation of tuberculous spondylitis even before any deformity of the spine is apparent.[59] General symptoms of malaise, fever, weight loss, night sweats, and fatigue precede the onset of neck pain and stiffness. Pain from lower neck involvement may refer to the shoulders and arms. Upper cervical spine disease may cause occipital or forehead referred pain. Pharyngeal symptoms may be present if an anterior abscess has formed in the retropharyngeal area. Heroin addicts may present with a more toxic picture associated with neck pain, fever, night sweats, weight loss, and neurologic dysfunction of rapid evolution.[45]

Infections secondary to *Actinomyces israelii*, *Nocardia asteroides*, and fungal organisms such as *C. immitis* are rare causes of vertebral osteomyelitis that may affect the cervical spine. Patients with actinomyces infection of the spine may develop lesions from extension of adjacent abscesses or from hematogenous spread.[60, 61] Actinomycosis may be the cause of anaerobic infection in patients with infected wounds of the face. The clinical course of these infections is similar to that of tuberculosis. These patients present with a history of constitutional symptoms over an extended period and complain of localized pain over the affected vertebral body.[62] *Nocardia*, an aerobic, gram-positive actinomycete, may cause hematogenous spread to vertebral bones in the patients with underlying immunodeficiency.[63] Cervical spine infection with *Nocardia* has been reported.[64] Coccidioidomycosis may affect the spine in 50% of the 0.5% of patients with disseminated disease.[65] Coccidioidomycosis may infect the upper cervical spine.[66]

Before the advent of penicillin, syphilis was a common cause of axial skeleton infection, but it is currently an extremely rare complication.[67, 68] Syphilis may affect the axial skeleton by direct infection of bone or by the loss of normal sensation.[69] Both forms are a result of tertiary syphilis, which is the form of the disease that occurs after the initial infection (primary) and hematogenous spread (secondary) of the organism. The pain is associated with arthritis in larger joints as well as other clinical manifestations of secondary syphilis. The growth of the organism in bone results in the formation of a gumma and bony destruction.[70] The cervical spine is the most frequently affected in the axial skeleton. The most common symptom is pain in the involved area, which is greatest at night, and is accompanied with stiffness and loss of normal spinal curvatures. Patients may develop neurologic symptoms including radicular pain secondary to nerve root impingement.[71] Patients with neurosyphilis, on the other hand, lose normal sensation; without this protective awareness, fractures and destruction of the bony skeleton result. This is called a neuropathic arthropathy or Charcot's disease. These patients feel little pain and are frequently symptom-free.

Echinococcus granulosus is a cestode worm of the dog.[72] Intermediate hosts for the ova of this worm are sheep, cattle, hogs, and humans. The ova attach to the intestinal mucosa and gain entrance to the blood stream where they disseminate, particularly to the liver and occasionally to bone where they form cysts (hydatid disease). The skeleton is affected in about 3% of patients with hydatid disease, and 50% of those cases are found in the spine.[73] The disease produces a slowly destructive lesion of bone that, in the spine, erodes through the vertebral bodies and can rupture into the neural canal. The cysts then migrate up and down the canal. Patients with hydatid disease of the spine have symptoms that can last from a few weeks to 5 years. Pain is a common symptom associated with swelling. Occasionally painless paraplegia of sudden onset may be the presenting sign of disease. Patients who develop paraplegia either die from the disease or are chronically disabled.[74]

Physical Examination

Physical findings in patients with vertebral osteomyelitis include a decreased range of motion, muscle spasm, and percussion tenderness over the involved bone. Patients with cervical osteomyelitis may have muscle spasm, torticollis, or Horner's syndrome.[75] They may also have tenderness over the midline and occiput, with pain exacerbation on head compression. An abscess anterior to the spine may be palpable near the throat. Some of the patients with bacterial vertebral osteomyelitis have a fever.[76, 77] A fever of greater than 100°F was calculated at 52% of one series of vertebral osteomyelitis patients.[78] Neurologic abnormalities, including paraplegia, are reported in a number of series of patients with vertebral osteomyelitis.[9, 79, 80] In one study, patients who developed paralysis had a period from symptoms to diagnosis of 3 months and were diabetic or had a urinary tract infection.[81] Patients with the more indolent infections of tuberculosis and coccidioidomycosis usually have less fever but greater spinal deformity than those with pyogenic vertebral osteomyelitis.

Laboratory Data

The commonly ordered blood tests (complete blood count, erythrocyte sedimentation rate [ESR], and serum chemistries) yield results that are normal or nonspecific. The ESR is abnormal in the majority of patients with vertebral osteomyelitis, particularly during the acute phase.[9, 76] In a study by Joughin and colleagues, ESR was better than fever or leukocytosis as a marker of vertebral osteomyelitis.[82] The hematocrit level may be normal, and there is a normal or slightly elevated white blood cell count. A small but significant number of patients have normal ESR and white blood cell counts.[83]

The most useful laboratory test for the diagnosis of vertebral osteomyelitis is the direct culture of blood and bone lesions. This may be abnormal in 50% of patients with acute osteomyelitis and negate the need for bone biopsy. In patients with normal blood cultures, bone aspiration or surgical biopsy produces material that on culture is often abnormal for the offending organism.[49] *S. aureus* is the bacterium associated with vertebral osteomyelitis in up to 60% of patients.[77, 80] Gram-negative organisms, *E. coli, Proteus,* and *Pseudomonas,* are often grown from elderly patients and parenteral drug abusers with vertebral osteomyelitis. When an infection in the cervical spine is secondary to penetrating trauma, cultures for multiple organisms are appropriate. In cases of stab wounds to the cervical spine, *Staphylococcus pyogenes* with *Bacteroides melaninogenicus* and *Streptococcus viridans* with *Candida albicans* have been identified on culture.[84] Cultures from peripheral sources of infection, such as urinary tract, skin, and respiratory tract, may be abnormal and should be obtained from the patient with suspected vertebral osteomyelitis. The diagnosis of brucellosis is associated with an abnormal bone culture or elevations in brucellar agglutinin titers of 1:32 or greater. Radioimmunoassay and enzyme-linked immunosorbent assay methods for *Brucella* antigens are also available.[85, 86] In general, immunoglobulin M (IgM) antibodies are associated with acute brucellosis, and IgG antibodies are associated with chronic infection.[87]

The purified protein derivative test is usually positive for patients with tuberculous spondylitis, unless they are anergic secondary to miliary disease. The number of organisms in an infected spine is less than 1 million bacteria. Therefore, it is appropriate to culture both purulent material and biopsy specimens to improve the potential for a positive culture.[88] Histologic evidence of granulomas suggests tuberculous or fungal infection. The ESR is rarely elevated in tuberculous spondylitis. As far as fungal infections are concerned, antibody titers may be raised or skin tests may be reactive, but none of these tests are as specific as the growth of organisms from either aspirated material or biopsy specimens. The laboratory abnormalities of tertiary syphilis include the presence of antibodies to nontreponemal (Venereal Disease Research Laboratory test) and treponemal (fluorescent treponemal antibody absorption test) antigens. Spirochetal organisms are not usually found in tertiary lesions on histologic examination. The histologic changes include a granulomatous necrotizing process with a prominent obliterative endarteritis.

Radiographic Evaluation

Radiographic changes follow the symptomatic onset of disease by 1 to 2 months (Table 12–4). The early abnormalities in pyogenic vertebral osteomyelitis include subchondral bone loss, narrowing of the disc space, and loss of definition of vertebral body. Continued dissemination of infection may produce soft tissue swelling associated with paravertebral abscesses. In the cervical spine, retropharyngeal swelling can lead to displacement and obliteration of contiguous prevertebral fat planes[89] (Fig. 12–1). Once the lesion starts to heal, bony regeneration appears and is characterized by osteosclerosis, which may finally result in bony fusion across the disc space. Conventional tomograms may be done to obtain better bony and soft tissue details than plain films.

Brucellar spondylitis causes narrowing of the intervertebral disc space and destruction of the contiguous vertebrae, which may be associated with a large paravertebral abscess. Bone sclerosis with parrot-beak exostosis is a late roentgenographic sign and usually indicates the stage of healing.[44]

The vertebral body is more commonly af-

TABLE 12–4. TIMETABLE FOR RADIOGRAPHIC FINDINGS IN BACTERIAL VERTEBRAL OSTEOMYELITIS

PERIOD	TIME OF APPEARANCE	OBSERVATIONS
1	3–6 weeks	Rarefaction of adjacent body end plates Widening of paraspinal lines Intervertebral space narrowing
2	6–10 weeks	Lytic scalloping and destruction of vertebral body end plates Compression of vertebral body as a result of central osteolysis Paravertebral soft tissue mass (abscess)
3	8–12 weeks	Reactive sclerosis
4	12–24 weeks	New bone formation with bony bridging of disc spaces
5	24 weeks and longer	Bony fusion of vertebral bodies

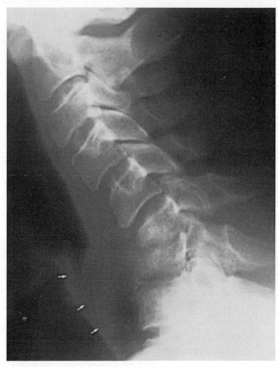

Figure 12–1. Vertebral osteomyelitis. A 41-year-old man with osteomyelitis involving C6 and C7. The infection has spread across the disc space, involving contiguous vertebral bodies. A soft tissue mass is noted anterior to the vertebral bodies *(arrows)*. (Courtesy of Anne Brower, M.D.)

fected than posterior elements in tuberculous spondylitis; they are affected in only 2% of spinal tuberculous cases. The infection causes erosion of the subchondral bone and invades the disc space. These changes occur much less rapidly with tuberculous spondylitis than with pyogenic spondylitis. The infection may also spread to soft tissue, forming paraspinal abscesses. In this form, the anterior cortex of the vertebral body is destroyed. Severe angular deformities occur from marked destruction of vertebral bodies. Vertebral bodies may appear wedge-shaped while the disc spaces are preserved. The lesion may look like a vertebra plana and may be confused with eosinophilic granuloma. The reactive sclerosis characteristic of healing pyogenic vertebral osteomyelitis does not occur with tuberculous spondylitis. In many patients the disease is limited to two contiguous vertebrae, although four or more segments may be involved.

Fungal infections of the spine spare the intervertebral discs, involve the anterior and posterior elements of the vertebral body, and rarely cause vertebral collapse, particularly with infections secondary to actinomycosis and coccidioidomycosis.[90] Actinomycosis causes

lytic lesions of bone surrounded by a rim of sclerotic new bone. The disc is spared although soft tissue abscesses may be present.[91] Coccidioidal spondylitis affects one or more vertebral bodies with paraspinal masses. This infection spares the discs and rarely causes vertebral collapse. The lesions are radiolucent and well demarcated. Periosteal new bone is seen, but sclerosis is infrequent.[92, 93]

Radiographic changes in the spine may include marked destruction and dissolution of bone in Charcot's arthropathy of the spine (neuropathic) and may show lysis and sclerosis in bone from gummatous osseous lesions (spirochetal infection).[69, 94] Periosteal changes may also be present.

In hydatid disease, the vertebral column is a common osseous location for this infection.[95] Hydatid disease is associated with single or multiple expansile osteolytic lesions containing altered trabeculae. Soft tissue calcification may also be seen, but periosteal new bone formation is unusual.[96]

Plain roentgenograms may be normal in patients with vertebral osteomyelitis. Plain roentgenograms might have the greatest opportunity to detect axial skeletal abnormalities in patients who are 50 years of age or older, have long duration of symptoms, and have point vertebral tenderness.[97] Others have suggested that younger people with risk factors, such as intravenous drug abuse, are appropriate candidates for plain roentgenographic evaluation.[98] Once again, good clinical judgment should guide the physician to the use of appropriate tests.

Bone scintigraphy demonstrates abnormalities in the area of infection at an earlier stage of disease than do plain radiographs. A bone scan may also demonstrate areas of involvement other than the one that is symptomatic. Technetium 99 bone scans become abnormal within 72 hours of infection and have about a 75% specificity for the diagnosis.[99] False-positive and false-negative results do occur, and increased uptake on bone scan may be caused by tumor, trauma, or arthritis. Normal bone scans may occur if the test is completed too early in the course of the disease.[100] The combination of technetium and indium scans can add specificity to the 90% sensitivity in the diagnosis of osteomyelitis.[101]

Computerized tomography (CT) may show bony changes prior to their appearance on routine radiographs. The extent of soft tissue abscesses is also more easily visualized by this method.[11, 102] CT may also be used to follow the course of illness after therapy is initiated.

Difficulties in the CT diagnosis of vertebral osteomyelitis can occur when the radiographic features believed to be pathognomonic of specific disease entities, such as vertebral malignancy and severe degenerative disc disease, are present that may be confused with characteristics of osteomyelitis.[101]

The value of magnetic resonance (MR) imaging in the diagnosis of vertebral infections continues to grow.[103] MR imaging changes correspond to the extent of the inflammatory process and increased water content in production of exudates containing white blood cells and fibrin. Variations in marrow signal are also noted with decreased T_1-weighted image and increased signal on T_2-weighted image. MR imaging has a high sensitivity for inflammatory processes in soft tissue or bone. It has a sensitivity exceeding that of plain films and CT scan and approaches that of scintiscans.[104] It is abnormal when other radiographic techniques, such as scintigraphic and CT scans, are normal.[105]

In patients with bacterial vertebral osteomyelitis, MR imaging is able to determine the involvement of the vertebral bodies and intervening disc and the extent of the extraosseous infection into the surrounding soft tissues.[105] The MR findings associated with tuberculous spondylitis that are different from bacterial vertebral osteomyelitis include the lack of abnormal signal of the intervertebral disc space, the involvement of the posterior elements rather than the end plates, and the presence of large paraspinal soft tissue masses[106] (Fig. 12–2). These findings are not specific for tuberculosis. Patients with fungal infection of the spine may also demonstrate similar MR findings, including preservation of disc height, destruction of posterior elements, and paravertebral masses.[107] Gadolinium-enhanced MR imaging has advantages over nonenhanced MR imaging in the evaluation of spinal infections.[108] Enhanced MR imaging detects the presence of epidural abscesses. This technique also localizes the portion of a lesion that is most active and documents a response to antibiotic therapy.

Differential Diagnosis

The definitive diagnosis of vertebral osteomyelitis is based on the recovery and identification of the causative organism from aspirated material or biopsy.[109] Clinical history, physical examination, and laboratory investigations are too nonspecific to ensure an accurate diagnosis.[110] A presumptive diagnosis may be accepted as indication for specific antibiotic therapy when the clinical and radiographic presentations are characteristic and abnormal blood cultures are obtained. When cultures are negative for growth, trochar aspiration from bone or needle aspiration from a retropharyngeal abscess may identify the source of

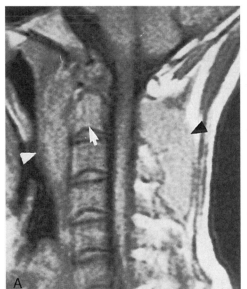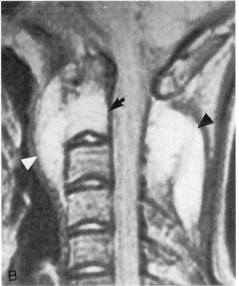

Figure 12–2. Tuberculous spondylitis: atlantoaxial destruction. In a 23-year-old man, sagittal T_1-weighted (TR/TE 450/30) *(A)* and T_2-weighted (TR/TE 1800/50) *(B)* spin echo magnetic resonance images reveal tuberculous involvement of the upper cervical spine. Findings include abnormalities of the axis *(arrows)* with anterior and posterior extension of the process *(arrowheads)*. (Courtesy of T. Mattsson, M.D., Riyadh, Saudi Arabia.)

the infection. Open vertebral biopsy may be required in the cervical spine because the chance for damage of the esophagus and vertebral artery with closed biopsy is real.[21] Conditions confused with vertebral osteomyelitis include discitis, metastatic tumors, multiple myeloma, eosinophilic granuloma, aneurysmal bone cyst, giant cell tumor of bone, and sarcoidosis. MR evaluation may help differentiate infection from other pathologic processes, but culture evidence of the causative organism is required.[111] The appropriate diagnosis is reached by careful review of biopsy material. If in doubt, biopsy of the lesions of the vertebral body must be performed. Only after biopsy is it possible to differentiate tuberculosis from sarcoidosis, myeloma, other tumors, and osteomyelitis.

On occasion more than one vertebral body is affected by osteomyelitis. Although in most instances simultaneous involvement occurs in contiguous vertebral bodies, involvement of distant vertebrae may occur. A bone scan showing two or more areas of increased uptake in the spine may be inappropriately attributed to metastases, compression fractures, or osteoarthritis.[77]

Treatment

Therapy for vertebral osteomyelitis includes antibiotics, bed rest, and immobilization. The goals for therapy for cervical osteomyelitis are eradication of the offending organism, mini-

mization of instability or deformity, and preservation of neurologic function. In patients with retropharyngeal abscess and no vertebral deformity, needle aspiration suffices to obtain culture material and for drainage. However, patients with bony destruction and deformity require an open biopsy from an anterior approach that allows for adequate drainage and definitive reconstruction.[21]

The choice of antibiotic therapy is decided by the organism causing the infection and its sensitivity to specific agents. Gram-positive bacteria such as *Staphylococcus* require penicillin or semisynthetic penicillin (nafcillin), and gram-negative bacteria are sensitive to aminoglycosides or to third-generation cephalosporins. Patients are treated for 4 to 6 weeks with parenteral antibiotics, followed by a course of oral antibiotics that may have a duration of as long as 6 months (Table 12–5). Others have suggested a shorter course of therapy of about 3 weeks to decrease the risk of antibiotic reactions.[112] In a study of 65 patients with vertebral osteomyelitis, 25% had relapse of infection when treated less than 28 days.[28] With more effective antibiotics, the need for prolonged therapy may be diminished. However, the correct duration of therapy depends on the results of ongoing studies and the clinical response of the individual patient with the infection. Bed rest is helpful in decreasing pain by limiting motion. Some patients require a collar as a temporary means to decrease neck pain.

Brucellosis may be treated with oral tetracy-

TABLE 12–5. ANTIMICROBIAL THERAPY FOR ADULT VERTEBRAL OSTEOMYELITIS

ORGANISM	PREFERRED INTRAVENOUS (IV) THERAPY	PREFERRED ORAL THERAPY	ALTERNATIVE THERAPY
Staphylococcus aureus (methicillin-sensitive)	Nafcillin, 2 g/4 h	Clindamycin, 300 mg/6 h	Clindamycin, 900 mg 8 h IV
S. aureus (methicillin-resistant)	Vancomycin, 1 g/12 h	NA	NA
Streptococcus A	Penicillin G, 3 million U/4 h	Penicillin-VK, 500 mg/ 6 h + probenecid	Clindamycin, 900 mg/8 h IV
Streptococcus D (enterococci)	Ampicillin, 2 g/4 h + Gentamicin, 1–1.5 mg/kg/ 8 h	NA	Vancomycin, 1 g/12 h IV + Gentamicin, 1–1.5 mg/kg/8 h
Escherichia coli	Ceftriaxone, 1 g/24 h or Cefazolin, 1 g/8 h	Trimethoprim/ sulfamethoxazole DS 12 h Ciprofloxacin, 500 mg/12 h	Trimethoprim/sulfamethoxazole 10 mg/kg/d 12 h IV Ciprofloxacin, 400 mg 12 h IV
Klebsiella pneumoniae	Ceftriaxone, 1 g/24 h	Trimethoprim/ sulfamethoxazole DS 12 h Ciprofloxacin, 500 mg/12 h	Trimethoprim/sulfamethoxazole 10 mg/kg/d 12 h IV Ciprofloxacin, 400 mg 12 h IV
Pseudomonas aeruginosa	Ceftazidime, 2 g 8 h IV or Ciprofloxacin, 400 mg/12 h	Ciprofloxacin, 750 mg/12 h	Imipenem, 500 mg/6 h
Bacteroides	Metronidazole, 500 mg/6 h	Clindamycin, 300 mg/6 h	Clindamycin, 900 mg/8 h IV

Choice of antibiotic should be matched to organism sensitivities determined with culture. Antibiotics listed in this table may be used as initial therapy until sensitivity results are available.

Modified from Norden C, Gillespie WJ, Nade S: Infections in Bones and Joints. Boston: Blackwell Scientific Publications, 1994, pp 211–230; Stausbaugh LJ: Vertebral osteomyelitis. In: Jauregui LE (ed): Diagnosis and Management of Bone Infections. New York: Marcel Dekker, 1995, pp 167–200; and Gary Simon, M.D.

cline at a dose of 2 gm/day. Therapy should continue for 3 to 4 weeks. In severe cases, 0.5 gm of streptomycin is injected twice a day for a similar period.

The current recommendation for treatment of tuberculosis in the United States is a first-line, three-drug regimen including isoniazid (300 mg/day), rifampin (600 mg/day), and pyrazinamide (up to 2 gm/day) for 2 months. Two drugs (rifampin and isoniazid) are continued for an extended period, usually 18 months. Drug-resistant tuberculosis is becoming an increasingly frequent problem.[113] Additional drugs for longer periods are required to control these infections. Patients may require a regimen of five to seven drugs for control of the drug-resistant organism.[114] The actual duration of therapy depends on the clinical response of the patient with osseous tuberculosis.[115]

Fungal osteomyelitis requires parenteral amphotericin B therapy at a dose that the patient can tolerate without developing renal dysfunction. A total dose of 2.5 gm is usually employed as the initial course of therapy. Bone lesions, however, may be resistant to chemotherapy and may require surgical débridement. Immobilization is required for these patients as well.

Patients with tertiary syphilis without neurologic involvement are effectively treated with penicillin. Long-acting penicillin, benzathine penicillin G at 2.4 million units intramuscularly weekly for 3 weeks, is usually used. Patients who are allergic to penicillin may take tetracycline or erythromycin.

Hydatid disease has been resistant to most anthelmintic therapy. Mebendazole has shown some efficacy in preliminary studies. Definitive therapy requires surgical excision of cysts, with care being taken to remove them totally. In patients with neurologic dysfunction and hydatid disease, anterior spinal decompression and fusion along with mebendazole therapy is associated with good neural recovery.[116]

Surgical procedures on the spine are needed in patients with vertebral osteomyelitis for abscess, spinal cord compression and neurologic defect, severe deformity, persistent symptoms and elevated ESR, and open biopsy to obtain culture material. Another indication for surgical intervention is the presence of spinal instability in association with osteomyelitis.[112] Many surgeons use an anterior approach to reach the cervical spine if multiple segments are affected. Laminectomy is not indicated in patients with vertebral osteomyelitis because the removal of bone results in increased spinal column instability, dislocation, and spinal cord compression.[117] A number of surgeons include interbody fusion along with anterior débridement as a means for obtaining neural decompression in combination with spinal stability.[118, 119]

Prognosis

The improvement in vertebral osteomyelitis may be monitored by following the decrease in a patient's symptoms, pain, and fever and the return of the ESR to normal. With early diagnosis and appropriate therapy, vertebral osteomyelitis resolves with minimal disability in the patient.[120] The case fatality rate in the antibiotic era is less than 5%.[121] Relapses may occur in 10% of individuals who receive inadequate type of duration of antibiotic. When the diagnosis is delayed and the infection spreads to involve the spinal cord by compression (resulting in epidural abscess and granulation tissue) or direct extension (meningitis), potentially life-threatening complications may occur.[10, 58] Anterior decompression is not free of risks in that osteomyelitis and vertebral artery injury may be complications of the operation.[122]

Epidural Abscess. A number of large series have been published reviewing the clinical manifestations, diagnostic evaluation, treatment modalities, prognostic indicators, and final outcomes of 112 patients with epidural abscesses.[123–125] In one large series, epidural abscess occurred in 1.2 per 10,000 hospital admissions.[10] A lower rate of 0.8 cases per 10,000 admissions was noted in another study.[118] Epidural infection occurs more commonly in men in most studies. Predisposing disorders include diabetes mellitus, alcoholism, intravenous drug abuse, and cirrhosis. Although osteoarthritis of the spine is present in a number of patients with epidural abscess, the degenerative abnormalities are not a risk factor for infection.[4] Although the source of an epidural infection may be distant (dental abscess) or local (decubitus ulcer), most often the source is unknown.[126] In a study of 45 patients the posterior epidural space in the cervical and cervicothoracic junction was the location for epidural abscess in 20% of cases.[123] Cervical epidural abscess is also described in occasional patients with osteomyelitis.[127–129]

The clinical manifestations of this infection occur secondary to direct compression by the abscess or granulation tissue or thrombosis of subarachnoid vessels. Neck pain is common but not universally seen in all patients who are unable to report their pain. The progression of symptoms goes from local spinal pain to root pain, then weakness, and finally quadriparesis. Neurologic findings appear with the onset of radicular symptoms. Spinal tenderness as well as fever, sweats, or rigors are present in the majority of patients. The course of symptoms may be days to several months.[130]

Laboratory data in the form of peripheral white blood cell counts and ESR are not helpful because they are normal or nonspecifically elevated. Blood cultures are positive for the infecting organism about 50% to 95% of the time, depending on the study group.[4, 123] In a study of 23 cases of cervical epidural abscess, a bacteriologic agent was identified in 91% of patients.[131] *S. aureus* is the predominant pathogen. The diagnosis is established by culture of cerebrospinal fluid (CSF). CSF is abnormal in 97% of patients, including elevated protein concentrations, low glucose levels, or pleocytosis. CSF cultures may be positive for bacterial growth in the setting of a normal CSF white blood cell count.

Radiographic evaluation of the spine is helpful in identifying the location and extent of the abscess. Roentgenograms of the spine reveal vertebral changes of osteomyelitis in 44%.[123] Technetium bone scan may be abnormal in most patients, and gallium scan may miss the location of the abscess in about one third of patients. Scintiscans are abnormal if underlying osteomyelitis is present in the setting of the epidural abscess. CT with intrathecal contrast establishes the presence of spinal cord encroachment in a majority. MR imaging is superior to CT/myelogram in defining the extent of the lesion. MR imaging is able to determine the extent of the cervical abscess in the spinal canal, the extraspinal extent of the lesion, the presence of intramedullary infection, and the presence of osteomyelitis in the contiguous vertebral bodies.[132] The use of gadolinium contrast for MR helps to delineate lesions that may be equivocal with plain MR testing.[133, 134] MR imaging is also able to document the response to therapy noninvasively.[134] In a study of 60 patients with epidural infection, 19 (32%) had cervical spine disease. MR imaging was able to locate the three vertebral bodies that showed abnormal bone marrow signal in the setting of epidural inflammation that extended an average of four levels. The most frequently involved levels in association with epidural abscess were C5 and C6. MR imaging documented spinal cord compression in 74% of patients.[135]

Therapy includes the use of antibiotics and

drainage of the abscess without causing instability of the spine. Speed in making the diagnosis is essential for obtaining a good outcome. Patients diagnosed within 36 hours of the onset of symptoms have minimal residual weakness. No recovery is observed in patients with paralysis for longer than 48 hours.[136] Mortality rates from epidural abscess range from 5% to 23%.[123, 136] These patients are significantly older than the rest of the patients who survive. Morbidity remains a significant problem when the cervical spinal cord is affected and the diagnosis is delayed.

References

VERTEBRAL OSTEOMYELITIS

1. Waldvogel FA, Vasey H: Osteomyelitis: the past decade. N Engl J Med 303:360, 1980.
2. Kulowski J: Pyogenic osteomyelitis of the spine: an analysis and discussion of 102 cases. J Bone Joint Surg 18A:343, 1936.
3. Sapico F, Montgomerie JZ: Pyogenic vertebral osteomyelitis: report of nine cases and review of the literatures. Rev Infect Dis 1:754, 1979.
4. Schwartz ST, Spiegel M, Ho G Jr: Bacterial vertebral osteomyelitis and epidural abscess. Semin Spine Surg 2:95, 1990.
5. Batson OV: The function of the vertebral veins and their role in the spread of metastases. Ann Surg 112:138, 1940.
6. Wiley AM, Trueta J: The vascular anatomy of the spine and its relationship to pyogenic vertebral osteomyelitis. J Bone Joint Surg 41B:796, 1959.
7. Adatepe MH, Parnell OM, Issacs GH, et al.: Hematogenous pyogenic vertebral osteomyelitis: diagnostic value of radionuclide bone imaging. J Nucl Med 27:1680, 1986.
8. Holzman RS, Bishko F: Osteomyelitis in heroin addicts. Ann Intern Med 75:693, 1971.
9. Garcia A Jr, Grantham SA: Hematogenous pyogenic vertebral osteomyelitis. J Bone Joint Surg 42A:429, 1960.
10. Baker AS, Ojemann RG, Swartz MN, Richardson EP Jr: Spinal epidural abscess. N Engl J Med 293:463, 1975.
11. Endress C, Guyot DR, Fata J, Salciccioli G: Cervical osteomyelitis due to IV heroin use: radiologic findings in 14 patients. AJR 155:3333, 1990.
12. Lloyd TV, Johnson JC: Infectious cervical spondylitis following traumatic endotracheal intubation. Spine 5:478, 1980.
13. Pinckney LE, Currarino G, Higgenboten CL: Osteomyelitis of the cervical spine following dental extraction. Radiology 135:335, 1980.
14. Barr RJ, Hannon DG, Adair IV, et al.: Cervical osteomyelitis after rigid esophagoscopy: brief report. J Bone Joint Surg 70B:147, 1988.
15. Parke WW, Rothman RH, Brown MD: The pharyngovertebral veins: an anatomic rationale for Grisel's syndrome. J Bone Joint Surg 66A:568, 1984.
16. Wetzel FT, La Rocca H: Grisel's syndrome: a review. Clin Orthop 240:141, 1989.
17. Ross PM, Fleming JL: Vertebral body osteomyelitis: spectrum and natural history: a retrospective analysis of 37 cases. Clin Orthop 118:190, 1976.

18. Kido D, Bryan D, Halpern M: Hematogenous osteomyelitis in drug addicts. AJR 118:356, 1973.

19. Lewis M, Grundy D: Vertebral osteomyelitis following manipulation of spondylitic necks: a possible risk. Paraplegia 30:788, 1992.

20. Compere EL, Garrison M: Correlation of pathologic and roentgenologic findings in tuberculosis and pyogenic infections of the vertebrae. Ann Surg 104:1038, 1936.

21. LaRocca SH, Eismont FJ: Other infectious diseases. In: Sherk HH, Dunn EJ, Eismont FJ, et al.: The Cervical Spine, 2nd ed. Philadelphia: JB Lippincott Co, 1989, pp 552–563.

22. Heary RF, Hunt CD, Wolansky LJ: Rapid bony destruction with pyogenic vertebral osteomyelitis. Surg Neurol 41:34, 1994.

23. De Wit D, Mulla R, Cowie MR, et al.: Vertebral osteomyelitis due to *Staphylococcus epidermidis*. Br J Rheumatol 32:339, 1993.

24. Lischke JH, McCreight PHB: Maternal group B streptococcal vertebral osteomyelitis: an unusual complication of vaginal delivery. Obstet Gynecol 76:489, 1990.

25. Hall M, Williams A: Group G streptococcal osteomyelitis of the spine. Br J Rheumatol 32:342, 1993.

26. Byrne FD, Thrall TM, Wheat LJ: Hematogenous vertebral osteomyelitis: *Pasteurella multocida* as the causative agent. Arch Intern Med 139:1182, 1979.

27. Redfern RM, Cottam SN, Phillipson AP: *Proteus* infection of the spine. Spine 13:439, 1988.

28. Charles RW, Mody GM, Govender S: Pyogenic infection of the lumbar vertebral spine due to gas-forming organisms. Spine 14:541, 1989.

29. Feng J, Austin TW: Anaerobic vertebral osteomyelitis. Can Med Assoc J 145:132, 1991.

30. Incavo SJ, Muller DL, Krag MH, Gump D: Vertebral osteomyelitis caused by *Clostridium difficile*. Spine 13:111, 1988.

31. Sapico FL, Montgomerie JZ: Vertebral osteomyelitis. Infect Dis Clin North Am 4:539, 1990.

32. Osenbach RK, Hitchon PW, Menezes AH: Diagnosis and management of pyogenic vertebral osteomyelitis. Surg Neurol 33:266, 1990.

33. Liebergall M, Chaimsky G, Lowe J, et al.: Pyogenic vertebral osteomyelitis with paralysis: prognosis and treatment. Clin Orthop 269:142, 1991.

34. Sapico FL, Montgomerie JZ: Vertebral osteomyelitis in intravenous drug abusers: report of three cases and review of the literature. Rev Infect Dis 2:196, 1980.

35. Ackerman G, Bayley JC: *Candida albicans* osteomyelitis in a vertebral body previously infected with *Serratia marcescens*. Spine 15:1362, 1990.

36. Young EJ: Human brucellosis. Rev Infect Dis 5:821, 1983.

37. Maguire JH: Case 37–1986. N Engl J Med 315:748, 1986.

38. Ariza J, Gudiol F, Valverde J, et al.: *Brucella spondylitis*: a detailed analysis based on current findings. Rev Infect Dis 7:656, 1985.

39. Torres-Rojas J, Taddonio RF, Sanders CV: Spondylitis caused by *Brucella abortus*. South Med J 72:1166, 1979.

40. El-Desouki M: Skeletal brucellosis: assessment with bone scintigraphy. Radiology 181:415, 1991.

41. Rajapakse CNA, Karin Al-Aska, Al-Orainey I, et al.: Spinal brucellosis. Br J Rheumatol 26:28, 1987.

42. Colmenero JD, Reguera JM, Fernandez-Nebro A, Cabrera-Franquelo F: Osteoarticular complications of brucellosis. Ann Rheum Dis 50:23, 1991.

43. Keenan JD, Metz CW Jr: Brucella spondylitis: a brief review and case report. Clin Orthop 82:87, 1972.

44. Kelley PJ, Martin WJ, Schirger A, Weed LA: Brucellosis of the bones and joints: experience with 36 patients. JAMA 174:347, 1960.

45. Forlenza SW, Axelrod JL, Grieco MH: Pott's disease in heroin addicts. JAMA 241:379, 1979.

46. Brashear HR Jr, Rendleman DA: Pott's paraplegia. South Med J 71:1379, 1978.

47. Friedman B: Chemotherapy of tuberculosis of the spine. J Bone Joint Surg 48A:451, 1966.

48. Goldblatt M, Cremin BJ: Osteoarticular tuberculosis: its presentation in the coloured races. Clin Radiol 29:669, 1978.

49. Chapman M, Murray RO, Stoker DJ: Tuberculosis of the bones and joints. Semin Roentgenol 14:266, 1979.

50. Seddon HJ: Pott's paraplegia: prognosis and treatment. Br J Surg 22:769, 1935.

51. Hsu LC, Yau ACMC: Tuberculosis. In: Sherk HH, Dunn EJ, Eismont FJ, et al.: The Cervical Spine, 2nd ed. Philadelphia: JB Lippincott Co, 1989, pp 544–551.

52. Dobson J: Tuberculosis of the spine. J Bone Joint Surg 33B:517, 1951.

53. Wurtz R, Quader Z, Simon D, et al.: Cervical tuberculous vertebral osteomyelitis: case report and discussion of the literature. Clin Infect Dis 16:806, 1993.

54. Lifeso R: Atlanto-axial tuberculosis in adults. J Bone Joint Surg 69B:183, 1987.

55. Corea JR, Tamimi TM: Tuberculosis of the arch of the atlas: case report. Spine 12:608, 1987.

56. Levin MF, Vellet AD, Munk PL, et al.: Tuberculosis of the odontoid bone: a rare but treatable cause of quadriplegia. J Can Assoc Radiol 43:199, 1992.

57. Hsu LES, Leong JEY: Tuberculosis of the lower cervical spine (C2–C7). J Bone Joint Surg 66B:1, 1984.

58. Gorse GJ, Pais MJ, Kusske JA, Cesario TC: Tuberculous spondylitis: a report of six cases and a review of the literature. Medicine 62:178, 1983.

59. Reeder MM, Palmer PCS: The Radiology of Tropical Diseases with Epidemiological, Pathological, and Clinical Correlation. Baltimore: Williams & Wilkins, 1981.

60. Simpson WM, McIntosh CA: Actinomycosis of the vertebrae (Actinomycotic Pott's disease). Arch Surg 14:1166, 1927.

61. Cope VZ: Actinomycosis of bone with special reference to infection of the vertebral column. J Bone Joint Surg 330:205, 1951.

62. Lane T, Goings S, Fraser D, et al.: Disseminated actinomycosis with spinal cord compression: report of two cases. Neurology 29:890, 1979.

63. Awad I, Bay JW, Petersen JM: Nocardial osteomyelitis of the spine with epidural cord compression: a case report. Neurosurgery 15:254, 1984.

64. Laurin JM, Resnick CS, Wheeler D, et al.: Cervical osteomyelitis related to *Nocardia asteroides*. J Infect Dis 149:824, 1984.

65. McGahan JP, Graves DS, Palmer PES: Coccidioidal spondylitis: usual and unusual radiographic manifestations. Radiology 136:5, 1980.

66. Resnick D, Niwayama G: Osteomyelitis, septic arthritis, and soft tissue infection: Organisms. In: Resnick D (ed): Diagnosis of Bone and Joint Disorders, 3rd ed. Philadelphia: WB Saunders Co, 1995, pp 2448–2558.

67. Reginato AJ: Syphilitic arthritis and osteitis. Rheum Dis Clin North Am 19:379, 1993.

68. Hunt JR: Syphilis of the vertebral column: its symptomatology and neural complications. Am J Med Sci 148:164, 1914.

69. Johns D: Syphilitic disorders of the spine: report of two cases. J Bone Joint Surg 52B:724, 1970.
70. Freedman E, Merschan I: Syphilitic spondylitis. AJR 49:756, 1943.
71. Karaharju EO, Hannuksela M: Possible syphilitic spondylitis. Acta Orthop Scand 44:289, 1973.
72. Alldred AJ, Nisbet NW: Hydatid disease of bone in Australia. J Bone Joint Surg 46B:260, 1964.
73. Morshed AA: Hydatid disease of the spine. Neurochirurgia 20:211, 1977.
74. Unger HS, Schneider LH, Sher J: Paraplegia secondary to hydatid disease: report of a case. J Bone Joint Surg 45A:1479, 1963.
75. Piercy EA, Smith JW: Vertebral osteomyelitis. In: Schlossberg D (ed): Orthopedic Infection. New York: Springer-Verlag, 1988, pp 21–38.
76. Collert S: Osteomyelitis of the spine. Acta Orthop Scand 48:283, 1977.
77. Digby JM, Kersley JB: Pyogenic non-tuberculous spinal infection: an analysis of thirty cases. J Bone Joint Surg 61B:47, 1979.
78. Sapico F, Montgomery JL: Pyogenic vertebral osteomyelitis: report of nine cases and review of the literature. Rev Infect Dis 5:754, 1979.
79. Freehafer AA, Furey JG, Pierce DS: Pyogenic osteomyelitis of the spine: resulting in spinal paralysis. J Bone Joint Surg 44A:710, 1962.
80. Griffiths HED, Jones DM: Pyogenic infection of the spine: a review of twenty-eight cases. J Bone Joint Surg 53B:383, 1971.
81. Liebergall M, Chaimsky G, Lowe J, et al.: Pyogenic vertebral osteomyelitis with paralysis: prognosis and treatment. Clin Orthop 289:142, 1991.
82. Joughin E, McDougall C, Parfitt C, et al.: Causes and clinical management of vertebral osteomyelitis in Saskatchewan. Spine 16:1049, 1991.
83. Schofferman L, Schofferman J, Zucherman J, et al.: Occult infections causing persistent low-back pain. Spine 14:417, 1989.
84. Craig JB: Cervical spine osteomyelitis with delayed onset tetraparesis after penetrating wounds of the neck. S Afr Med J 69:197, 1986.
85. Parrett D, Neilsen KII, White RG: Radioimmunoassay of IgM, IgG, and IgA *Brucella* antibodies. Lancet 1:1075, 1977.
86. Sippel JD, Masry NA, Farid Z: Diagnosis of human brucellosis with ELISA. Lancet 2:19, 1982.
87. Neinstein LS, Goldenring J: *Brucella* sacroiliitis. Clin Pediatr 22:645, 1983.
88. David PT, Horowitz T: Skeletal tuberculosis: a review with patient presentations and discussion. Am J Med 48:77, 1970.
89. Stauffer RN: Pyogenic vertebral osteomyelitis. Orthop Clin North Am 6:1015, 1975.
90. Pritchard DJ: Granulomatous infections of bones and joints. Orthop Clin North Am 6:1029, 1975.
91. Young WB: Actinomycosis with involvement of the vertebral column: case report and review of the literature. Clin Radiol 11:175, 1960.
92. Dalinka MK, Greendyke WH: The spinal manifestations of coccidioidomycosis. J Can Assoc Radiol 22:93, 1971.
93. Halpern AA, Rinsky LA, Fountains S, Nagel DA: Coccidioidomycosis of the spine: unusual roentgenographic presentation. Clin Orthop 140:78, 1979.
94. Cleveland M, Wilson HJ: Charcot disease of the spine: a report of two cases treated by spine fusion. J Bone Joint Surg 41A:336, 1959.
95. Stewart GR, Loewenthal J: Vertebral hydatidosis. Aust NZ J Surg 36:175, 1967.
96. Hutchinson WF, Thompson WB, Derian PS: Osseous hydatid (echinococcus) disease. JAMA 182:81, 1962.
97. Deyo RA: Plain roentgenography for low-back pain: finding needles in a haystack. Arch Intern Med 149:27, 1989.
98. Chandrasekar P: Low back pain and intravenous abusers. Arch Intern Med 150:1125, 1990.
99. Schauwecker DS: The scintigraphic diagnosis of osteomyelitis. AJR 158:9, 1992.
100. Schlaeffer F, Mikolich DJ, Mates SM: Technetium Tc 99m diphosphonate bone scan: false-normal findings in elderly patients with hematogenous vertebral osteomyelitis. Arch Intern Med 147:2024, 1987.
101. Smith AS, Blaser SI: Infectious and inflammatory processes of the spine. Radiol Clin North Am 29:809, 1991.
102. Kattapuram SV, Phillips WC, Boyd R: CT in pyogenic osteomyelitis of the spine. AJR 140:1199, 1983.
103. Modic MT, Pelanze W, Feiglin DHI, Belbobek G: Magnetic resonance imaging of musculoskeletal infections. Radiol Clin North Am 24:247, 1986.
104. Modic MT, Feiglin DH, Piraino DW, et al.: Vertebral osteomyelitis: assessment using MR. Radiology 157:157, 1985.
105. Meyers SP, Weiner SN: Diagnosis of hematogenous pyogenic vertebral osteomyelitis by magnetic resonance imaging. Arch Intern Med 151:683, 1991.
106. Smith AS, Weinstein MA, Mizushima A, et al.: MR imaging characteristics of tuberculous spondylitis vs vertebral osteomyelitis. AJR 153:399, 1989.
107. Cure JK, Mirich DR: MR imaging in cryptococcal spondylitis. AJNR 12:1111, 1991.
108. Post MJ, Sze G, Quencer RM, et al.: Gadolinium-enhanced MR in spinal infection. J Comput Assist Tomogr 14:721, 1990.
109. Musher DM, Thorsteinsson SB, Minuth JN, Luchi RJ: Vertebra osteomyelitis: still a diagnostic pitfall. Arch Intern Med 136:105, 1976.
110. Kornberg M, Rechtine GR, Dupuy TE: Unusual presentation of spinal osteomyelitis in a patient taking propylthiouracil: a case report. Spine 10:104, 1985.
111. Borges LF: Case records of the Massachusetts General Hospital. N Engl J Med 320:1610, 1989.
112. Patzakis MJ, Rao S, Wilkins J, et al.: Analysis of 61 cases of vertebral osteomyelitis. Clin Orthop 264:178, 1991.
113. Freiden TR, Sterling T, Pascal-Mendez A, et al.: The emergence of drug resistant tuberculosis in New York City. N Engl J Med 328:521, 1993.
114. Norden C, Gillespie WJ, Nade S: Mycobacterial infections of the musculoskeletal system. In: Infections in Bones and Joints. Boston: Blackwell Scientific Publications, 1994, pp 211–230.
115. Barnes PF, Barrows SA: Tuberculosis in the 1990s. Ann Intern Med 119:400, 1993.
116. Charles RW, Govender CS, Naidoo KS: Echinococcal infection of the spine with neural involvement. Spine 13:47, 1988.
117. Kemp HBS, Shaw NC: Laminectomy in paraplegia due to infective spondylosis. Br J Surg 61:66, 1974.
118. Emery SE, Chan DPK, Woodward HR: Treatment of hematogenous pyogenic vertebral osteomyelitis with anterior debridement and primary bone grafting. Spine 14:284, 1989.
119. Lifeso RM: Pyogenic spinal sepsis in adults. Spine 15:1265, 1990.
120. Thacker AK, Radhakrishnan K, Maloo JC: Pyogenic cervical vertebral osteomyelitis. Br J Clin Prac 44:763, 1990.
121. Stausbaugh LJ: Vertebral osteomyelitis. In: Jauregui

LE (ed): Diagnosis and Management of Bone Infections. New York: Marcel Dekker, 1995, pp 167–200.

122. Smith MD, Emery SE, Dudley A, et al.: Vertebral artery injury during anterior decompression of the cervical spine: a retrospective review of ten patients. J Bone Joint Surg 75B:410, 1993.

123. Darouiche RO, Hamill RJ, Greenberg SB, et al.: Bacterial spinal epidural abscess: review of 43 cases and literature survey. Medicine 71:369, 1992.

124. Curling OD, Gower DJ, McWhorter JM: Changing concepts in spinal epidural abscess: a report of 29 cases. Neurosurgery 27:185, 1990.

125. Hlavin ML, Kaminski HJ, Ross JS, Ganz E: Spinal epidural abscess: a ten-year perspective. Neurosurgery 27:177, 1990.

126. Guerrero IC, Slap GB, MacGregor RB, et al.: Anaerobic spinal epidural abscess. J Neurosurg 48:465, 1978.

127. McKnight P, Friedman J: Torticollis due to cervical epidural abscess and osteomyelitis. Neurology 42:696, 1992.

128. Levy ML, Wieder BH, Schneider J, et al.: Subdural empyema of the cervical spine: clinicopathological correlates and magnetic resonance imaging. J Neurosurg 79:929, 1993.

129. Auten GM, Levy CS, Smith MA: *Haemophilus parainfluenzae* as a rare cause of epidural abscess: case report and review. Rev Infect Dis 13:609, 1991.

130. Eismont FJ, Montero C: Infections of the Spine. In: Davidoff RA (ed): Handbook of the Spinal Cord. New York, Marcel Dekker, 1987, pp 411–449.

131. Rigamonti D, Liem L, Wolf AL, et al.: Epidural abscess in the cervical spine. Mt Sinai J Med 61:357, 1994.

132. Kricun R, Shoemaker EI, Chovanes GI, Stephens HW: Epidural abscess of the cervical spine: MR findings in five cases. AJR 158:1145, 1992.

133. Sandhu FS, Dillon WP: Spinal epidural abscess: evaluation with contrast-enhanced MR imaging. AJNR 12:1087, 1992.

134. Sadato N, Numaguchi Y, Rigamonti D, et al.: Spinal epidural abscess with gadolinium-enhanced MRI: serial follow-up studies and clinical correlations. Neuroradiology 36:44, 1994.

135. Friedmand DP, Hillis JR: Cervical epidural spinal infection: MR imaging characteristics. AJR 163:699, 1994.

136. Heusner AP: Nontuberculous spinal epidural infections. N Engl J Med 239:845, 1948.

MENINGITIS

Capsule Summary

Frequency of neck pain—very common

Location of neck pain—cervical spine, occiput

Quality of neck pain—sharp ache

Symptoms and signs—fever, meningismus, mental status changes

Laboratory and x-ray tests—leukocytosis, increased erythrocyte sedimentation rate; abnormal cerebrospinal fluid

Treatment—antibiotics

Prevalence and Pathogenesis

Meningitis is an infection of the lining of the central nervous system, the meninges. Meningitis may be caused by the following bacteria: *Streptococcus pneumoniae, Neisseria meningitidis,* and *Haemophilus influenzae;* viruses: retrovirus, Coxsackie, and enteric cytopathogenic human orphan (ECHO); mycobacteria: *Mycobacterium tuberculosis;* fungi: *Coccidioides immitis, Cryptococcus neoformans;* spirochetes: *Treponema pallidum;* and protozoa: *Toxoplasma gondii.* Meningitis usually develops from hematogenous spread through the blood stream from a distant, infected location to the choroid plexus; from septic emboli to small arteries; or by contiguous spread from local structures, such as the nasopharynx and mastoid bone. Recurrent episodes of meningitis suggest an opening of the central nervous system (CNS) to the outside environment, such as a dural tear, a skull fracture, or an immunocompromised state.[1] The infection causes an exudation of cells and protein into the subarachnoid space. The meningeal reaction spreads through the CNS, involving the meninges covering the spinal cord, as well as the brain. The clinical symptoms and course of the infection depend on the infecting organism and host inflammatory response. Bacterial and viral infections are characterized by constitutional symptoms including fever and change in mentation. Cerebral irritation results in headache, seizures, photophobia, and cranial nerve palsies. A more indolent course associated with gradual changes in mentation is more closely associated with tuberculous, fungal, spirochetal, and protozoal infections.

The diagnosis of bacterial or viral meningitis in the patient with acute symptoms is made without difficulty because of the high index of suspicion of the physician. The diagnosis of chronic meningitis is more difficult because symptoms and signs develop more gradually. The inflammatory response with bacterial infection results in the exudation of polymorphonuclear (PMN) leukocytes into the subarachnoid space. The cellular changes are accompanied by the seepage of proteins, which are usually excluded by the blood-brain barrier, into the meninges. The cerebrospinal fluid (CSF) becomes thick with the protein, eventually slowing the usual flow from the basal cisterns through Luschka's and Magendie's foramina to the lower spinal canal. Increasing CSF pressure, in an acute state, results in the clinical symptoms of meningismus and altered cerebral function.

The definitive diagnosis of meningitis is confirmed by culturing the offending organism from CSF obtained by lumbar puncture. The cornerstone of therapy for meningitis is antibiotics that are selected for their ability to kill the infecting organisms and their diffusing capacity across the meninges. When diagnosed expeditiously and treated aggressively, meningitis can be cured with no residual deficit. Delay in diagnosis is associated with increased neurologic morbidity and mortality.

Meningitis remains a significant health problem despite the use of bacterial and viral vaccines and antibodies. The yearly attack rate is 3 to 10 cases per 100,000 population in the United States.[2] A significant proportion of infections occur in children younger than 12 years of age. Higher yearly attack rates are found in developing countries.

Certain characteristics of the subarachnoid space allow for the development of meningitis.[3] In its normal state, the subarachnoid space contains lower concentrations of immunoglobulins and complement than the serum.[4] Organisms that gain entry into the subarachnoid space face less intense defense mechanisms than those present in the serum. Certain of these same factors may predispose certain individuals to infection with specific organisms. Otitis media, mastoiditis, and pneumonia predispose to *S. pneumoniae. Staphylococcus aureus* is associated with neurosurgical procedures, and *Staphylococcus epidermidis* may be associated with infected ventriculoperitoneal shunts.[5, 6] Factors that may play a role include the patient's age, immunologic status, trauma, and exposure to carrier of an organism (*N. meningitidis*). For example, patients who lack the terminal components of the complement system are at increased risk of *N. meningitidis* infection.[7] Adult bacterial meningitis is caused by *S. pneumoniae, N. meningitidis,* and *H. influenzae* in more than 80% of the infections (Table 12–6).[8] Meningitis secondary to *H. influenzae* occurs less frequently than infection

secondary to the other organisms. *H. influenzae* occurs in adults exposed to children with the infection.[9] Meningitis in children may be caused by additional organisms, including group B streptococcus, *Escherichia coli,* and other coliform organisms.[10, 11] *Listeria monocytogenes* is a gram-positive bacillus that causes 2% of meningitis in the United States. The most common hosts are neonates and immunocompromised adults. Most occurrences are associated with consumption of contaminated food, mostly dairy products.[8]

Clinical History

The primary symptoms of patients with meningitis include head and neck pain along with neck stiffness (meningismus). Patients with bacterial meningitis usually have associated fever. Changes in mental status ranging from mild confusion to frank coma occur in a majority of patients. The onset of symptoms with bacterial meningitis is usually acute and develops over 24 to 36 hours. In a minority of patients, the progression of symptoms may occur over 3 to 5 days. The course of symptoms is from headache and neck stiffness to confusion, obtundation, and coma.

Of the 4,000 cases of aseptic (nonbacterial) meningitis that occur each year in the United States, 25% have a defined etiology.[12] Of these, ECHO virus and Coxsackie virus are enteroviruses and are the most common cause of aseptic meningitis.[13] After the virus enters the body through the gastrointestinal or respiratory tract, the virus enters the meninges after a generalized viremia through the blood stream. The incubation period for growth of the virus may range from a few days to several weeks. The patient develops fever, sore throat, and myalgias, followed by frontal headache, photophobia, neck pain, neck stiffness, and fever. Human immunodeficiency virus (HIV) can also cause an acute or chronic aseptic meningitis associated with headache, fever, meningismus, and cranial neuropathies. This infection may be prior to the appearance of acquired immunodeficiency syndrome (AIDS).[14] Other forms of aseptic meningitis involve intracranial tumors, medications, and systemic illnesses (Table 12–7).

Tuberculous meningitis, once a disease of children, occurs more commonly in the elderly.[15] *M. tuberculosis* enters the body through the respiratory tract and grows in regional lymph nodes. Hematogenous seeding of the meninges may occur at that time. The infec-

TABLE 12–6. ORGANISMS CAUSING ADULT BACTERIAL MENINGITIS

Streptococcus pneumoniae	30%–50%
Neisseria meningitidis	10%–35%
Staphylococcus aureus/epidermidis	5%–15%
Gram-negative bacilli	1%–10%
Streptococci	5%
Listeria	5%
Haemophilus influenzae	1%–3%

Modified from Wispelwey B, Tunkel AR, Scheld WM: Bacterial meningitis in adults. Infect Dis Clin North Am 4:645, 1990.

TABLE 12–7. ACUTE ASEPTIC MENINGITIS

SYSTEMIC ILLNESSES

Systemic lupus
   erythematosus
Sjögren's syndrome
Rheumatoid arthritis
Polymyositis
Behçet's syndrome
Sarcoidosis
Vogt-Koyanagi-Harada
   syndrome

INTRACRANIAL TUMORS

Pharyngioma
Pituitary adenoma
Astrocytoma
Glioblastoma multiforme
Medulloblastoma
Ependymoma

MISCELLANEOUS

Postseizure
Postmigraine
Serum sickness
Heavy metal poisoning
Recurrent benign
   meningitis (Mollaret's)

VIRUSES

Enteroviruses
Mumps
Herpes simplex
Lymphocytic
   choriomeningitis

MEDICATIONS

Trimethoprim-
   sulfamethoxazole
Ibuprofen
Sulindac
Naproxen
Tolmetin
Azathioprine
Isoniazid

PROCEDURE-RELATED

Postneurosurgery
Spinal anesthesia
Intrathecal injections
Chymopapain injection

Modified from Connolly KJ, Hammer SM: The acute aseptic meningitis syndrome. Infect Dis Clin North Am 4:599, 1990.

tion may remain dormant for an extended period, only to become activated at a time of diminished host resistance to infection. The organisms grow in the meninges, which elicits an intense inflammatory reaction that is most prominent at the base of the brain. The inflammation in this location may result in inflammatory tissue that compresses cranial nerve blood vessels. This inflammation results in vessel thrombosis and infarction of tissue supplied by that vessel or in a blockage of the free flow of CSF around the brain, leading to increased intracranial pressure and hydrocephalus. Once the infection has started, the clinical manifestations of the infection progress throughout a 2- to 3-week period. Patients develop an insidious prodrome of malaise, lassitude, low-grade fever, and intermittent headache. During the next 2 to 3 weeks, there are protracted headache, neck pain, neck stiffness, fever, vomiting, and alterations in mental status. In untreated patients, seizures, coma, and death occur within 5 to 8 weeks.[16, 17]

Fungal infection with *C. immitis* or *C. neoformans* causes similar symptoms as those of tuberculous meningitis.[18] Approximately 30% of patients with extrapulmonary *C. immitis* infection develop meningitis. The pulmonary infection is asymptomatic or self-limited. Other extrapulmonary sites of infection include the skin and musculoskeletal systems. Meningitis

affects the base of the brain with a granulomatous inflammatory response that blocks the flow of CSF, resulting in hydrocephalus and cranial nerve palsies. The onset of these symptoms is gradual. Headache is the most prominent symptom of patients with fungal meningitis. Meningismus, personality changes, and fever are less prominent symptoms.[19]

Cryptococcal meningitis is an important and potentially life-threatening form of this infection.[20] *C. neoformans* is a ubiquitous yeast-like fungus found in association with pigeons, fruits, vegetables, and soil. In light of frequent exposure of humans to this fungus, natural resistance to this organism is substantial.[21] Cryptococcosis develops after inhalation and a mild pulmonary infection. Hematogenous dissemination results in an exposure of a number of organs and a predilection to the CNS.[19] The onset of disease is usually gradual, with intermittent episodes of persistent headache and fever. Headache is the most common symptom. The organism grows in the meninges and brain with a minimal inflammatory response. As the infection progresses over months, patients complain increasingly of impaired mentation, irritability, dizziness, weakness, and changes in vision. A stiff, painful neck is a frequent symptom but may be absent. If left untreated, both coccidioidal and cryptococcal meningitis may result in increasing neurologic deficits, coma, and death. Cryptococcal meningitis is a common manifestation of AIDS, affecting from 6% to 66% of patients.[22, 23] It may be the first opportunistic infection affecting AIDS patients.

T. pallidum is the spirochete that causes syphilis. Invasion of the CNS occurs during the primary and secondary stages of the illness. *T. pallidum* may be isolated from CSF in patients during the primary and secondary stages of the illness.[24] *T. pallidum* gains entrance to the blood stream during the primary stage of the infection after direct exposure of the genitourinary tract or oropharynx. During dissemination, or secondary phase, meningitis and cranial nerve palsies may occur. However, the frequency of acute meningitis is only 1% to 2%. More commonly, dissemination is associated with vague symptoms including headache, stiff neck, photophobia, and myalgias without fever. Progressive lesions associated with arteritis cause mental confusion, seizures, and focal deficits. If untreated, tertiary syphilis causes a wide range of neurologic dysfunctions, including general paresis, tabes dorsalis, space-occupying lesions (gummas), and meningovascular disease.[25] Patients with HIV infection may be at increased risk of following a more rapid course to symptomatic neurosyphilis.[26]

A more unusual form of meningitis is caused by the protozoan *T. gondii.* CNS toxoplasmosis occurs most commonly in the immunosuppressed host who has a lymphoreticular malignancy, has taken immunosuppressive drugs, or has a viral infection that impairs cellular immune function (AIDS).[27] Patients with CNS toxoplasmosis may present with an acute or subacute course, including headache, stiff neck, and seizures. If brain tissue is also infected (encephalitis), the patient may develop focal neurologic deficits that progress to cause changes in mentation as well as coma. Patients with AIDS frequently have intracranial mass lesions in association with their toxoplasmosis. Toxoplasmosis may be the most frequent cause of that cerebral lesion in HIV patients.[28]

Physical Examination

The patient with meningitis may manifest abnormalities in a number of organ systems during the physical examination. Patients with meningitis of any cause are frequently febrile. Patients with meningeal irritation develop reflex contraction of neck muscles (nuchal rigidity), Kernig's sign (pain in the hamstrings with knee extension in the supine position), and Brudzinski's sign (involuntary flexion of the hips with neck flexion). These signs are abnormal in 50% of bacterial meningitis patients.[29] A maculopetechial or purpuric rash may be present in the patients with meningococcal meningitis or other bacterial infections. About 50% of meningococcal patients have a rash.[8] ECHO virus may cause a maculopapular rash that appears on the face before other parts of the body are affected. Funduscopic examination may demonstrate papilledema (swelling of the head of the optic nerve), which is secondary to increased intracranial pressure. Infection of the middle ear (otitis media), a possible local source of infection, would be noted on examination of the ear. Chest examination may be positive for decreased breath sounds indicative of a pneumonic process secondary to bacteria (*S. pneumoniae*), mycobacteria (*M. tuberculosis*), or fungi (*C. immitis*). Murmurs on cardiac examination suggest endocarditis, which may be the source of the primary infection, including *S. aureus*.

The range of neurologic abnormalities is wide. Loss of mental function in the form of memory loss or inability to perform calculations occurs with all forms of meningitis. A change in mental status or coma is found in 50% or more of bacterial meningitis patients and is a strong indicator of this type of infection.[30]

Elderly patients with bacterial meningitis are frequently confused and have severe mental status changes in the setting of pneumonia. Confusion occurs in 92% with pneumococcal meningitis and in 78% with gram-negative bacillary meningitis.[31, 32] Fever may be absent. Neck stiffness must be differentiated from that of osteoarthritis of the cervical spine.

Neurologic abnormalities are also associated with meningitis caused by other organisms, including *M. tuberculosis, C. immitis,* and *T. pallidum.*[33–35] Abnormalities of cranial nerves (eyes, facial, and tongue movements) occur most commonly in patients with granulomatous meningitis, which affects the base of the brain.

Laboratory Data

Nonspecific findings, such as elevation in peripheral white blood cells (WBCs) and erythrocyte sedimentation rate, are not helpful in making a diagnosis of meningitis but are useful in following the response of patients to therapy.

The diagnosis of meningitis is made by the examination of CSF. This fluid is obtained by lumbar puncture. In most circumstances, a lumbar puncture can be completed without complication. Contraindications for this procedure are signs of increased intracranial pressure or skin infection overlying the needle entry point. Lumbar puncture in the face of increased intracranial pressure may cause the brain to be pressed against the base of the skull, causing acute compression of the brain stem, which controls autonomic functions of the lungs and heart. Patients who "cone" develop cardiopulmonary arrest. Attempting an injection through an area of cellulitis may result in inoculating organisms into the CNS, causing meningitis or vertebral osteomyelitis.

The definitive diagnosis of meningitis is based on the growth of the offending organism from CSF or blood. Unfortunately, cultures take time to become positive, leaving the diagnosis of meningitis to be based on other characteristic changes in CSF. Bacterial meningitis causes WBC counts greater than 1,000 cells/mm, a predominance of PMN leukocytes, a decreased glucose level that is less than

50% of the serum level, an elevated protein level of greater than 100 mg/dL, and positive Gram's stain smear of organisms from a spun specimen in 80% of patients.[30, 36] Gram's stain smear is positive in 90% of *S. pneumoniae* and *S. aureus,* 86% in *H. influenzae,* 75% in *N. meningitidis,* and 50% or less in other gram-negative organisms.[37] CSF cultures are positive for growth of the causative organism in the majority of patients if the samples are cultured promptly to minimize the loss of fastidious organisms such as *H. influenzae, N. meningitidis,* and anaerobes. The presence of bacteria in CSF may also be detected through identification of bacterial antigens with coagglutination and latex agglutination tests. These tests are less sensitive than CSF culture and are not a substitute for it.[38]

Viral meningitis causes less of a leukocytosis (less than 500 WBC/mm), predominantly lymphocytic in character, with normal glucose and slightly elevated protein levels.[39] CSF obtained early in the course of aseptic meningitis may reveal an increased number of PMN leukocytes. A repeat CSF examination is warranted because subsequent evaluations reveal a switch to a predominance of lymphocytes.[40] The measurement of CSF pressure is not associated with a specific form of meningitis. CSF protein concentrations are also nondiagnostic.

Tuberculous and fungal meningitis cause a CSF WBC count of less than 500 cells/mm, with a predominance of lymphocytes. Tuberculous meningitis causes a marked reduction in glucose and marked increased in protein levels. Organisms are rarely seen on smear. Culture may be positive in 78% of patients.[37] Culture may require up to 8 weeks before growth is detected. Fungal meningitis is associated with a slight reduction of glucose level, moderate increase in protein level and, in the case of *Cryptococcus,* the presence of organisms by india ink examination. In toxoplasmosis, CSF examination may be normal or demonstrate mild WBC elevation with lymphocytes.

Other ancillary laboratory tests may detect the presence of pathogenic organisms in locations other than the CNS. Blood cultures detect bacteremia with *H. influenzae, S. pneumoniae,* and *N. meningitidis,* in 80%, 50%, and 40% of patients, respectively.[41] Respiratory tract cultures are useful for organisms that are associated with pulmonic infections.

Radiographic Evaluation

Radiographic examination is not useful in the diagnosis or management of uncompli-

cated meningitis.[42] Computerized tomography (CT) in meningitis may detect widening of the subarachnoid space. Radiographic techniques are most useful in the patient with meningitis who has an associated abnormality such as a parameningeal focus of infection or brain abscess. CT can localize the space-occupying lesion in the patient with focal cerebral signs who does not respond to usual therapy. CT scan may demonstrate contrast enhancement of the leptomeninges, widening of the subarachnoid space, and patchy areas of diminished density in the brain.[43] Magnetic resonance (MR) imaging may also be useful to document intracranial lesions that may be associated with meningeal infection.[44]

Differential Diagnosis

The diagnosis of meningitis is based on the results of cultures of CSF. The clinical course, CSF abnormalities, along with culture results, help differentiate the various forms of meningitis (pyogenic versus granulomatous versus protozoan). Parameningeal infection, such as epidural abscess, subdural empyema, and brain abscess, may cause meningeal symptoms and neurologic signs. Radiographic evaluation should differentiate these entities from meningitis alone.

Treatment

The treatment for bacterial meningitis is intravenous or intrathecal antibiotic that is bactericidal for the infecting organisms. Bacterial meningitis represents an infection in a location of impaired host defenses. Factors including inefficient surface phagocytosis in a body fluid, lack of immunoglobulin and complement opsonic, and bactericidal activity require bactericidal antibiotics. A problem obtaining and maintaining adequate concentrations of antibiotic in CSF is the blood-brain barrier. The blood-brain barrier excludes proteins and antibiotics from the brain and CNS. When inflamed, the integrity of the blood-brain barrier is lost, allowing the ingress of antibiotics. Antibiotics are administered intravenously, in high, divided doses, every few hours (Table 12–8). Penicillin, nafcillin, ampicillin, cefotaxime, and ceftriaxone are antibiotics used with gram-positive and gram-negative infections. Some gram-negative meningitis requires aminoglycoside (gentamicin) therapy. Aminoglycosides do not cross the blood-brain barrier

TABLE 12–8. ANTIBIOTIC THERAPY FOR BACTERIAL MENINGITIS

ORGANISM	ANTIBIOTIC	ADULT 24-HOUR DOSE	ALTERNATE THERAPY 24-HOUR DOSE
Streptococcus pneumoniae	Ceftriaxone +/− vancomycin 2 g intravenous (IV)	4 g	NA
Streptococcus groups A and B	Penicillin G	24 million U IV	Ceftriaxone, 4 g IV
Group D (enterococci)	Penicillin G + gentamicin	24 million U IV + gentamicin intrathecal (IT)	Vancomycin, 2 g IV + gentamicin IV and IT
Neisseria meningitidis	Penicillin G	24 million U IV	Ceftriaxone 4 g IV
Haemophilus influenzae (Beta-lactamase negative)	Ampicillin IV	12 g	Ceftriaxone 4 g IV
(Beta-lactamase positive)	Ceftriaxone	4 g IV	Chloramphenicol 4 g IV
Staphylococcus aureus	Nafcillin	12 g IV	Vancomycin 2 g IV
Gram-negative	Ceftazidime	6–9 g IV	Gentamicin 4–10 mg IT

Choice of antibiotic should be matched to organism sensitivities determined with culture. Antibiotics listed in this table may be used as initial therapy until sensitivity results are available.
IT = Intrathecal
Courtesy of Gary Simon, M.D.

and require intrathecal administration (lumbar puncture, ventricular pump).[45]

The therapy for aseptic meningitis is symptomatic. There is no effective antiviral therapy that shortens the course of the infection. Recovery begins within days and is usually complete in a few weeks. Patients with HIV meningitis also have a self-limited illness that resolves without specific treatment in 4 weeks.[14]

Tuberculous meningitis requires three drug therapies, including isoniazid, rifampin, and ethambutol or pyrazinamide. This therapy must be continued for 12 months. Drug-resistant tuberculosis is becoming an increasingly frequent problem. Additional drugs for longer periods are required to control these infections. These patients may require five to seven drugs for periods up to 24 months. Patients with hydrocephalus, or cranial nerve dysfunction secondary to tuberculous meningitis, may benefit from a course of corticosteroids.[46]

Patients with fungal meningitis require amphotericin B therapy. Cryptococcal meningitis may be cured with intravenous therapy, which is given in increments of 20 to 30 mg/day up to a total of 2 to 3 gm. Patients with HIV-related cryptococcal meningitis may require a 6-week course of amphotericin B and flucytosine, followed by long maintenance therapy.[25, 47] In coccidioidal meningitis, amphotericin B therapy given by an intravenous route does not reach adequate levels in CSF. Intrathecal administration is necessary for control of the infection.

Neurosyphilis requires treatment with intravenous penicillin. The recommended dose is 2 to 4 million units IV every 4 hours.[25]

CNS toxoplasmosis requires prolonged therapy with pyrimethamine and sulfonamides. In adults, 25 mg of pyrimethamine is given daily along with four 1-gm doses of sulfadiazine daily. Therapy must be continued for a minimum of 6 weeks.

Prognosis

The course and outcome of meningitis depend on the agent that causes the infection and the immunologic status of the patient. Patients who have a compromised immune system are at risk of developing tuberculous or fungal meningitis and have a poorer prognosis than those patients who have an episode of aseptic, viral meningitis. Patients with bacterial meningitis will have a full recovery if the diagnosis is made expeditiously and appropriate therapy is given. Antibiotic therapy is given for 2 weeks, with the response to therapy monitored by the return of CSF abnormalities to normal. Patients with parameningeal foci of infection may not improve until the focus is drained.

Tuberculous meningitis is associated with a 20% mortality rate even in patients who receive drug therapy. The improvement with therapy may be slow, with survivors continuing with neurologic dysfunction.

Patients with fungal meningitis may have relapses of their disease despite receiving long courses of amphotericin B therapy. Patients who have a poor clinical outcome with cryptococcal meningitis have an underlying lymphoreticular malignancy, continued abnormal CSF white blood cells, or cryptococci on smear.[20]

CNS toxoplasmosis is uniformly fatal unless aggressively treated. Patients with AIDS or other immunocommpromised states may have a poor outcome despite maximum therapy.

References

MENINGITIS

1. Critchley EMR: Meningitis disorders and myelopathies. In: Critchley E, Eisen A (eds): Diseases of the Spinal Cord. London: Springer-Verlag, 1992, pp 209–233.
2. Schlech WF III, Ward JI, Band JD, et al.: Bacterial meningitis in the United States, 1978 through 1981: the national bacterial meningitis surveillance study. JAMA 253:1749, 1985.
3. Tunkel AR, Wispelwey B, Scheld WM: Pathogenesis and pathophysiology of meningitis. Infect Dis Clin North Am 4:555, 1990.
4. Smith H, Bannister B, O'Shea MJ: Cerebrospinal fluid immunoglobulins in meningitis. Lancet 1:591, 1973.
5. Chernick NL, Armstrong D, Posner JB: Central nervous system infections in patients with cancer. Medicine 52:563, 1973.
6. Schoenbaum SC, Gardner P, Shillito J: Infections of cerebrospinal fluid shunts: epidemiology, clinical manifestations, and therapy. J Infect Dis 131:543, 1975.
7. Ross SC, Densen P: Complement deficiency states and infection: epidemiology, pathogenesis, and consequences of neisserial and other infections in an immune deficiency. Medicine 63:243, 1984.
8. Wispelwey B, Tunkel AR, Scheld WM: Bacterial meningitis in adults. Infect Dis Clin North Am 4:645, 1990.
9. Ward JL, Fraser DW, Baraff LJ, et al.: *Haemophilus influenzae* meningitis: a national study of secondary spread in household contact. N Engl J Med 301:122, 1979.
10. Shelton MM, Marks WA: Bacterial meningitis. Neurol Clin 8:605, 1990.
11. Saez-Llorens X, McCracken GH Jr: Bacterial meningitis in neonates and children. Infect Dis Clin North Am 4:623, 1990.
12. Meyer HM, Johnson RT, Crawford IP, et al.: Central nervous system syndromes of "viral" etiology: a study of 713 cases. Am J Med 29:334, 1960.
13. Connolly KJ, Hammer SM: The acute aseptic meningitis syndrome. Infect Dis Clin North Am 4:599, 1990.
14. McArthur J: Neurologic manifestations of AIDS. Medicine 66:407, 1987.
15. Hinman AR: Tuberculous meningitis at Cleveland Metropolitan General Hospital 1959 to 1963. Am Rev Respir Dis 95:670, 1967.
16. Molavi A, LeFrock JL: Tuberculous meningitis. Med Clin North Am 69:315, 1985.
17. Leonard JM, Des Prez RM: Tuberculous meningitis. Infect Dis Clin North Am 4:769, 1990.
18. Ellner JJ, Bennett JE: Chronic meningitis. Medicine 55:341, 1976.
19. Treseler CB, Sugar AM: Fungal meningitis. Infect Dis Clin North Am 4:789, 1990.
20. Diamond RD, Bennett JE: Prognostic factors in cryptococcal meningitis: a study in 111 cases. Ann Intern Med 80:176, 1974.
21. Armstrong D: Problems in management of opportunistic fungal diseases. Rev Infect Dis 11:S1591, 1989.
22. Kovacs JA, Kovacs AA, Polis M, et al.: Cryptococcosis in the acquired immunodeficiency syndrome. Ann Intern Med 103:533, 1985.
23. Levy RM, Bresden DE, Rosenblum ML: Neurological manifestations of acquired immunodeficiency syndrome (AIDS). J Neurosurg 62:475, 1985.
24. Lukehart SA, Hook EW, Baker-Zander SA, et al.: Invasion of the central nervous system by *Treponema pallidum*: implications of diagnosis and treatment. Ann Intern Med 109:855, 1988.
25. Coyle PK, Dattwyler R: Spirochetal infection of the central nervous system. Infect Dis Clin North Am 4:731, 1990.
26. Johns DR, Tierney M, Felsenstein D: Alteration in the natural history of neurosyphilis by concurrent infection with the human immunodeficiency virus. N Engl J Med 316:1569, 1987.
27. Townsend JJ, Wolinsky JS, Baunger JR, Johnson PC: Acquired toxoplasmosis: a neglected cause of treatable nervous system disease. Arch Neurol 32:335, 1975.
28. Novia BA, Petito CK, Gold JWM: Cerebral toxoplasmosis complicating the acquired immune deficiency syndrome. Ann Neurol 19:224, 1985.
29. Carpenter RR, Petersdorf RG: The clinical spectrum of bacterial meningitis. Am J Med 33:262, 1962.
30. Geiseler PJ, Nelson KE, Levin S, et al.: Community-acquired purulent meningitis: a review of 1216 cases during the antibiotic era, 1954–1976. Rev Infect Dis 2:725, 1980.
31. Behrman RE, Meyer BR, Mendelsohn MH, et al.: Central nervous system infections in the elderly. Arch Intern Med 149:1596, 1989.
32. Gorse GJ, Thrupp LD, Nudlenan KL, et al.: Bacterial meningitis in the elderly. Arch Intern Med 144:1603, 1984.
33. Kennedy DH, Fallon RJ: Tuberculous meningitis. JAMA 241:64, 1979.
34. Bouza E, Dreyer JS, Hewitt WL, et al.: Coccidioidal meningitis: an analysis of thirty-one cases and review of the literature. Medicine 60:139, 1981.
35. Jordan KG: Modern neurosyphilis: critical analysis. West J Med 149:47, 1988.
36. Karandanis D, Shulman JA: Recent survey of infectious meningitis in adults: review of laboratory findings in bacterial, tuberculous, and aseptic meningitis. South Med J 68:449, 1976.
37. Greenlee JE: Approach to diagnosis of meningitis: cerebrospinal fluid evaluation. Infect Dis Clin North Am 4:583, 1990.
38. Yogev R: Advances in diagnosis and treatment of childhood meningitis. Pediatr Infect Dis J 4:321, 1985.
39. Lepow ML, Carver DH, Wright HT Jr, et al.: A clinical, epidemiologic, and laboratory investigation of aseptic meningitis during the four-year period 1955–58. N Engl J Med 266:1181, 1962.
40. Feigin RD, Shackelford PG: Value of repeat lumbar puncture in the differential diagnosis of meningitis. N Engl J Med 304:1278, 1973.
41. Swartz MN, Dodge PR: Bacterial meningitis: a review of selected aspects. I. General clinical features, special problems and unusual meningeal reactions mimicking bacterial meningitis. N Engl J Med 272:725, 1965.
42. Weisberg LA: Computed tomography in the diagnosis of intracranial disease. Ann Intern Med 91:87, 1979.
43. Weisberg LA: Cerebral computerized tomography in

intracranial inflammatory disorders. Arch Neurol 37:137, 1980.

44. Krol G, Becker R, Zimmerman R, et al.: Contribution of MRI to the diagnosis of intracranial complications of acquired immune deficiency syndrome. Neuroradiology 86:99, 1985.

45. Tauber MG, Sande MA: General principles of therapy of pyogenic meningitis. Infect Dis Clin North Am 4:661, 1990.

46. O'Toole RD, Thorton GF, Mukherjee MK, Nath RL: Dexamethasone in tuberculous meningitis: relationship of cerebrospinal fluid effects to therapeutic effects to therapeutic efficacy. Ann Intern Med 70:39, 1969.

47. Dismukes WE, Cloud G, Gallis HA, et al.: Treatment of cryptococcal meningitis with combination amphotericin B and flucytosine for four as compared with six weeks. N Engl J Med 317:334, 1987.

INTERVERTEBRAL DISC SPACE INFECTION

Capsule Summary

Frequency of neck pain—very common

Location of neck pain—cervical spine, disc space

Quality of neck pain—severe, sharp

Symptoms and signs—percussion tenderness, decreased motion

Laboratory and x-ray tests—increased erythrocyte sedimentation rate, blood cultures, disc space narrowing on plain roentgenogram, magnetic resonance imaging for early infection

Treatment—antibiotics, immobilization

Prevalence and Pathogenesis

Infection of the intervertebral disc (IVD) is an uncommon but potentially disabling cause of neck pain. Once thought to be exclusively a complication of vertebral osteomyelitis, IVD infection also can develop secondary to hematogenous invasion through the blood stream and by direct penetration during disc surgery. A significant clinical feature of this illness is the long delay between the onset of symptoms of neck pain, muscle spasm, and limitation of motion and the establishment of the diagnosis.

IVD infection is an uncommon disease in adults, occurring with an incidence of two patients per year at an orthopedic hospital in one study.[1] IVD infection occurs more commonly in the lumbar spine compared with the frequency of infection in the cervical spine.[2] Approximately 2.8% of patients who have lumbar disc surgery develop IVD infection.[3] Men are more frequently affected, and the disease has been diagnosed in patients as old as 63 years of age.[1]

The pathogenesis of IVD infection in adults in the absence of a surgical or diagnostic procedure remains in doubt. In children, blood vessels supply the IVDs. Infection occurs secondary to hematogenous spread of organisms. Other researchers consider discitis in children a noninfectious disease, an inflammatory or traumatic disorder. The course in children is relatively benign.[4]

Although it is generally believed that the IVDs are avascular in adult life, some investigators have demonstrated blood flow in adults.[5, 6] Although there is a decrease in the number of vessels that enter the nucleus pulposus with aging, an adequate circumferential supply is maintained from the periphery.[7] The blood supply to IVDs is greater in children, and this may explain the increased frequency of IVD infection in the pediatric age group when compared with adults.[4]

There is evidence supporting the importance of the venous and arterial systems in the development of IVD infection. Patients with pelvic and urinary tract infections may develop involvement of disc spaces with the identical organism, and it is postulated that these organisms may spread by means of the vertebral venous Batson's plexus.[8–10] Batson's plexus is a network of veins that surrounds the vertebral column, and it is connected to the major veins that return blood to the heart, the inferior and superior venae cavae. However, other investigators believe that the reversal of flow in the venous system, which would allow infected blood to enter Batson's plexus, does not occur under usual circumstances. Instead, they suggest hematogenous spread through the arterial system as the source of infection.[6, 11] It is probable that either route may be involved in appropriate circumstances.

The IVDs are infected by hematogenous spread, most commonly through the blood stream. A variety of infections of the skin, urinary tract, and soft tissues in compromised hosts have been associated with disc infection.[12] However, other mechanisms may play a role in other circumstances. A few patients have been reported to have developed IVD infection following trauma, resulting from lifting objects at work or heavy physical labor.[13, 14] Trauma in the area of the IVD may result in the formation of a hematoma, which is then infected by blood-borne organisms, but the likelihood of this occurrence is not great. In fact, most patients with IVD infection deny previous trauma.[1] Therefore, the association of this infection and trauma is unlikely. Patients who undergo operative procedures, needle biopsy, discography, or puncture of a disc during an aspiration to obtain cerebrospinal fluid can develop infection by direct inoculation of the organism at the time of the procedure.[3] In the cervical spine, IVD infection has been reported to occur spontaneously with cervical discography and subsequent to cerebral angiography.[15–17] Spinal infection associated with lumbar disc surgery occurs less than 1% of the time whether an anterior, posterior, or percutaneous route is used.[18] Other people may develop IVD infection from organisms that arise from contiguous abscesses.[19]

Clinical History

Patients with IVD infection of the cervical spine have symptoms of localized neck pain. In some, the onset of pain is acute and severe. In other patients, pain may be more insidious and milder. The duration of pain before diagnosis ranges from 1 month to 2 years.[14] It becomes chronic and may be associated with radiation into the arms and hands. Pain is exacerbated by movement and relieved by absolute rest. Motion may initiate paroxysms of paravertebral muscle spasm, and patients usually have great difficulty moving their neck. Loss of motor strength or sensory symptoms in the upper and lower extremities suggests spinal cord compression with the development of epidural abscess.[16]

In one study, 77% of cases affected the lumbar disc, 15% the cervical spine, and 8% the thoracic spine.[14] In one group of patients, 3 of 13 had neurologic deficits at time of diagnosis.

Discitis may also be a complication of invasive procedures, including discography and discectomy. Patients who have postoperative infection develop a significant increase in neck pain after a period of initial relief with no significant increase in radicular pain initially. Radicular or myelopathic symptoms may appear as the infection spreads from the disc to the bone to the epidural space.

Physical Examination

Physical findings in patients with IVD infection include localized tenderness on palpation, limitation of motion of the cervical spine, and paravertebral muscle spasm. Fever is rarely present.[14, 20] Patients prefer to remain motionless in bed. Examination of the skin, respiratory system, gastrointestinal system, and genitourinary system may demonstrate the primary source of infection. Neurologic examination may demonstrate evidence of myelopathy (spasticity, sensory level, hyperreflexia, and positive extensor response) in patients with spinal cord compression in the cervical area.[15]

Laboratory Data

The laboratory findings are nonspecific in IVD infection. The most commonly abnormal test is the erythrocyte sedimentation rate (ESR). It is increased in up to 75% of patients.[1] The ESR is increased in lumbar spine surgery patients for 2 weeks postoperatively. Rates remain increased in patients with IVD infection for longer periods.[21] C-reactive protein (CRP) levels return to normal more rapidly than ESR after uncomplicated lumbar spine surgery. A persistently elevated CRP level may be associated with a postoperative infection.[22] A mild leukocytosis with a normal differential is also seen.[14] Occasionally, blood cultures are positive during the acute phases of the illness,[14] but culture of fluid obtained by needle aspiration of the IVD space or at surgery is usually positive.[14, 23] The most frequently cultured organism that causes IVD infection is *Staphylococcus aureus*. Other gram-positive organisms include *Staphylococcus epidermidis* as well as streptococcal species, including *Streptococcus milleri*.[24, 25] Gram-negative organisms have also been implicated, particularly *Pseudomonas aeruginosa,* in intravenous drug abusers.[23, 26] Gram-negative organisms, *Enterobacter cloacae* and *Escherichia coli,* have been the source of infection in other immunocompromised patients, including the elderly and patients with urosepsis.[27, 28] Gram-negative organisms, including *Campylobacter fetus,* group Ve-1, and *Kingella kingae,* have caused discitis in otherwise immunocompetent patients.[29–31] Anaerobic organisms have been implicated in rare circumstances, as have fungal organisms.[32, 33] The list of anaerobes and fungal organisms that are associated with discitis has been expanded to include *Eikenella corrodens* and *Aspergillus fumigatus,* respectively.[34–36]

Radiographic Evaluation

The radiographic features of IVD infection are distinctive and help differentiate them from that of vertebral osteomyelitis; however, they may lag behind clinical symptoms by 6 weeks or more.[1] The earliest change is a decrease in the height of the affected IVD space. Two months after the appearance of IVD space narrowing, reactive sclerosis of subchondral bone appears in the adjoining vertebral bodies. Subsequently, progressive irregularity of the vertebral end plates develops and indicates a local extension of the inflammatory process and an osteomyelitis. At this juncture, the loss of vertebral bone may be associated with a "ballooning" of the IVD space.[1] This increase in apparent IVD space is usually associated with involvement of the vertebral body posteriorly. Repair may occur at any stage of infection, and it is manifested by bony proliferation about the outside margin of the disc. The process may heal with bony ankylosis across the affected IVD space of the adjacent vertebral bodies.

Bone scintiscans are useful in rapidly identifying increased bone activity in areas contiguous to infected IVDs. The bone scan may be abnormal in an area of infection that appears normal on plain radiographs.[37] Both technetium 99m and gallium 67 citrate scans are more sensitive than plain roentgenograms in detecting early disc infections.[38, 39] The use of single photon emission computerized tomography has increased the sensitivity of bone scintigraphy in the diagnosis of infectious processes in the axial skeleton. Indium leukocyte imaging has not proved to be adequately sensitive to be clinically useful in patients with IVD infections.[40]

Computerized tomography (CT) is helpful in assessing bony alterations and soft tissue involvement to a greater extent than scintiscan. Sensitivity is increased if CT technique includes soft tissue and bone windows. CT findings consistent with discitis include disc narrowing and end-plate erosion. CT is unable to detect early changes of discitis during the first 14 days of symptoms and cannot differentiate postoperative changes from infection.[41, 42]

Magnetic resonance (MR) imaging is a sensitive method for the early detection of inflammation in infected tissues. MR imaging is able to detect early disc infection before changes occur on plain roentgenograms[43] (Fig. 12–3). MR imaging with gadolinium enhancement is a useful test for the differentiation of normal postoperative healing changes from those related to septic discitis. Gadolinium-enhanced MR findings associated with infection include decreased signal intensity on T_1-weighted images in the bone marrow adjacent to the disc, increased signal intensity

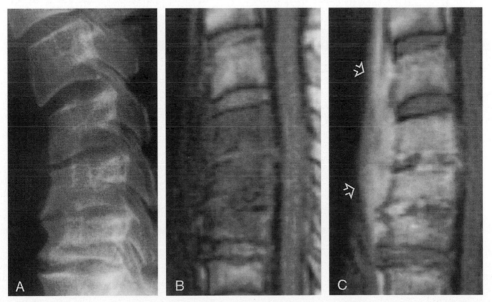

Figure 12–3. Spinal infection: magnetic resonance (MR) imaging. Pyogenic spondylitis. This 40-year-old man developed infective spondylitis after multilevel cervical discography. *A,* Routine radiography shows narrowing of the intervertebral discs at the C4–C5 and the C5–C6 levels. Prevertebral soft tissue swelling was also evident. *B,* Sagittal T_1-weighted (TR/TE 500/12) spin echo MR image reveals low-signal intensity of the marrow of the fourth, fifth, and sixth cervical vertebral bodies. *C,* After intravenous administration of gadolinium contrast agent, a sagittal T_1-weighted (TR/TE 500/12) spin echo MR image shows hyperintensity in the prevertebral soft tissues *(arrows).* In comparison with the findings in *B,* the marrow involvement is less apparent. (From Resnick D, Niwayama G: Osteomyelitis, septic arthritis, and soft tissue infection: Axial skeleton. In: Resnick D [ed]: Diagnosis of Bone and Joint Disorders, 3rd ed. Philadelphia: WB Saunders Co, 1995, p 2434.)

with loss of the intranuclear cleft in the disc space, and posterior annulus on T_2-weighted sequences.[44]

Differential Diagnosis

The diagnosis of IVD infection is often overlooked because of nonspecific symptoms and IVD's relative infrequency as a cause of neck pain compared with mechanical disorders and the spondyloarthropathies. Nonetheless, physicians should be aware of this treatable entity so that an appropriate diagnosis is made expeditiously. The definitive diagnosis of an IVD infection depends on the aspiration or biopsy of the infected site, with subsequent confirmation by culture of the causative organism. A bone scan may help identify the patient with this entity who has normal roentgenograms.

The differential diagnosis of septic discitis and mechanical discitis is a problem in patients who have undergone invasive procedures (discography and discectomy) involving the IVD.[45, 46] The frequency of discitis after discography ranges from 1% to 4% of procedures.[47] Patients with septic discitis (culture positive or negative) have elevated ESR and CRP levels and evidence of large infiltrates of lymphoplasmocytic cells.[45] Patients who develop discitis postoperatively present with new

onset of pain as early as 3 days and as late as 20 months after their surgery. The pain occurs after resolution of the preoperative pain and may be of a different quality and radiation. The organism that causes this infection is *S. epidermidis,* a skin contaminant, suggesting seeding at the time of operation.[48] The pain is severe and may be ascribed to a recurrent herniated disc or hysteria.[49] Diagnosis of discitis including postoperative infections may be confirmed by the use of an automated percutaneous biopsy.[50]

Other diseases that may be associated with IVD narrowing accompanied by lysis or sclerosis of adjacent vertebrae include osteomyelitis of a vertebral body, degenerative disease, calcium pyrophosphate dihydrate crystal deposition, neuroarthropathy, and trauma.[51] Sarcoidosis may cause similar changes on occasion. MR imaging is able to detect the presence of sarcoid spondylodiscitis but cannot differentiate pyogenic from granulomatous inflammation. Biopsy of the IVD space is required.[52] Patients with chronic renal failure may develop spinal erosive changes that simulate IVD space infections. IVD changes range from superficial erosions at the anterosuperior margins and anteroinferior margins of the vertebral bodies to large resorptive defects mimicking IVD infection.[53] These changes occur after 3 years on dialysis. Table 12–9 describes the

TABLE 12–9. DIFFERENTIAL DIAGNOSIS OF SOME DISORDERS PRODUCING DISCAL NARROWING

DISORDER	DISCOVERTEBRAL MARGIN	SCLEROSIS	VACUUM PHENOMENA	OSTEOPHYTOSIS	OTHER FINDINGS
Infection	Poorly defined	Variable[1]	Rare[2]	Absent	Vertebral lysis, soft tissue mass
Intervertebral osteochondrosis	Well defined	Prominent	Present	Variable	Cartilaginous nodes
Rheumatoid arthritis	Poorly or well defined with "erosions"	Variable	Absent	Absent or mild	Apophyseal joint abnormalities, subluxation
Calcium pyrophosphate dihydrate crystal deposition disease	Poorly or well defined	Prominent	Variable	Variable	Fragmentation, subluxation
Neuropathic osteoarthropathy	Well defined	Prominent	Variable	Prominent	Fragmentation, subluxation, disorganization
Trauma	Well defined	Prominent	Variable	Variable	Fracture, soft tissue mass
Sarcoidosis	Poorly or well defined	Variable, may be prominent	Absent	Absent	Soft tissue mass

[1]Usually evident in pyogenic infections and in tuberculosis in the black patient.
[2]Vacuum phenomena initially may be evident when intervertebral osteochondrosis also is present or, rarely, when a gas-forming microorganism is responsible for the infection.
From Resnick D, Niwayama G: Osteomyelitis, septic arthritis, and soft tissue infection: Axial skeleton. In: Resnick D (ed): Diagnosis of Bone and Joint Disorders, 3rd ed. Philadelphia: WB Saunders Co, 1995, p 2436.

characteristic alterations that help differentiate these possible diagnoses. Primary or metastatic tumor in the spine does not lead to significant loss of IVD space. An intact IVD space with adjacent vertebral body lysis is more characteristic of a tumor than infection. On occasion, myeloma and chordoma can extend across or around the IVD to involve contiguous vertebrae.[54] It is also possible for intraosseous disc herniation to occur secondary to vertebral body bone weakening secondary to invasion.[55]

Treatment

Therapy of IVD infection in adults includes antibiotics and immobilization by bed rest, casts, or bracing. There is little agreement in the literature as to just what component of therapy is most effective in this disease. Some authors suggest that bed rest and immobilization are adequate and that antibiotics are not necessary[56]; however, most patients receive a 4- to 6-week course of antibiotic therapy.[14] The response to treatment is monitored by a relief of pain, return of the ESR to normal, and radiographic evidence of IVD space restoration or bony ankylosis of adjacent vertebral bodies. Five French immunosuppressed patients with *Aspergillus* discitis were treated with itraconazole alone or in combination with 5-flucytosine and amphotericin B. Surgical débridement was not necessary in these patients with fungal discitis.[57] Surgical exploration is not indicated unless there are signs of spinal cord compression.[15] Surgical fusion is unnecessary.

Prognosis

Most patients with IVD infection have a benign course and recover fully without disability. Patients usually have fusion of the IVD space with full range of motion on healing and are asymptomatic.[14] In the cervical spine, spontaneous fusion occurs in 6 to 7 weeks after discitis secondary to discography.[45]

When discitis is suspected early and antibiotics are given in high doses until normalization of ESR, discitis resolves in a few weeks and mild or no vertebral erosions occur. When antibiotic therapy is delayed or is inadequate in regard to the sensitivity of the organism, dosage, or duration, infection may last months and be associated with marked destruction of the vertebral bodies.[58]

The most serious complication of IVD space infection was reported by Kemp and colleagues.[1] In their group of 13 patients, 3 were hemiplegic and 3 were paraplegic, and all required surgical decompression. At operation, direct extension of inflammatory granulation tissue was identified growing posteriorly and involving the meninges and spinal cord. Cord damage was secondary to compression of the cord by edema, by inflammatory tissue, or from thrombosis of spinal cord vessels. Of the six patients with neurologic symptoms, two had complete recovery, two had partial recovery, and two had no recovery after surgical decompression. The appearance of neurologic symptoms was rapid in these patients, although most of them had back pain for longer than 4 months. Accurate diagnosis and the prompt institution of appropriate therapy should prevent the emergence of this complication of disc infection.

References

INTERVERTEBRAL DISC SPACE INFECTION

1. Kemp HBS, Jackson JW, Jeremiah JD, Hall AJ: Pyogenic infections occurring primarily in intervertebral discs. J Bone Joint Surg 55B:698, 1973.
2. McCain GA, Harth M, Bell DA, et al.: Septic discitis. J Rheumatol 8:100, 1981.
3. Pilgaard S: Discitis (closed space infection) following removal of lumbar intervertebral disc. J Bone Joint Surg 51A:713, 1969.
4. Boston HC Jr, Bianco AJ Jr, Rhodes KH: Disk space infections in children. Orthop Clin North Am 6:953, 1975.
5. Smith NR: The intervertebral discs. Br J Surg 18:358, 1931.
6. Wiley AM, Trueta J: The vascular anatomy of the spine and its relationship to pyogenic vertebral osteomyelitis. J Bone Joint Surg 41B:796, 1959.
7. Hassler O: The human intervertebral disc. Acta Orthop Scand 40:765, 1970.
8. Batson OV: The function of the vertebral veins and their role in the spread of metastasis. Ann Surg 112:138, 1940.
9. Doyle JR: Narrowing of the intervertebral disc space in children. J Bone Joint Surg 42A:1191, 1960.
10. Griffiths HED, Jones DM: Pyogenic infection of the spine. J Bone Joint Surg 53B:383, 1971.
11. Ghormley RK, Bickel WH, Dickson DD: A study of acute infectious lesions of the intervertebral discs. South Med J 33:347, 1940.
12. Lundstrom TS, Levine DP: Disk space infections. In: Jauregui LE (ed): Diagnosis and Management of Bone Infections. New York: Marcel Dekker, 1995, pp 151–166.
13. Ettinger WH Jr, Arnett FC Jr, Stevens MB: Intervertebral disc space infections: another low back syndrome of the young. Johns Hopkins Med J 141:23, 1977.
14. Onofrio BM: Intervertebral discitis: incidence, diagnosis and management. Clin Neurosurg 27:481, 1980.
15. Oliff JFC, Gwyther SJ, Hart G: Case of the month: a case of postoperative paresis. Br J Radiol 63:819, 1990.

16. Lownie SP, Ferguson GG: Spinal subdural empyema complicating cervical discography. Spine 14:1415, 1989.

17. Cashion EL: Cervical intervertebral disc space infection following cerebral angiography. Neuroradiology 2:176, 1971.

18. Abramovitz JN: Complications of surgery for discogenic disease of the spine. Neurosurg Clin North Am 4:167, 1993.

19. Gordon EJ: Infection of disc space secondary to fistula from pelvic abscess. South Med J 70:114, 1977.

20. Boscamp JR, Steigbigel NH: Disk space infection. In: Schlossberg D (ed): Orthopedic Infection. New York: Springer-Verlag, 1988, pp 49–68.

21. Jonsson B, Soderholm R, Stromqvist B: Erythrocyte sedimentation rate after lumbar spine surgery. Spine 16:1049, 1991.

22. Thielander U, Larsson S: Quantification of C-reactive levels and erythrocyte sedimentation rate after spinal surgery. Spine 17:400, 1992.

23. Scherbel AL, Gardner JW: Infections involving the intervertebral discs: diagnosis and management. JAMA 174:370, 1960.

24. Rawlings CE III, Wilkins RH, Gallis HA, et al.: Postoperative intervertebral disc space infection. Neurosurgery 13:371, 1983.

25. Meyes E, Flipo R, Van Bosterhaut B, et al.: Septic *Streptococcus milleri* spondylodiscitis. J Rheumatol 17:1421, 1990.

26. Selby RC, Pillary KV: Osteomyelitis and disc infection secondary to *Pseudomonas aeruginosa* in heroin addiction: case report. J Neurosurg 37:463, 1972.

27. Ponte CD, McDonald M: Septic discitis resulting from *Escherichia coli* urosepsis. J Fam Pract 34:767, 1992.

28. Solans R, Simeon P, Cuenca R, et al.: Infectious discitis caused by *Enterobacter cloacae*. Ann Rheum Dis 51:906, 1992.

29. Mathieu E, Koeger A, Rozenberg S, Bourgeois P: *Campylobacter* spondylodiscitis and deficiency of cellular immunity. J Rheumatol 18:1929, 1991.

30. Levy DI, Bucci MN, Hoff JT: Discitis caused by the Centers for Disease Control microorganism group Ve-1. Neurosurgery 25:655, 1989.

31. Meis JF, Sauerwein RW, Gyssens IC, et al.: *Kingella kingae* intervertebral diskitis in an adult. Clin Infect Dis 15:530, 1992.

32. Pate D, Katz A: Clostridia discitis: a case report. Arthritis Rheum 22:1039, 1979.

33. Pennisi AK, Davis DO, Wiesel S, Moskovitz P: CT appearance of *Candida* diskitis. J Comput Assist Tomogr 9:1050, 1985.

34. Noordeen MHH, Godfrey LW: Case report of an unusual cause of low back pain: intervertebral diskitis caused by *Eikenella corrodens*. Clin Orthop 280:175, 1992.

35. Sugar AM: Case records of the Massachusetts General Hospital. N Engl J Med 324:754, 1991.

36. Castelli C, Benazzo F, Minoli L, et al.: *Aspergillus* infection of the L3–L4 disc space in an immunosuppressed heart transplant patient. Spine 15:1369, 1988.

37. Norris S, Ehrlich MG, Keim DE, et al.: Early diagnosis of disc-space infection using gallium-67. J Nucl Med 19:384, 1978.

38. Choong K, Monaghan P, McGuigan L, McLean R: Role of bone scintigraphy in the early diagnosis of discitis. Ann Rheum Dis 49:932, 1990.

39. Nolla-Sole JM, Mateo-Soria L, Rozadilla-Sacanell A, et al.: Role of technetium-99m diphosphonate and gallium-67 citrate bone scanning in the early diagnosis of infectious spondylodiscitis: a comparative study. Ann Rheum Dis 51:665, 1992.

40. Whalen JL, Brown ML, McLeod R, Fitzgerald RH: Limitations of indium leukocyte imaging for the diagnosis of spine infections. Spine 16:193, 1991.

41. Nielsoen VAH, Iversen E, Ahlgren P: Postoperative discitis: radiology of progress and healing. Acta Radiol 31:559, 1990.

42. Dall BE, Rowe DE, Odette WG, Batts DH: Postoperative discitis: diagnosis and management. Clin Orthop 224:138, 1987.

43. Morgenlander JC, Rozear MP: Disc space infection: a case report with MRI diagnosis. Am Fam Physician 42:984, 1990.

44. Boden SD, David DO, Dina T, et al.: Postoperative diskitis: distinguishing early MR imaging findings from normal postoperative disk space changes. Radiology 184:765, 1992.

45. Guyer RD, Collier R, Stith WJ, et al.: Discitis after discography. Spine 13:1352, 1988.

46. Fouquet B, Goupille P, Jattiot F, et al.: Discitis after lumbar disc surgery: features of "aseptic" and "septic" forms. Spine 17:356, 1992.

47. Osti OL, Fraser RD, Vernon-Roberts B: Discitis after discography. J Bone Joint Surg 72B:271, 1990.

48. Taylor TKF, Bye WA: Role of antibiotics in the management of postoperative disc space infections. Aust NZ J Surg 48:74, 1978.

49. Teplick JG, Haskin ME: Intravenous contrast-enhanced CT of the postoperative lumbar spine: improved identification of recurrent disk herniation, scar, arachnoiditis, and diskitis. AJR 143:845, 1984.

50. Onik G, Shang Y, Maroon JC: Automated percutaneous biopsy in postoperative diskitis: a new method. AJNR 11:391, 1990.

51. Patton JT: Differential diagnosis of inflammatory spondylitis. Skeletal Radiol 1:77, 1976.

52. Kenney CM III, Goldstein SJ: MRI of sarcoid spondylodiskitis. J Comput Assist Tomogr 16:660, 1992.

53. Sundaram M, Seelig R, Pohl D: Vertebral erosions in patients undergoing maintenance hemodialysis for chronic renal failure. AJR 149:323, 1987.

54. Resnick D, Niwayama G: Osteomyelitis, septic arthritis, and soft-tissue infection: The axial skeleton. In: Resnick D (ed): Diagnosis of Bone and Joint Disorders, 3rd ed. Philadelphia, WB Saunders Co, 1995, pp 2419–2447.

55. Resnick D, Niwayama G: Intervertebral disc abnormalities associated with vertebral metastasis: observations in patients and cadavers with prostate cancer. Invest Radiol 13:182, 1978.

56. Sullivan CR: Diagnosis and treatment of pyogenic infections of the intervertebral disc. Surg Clin North Am 41:1077, 1961.

57. Cortet B, Deprez X, Trili R, et al.: *Aspergillus* discitis: a report of five cases. Rev Rhum Ed Fr (Eng. Abstr.) 60:38, 1993.

58. Postacchini F, Cinotti G: Iatrogenic lumbar discitis. J Bone Joint Surg 74B:(suppl 1) 70, 1992.

HERPES ZOSTER

Capsule Summary

Frequency of neck pain—very common
Location of neck pain—cervical dermatomes
Quality of neck pain—burning, tingling, sharp, deep, boring

Symptoms and signs—vesicular dermatomal rash, fever

Laboratory and x-ray tests—lymphocytosis, increased antibody response, lesional culture

Treatment—analgesics, corticosteroids, antiviral agents

Prevalence and Pathogenesis

Herpes zoster (shingles) is a late complication of a varicella infection (chickenpox) during childhood. The disease is characterized by an erythematous, papular rash accompanied by pain in the distribution of a peripheral sensory nerve. Pain may antedate the skin lesions by 4 to 7 days and confuse the diagnosis. The process may resolve without any residual symptoms but, in older patients, the infection may result in scarring and persistent pain that is resistant to treatment. In some patients, the pain is severe enough to cause considerable disability.

The varicella-zoster virus (VZV) belongs to the herpesvirus group, which includes herpes simplex virus, cytomegalovirus, and Epstein-Barr virus. These viruses contain deoxyribonucleic acid (DNA) in a viral capsid surrounded by an envelope that allows the VZV to gain entrance into the host cells. The VZV can replicate itself only within host cells. It incorporates variable amounts of host membrane into its envelope, allowing it to lie dormant in a normal cell. Clinical expression of the disease occurs when immune surveillance diminishes, allowing the virus to emerge from its hiding place.

The initial infection with VZV is varicella (chickenpox), at which time patients develop a viremia with dissemination of the virus throughout the body. The termination of this illness corresponds with the development of both humoral and cellular immune mechanisms. The VZV is sequestered in the posterior spinal sensory ganglia in the spinal cord where it remains dormant for an unspecified time. During a period of low host resistance, the viruses grow in a ganglion or nerve, resulting in skin lesions and pain. These patients are infectious and can transmit a varicella infection to previously unexposed people. Evidence suggests that zoster is a reactivation of a previous infection and is not the result of a new exposure: a varicella infection in a patient does not give herpes zoster to someone who has previously had chickenpox.[1]

The factors that initiate the resurgence of infection are not known, but advancing age and diminished immune competence play a role. Herpes zoster has increased incidence in patients older than 50 years of age. Hope-Simpson reported in a study of 182 herpes zoster patients a rate of 2 to 3 cases per 1,000 for patients 20 to 50 years of age, 5 cases per 1,000 for patients 50 years of age, and more than 10 cases per 1,000 for those 80 years of age.[2] In another study, herpes zoster also occurred more frequently in an elderly population.[3] Herpes zoster occurs in 10% to 20% of the population.[4] Herpes zoster also occurs more commonly in patients with impaired immune function. This may be particularly true in patients with diminished cell-mediated immunity to VZV; lesional interferon concentrations are decreased in those with more widespread disease.[5] Herpes zoster was associated with lymphoreticular malignancies with VZV infection occurring in 25% of patients with Hodgkin's disease and 10% of non-Hodgkin's lymphoma patients during a 2-year study.[6] Patients who are receiving chemotherapy or radiotherapy may also have an increased risk of developing herpes zoster. However, people who are otherwise normal who develop herpes zoster are not more likely to develop a malignancy than any other healthy person.[7] Often, there is no identifiable precipitating cause for the reactivation of the virus, although trauma to an area of skin may precede the appearance of lesions. Herpes zoster exhibits no sexual or racial predilection and has no seasonal variation or relation to varicella epidemics. A study of 1,019 herpes zoster patients reported 60% women, with a mean age of 58 years, with a prevalence varying between 1.3 to 1.6 per 1,000 per year.[8] This study also reported a statistically significant seasonal variation, with the lesions appearing most often in summer and least often in spring.[8]

Herpes zoster starts in an individual with a history of chickenpox with replication of virus in the cell body of a cutaneous sensory neuron lying in the dorsal root ganglion. The virus spreads within the sensory nerve centrally and peripherally. Histologic examination of the central nervous system reveals inflammation, hemorrhage, and necrosis in the dorsal root ganglion, the posterior horn and, occasionally, the corresponding motor neuron in the adjacent anterior horn. (This finding correlates with the occasional patient with motor loss associated with herpes zoster lesions.) The large, myelinated sensory fibers are preferentially affected; this results in a decreased ratio of large position to small pain fibers, diminishing pain modulation at the spinal cord level. The virus reaches the skin and replicates in the lower epidermal layers with ballooning degeneration of cells and development of multinucleated giant cells and intranuclear inclusion bodies. Inflammation in the skin causes erythema, edema, vesicular eruptions, hemorrhage, and necrosis. Healing in the skin results in depigmentation, atrophy, and permanent scarring. The virus can be grown from early vesicles, but that is unlikely once the lesion becomes pustular and develops a crust.

In patients who are immunocompromised, herpes zoster may cause damage to the spinal cord (myelitis) and brain (encephalitis).[9, 10] These patients have symptoms and signs that extend beyond the dermatome that was initially affected.

Clinical History

Herpes zoster presents with a 4- to 28-day prodrome of constitutional symptoms including fever, malaise, chills, lethargy, and gastrointestinal symptoms, particularly in the elderly. The first local symptom is usually pain in the nerve segment, which is burning or shooting in character, and is often associated with dysesthesias in the area of skin supplied by the affected nerve root. Within a week after the onset of pain, an eruption appears as a series of localized erythematous papules that develop into vesicles grouped together on an erythematous base and follow a segmental distribution. Rarely, the pain may be followed by minimal erythema or no skin changes at all (zoster sine herpete).[11] In this situation, the central nervous system is damaged without producing skin ulcers. This form of the disease may cause extensive neurologic disease and may be fatal in patients who are immunocompromised.[12] Within days, the eruption fades and the vesicles dry with crusts, leaving small scars in the skin. The skin may become partially or completely analgesic. Pain usually resolves with the skin lesion; however, it may persist for years. This postherpetic neuralgia is more likely to occur in elderly patients.

The course of pain of herpes zoster follows a characteristic pattern. Once the rash appears, pain of the prodrome period recedes. As the rash evolves, the sensory and pain disturbances disappear, especially in people younger than 40 years of age. In people older than 50 years of age, the pain is more pronounced and is usually associated with unpleasant dysesthesias, the most distressing of which is pressure sensi-

tivity of the skin to any touch. When the rash is at its greatest extent, pain is minimal. As the rash crusts, pain recurs, usually with an intense, lancinating quality. Pain becomes constant, deep, and boring. The skin feels increasingly tightened. The course of the rash and the pain are clearly not synchronous. Patients with resolution of the rash but continued pain are considered to have postherpetic neuralgia.

The frequency and severity of postherpetic neuralgia increase with age, with 35% of patients 60 years of age and 50% of patients older than 70 years of age developing herpes zoster.[13] The symptoms may last weeks to years. Pain has an unrelenting, deep, boring quality that is intensified by paroxyms of lancinating pain. Patients try to keep clothes off the area to diminish the dysesthesias. Others may complain of a feeling of worms under the skin or ants crawling on the skin (formication). Patients may become clinically depressed because of the pain.

The dermatomes over the whole back are frequently affected. The thoracic spinal nerves are affected in 50% to 55% of cases, the cervical nerves in 15% to 24%, the lumbar and sacral nerves in 10% to 15%, and cranial nerves in 10% to 15%.[8, 14] The upper cervical segments (C2–C4) are more commonly affected than the lower segments.[14] The same segment may be involved with herpes zoster on two or three occasions.[2]

Physical Examination

The skin lesions may be found in any segmental sensory nerve distribution. They have a characteristic appearance that helps distinguish this lesion from other skin diseases. The lesions begin as an erythematous patch or indurated plaque. Scattered, grouped vesicles (1 to 3 mm) on an erythematous base are usual. The distal end of a skin dermatome is affected initially, and new lesions appear in a more central location for a week. The lesions tend to coalesce and form a linear array but remain unilateral and do not cross the midline. Occasionally, patients do develop bilateral disease and a few scattered extradermatomal vesicles. This is not necessarily a sign of disseminated disease associated with a worse prognosis.[15]

The vesicles initially clear, then grow cloudy, crust, and desquamate for 3 weeks. Once crusts appear, the lesions are no longer contagious. The lesions heal with postinflammatory hypopigmented macules or patches. If secondarily infected, lesions may have depressed scars. A number of areas of cutaneous lesions suggest disseminated disease.

In addition to cutaneous manifestations, patients with herpes zoster may demonstrate other manifestations of neurologic dysfunction. Patients may have mild motor paresis in the motor nerve that corresponds to the spinal root level of the involved cutaneous nerve. The paresis is usually temporary.[16] Visceral involvement as well as autonomic nerve involvement occurs. Patients with cervical herpes zoster may develop diaphragmatic paralysis and respiratory insufficiency.[17] Hoarseness secondary to spinal cord involvement may be a complication. Other rare signs of central nervous system involvement include transverse myelitis, encephalitis, and cerebral vasculitis.[18, 19] Patients with cervical herpes zoster may develop brain-stem infarction with associated hemiplegia.[20]

Physical examination may reveal fever and localized lymphadenopathy during the initial phase of disease. A nonimmunosuppressed patient with no known underlying disease who develops disseminated lesions warrants a careful physical examination for lymphadenopathy and splenomegaly and laboratory tests (complete blood count, renal function, and anergy panel) to screen for a hidden lymphoproliferative malignancy. People who are younger than 50 years who develop herpes zoster in the cervical distribution should be examined for signs of acquired immunodeficiency syndrome. These people may have signs of other infections, including herpes simplex and candidiasis as well as oral hairy leukoplakia or lymphoma.[21]

Laboratory Data

Cerebrospinal fluid examination may demonstrate an increase in white blood cells in up to one third of patients with herpes zoster. Viral cultures may be positive for virus if fluid from acute vesicular lesions is cultured. Gel-precipitin techniques can also be used to demonstrate specific antigens in fluid and crusts of lesions. Herpes zoster antibodies may show a fourfold rise during an infection.[22]

Dermal epithelial cells obtained from scraping the early lesions may show giant cells and intranuclear inclusion bodies. Tzanck's test findings are compatible but not diagnostic of herpes zoster infection because herpes simplex may show similar abnormalities.

Radiographic Evaluation

Magnetic resonance (MR) imaging of the cervical spinal cord may demonstrate enlargement of the cord with noncontiguous areas of increased intramedullary signal in herpes zoster patients. These enhanced images may extend beyond the level of the involved dermatome. Gadolinium enhancement may highlight the dorsal root entry zone as well as the spinal cord. Repeat MR imaging may demonstrate a return of the spinal cord to normal size, but continued increased signal in the dorsal and intramedullary zones is suggestive of glial scarring.[23]

Differential Diagnosis

The diagnosis of herpes zoster offers little difficulty when the characteristic pain and vesicular eruption are present. The diagnosis is more difficult in the pre-eruptive stage. Herpes zoster should be considered in patients with sudden onset of burning pain in a segmental distribution. Following these patients for a short time until the appearance of vesicles helps establish the correct diagnosis. Herpes zoster needs to be considered in the differential diagnosis of radiculopathy, even in the absence of rash.[24]

Other skin lesions may be confused with herpes zoster infection. Herpes simplex does not usually affect an entire dermatome like herpes zoster. Culture of lesions should help make the distinction. Contact dermatitis may appear in linear band but lacks the painful prodrome. It is pruritic as opposed to painful, may cross the midline, and does not cause paresthesias. Superficial pyoderma, like impetigo, has fewer lesions, is not linear, and has no associated paresthesias. The radiation of pain may be confused with muscle strain or a herniated intervertebral disc.[25] The appearance of the skin rash helps differentiate these individuals.

Treatment

The treatment of herpes zoster is mainly supportive and directed at controlling pain; antibiotic therapy is indicated only for patients who develop bacterial superinfection. Patients with vesicles are infectious and should limit contact with people who have not had varicella; they are no longer infectious once the lesions crust over.

The therapeutic goals are to limit segmental infection and prevent general dissemination, tissue injury, and postherpetic neuralgia (Table 12–10). The first two deal with limiting viral replication, and the second two deal with limiting inflammation that causes tissue injury.[26] Herpes zoster is a self-limited disease such that treatment must be tailored specifically to the patient's age and status of immune function. In healthy patients younger than 50 years of age, therapy may be limited to analgesics, mild sedatives, antipruritics, and antibacterial ointments. In healthy patients older than 50 years of age, the goal is to prevent postherpetic neuralgia. Corticosteroids in short-course therapy have been shown to prevent the development of postherpetic pain in a significant percentage of patients.[27, 28] A study of oral high-dose acyclovir (an inhibitor of herpes virus DNA polymerase) in 205 immunocompetent patients older than 60 years of age demonstrated faster healing when the drug was given early in the course of the eruption.[29] Adenosine phosphate, 100 mg administered intramuscularly three times a week for 4 weeks, has improved healing and decreased pain compared to a placebo group.[30] Additional studies are needed to clarify the role of all these drugs in herpes zoster infection in normal hosts. Epidural or sympathetic blockade in patients with herpes zoster for 28 days or less does not prevent the onset of postherpetic neuralgia.[31, 32] Review of all the studies of drugs used for the prevention of postherpetic neuralgia demonstrates deficiencies in study design.[33]

Appropriate therapy for immunocompromised patients, young and old, is associated with greater potential toxicities. The therapy is instituted to prevent the dissemination of virus beyond the primary dermatome. Vidarabine, a purine analogue that blocks viral replication through its effects on viral DNA polymerase, when given within 3 days of the onset of skin rash, accelerates healing and decreases dissemination and postherpetic neuralgia when compared with control subjects.[34] The disadvantages of the drug include the need for 12-hour continuous intravenous infusion and renal toxicity. Zoster immune globulin has not been shown to be better than serum gamma globulin for prevention of dissemination and postherpetic neuralgia in immunocompromised patients and has not been recommended for this purpose.[35]

Intravenous acyclovir has become the recommended therapy for immunocompromised patients. The recommended intravenous dosage of 500 mg/m² of body surface area administered for 1 hour three times a week for 1 week at the earliest sign of the rash has reduced pain and dissemination and increased the rate of healing. Acyclovir is more selective an antiviral agent and has less host toxicity. Oral acyclovir is used in ambulatory patients. Oral acyclovir, 800 mg five times a day for 7 days, is recommended for herpes zoster in normal hosts.[36]

The role of corticosteroids in the immunocompromised group is limited. Corticosteroids may promote dissemination and not prevent postherpetic pain. Therefore, they have not been recommended for this group of patients.

Postherpetic neuralgia, once established, is a difficult problem to treat. Oral acyclovir is no better than placebo in relieving pain secondary to postherpetic neuralgia.[37] Therapy is directed at controlling pain, not at killing virus. Some of the therapies that have been tried include amitriptyline (25 mg nightly, with maintenance doses of 100 mg), oral corticosteroids, intralesional triamcinolone, cutaneous nerve stimulation, anesthetic nerve blocks, and topical medications including capsaicin.[38] Niv and colleagues have suggested that different components of postherpetic pain be treated with specific agents.[39] Burning pain may best respond to tricyclic antidepressants. Lancinating pain responds to anticonvulsant drugs (valproic acid). Dysesthetic pain responds to neuroleptic medication (fluphenazine). Patients with intact skin sensitivity respond to transcutaneous electrical nerve stimulator therapy. Patients with intact sensation may respond to dry

TABLE 12–10. THERAPY FOR HERPES ZOSTER

Immunocompetent	
Younger than 50 years of age	Analgesics, sedatives, topical antibacterial ointment for ulcerations
Older than 50 years of age	Corticosteroids (60 mg/d for 3-week period)
	Acyclovir (?)
	Adenosine monophosphate (?)
Immunocompromised	Intravenous acyclovir 500 mg/m² for 1 hour three times daily for 1 week
	or
	Oral acyclovir 800 mg five times daily for 1 week
Postherpetic neuralgia	Amitriptyline up to 100 mg daily, cutaneous nerve stimulation, local nerve blocks, capsaicin (?)

needling to the level of the underlying muscle. The majority of the 97 consecutive patients treated with components of this conservative therapy had significant pain relief.[39]

A study of oral corticosteroids demonstrated no definite improvement compared with placebo for postherpetic neuralgia.[40] Antidepressants—amitriptyline and desipramine but not lorazepam—have been associated with relief of postherpetic pain.[41, 42] Topical capsaicin is more effective than the cream's vehicle for pain relief when applied daily for 6 weeks.[43] On a single-dose basis, 0.2 mg of clonidine has greater pain relief than 120 mg of codeine, 800 mg of ibuprofen, and placebo for postherpetic neuralgia.[44] Mexiletine, an oral lidocaine-like antiarrhythmic agent, has been helpful in the treatment of diabetic neuropathy.[45] Mexiletine, administered 450 to 900 mg in divided doses, has been effective in decreasing pain associated with peripheral nerve injuries.[31] This drug may also have the potential to be an effective agent for the treatment of neuralgia secondary to herpes virus reactivation. Studies involving herpes zoster patients need to be completed before the efficacy is documented. In general many patients with neuralgia remain resistant to these therapies and continue with pain.

Prognosis

Herpes zoster is usually a disease of short duration resulting in little permanent disability; however, the patient who is older and has an underlying disease may be left with permanent residual effects. These may include postherpetic neuralgia, paralysis, and widespread dissemination. Postherpetic neuralgia is rare in patients younger than 40 years of age but occurs in up to 75% of patients older than 60 years of age.[28] Disseminated herpes zoster with at least 20 or more vesicles outside the primary dermatome occurs up to 10 days after the onset of rash and affects up to 10% of herpes zoster infections. Approximately 30% of these patients are immunocompromised, particularly those with lymphoproliferative malignancy, immunosuppressive therapy, and poor cell-mediated immunity.[46, 47] Most patients have resolution of disseminated herpes zoster without sequelae. However, the immunocompromised patient has a worse prognosis. Patients with cervical herpes zoster may develop myelitis. These patients have more neurologic dysfunction that may not return to normal. These individuals are at risk for a worse prognosis.

Those patients left with persistent and intractable postherpetic pain may suffer significant disability. Available therapy to prevent this component of herpes zoster infection or to manage its aftereffects is inadequate.

References

HERPES ZOSTER

1. Miller LH, Brunell PA: Zoster, reinfection or activation of latent virus? Observations on the antibody response. Am J Med 49:480, 1970.
2. Hope-Simpson RE: The nature of herpes zoster: a long-term study and a new hypothesis. Proc Ro Soc Med 58:9, 1965.
3. Weller TH: Varicella and herpes zoster: changing concepts of the natural history, control, and importance of a not-so-benign virus. N Engl J Med 309:1362, 1983.
4. Strauss SE, Ostrove JM, Inchauspe G, et al.: Varicella-zoster virus infections: biology, natural history, treatment, and prevention. Ann Intern Med 108:221, 1988.
5. Stevens DA, Merigan TC: Interferon, antibody, and other host factors in herpes zoster. J Clin Invest 51:1170, 1972.
6. Schimpff S, Serpick A, Stoler B, et al.: Varicella-zoster infection in patients with cancer. Ann Intern Med 76:241, 1972.
7. Ragozzino MW, Melton LJ, Kurland LT, et al.: Risk of cancer after herpes zoster: a population-based study. N Engl J Med 307:393, 1982.
8. Glynn C, Crockford G, Gavaghan D, et al.: Epidemiology of shingles. J R Soc Med 83:617, 1990.
9. Devinsky O, Cho E, Petito CK, Price RW: Herpes zoster myelitis. Brain 114:1181, 1991.
10. Jemesek J, Greenberg SB, Taber L, et al.: Herpes zoster-associated encephalitis: clinicopathologic report of 12 cases and review of the literature. Medicine 52:81, 1983.
11. Burgoon CF, Burgoon JS, Baldridge GD: The natural history of herpes zoster. JAMA 164:265, 1957.
12. Dueland AN, Devlin M, Martin JR, et al.: Fatal varicella-zoster virus meningoradiculitis without skin involvement. Ann Neurol 29:569, 1991.
13. de Moragas JM, Kierland RR: The outcome of patients with herpes zoster. Arch Dermatol 75:193, 1957.
14. Watson CPN: Postherpetic neuralgia. Neurol Clin 7:231, 1989.
15. Juel-Jensen BE: Herpes simplex and zoster. Br Med J 1:406, 1973.
16. Thomas JE, Howard FM Jr: Segmental zoster paresis: a disease profile. Neurology 22:459, 1972.
17. Stowasser M, Cameron J, Oliver WA: Diaphragmatic paralysis following cervical herpes zoster. Med J Aust 153:555, 1990.
18. Hogan EL, Krigman MR: Herpes zoster myelitis: evidence for viral invasion of the spinal cord. Arch Neurol 29:309, 1973.
19. Horte B, Price RW, Jiminez D: Multifocal varicella-zoster virus leukoencephalitis temporally remote from herpes zoster. Ann Neurol 9:251, 1981.
20. Willeit J, Schmutzhard E: Cervical herpes zoster and delayed brainstem infarction. Clin Neurol Neurosurg 93:245, 1991.
21. Corey JP, Seligman I: Otolaryngology problems in the

immune compromised patient: an evolving natural history. Otolaryngol Head Neck Surg 104:196, 1991.

22. Williams V, Gershon A, Brunnel PA: Serologic response varicella-zoster membrane antigens measured by indirect immunofluorescence. J Infect Dis 130:669, 1974.

23. Esposito MB, Arrington JA, Murtaugh FR, et al.: MR of the spinal cord in a patient with herpes zoster. AJNR 14:203, 1993.

24. Burkman KA, Gaines RW Jr, Kashani SR, Smith RD: Herpes zoster: A consideration in the differential diagnosis of radiculopathy. Arch Phys Med Rehabil 69:132, 1988.

25. Rash MR: Herpes zoster complicating a herniated-thoracic disc. Orthop Rev 11:91, 1982.

26. Price RW: Herpes zoster: an approach to systemic therapy. Med Clin North Am 66:1105, 1982.

27. Eaglestein WH, Katz R, Brown JA: The effects of early corticosteroid therapy on skin eruption and pain of herpes zoster. JAMA 211:1681, 1970.

28. Keczkes K, Basheer AM: Do corticosteroids prevent post-herpetic neuralgia? Br J Dermatol 102:551, 1981.

29. McKendrick MW, McGill JI, White JE, Wood MJ: Oral acyclovir in acute herpes zoster. Br Med J 293:1529, 1986.

30. Sklar SH, Blue WT, Alexander EJ, Bodian CA: Herpes zoster: the treatment and prevention of neuralgia with adenosine monophosphate. JAMA 253:1427, 1985.

31. Yanagida H, Suwa K, Corssen G: No prophylactic effect of early sympathetic blockade on postherpetic neuralgia. Anesthesiology 66:73, 1987.

32. Nurmikko TJ, Rasanen A, Hakkinen V: Clinical and neurophysiological observations on acute herpes zoster. Clin J Pain 6:284, 1990.

33. Schmader KE, Studenski S: Are current therapies useful for the prevention of postherpetic neuralgia? A critical analysis of the literature. J Gen Intern Med 4:83, 1989.

34. Whitley RJ, Soong SJ, Dolin R, et al.: NIAID collaborative antiviral study group: early vidarabine therapy to control the complications of herpes zoster in immunocompromised patients. N Engl J Med 307:971, 1982.

35. Stevens D, Merigan T: Zoster immune globulin prophylaxis of disseminated zoster in compromised hosts. Arch Intern Med 140:52, 1980.

36. Whitley RJ, Gnann JW Jr: Acyclovir: a decade later. N Engl J Med 327:782, 1992.

37. Surman OQ, Flynn T, Schooley RT, et al.: A double-blind, placebo-controlled study of oral acyclovir in postherpetic neuralgia. Psychosomatics 31:287, 1990.

38. Waston CP, Evans RJ, Reed K, et al.: Amitriptyline vs placebo in postherpetic neuralgia. Neurology 32:671, 1982.

39. Niv D, Ben-Ari S, Rappaport A, et al.: Postherpetic neuralgia: clinical experience with a conservative treatment. Clin J Pain 5:295, 1989.

40. Post BT, Philbrick JT: Do corticosteroids prevent postherpetic neuralgia? J Am Acad Dermatol 18:605, 1988.

41. Max MB, Schafer SC, Culnane M, et al.: Amitriptyline, but not lorazepam, relieves postherpetic neuralgia. Neurology 38:1427, 1988.

42. Kishore-Kumar R, Max MB, Schafer SC, et al.: Desipramine relieves postherpetic neuralgia. Clin Pharmacol Ther 47:305, 1990.

43. Bernstein JE, Korman NJ, Bickers DR, et al.: Topical capsaicin treatment of chronic postherpetic neuralgia. J Am Acad Dermatol 21:265, 1989.

44. Max MB, Schafer SC, Culnane M, et al.: Association of pain relief with drug side effects in postherpetic neuralgia: a single-dose study of clonidine, codeine, ibuprofen, and placebo. Clin Pharmacol Ther 43:363, 1988.

45. Dejgard A, Petersen P, Kastrup J: Mexiletine for the treatment of chronic painful diabetic neuropathy. Lancet 1:9, 1988.

46. Merselis J, Kaye D, Hook E: Disseminated herpes zoster: a report of 17 cases. Arch Intern Med 113:679, 1964.

47. Mazur W, Whitley R, Dolin R: Serum antibody levels as risk factors in the dissemination of herpes zoster. Arch Intern Med 139:1341, 1979.

LYME DISEASE

Capsule Summary

Frequency of neck pain—uncommon

Location of neck pain—cervical spine

Quality of neck pain—ache

Symptoms and signs—erythema migrans, general malaise, neck stiffness, radiculoneuritis

Laboratory and x-ray tests—increased erythrocyte sedimentation rate, *Borrelia* antibodies, cerebrospinal fluid pleocytosis

Treatment—antibiotics: oral for early disease, intravenous for late disease

Prevalence and Pathogenesis

Lyme disease is an infectious disease caused by the spirochete *Borrelia burgdorferi*. The organism was identified by Willie Burgdorfer and colleagues in 1982.[1] The organism is transmitted to humans by a tick vector. The clinical manifestations of the disease appear as the *Borrelia* disseminate through the organs of the body and the immune system mounts a cellular and humoral response to the organism. A generalized malaise mimicking a flu-like state, including neck pain and stiffness, occurs simultaneously with the appearance of a characteristic rash, erythema migrans (formerly known as erythema chronicum migrans). In later stages of the disease, cardiac and neurologic manifestations become prominent. Polyradiculitis, including the upper and lower extremities, is associated with this stage of the disease. Chronic arthritis, chronic fatigue, and encephalomyelitis are potential manifestations of late disease. The diagnosis of Lyme disease is suspected in an individual exposed to ticks, who develops an appropriate array of symptoms and signs, and who is confirmed by the presence of immunoglobulin M (IgM) or IgG antibodies to the *Borrelia*. All stages of the disease are treated with antibiotics, which are most successful in the early stages.

Lyme disease is the most common vector-transmitted disease in the United States.[2] Over 40,000 cases were reported to the Centers for Disease Control and Prevention from 1982 to 1991.[3] The disease is endemic in three areas of the United States: the Northeast, from Maryland to northern Massachusetts; the upper Midwest, in Minnesota and Wisconsin; and the West, primarily the coast of California and Oregon. Approximately 85% of human Lyme disease cases are reported from the endemic areas of the Northeast and Midwest.[4] The 10 states with 88% of the patients are New York, Connecticut, New Jersey, Pennsylvania, Rhode Island, Massachusetts, Maryland, Wisconsin, Minnesota, and California. These locations correspond to areas associated with large deer populations. Deer are the primary hosts for the deer tick, the vector for transmission of Lyme disease. The tick species responsible for transmitting *B. burgdorferi* to humans is restricted to *Ixodes persulcatus*.[5] In the East, *Ixodes scapularis* and, in the West, *Ixodes pacificus* are the tick vectors associated with Lyme disease. The populations of *I. scapularis* occurring in the Northeast and upper Midwest were formerly referred to as a separate third species *Ixodes dammini* because of important ecological and behavioral attributes that differ from those of populations occurring in the middle and southern states.[5, 6] The disease is not exclusively limited to these areas of the United States; cases have been reported in 46 of the contiguous states and Hawaii.[4] The geographic spread of the disease in individual states has increased.[7] The disease has also been reported in Europe, Russia, Japan, and Australia. Lyme disease affects people in all age groups. A significant number of children are affected up to the age of 9 years. Females and males are almost equally affected (53% and 47%, respectively).[3] The disease occurs primarily in whites, reflecting the exposure of this group to nonurban settings.

The disease is spread to the geographic areas by the tick vector. Other ticks and biting insects may be secondary vectors of infection. Other types of ticks and horse flies, deer flies, and mosquitoes have been reported to carry *B. burgdorferi*.[8, 9] The tick has a four-stage, 2-year life cycle. The life cycle includes an egg, larval, nymphal, and adult stage of development. Each of the three motile stages feeds only once before molting into the next stage. The usual host for the larval and nymph stage is the white-footed mouse, *Peromyscus leucopus*. The mouse is the primary reservoir for *B. burgdorferi*. The *Borrelia* parasitize the mice without causing any illness. The host is disease-free from the *Borrelia* for the remainder of its life.

The life cycle of the tick is a complex process. Eggs are deposited in the early summer. Larvae do not hatch until July. Larvae that feed before September molt to become nymphs. Those that do not feed will feed the following spring. Nymphs must feed again before they molt to become adults. Adult females attach to large vertebrates to feed and mate. After mating, the females are able to lay eggs to start a new cycle. White-tailed deer are the favorite host for the adult ticks. Each stage of the life cycle is a balance between death from the environment or survival with host contact. The balance between these two outcomes determines the number of ticks in any given geographic area. The frequency of Lyme disease infections relates, to a significant extent, to the size of the local deer population.

Larval and nymphal ticks feed on the infected mice and become colonized with *B. burgdorferi*. The ticks become vectors of the disease for humans when the ticks feed in a later developmental stage. The *B. burgdorferi* reside in the midgut of the tick. With attachment of the tick to a host, the *Borrelia* are mobilized to the salivary glands, where they infect the vertebrate.[10] This process requires approximately 24 hours to complete. Adult ticks do not transfer *B. burgdorferi* to their offspring. Larvae typically become infected with *Borrelia* by feeding on a reservoir host rather than from congenital transmission. The passage of *B. burgdorferi* between ticks and mice maintains the high rate of infection of the tick vectors in an endemic area.

The pathogenesis of Lyme disease is not entirely clear.[11] The currently accepted theory is that the organisms persist throughout the course of the disease. Organisms, although few in number, have been detected in affected organ systems long after the onset of the disease.[12, 13] Further evidence for the persistence of organisms is the variety of new IgG antibodies that emerge over time with prolonged disease. Amplification of the B-cell response would be unlikely without a changing antigenic stimulus.[14] In addition, antibiotics have a beneficial effect on the course of the disease at all of its stages.[15] In regard to genetic predisposition to particular manifestations of the disease, people with histocompatibility typing DR4 are susceptible to chronic Lyme arthritis.[16]

Clinical History

The clinical manifestations of Lyme disease may be dermatologic, cardiac, neurologic, or

TABLE 12–11.   CLINICAL STAGES OF LYME DISEASE

EARLY INFECTION		LATE INFECTION
Localized	*Disseminated*	*Persistent*
Erythema migrans	Multiple annular lesions	Chronic arthritis
Local lymphadenopathy	Bell's palsy	Encephalomyelitis
	Meningitis	Chronic fatigue
	Radiculoneuritis	Acrodermatitis chronica atrophicans
	Atrioventricular nodal block	
	Migratory arthralgias	
	Severe fatigue	
	Generalized lymphadenopathy	

musculoskeletal during the course of the illness (Table 12–11). The disease is best described by a classification system that divides it into early and late infection. The affected organ systems manifest a variety of abnormalities, depending on the duration of the infection.

Early infection is characterized by the emergence of pathognomonic skin lesions, localized lymphadenopathy, and a flu-like syndrome (Fig. 12–4). This stage corresponds to the local invasion of the skin and associated lymph nodes by the organisms, along with systemic response manifested by a flu-like syndrome. Erythema migrans (EM) is the most common and distinctive cutaneous manifestation of Lyme disease. EM appears at the site of the tick bite. The lesions are identified in 60% to 80% of Lyme disease patients.[15, 17] Skin lesions appear 2 to 28 days after the bite of an infected tick. The lesion starts as a single,

expanding red macule and expands in an annular fashion. In the United States, most EM lesions occur within 2 weeks of onset and lack central clearing.[18] The central area may clear, forming a target lesion. Central clearing may be a characteristic of EM lesions lasting 5 to 6 weeks. The skin lesion is usually asymptomatic but may be tender, warm, or pruritic. The lesion may become 15 cm or larger. A small number (less than 5%) may have a vesicular center. The EM lesion is located at the site of attachment of the tick. Only 32% of patients may recall a tick bite. The lack of awareness may be related to the small size of the nymphal *I. scapularis* tick, the lack of local tenderness or pruritus, and areas that may be difficult to visualize.[18] *B. burgdorferi* may be isolated occasionally from skin biopsies obtained from the advancing front of the lesion but are rarely needed to identify the origin of the skin le-

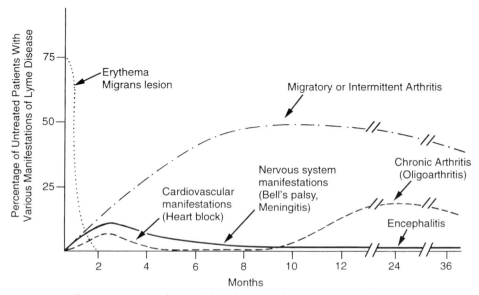

Figure 12–4. Lyme disease. Clinical course of organ system involvement.

sion.[19] Skin lesions appear most commonly on the trunk (38%), lower extremities (38%), upper extremities (11%), pelvic region (7%), and head and neck (6%).[20] Skin folds are preferred areas for tick attachment.

The flu-like syndrome is characterized by fatigue, fever, chills, malaise, headache, stiff neck, and arthralgias. Neck stiffness and pain occur in approximately 26% of patients.[21, 22] These constitutional symptoms may be the only clues to the diagnosis of Lyme disease when skin lesions are absent. Less common manifestations include malar rash, sore throat, nausea, and vomiting.

As the B. burgdorferi organisms escape to the systemic circulation, the disseminated phase of early infection occurs. Additional organ systems are affected. Within a few weeks of disease onset, up to 48% of untreated patients develop multiple annular skin lesions.[23] Other studies have reported the incidence of secondary lesions in less than 25% of patients.[18] Hematogenous spread of the Borrelia causes these lesions, which resemble EM, to appear. The lesions may vary in number up to 20, are smaller than EM lesions, and are less expansive. Secondary lesions may be evanescent, appear suddenly during an examination, then fade. Lesions may become more prominent with heating associated with bathing.[18]

Cardiac manifestations of early disseminated disease appear 4 days to 7 months after the onset of disease.[24] Cardiac disease has been reported in 4% to 20% of Lyme disease patients. Heart block is the primary manifestation of cardiac involvement.[25] First-degree to complete heart blocks have been reported. Cardiac conduction abnormalities are temporary, lasting a few weeks. Temporary pacing is occasionally required for high-grade atrioventricular block. Atrial arrhythmias occur in association with Lyme pericarditis, and ventricular arrhythmias are associated with myocarditis.

Neurologic system involvement complicates early disseminated disease in 20% of patients.[26] Throughout the disease, 40% of symptomatic infections have neurologic involvement.[27] Neurologic symptoms and signs develop weeks to 12 months after the resolution of EM. Both the peripheral nervous system (PNS) and the central nervous system (CNS) may be involved. The manifestations of nervous system disease include one or more of six neurologic syndromes: lymphocytic meningitis, cranial nerve palsies, and radiculoneuritis (early infection); and encephalopathy, polyneuropathy, and meningoencephalomyelitis (late infection).[27, 28] Lyme meningitis, the most common CNS man-

ifestation of Lyme disease, is associated with severe headache, stiff neck, photophobia, nausea, vomiting, and irritability.[29] Meningitis is the result of direct invasion of the CNS by B. burgdorferi. Meningitis may be acute, relapsing, or chronic. Most patients describe a fluctuating, mild headache. Meningismus, in the form of a stiff neck, is minimal to mild.[30] Patients with meningitis may also have significant myalgias. Approximately 50% of patients with Lyme meningitis have associated encephalitis. Concentration deficits, emotional lability, and persistent fatigue are manifestations of encephalitis. A majority of patients, up to 80%, may develop facial (Bell's) palsy.[30] Other cranial nerves, including the third, fifth, and eighth, have also been affected. A minority of patients (31% to 44%) develop radiculoneuritis, usually in the setting of cranial neuropathy.[28, 29] The peripheral nervous system is also involved. Peripheral neuritis; sensory radiculitis; brachial, lumbar, or sacral plexitis; and sensorimotor radiculoneuritis may occur within the first months of the disease.[1] These neurologic disorders may present with a variety of symptoms and signs including burning pain, paresthesia, loss of reflexes, and focal motor weakness. Rarely does the neuropathy result in atrophy or marked weakness.[30] Upper extremity abnormalities are more common than lower extremity abnormalities. Involvement of the sensory and motor nerves of the lower extremities may occur in the setting of similar disease in the upper extremities. The patients with lower extremity disease have severe radicular pain, dyesthesias, sensory loss, leg weakness, and mononeuritis multiplex. Pain is the first symptom, followed within 4 weeks by motor weakness. Weakness begins gradually and may progress to mild atrophy of the muscle. Sensory loss follows pain in a similar period in 50% of patients.[26] The sensory loss is dermatomal in distribution in the upper extremities. In the lower extremities a symmetrical distal sensory loss may also occur. The occurrence simultaneously of radiculoneuritis and cerebrospinal fluid pleocytosis is common in Europe and is known as Bannwarth's syndrome or tick-borne meningopolyneuritis.[31]

Musculoskeletal manifestations of early disease are primarily arthralgias and myalgias that occur within 8 weeks of infection.[32] Pain occurs in one or two sites at a time and migrates to other musculoskeletal structures. These locations may be affected for hours to days, with spontaneous resolution of symptoms lasting for months. Fatigue is the most common associated symptom. Subsequently, a majority of untreated patients develop intermittent episodes of frank arthritis 4 days to 2 years after disease onset.[32] The large joints, particularly the knee, become swollen and warm but not significantly painful. Other joints affected include the shoulder, ankle, elbow, temporomandibular, wrist, and hip.[33] The pattern of involvement is asymmetrical. Small joint involvement, independent of large joint disease, is unusual. The most frequently affected extra-articular locations as reported in 28 patients with Lyme disease are the back and neck in 32% and 21% of cases, respectively.[33] Periarticular involvement may occur, interspersed with episodes of arthritis in other locations of the musculoskeletal system. In most circumstances, only one periarticular structure is affected at a time, with pain lasting weeks to months in a given location.

Late infection manifestations occur as the *Borrelia* persist in organ systems infected during earlier stages. Acrodermatitis chronica atrophicans is the skin manifestation of persistent infection in Lyme borreliosis.[34] The lesion occurs predominantly in women from 40 to 70 years of age. It begins insidiously with bluish-red discoloration and swollen skin on an extremity, usually the lower leg or foot. The inflammatory stage of the lesion may persist for years. Subsequently, the skin in the involved area becomes atrophic and develops a wrinkled appearance. EM may have been present at the same site years earlier. *B. burgdorferi* may be cultured from these lesions as long as 10 years after their onset.[35]

A range of CNS and PNS abnormalities has been described in late disease that occurs more than 1 year after the onset of disease. These disease manifestations are uncommon. Patients with late symptomatic neurologic disease may have both an encephalopathy and polyneuropathy syndrome. The most clearly defined syndrome is progressive encephalomyelitis, which is characterized by spastic paresis, bladder dysfunction, ataxia, cranial nerve deficits, and dementia.[36] Late polyneuropathy may be manifested by sensory or motor abnormalities. Tingling paresthesias may occur in 50% of patients with late Lyme borreliosis.[37] The paresthesias are located distally in the arms, legs, or both and are asymmetrical and patchy in distribution. Radicular pain in the legs occurs in 25% of patients, with onset corresponding with the onset of paresthesias.[38] Median nerve entrapment (carpal tunnel syndrome) has been reported in up to 25% of patients with late symptomatic infections.[39] Other rare syndromes associated with Lyme disease include pseudotumor cerebri, stroke-like syndromes, hallucinations, and myositis.[27]

Monarticular or oligoarticular arthritis involving the knee is the most common musculoskeletal manifestation of late Lyme borreliosis.[32] Approximately 11% of untreated people with EM develop arthritis that persists for 1 year or longer. Synovitis appears 4 months to 4 years after EM. In addition to the knee, the shoulder or hip is affected. Joint involvement is a more frequent manifestation of illness in Europe than in the United States. The arthritis may persist for 4 years or longer or resolve spontaneously.[40] Figure 12–4 depicts the course of organ system involvement throughout time.

Physical Examination

Physical findings in the initial stages of the disease include the presence of EM and regional lymphadenopathy. Musculoskeletal pain may occur at rest or with motion. The cervical spine may be painful on palpation. Pain occurs in only one or two regions at a time. Episodes may resolve in hours to several days. This syndrome has been referred to as localized, intermittent musculoskeletal pain (LIMP).[41] Irregular pulse may be noticed in patients with cardiac involvement. Neurologic abnormalities may include cranial nerve dysfunction (Bell's palsy), sensory or motor nerve impairment (including brachial nerve), and mental confusion or impaired memory. Patients with late disease may have patches of atrophic skin, persistent monarticular arthritis, spastic paresis, or organic brain syndrome.

Laboratory Data

The commonly ordered screening blood tests, including complete blood count, erythrocyte sedimentation rate (ESR), and serum chemistries, yield results that are normal or nonspecific during early disseminated disease.[42] The ESR is elevated in a majority of patients. A smaller proportion of patients have abnormal levels of immunoglobulins, cryoglobulins, liver enzymes, and microscopic hematuria.[43] In patients with neurologic involvement, the cerebrospinal fluid (CSF) is found to have a lymphocytic pleocytosis and elevated protein concentration.[26] CSF is invariably abnormal in Lyme meningitis and patients with acute radicular syndromes. Patients with PNS disease, encephalopathy, and cranial neuropathy frequently have normal CSF findings. Normal CSF tests do not rule out the possibility of *B. burgdorferi* infection of the nervous system.[27] Antibodies against *Borrelia* may be locally produced and detected in CSF. The most useful CSF test is the detection of antibody to *B. burgdorferi* by Western blot analysis. This test is able to differentiate individuals with false-positive enzyme-linked immunosorbent assay (ELISA) serum assays for antibody.[30] It is essential to compare serum with CSF antibody levels to estimate the amount of intrathecal production. Synovial fluid analysis reveals findings consistent with an inflammatory arthropathy, including leukocyte counts of 5,000 to 100,000/mm³ predominantly polymorphonuclear leukocytes, with elevated protein and normal glucose concentrations.[15] Culture of skin, blood, or synovial fluid rarely renders a positive result for *B. burgdorferi* and is rarely obtained in the clinical setting.

Histopathologic evaluation of tissue biopsies has the potential to identify the presence of organisms in affected organs.[44] The organisms are most easily identified in the skin when the organisms are most abundant before dissemination. Inflammatory infiltrates may be identified in a variety of tissue samples but are not specific enough in the absence of organisms to permit a specific diagnosis. For example, synovial biopsy specimens reveal histopathologic changes that are similar to rheumatoid arthritis and Reiter's syndrome.[45]

Serologic tests are helpful in detecting the antibody response, including IgM and IgG antibodies, to epitopes on the surface structures of *B. burgdorferi*.[46] Within the first 2 to 4 weeks of infection, IgM antibodies directed against the flagellar antigen of *B. burgdorferi* appear. IgM antibodies peak after 6 to 8 weeks of disease. IgG antibodies appear over the next few weeks, corresponding with the gradual 4- to 6-month decrease in IgM antibody titer. Patients with persistent disease have IgG antibodies exclusively that remain indefinitely. Successful antibiotic therapy may result in a fall in IgG titer, but only throughout several months. Some patients have persistently elevated antibodies despite eradication of the organism. These antibodies are most effectively detected by the ELISA test. The ELISA test is more sensitive and reproducible than immunofluorescence assays. Most ELISA tests use extracts of sonicated whole *B. burgdorferi* as antigen. The ELISA test is associated with false-negative and false-positive results. False-negative results occur during the first few weeks of infection before antibodies develop or in

individuals who receive an inadequate course of antibiotic therapy early in the course of the disease and remain infected with live organisms. False-positive results occur in patients with a variety of spirochetal illnesses, including gingivitis, syphilis, Rocky Mountain spotted fever, mononucleosis, and autoimmune disorders such as rheumatoid arthritis and systemic lupus erythematosus. Although poor reproducibility of results is a major concern in interpreting Lyme antibody titers, the standardization of ELISA tests along with a relative high titer level has helped to differentiate true positive tests from sources of background cross-reactivity.

Western blot analysis is an immunoblotting technique used to confirm ELISA results or to detect antibodies early in the clinical course of the disease that may not be detected by the ELISA method.[47] Western blot analysis is able to detect antibodies to a number of specific *Borrelia* antigens. Although the ELISA method and Western blot analyses are helpful, great diversity exists in the results of laboratories when testing the same samples.[48] These inconsistencies emphasize the utility of serologic tests as adjuncts in the clinical diagnosis of Lyme disease.

In rare circumstances, when the diagnosis of Lyme disease is suspected but serologic tests are inconclusive, T lymphocyte assays for reactivity to *Borrelia*-specific antigens may be helpful.[49] The subset of patients with late Lyme disease who have negative or indeterminate antibody responses are the best candidates for the T cell proliferative assay.[50] T cells from infected patients proliferate when exposed to whole organisms. This assay is time-consuming and should be completed in patients who elicit a strong suspicion for the diagnosis without abnormal serologic tests.

A test that should be available soon for the diagnosis of Lyme disease uses polymerase chain reaction (PCR) technology.[51] PCR is able to detect the presence of a small amount of genomic DNA of *B. burgdorferi*. The PCR is superior to the ELISA or the Western blot analysis because it relies on the presence of the organism itself for a positive result. The PCR assay is very specific because particular parts of the *Borrelia* genome may be chosen for replication. The PCR of CSF of patients with Lyme meningitis is positive in about 50% of samples tested.[52] The 50% yield is consistent with the absence of *Borrelia* in organs other than the skin, and the perivascular location, and absence in body fluids, of the organisms in chronic infections.[30] The PCR has also been used for the rapid identification of *B. burgdorferi* in the serum. The PCR is three times more sensitive than culture for identifying *Borrelia* in serum for early diagnosis of Lyme disease.[53]

Radiographic Evaluation

Radiographic findings of the cervical spine are normal in patients with Lyme disease. Radiographic abnormalities, when they occur, are located in the peripheral joints, primarily the knee. Abnormalities include soft tissue swelling, loss of articular cartilage, chondrocalcinosis, and periarticular osseous erosions.[54]

Neuroimaging of the brain is abnormal in 25% of patients with neuroborreliosis. The most common finding is scattered white-matter lesions that do not enhance on MR evaluation. These lesions are smaller than those associated with demyelinating diseases. Occasionally, MR imaging reveals enhancing lesions of cranial nerves and meninges.[55]

Differential Diagnosis

The diagnosis of Lyme disease is based on the presentation of appropriate clinical symptoms in a patient who lives in or has visited an endemic area. The history of a tick bite is helpful but not essential for the diagnosis. Culture of the organism from skin or viewing it on histologic sections of biopsies from affected organs is usually unrevealing. Serologic tests are useful adjuncts in diagnosis, but abnormal findings may be present in people previously exposed to the organisms but who have cleared the infection. Basing a diagnosis solely on the presence of antibodies reactive to *B. burgdorferi* is to be discouraged.

The differential diagnosis as it affects neck pain is related to the muscle pain syndromes and neurologic disorders that cause radiculopathy and plexopathy. Fibromyalgia has been associated with Lyme disease. Patients may develop tender points in the setting of Lyme disease.[56, 57] More often, patients develop the LIMP syndrome confined to one or two joint areas in clear distinction of the multiple areas affected with fibromyalgia.

The differential diagnosis of radiculopathy includes mechanical, neoplastic, and autoimmune disorders. Patients with mechanical disorders describe radiating pain that is affected by body position. Assuming a comfortable position frequently relieves pain in patients with a mechanical cause of radiculopathy. Patients

with neoplastic disorders frequently have associated systemic symptoms that are rapidly progressive and disabling. Autoimmune disorders, such as systemic lupus erythematosus and systemic vasculitis, are associated with characteristic abnormalities in a variety of organ systems (malar rash and nodose lesions). These abnormalities help separate those patients with autoimmune disorders who may have false-positive serologic tests for Lyme disease from patients infected with *B. burgdorferi*.

Treatment

The risk of tick bites can be reduced in endemic areas. Lyme disease starts in late May when tick nymphs start searching for hosts. About 25% of nymphs contain *Borrelia* but are responsible for 90% of Lyme disease patients.[5] The association between the nymphs and disease relates to their greater abundance, their small size, and the temporal coincidence of their peak feeding activity with human outdoor activity.[5] Therefore, starting in late spring, proper dress should be encouraged by covering the skin, including tucking trousers into socks to block attachment of ticks on the lower extremities. Clothes may be impregnated with N,N-diethylmetatoluamide or permethrin to deter ticks. However, exposure of the skin to these chemicals must be limited to decrease toxicities from these agents. During periods of feeding by the various forms of the tick from spring to late summer, individuals should be examined daily for the presence of ticks. The transmission of disease is diminished by the daily removal of ticks because the inoculation of *B. burgdorferi* requires 24 hours or longer.

Randomized studies have demonstrated that the probability of developing symptoms of Lyme disease after an *Ixodes* tick bite is low and equals the rate of toxicity of the antibiotics used to treat the illness.[58] Prophylactic antibiotics should not be given routinely for tick bites.

Therapy for Lyme disease is based on antibiotics effective in eradicating *B. burgdorferi* from infected patients when clinical symptoms appear. *B. burgdorferi* is highly sensitive to tetracyclines, semisynthetic penicillins, and second- and third-generation cephalosporins. Erythromycin is an alternative agent but is less desirable than amoxicillin or doxycycline.[59] The choice of agent and its formulation, oral or intravenous, depend on the stage and organ involvement of the illness[60] (Table 12–12). The

TABLE 12–12. ANTIBIOTIC THERAPY FOR LYME DISEASE

Early local infection	
Erythema migrans	Tetracycline 500 mg four times daily 10–30 days
	Doxycycline 100 mg twice daily 10–30 days
Children	Amoxicillin 500 mg four times daily 10–30 days
Penicillin-allergic	Erythromycin 500 mg three times daily 10–30 days
Early disseminated infection	
Flu syndrome, Bell's palsy, first-degree heart block	Oral regimens
Meningitis, radiculopathy, complete heart block, arthritis	Ceftriaxone 2 g IV four times daily 14–28 days
or	Cefotaxime 3 g IV twice daily 14–28 days
Late persistent infection	Benzylpenicillin
	5 million U IV four times daily 14–28 days

treatment of choice for early local disease including EM is doxycycline or tetracycline. Amoxicillin is used for children and pregnant women. Erythromycin is less effective but is an alternative for patients allergic to penicillin. The duration of therapy is 10 days. If patients have early disseminated disease, therapy may be continued for 30 days. Patients with facial palsy or first-degree heart block can be treated with oral antibiotics.

Patients with evidence of meningitis, radiculitis, or complete heart block have been treated with intravenous antibiotics. No ideal antibiotic regimen has been determined. Intravenous antibiotics used to treat Lyme borreliosis include ceftriaxone and penicillin. Cefotaxime is also effective for disseminated disease. Therapy is continued for 14 to 28 days. Patients with Lyme arthritis are also treated with intravenous antibiotics. Although no controlled studies have been completed for persistent late infection including CNS or PNS disease, intravenous antibiotics are given for 28 days. The symptoms may not rapidly respond to the course of antibiotics. Clinical response may be delayed for as long as 6 to 8 months.[61] In a comparison of intravenous penicillin and ceftriaxone, ceftriaxone was significantly more effective with an 85% cure rate.[62] There is no scientific evidence to date supporting repeated courses of antibiotics for extended periods in the treatment of Lyme disease.

Prognosis

The prognosis of patients with Lyme disease and neck pain is excellent if these patients receive an appropriate course of antibiotics. They usually have no residual neck pain or stiffness. Patients who have radiculopathy have neuroborreliosis. These patients may also respond to antibiotics but may require intravenous medicines to improve. Clinical awareness of the symptoms and signs of Lyme disease in patients who are exposed to ticks should result in the rapid identification of the patient at risk for this disease. This is the most important way to prevent the dissemination of the organisms resulting in more serious forms of this disease. Radiculoneuropathy and peripheral neuropathy may resolve slowly for 24 months. The slow recovery may correspond to the slow healing of axonal damage. Prolonged courses of antibiotics do not influence the rate of recovery.

References

LYME DISEASE

1. Burgdorfer W, Barbour AG, Hayes SF, et al.: Lyme disease: a tick-borne spirochetosis? Science 216:1317, 1982.
2. Rahn DW: Lyme disease: clinical manifestations, diagnosis, and treatment. Semin Arthritis Rheum 20:201, 1991.
3. Dennis DT: Epidemiology. In: Coyle PK (ed): Lyme Disease. St Louis: Mosby-Year Book, 1993, pp 27–37.
4. CDC Lyme Disease—United States, 1993. MMWR 43:564, 1993.
5. Fish D: Environmental risk and presentation of Lyme disease. Am J Med 98 (suppl 4A):2S, 1995.
6. Oliver JH Jr, Owsley MR, Hutcheson HJ, et al.: Conspecificity of the ticks *Ixodes scapularis* and *I. dammini* (Acari:Ixodidae). J Med Entomol 30:54, 1993.
7. White DJ, Chang H, Benach JL, et al.: The geographic spread and temporal increase of the Lyme disease epidemic. JAMA 266:1230, 1991.
8. Anderson JF, Magnarelli LA: Avian and mammalian hosts for spirochete-infected ticks and insects in a Lyme disease focus in Connecticut. Yale J Biol Med 57:621, 1984.
9. Magnarelli LA, Anderson JF, Barbour AG: The etiologic agent of Lyme disease in deer flies, horse flies and mosquitoes. J Infect Dis 154:355, 1986.
10. Burgdorfer W: Vector/host relationships of Lyme disease spirochete, *Borrelia burgdorferi*. Rheum Dis Clin North Am 15:775, 1989.
11. Garcia-Monco JC, Benach JL: The pathogenesis of

Lyme disease. Rheum Dis Clin North Am 15:711, 1989.

12. Asbrink E, Hovmark A, Hederstedt B: The spirochetal etiology of acrodermatitis chronica atrophicans herxheimer. Acta Derm Venereol 64:506, 1984.

13. Johnston YE, Duray PH, Steere AC, et al.: Lyme arthritis: spirochetes found in synovial microangiopathic lesions. Am J Pathol 118:26, 1985.

14. Craft JE, Fischer DF, Shimamoto GT, Steere AC: Antigens of *Borrelia burgdorferi* recognized during Lyme disease: appearance of a new immunoglobulin M response and expansion of the immunoglobulin G response late in the illness. J Clin Invest 78:934, 1986.

15. Steere AC: Lyme disease. N Engl J Med 321:586, 1989.

16. Steere AC, Dwyer E, Winchester R: Association of chronic arthritis with increased DR4 and DR3. N Engl J Med 323:219, 1990.

17. Berger BW: Cutaneous manifestations of Lyme borreliosis. Rheum Dis Clin North Am 15:627, 1989.

18. Nadelman RB, Wormser GP: Erythema migrans and early Lyme disease. Am J Med 98 (suppl 4A):15S, 1995.

19. Steere AC, Grodzicki RL, Kornblatt AN, et al.: The spirochetal etiology of Lyme disease. N Engl J Med 308:733, 1983.

20. Berger BW: Dermatologic aspects. In: Coyle PK (ed): Lyme Disease. St Louis: Mosby-Year Book, 1993, pp 69–72.

21. Steere AC, Bartenhagen NH, Craft JE, et al.: The early clinical manifestations of Lyme disease. Ann Intern Med 99:76, 1983.

22. Reik L Jr: Lyme Disease and The Nervous System. New York: Thieme Medical Publishers, 1991, pp 1–130.

23. Berger BW: Erythema chronicum migrans of Lyme disease. Arch Dermatol 120:1017, 1984.

24. Steere AC, Batsford WP, Weinberg M, et al.: Lyme carditis: cardiac abnormalities of Lyme disease. Ann Intern Med 93:8, 1980.

25. McAlister HF, Klementowicz PT, Andrews C, et al.: Lyme carditis: an important cause of reversible heart block. Ann Intern Med 110:339, 1989.

26. Reik L Jr: Neurologic aspects of North American Lyme disease. In: Coyle PK (ed): Lyme Disease. St. Louis: Mosby-Year Book, 1993, pp 101–112.

27. Coyle PK: Neurologic complications of Lyme disease. Rheum Dis Clin North Am 19:993, 1993.

28. Pachner AR, Steere AC: The triad of neurologic manifestations of Lyme disease: meningitis, cranial neuritis, and radiculoneuritis. Neurology 35:47, 1985.

29. Reik L, Steere AC, Bartenhagen NH, et al.: Neurologic abnormalities of Lyme disease. Medicine 58:281, 1979.

30. Pachner AR: Early disseminated Lyme disease: Lyme meningitis. Am J Med 98 (suppl 4A):30S, 1995.

31. Ackerman R, Horstrup P, Schmidt R: Tick-borne meningopolyneuritis (Garin-Boujadoux, Bannwarth). Yale J Biol Med 57:485, 1984.

32. Steere AC, Schoen RT, Taylor E: The clinical evolution of Lyme arthritis. Ann Intern Med 197:725, 1987.

33. Steere AC: Musculoskeletal manifestations of Lyme disease. Am J Med 98 (suppl 4A):44S, 1995.

34. Asbrink E, Hovmark A: Early and late cutaneous manifestations of *Ixodes*-borne borreliosis (erythema migrans borreliosis, Lyme borreliosis). Ann N Y Acad Sci 539:4, 1988.

35. Asbrink E, Hovmark A: Successful cultivation of spirochetes from skin lesions of patients with erythema chronicum migrans Afzelius and acrodermatitis chronica atrophicans. Acta Pathol Microbiol Immunol Scand 66:161, 1985.

36. Ackermann R, Rehse-Kupper B, Gollmer E, Schmidt

R: Chronic neurologic manifestations of erythema migrans borreliosis. Ann N Y Acad Sci 539:16, 1988.

37. Logigian EL, Steere AC: Clinical and electrophysiologic findings in chronic neuropathy of Lyme disease. Neurology 42:303, 1992.

38. Logigian EL, Kaplan RF, Steere AC: Chronic neurologic manifestations of Lyme disease. N Engl J Med 323:1438, 1990.

39. Halperin JJ, Volkman DJ, Luft BJ, et al.: CTS in Lyme borreliosis. Muscle Nerve 12:397, 1989.

40. Kaell AT, Bennett RS, Hamburger MI: Rheumatic manifestations. In: Coyle PK (ed): Lyme Disease. St. Louis: Mosby-Year Book, 1993, pp 73–85.

41. Kolstoe J, Messner RP: Lyme disease: musculoskeletal manifestations. Rheum Dis Clin North Am 15:649, 1989.

42. Rahn DW, Malawista SE: Lyme disease: recommendations for diagnosis and treatment. Ann Intern Med 114:472, 1991.

43. Kujala GA, Steere AC, Davis JS IV: IgM rheumatoid factor in Lyme disease: correlation with disease activity, total serum IgM and IgM antibody to *Borrelia burgdorferi*. J Rheumatol 14:772, 1987.

44. Duray PH: Histopathology of human borreliosis. In: Coyle PK (ed): Lyme Disease. St. Louis: Mosby-Year Book, 1993, pp 49–58.

45. Duray PH: The surgical pathology of human Lyme disease: an enlarging picture. Am J Surg Pathol 11:47, 1987.

46. Magnarelli LA: Laboratory diagnosis of Lyme disease. Rheum Dis Clin North Am 15:735, 1989.

47. Ma B, Christen B, Leung D, Vigo-Pelfrey C: Serodiagnosis of Lyme borreliosis by western immunoblot: reactivity of various significant antibodies against *Borrelia burgdorferi*. J Clin Microbiol 30:370, 1992.

48. Corpuz M, Hilton E, Lardis P, et al.: Problems in the use of serologic tests for the diagnosis of Lyme disease. Arch Intern Med 151:1837, 1991.

49. Dattwyler RJ, Volkman DJ, Luft BJ, et al.: Seronegative Lyme disease: dissociation of specific T- and B-lymphocyte responses to *Borrelia burgdorferi*. N Engl J Med 319:1441, 1988.

50. Dressler F, Yoshinari NH, Steere AC: The T-cell proliferative assay in the diagnosis of Lyme disease. Ann Intern Med 115:533, 1991.

51. Rosa PA, Schwan TG: A specific and sensitive assay for the Lyme disease spirochete *Borrelia burgdorferi* using the polymerase chain reaction. J Infect Dis 160:1018, 1989.

52. Pachner AR, Delaney E: The polymerase chain reaction (PCR) in the diagnosis of Lyme neuroborreliosis. Ann Neurol 34:544, 1993.

53. Goodman JL, Bradley JF, Ross AE, et al.: Bloodstream invasion in early Lyme disease: results from a prospective, controlled, blinded study using the polymerase chain reaction. Am J Med 99:6, 1995.

54. Lawson JP, Rahn DW: Lyme disease and radiologic findings in Lyme arthritis. AJR 158:1065, 1992.

55. Nelson JA, Wolf MD, Yah WTC, et al.: Cranial nerve involvement with Lyme borreliosis demonstrated by MRI. Neurology 42:671, 1992.

56. Dinerman H, Steere AC: Lyme disease associated with fibromyalgia. Ann Intern Med 117:281, 1992.

57. Sigal L: Summary of the first 100 patients seen at a Lyme disease referral center. Am J Med 88:577, 1990.

58. Costello CM, Steere AC, Pinkerton RE, Feder HM: A prospective study of tick bites in an endemic area of Lyme disease. J Infect Dis 159:136, 1989.

59. Johnson RC, Kodner C, Russell M: In vitro and in vivo susceptibility of the Lyme disease spirochete *Borrelia*

burgdorferi to four antimicrobial agents. Antimicrob Agents Chemother 31:164, 1987.

60. Sigal LH: Current recommendations for the treatment of Lyme disease. Drugs 43:683, 1992.

61. Steere AC, Green J, Schoen RT, et al.: Successful parenteral penicillin therapy for established Lyme arthritis. N Engl J Med 312:869, 1984.

62. Dattwyler RJ, Halperin JJ, Volkman DJ, et al.: Treatment of late Lyme disease: randomized comparison of ceftriaxone and penicillin. Lancet 2:1191, 1988.

13

Tumors and Infiltrative Lesions of the Cervical Spine

Tumors and infiltrative lesions of the cervical spine are unusual causes of neck pain: however, of all causes, these diseases are associated with the greatest dysfunction, morbidity, and mortality. The differential diagnosis of neck pain should include the possibility of a neoplastic lesion. Patients with tumors of the cervical spine usually have neck pain as a presenting or early symptom of their disease. A mild traumatic event, such as a mild whiplash injury, may be thought to be the cause of the patient's pain. Only as the pain persists and increases in intensity does it become clear the trauma was an incidental event unassociated with the underlying disease process.

As with lesions in the lumbar spine, a history of nocturnal pain or pain that increases with recumbency is a hallmark of tumors of the vertebral column, spinal cord, and nerve roots. Some lesions of the spinal cord may be painless although associated with abnormal neurologic signs. Lesions in the cervical spine cause more extensive lesions of the spinal cord resulting in myelopathy (quadriparesis, difficult breathing, and spasticity) than lesions in the lumbar spine. Physical examination demonstrates localized tenderness as well as neurologic dysfunction in the spinal cord or nerve roots that are compressed. Most laboratory findings are nonspecific, although evaluation of cerebrospinal fluid is helpful in identifying the presence of intradural tumors or myelitis. In contrast, radiographic evaluation is useful in identifying characteristic changes in the bony and soft tissue areas of the spine that help identify the location and type of neoplastic lesion. In general, benign tumors are located in the posterior elements of vertebrae

(spinous and transverse process), and malignant (both primary and metastatic) tumors are located in the anterior components of vertebrae (body) (Fig. 13–1). Radiographic techniques include plain roentgenograms and computerized tomography for evaluating bony architecture and myelography and magnetic resonance imaging for evaluating soft tissue structures. The definitive diagnosis of a tumor, including intraspinal lesions, must be derived from histologic examination of biopsy material obtained from the lesion (tissue diagnosis). The most effective therapy for benign and malignant tumors is the total removal of the lesions that are accessible to surgical excision. When excision is not possible, partial resection, radiation therapy, corticosteroids, or chemotherapy may be indicated to control symptoms and compression of the spinal cord and nerve roots. In general, patients with malignant tumors have a poorer prognosis than those with benign neoplasms.

BENIGN TUMORS

OSTEOBLASTOMA

Capsule Summary

Frequency of neck pain—very common
Location of neck pain—cervical spine
Quality of neck pain—dull ache
Symptoms and signs—nocturnal pain, localized tenderness
Laboratory and x-ray tests—posterior element expansile lesion on plain roentgenogram
Treatment—en bloc or partial excision

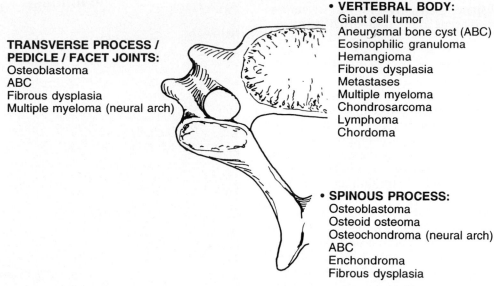

• VERTEBRAL BODY:
Giant cell tumor
Aneurysmal bone cyst (ABC)
Eosinophilic granuloma
Hemangioma
Fibrous dysplasia
Metastases
Multiple myeloma
Chondrosarcoma
Lymphoma
Chordoma

**TRANSVERSE PROCESS /
PEDICLE / FACET JOINTS:**
Osteoblastoma
ABC
Fibrous dysplasia
Multiple myeloma (neural arch)

• SPINOUS PROCESS:
Osteoblastoma
Osteoid osteoma
Osteochondroma (neural arch)
ABC
Enchondroma
Fibrous dysplasia

Figure 13–1. Tumors associated with posterior components (transverse and spinous processes) and anterior component (body) of vertebrae.

Prevalence and Pathogenesis

Osteoblastoma is a rare, benign neoplasm of bone that comprises about 3% of all benign bone tumors and about 0.5% of all biopsied bone tumors.[1, 2] A majority of the lesions appear from the second to the third decade of life. Nearly 90% of patients diagnosed with osteoblastoma are 30 years of age or younger.[3, 4] The tumor has a predilection for the spine. Approximately 40% of lesions are located in the axial skeleton.[5] In reported series of osteoblastoma patients with axial skeletal involvement, the frequency of cervical spine lesions varies from 20% to 38%.[6–8] The male-to-female ratio is 2.5:1.[6]

In the past, osteoblastoma has been referred to as osteogenic fibroma, giant osteoid osteoma, spindle-cell variant of giant cell tumor, and osteoblastic osteoid tissue-forming tumor. Jaffe and Mayer in 1932 described a "benign" osteoblastic tumor of bone, but it was Lichtenstein in 1956 who designated the lesion a benign osteoblastoma, which is now the accepted terminology.[9, 10] Osteoblastoma has subtypes including those that resemble osteoid osteoma, both the aggressive and "malignant" forms.[11] The pathogenesis of osteoblastoma is unknown.

Clinical History

The major clinical symptom of osteoblastoma is dull, aching, localized pain over the involved bone. The pain is insidious in onset and may have a duration of months to years before diagnosis. The duration of pain before diagnosis averages about 14 months. As opposed to the pain of osteoid osteoma, the pain of osteoblastoma is less severe, not nocturnal, and not relieved by salicylates. In the studies by Nemoto and colleagues, only 27% of patients had pain relief with aspirin therapy.[6] Pain is continuous and may be aggravated by activity. Torticollis may be a presenting feature in a minority of patients with cervical involvement.[6, 7] Radicular pain and spinal cord compression are more likely to occur in osteoblastoma than in osteoid osteoma because of the former's larger size, the erosion of bone cortex, and the formation of soft tissue masses. Osteoblastoma may invade the spinal canal and completely encircle nerve roots, resulting in corresponding neurologic symptoms.[7]

Physical Examination

Physical examination may demonstrate local tenderness on palpation with mild swelling over the spine. Pain may be exacerbated by spine extension.[12] Osteoblastoma associated with spinal cord compression results in abnormalities on sensory and motor examination of the upper and lower extremities corresponding to the level of the lesion. Reflexes may also be abnormal in the upper extremity with cervical spine lesions. Atrophy of surrounding muscles adjacent to the tumor may be seen.

Laboratory Data

This benign neoplasm does not have any associated abnormal screening blood tests. Characteristic abnormalities are present on pathologic examination. On gross examination, tumors are well circumscribed and are composed of hemorrhagic granular tissue with variable calcification. The tumors range from 2 to 10 cm in length.

Histologically, osteoblastoma may demonstrate cellular osteoblastic tissue with large amount of osteoid material and the absence of chondrocytes and cartilage. Multinucleated giant cells may be present. Mitotic figures may be seen but atypical ones are not.[12] The tumor appears loosely arranged because of the large number of capillaries between the trabeculae of bone. The vascular character of the tumor shows features similar to those seen with aneurysmal bone cyst. The borders of the tumor are well demarcated and do not permeate the surrounding normal bone.

Difficulties exist in the differentiation of benign and aggressive, premalignant forms of osteoblastoma.[11] Flow cytometry may become more useful as a means of quantifying neoplastic cells harvested from the tumor. Additional studies are needed to correlate the aneuploidy of cells with the biologic behavior of the tumor.[13]

Radiographic Evaluation

Radiographic findings of osteoblastoma are variable and nonspecific. In the spine, lesions are most commonly located in the posterior elements of the vertebrae, including pedicles, laminae, and transverse and spinous processes (Fig. 13–2).[14] The vertebral body is rarely primarily involved.[15] Osteoblastoma is located in the cervical spine in 36% of lesions, the sacrum or lumbar spine in 40%, and the thoracic spine in 24%.[1] In a study of 98 patients with osteoblastoma, 32 had spinal involvement. The distribution of lesions was 10 (31%) in the lumbar spine, 11 (34%) in the thoracic spine, 10 (31%) in the cervical spine, and 1 (3%) in the sacrum.[16] The cervical spine was the site of osteoblastoma in 31% of 32 patients reported with this tumor in the axial skeleton.[7] Osteoblastoma has been reported affecting the atlas.[17] Osteoblastoma is expansile and may

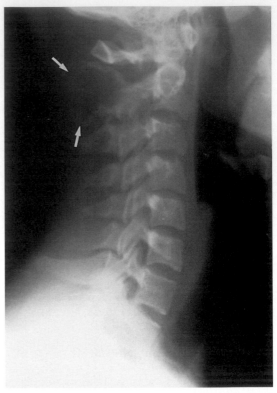

Figure 13–2. Osteoblastoma. A 14-year-old female developed a painless neck mass. Lateral view of cervical spine reveals a large expansile lesion, with well-circumscribed margins, growing from the spinous process of C2 *(arrows)*. (Courtesy of Anne Brower, M.D.)

grow rapidly as measured by serial radiographic studies. Characteristically, the lesion is well delineated and is covered by a thin layer of periosteal new bone. The extent of reactive new bone formation is much less than that associated with osteoid osteoma.[16] The center of the lesion may be radiolucent or radiopaque. A bone scan is helpful in localizing the lesion, but the finding of localized increased uptake is nonspecific. Bone scintigraphy may identify the location of an osteoblastoma even in the absence of abnormalities on plain roentgenograms.[18]

Computerized tomography (CT) may provide better localizations of the tumor, particularly when the lesion is obscured on plain roentgenogram.[19] CT scan helps determine the extent of the lesion and assess the extent of tumor matrix mineralization.[6] The relationship of the tumor to the spinal cord is better visualized in all circumstances with CT.[20] Angiography of the lesion does not help make a specific diagnosis, but it highlights the vascular nature of the tumor.[21]

CT scan is the best radiographic method

for determining the bony architecture of an osseous lesion of the cervical spine. However, magnetic resonance (MR) imaging is better than CT scanning in demonstrating the extent of bone sclerosis and in differentiating the tumor from adjacent soft tissue structures and bone marrow.[22] Increased signal intensity in soft tissue surrounding the tumor is secondary to edema.[20] On occasion, low signal intensity is noted in a wide area beyond the osteoblastoma. This pattern may be confused with a malignant process. A marked inflammatory response to the tumor results in this MR appearance. The extent of the process may be overestimated by MR imaging, and a biopsy may be taken from outside the tumor. This circumstance is evidence for the use of CT scan as the modality of choice to determine the appropriate site for biopsy of a bone tumor.[23] A biopsy of lesions in the cervical spine may be done with CT guidance in a safe manner without the need for surgery.[24]

Differential Diagnosis

The diagnosis of osteoblastoma is made by the thorough examination of biopsied samples. This lesion may be confused with a wide variety of other bone growths.

Osteoid Osteoma. Osteoid osteoma is a lesion that has similar characteristics to osteoblastomas. Osteoid osteoma comprises about 2.6% of all excised primary tumors of bone and about 12.1% of all benign tumors.[25, 26] Young adults 20 to 30 years of age are at greatest risk of developing this benign tumor. The ratio of men to women is 2:1.[27] Seven percent to 18% of all osteoid osteomas are located in the spine, with the lumbar area being the most common location in the axial skeleton (lumbar 40%, thoracic 30%, and cervical 30%).[27, 28] In another series of patients with osteoid osteoma, spine involvement oc-

curred in 27%.[8] In general, the cervical spine is second to the lumbar spine as the most common location for osteoid osteoma in the axial skeleton.[29] Osteoid osteoma must be differentiated from osteoblastoma. Table 13–1 shows the features that differentiate these tumors. In brief, osteoid osteoma has more intense, nocturnal pain, a lesion that is less than 2 cm in diameter, no associated soft tissue mass, and a histologic appearance demonstrating osteoid trabeculae with continuous and regular bone formation. In the cervical spine, osteoid osteoma is found almost exclusively in the pedicles and the posterior elements, including spinous processes.[30] Patients with osteoid osteoma of the cervical spine describe deep, boring pain localized to the area of the bone lesion. Associated muscle spasm may result in a torticollis of the neck.[31] Symptoms of osteoid osteoma may be present before the lesion, a dense area of sclerosis surrounding a small central nidus, is visualized on plain roentgenogram. A bone scintiscan may detect the tumor that is not visible on plain roentgenogram. A CT scan is the best radiographic method for detecting the extent of the bone lesion (Fig. 13–3). Treatment is total excision of the central nidus.[31, 32] Methods for confirming the complete removal of the lesion include the preoperative injection of radionuclide and intraoperative localization with a scintillation probe. Another method uses preoperative dosing with tetracycline and pathologic examination of the biopsy specimen with ultraviolet light, revealing nidus fluorescence.[33] Removal of osteoid osteoma in a pedicle must be done with care to prevent damage to the vertebral artery and maintain the apophyseal joint.[34] Fusion of the cervical spine may be required depending on the tumor.[35]

Osteosarcoma. Osteosarcoma at presentation may be easily confused clinically, radiographically, and histologically with osteoblastoma.[36] The presence of an outer rim of

---

TABLE 13–1.   DIFFERENTIATION OF OSTEOBLASTOMA AND OSTEOID OSTEOMA

	OSTEOBLASTOMA	OSTEOID OSTEOMA
Clinical presentation	Moderate nocturnal pain	Intense nocturnal pain
	Lesion greater than 2 cm	Limited growth less than 1.5 cm
	Rapid increase in size	Limited growth potential
Radiography	Minimal perifocal sclerosis	Marked perifocal sclerosis
	Associated soft tissue mass	No soft tissue mass
Histology	Osteoid trabeculae—discontinuous and irregular	Osteoid trabeculae—continuous and regular
	Stromal reaction—abundant	Stromal reaction—scant
	Osteoblastic giant cells—abundant	Osteoblastic giant cells—scant

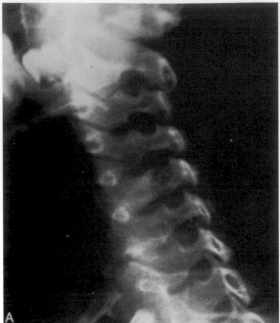

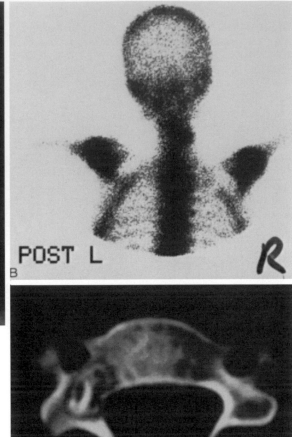

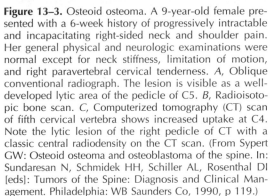

Figure 13–3. Osteoid osteoma. A 9-year-old female presented with a 6-week history of progressively intractable and incapacitating right-sided neck and shoulder pain. Her general physical and neurologic examinations were normal except for neck stiffness, limitation of motion, and right paravertebral cervical tenderness. *A*, Oblique conventional radiograph. The lesion is visible as a well-developed lytic area of the pedicle of C5. *B*, Radioisotopic bone scan. *C*, Computerized tomography (CT) scan of fifth cervical vertebra shows increased uptake at C4. Note the lytic lesion of the right pedicle of CT with a classic central radiodensity on the CT scan. (From Sypert GW: Osteoid osteoma and osteoblastoma of the spine. In: Sundaresan N, Schmidek HH, Schiller AL, Rosenthal DI [eds]: Tumors of the Spine: Diagnosis and Clinical Management. Philadelphia: WB Saunders Co, 1990, p 119.)

bone on radiographic examination and the absence of cartilage and anaplastic cells on biopsy help differentiate osteoblastoma from a malignant process. Osteosarcoma is the most common primary bone tumor, accounting for 20% to 35% of bone tumor cases.[37, 38] The relative incidence of tumors arising in the spine ranges from 0.85% to 3%.[37] The second decade of life is associated with the peak incidence of this tumor. The other group at risk for osteoasarcoma comprises people older than 50 years of age.[39] Approximately 50% of osteosarcomas are secondary to other conditions, including Paget's disease of bone, or bony infarcts secondary to radiation exposure.[40] Primary osteosarcomas involving the cervical spine have been reported.[36, 41, 42] In the spine, 14% of patients with osteosarcoma have cervical spine involvement.[43] However, in other studies of adults with osteosarcoma, the

spine is spared.[44] Ewing's sarcoma is a malignant tumor that rarely affects the cervical spine. Patients who develop this tumor are younger than those affected by osteoblastoma.[38, 45] The proximity of the tumor to the spinal cord and nerve roots results in early onset of symptoms, even with small tumors. Therapy for osteosarcoma is directed at the resection of the vertebral body. Subsequent therapy may include chemotherapy and radiation therapy.[46] The overall 5-year survival rate of 922 osteosarcoma patients, studied from 1973 to 1987, was 41%.[38]

Giant cell tumor of bone may contain areas of woven bone like an osteoblastoma. However, this lesion contains areas of solidly packed giant and stromal cells without intervening osteoid. Osteoblastoma contains areas of intervening bone and osteoid between collections of giant cells. Rarely, brown tumor of hyperparathyroidism may appear histologically like an osteoblastoma because of the presence of giant cells. Serum determinations of calcium and phosphorus levels should differentiate elevated concentrations of these serum factors associated with hyperparathyroidism from the normal levels associated with osteoblastoma.

Treatment

Local excision of the entire lesion is the treatment of choice if bone can be sacrificed without loss of function or excessive risk for neurogenic dysfunction. Osteoblastoma in the posterior elements of the spine is usually inaccessible for complete excision in up to 40% of lesions in the spine. Partial curettage of these lesions may be associated with cessation of growth and relief of symptoms for an extended period.[5] Osteoblastomas that rapidly expand or recurrent lesions may be controlled with radiation therapy. However, radiation therapy may be ineffective and is not completely free of risk in the form of malignant transformation, spinal cord necrosis, and aggravation of spinal cord compression. Chemotherapy, including high-dose methotrexate and doxorubicin, has been reported to slow the growth of aggressive osteoblastomas that are inaccessible to surgical removal.[47]

Prognosis

The course of osteoblastoma is usually benign. Bohlman and colleagues reported the resolution of neck pain and neurologic symptoms and signs after excision of the tumor.[35] However, tumors affecting the axial skeleton have greater morbidity and mortality.[48] The lesion is responsive to partial curettage and low-dose radiation therapy. Marsh and colleagues reported a series in which 1 of 13 spinal osteoblastomas had a recurrence resulting in paraplegia 7 months after surgery.[5] Laminectomy and postoperative radiation were the treatment for this complication. Recurrences occur in less than 5% of osteoblastomas; however, multiple recurrences have been described.[49] Recurrences may occur after symptom-free periods of up to 17 years.[50] Malignant changes occur in a very few lesions considered to be correctly diagnosed as benign osteoblastomas.[51]

References

OSTEOBLASTOMA

1. Dahlin DC, Unni KK: Bone Tumors: General Aspects and Data on 8,542 Cases, 4th ed. Springfield, Illinois: Charles C Thomas, Publisher, 1986, pp 102–118.
2. Mirra JM: Bone Tumors: Clinical, Radiologic, and Pathologic Correlations. Philadelphia: Lea & Febiger, 1989, pp 389–430.
3. McLeod RA, Dahlin DC, Beabout JW: The spectrum of osteoblastoma. AJR 126:321, 1976.
4. Schajowicz F: Tumors and Tumorlike Lesions of Bone: Pathology, 2nd ed. Berlin: Springer-Verlag, 1994, pp 48–71.
5. Marsh BW, Bonfiglio M, Brady LP, Enneking WF: Benign osteoblastoma: range of manifestations. J Bone Joint Surg 57A:1, 1975.
6. Nemoto O, Moser RP, Van Dam BE, et al.: Osteoblastoma of the spine: a review of 75 cases. Spine 15:1272, 1990.
7. Boriani S, Capanna R, Donati D, et al: Osteoblastoma of the spine. Clin Orthop 278:37, 1992.
8. Sypert GW: Osteoid osteoma and osteoblastoma of the spine. In: Sundaresan N, Schmidek HH, Schiller AL, Rosenthal DI (eds): Tumors of the Spine: Diagnosis and Clinical Management. Philadelphia: WB Saunders Co, 1990, pp 117–127.
9. Jaffe HL, Mayer L: An osteoblastic osteoid tissue–forming tumor of a metacarpal bone. Arch Surg 24:550, 1932.
10. Lichtenstein L: Benign osteoblastoma: a category of osteoid and bone-forming tumors other than classical osteoma, which may be mistaken for giant cell tumor or osteogenic sarcoma. Cancer 9:1044, 1956.
11. Schajowicz F: Osteoid osteoma and osteoblastoma. Orthop Clin North Am 20:313, 1989.
12. Huvos AG: Bone Tumors: Diagnosis, Treatment, and Prognosis, 2nd ed. Philadelphia: WB Saunders Co, 1991, pp 67–83.
13. Schajowicz F, McGuire MH: Diagnostic difficulties in skeletal pathology. Clin Orthop 240:281, 1989.
14. DeSouza-Dias L, Frost HM: Osteoblastoma of the spine: a review and report of eight new cases. Clin Orthop 91:141, 1973.
15. Alp H, Ceviker N, Baykaner K, et al: Osteoblastoma of the third lumbar vertebra. Surg Neurol 19:276, 1983.
16. Pochaczevsky R, Yen YM, Sherman RS: The roentgen appearance of benign osteoblastoma. Radiology 75:429, 1960.
17. Gelberman RH, Olson CO: Benign osteoblastoma of the atlas: a case report. J Bone Joint Surg 56A:808, 1974.
18. Makhija MC, Stein IH: Bone imaging in osteoblastoma. Clin Nucl Med 8:141, 1983.
19. Tonai M, Campbell CT, Ahn GH, et al: Osteoblastoma: classification and report of 16 patients. Clin Orthop 167:222, 1982.
20. Kroon HM, Schurmans J: Osteoblastoma: clinical and radiologic findings in 98 new cases. Radiology 175:783, 1990.
21. Banna M: Angiography of spinal osteoblastoma. J Can Assoc Radiol 30:118, 1974.
22. Syklawer R, Osborn RE, Kerber CW, Glass RF: Magnetic resonance imaging of vertebral osteoblastoma: a report of two cases. Surg Neurol 34:421, 1990.
23. Crim JR, Mirra JM, Eckardt JJ, Seeger LL: Widespread inflammatory response to osteoblastoma: the flare phenomenon. Radiology 177:835, 1990.
24. Babu NV, Titus VTK, Chittaranjan S, et al: Computed

tomographically guided biopsy of the spine. Spine 19:2436, 1994.

25. Mirra JM: Bone Tumors: Radiologic, and Pathologic Correlations. Philadelphia: Lea & Febiger, 1989, pp 226–248.

26. Dahlin DC, Unni KK: Bone Tumors: General Aspects and Data on 8,542 Cases, 4th ed. Springfield, Illinois: Charles C Thomas, Publisher, 1986, pp 88–101.

27. Cohen MD, Harrington TM, Ginsburg WW: Osteoid osteoma: 95 cases and a review of the literature. Semin Arthritis Rheum 12:265, 1983.

28. Freiberger RH: Osteoid osteoma of the spine: a cause for back-ache and scoliosis in children and young adults. Radiology 75:232, 1983.

29. Dunn EJ, Davidson RI, Desai S: Tumors of the cervical spine. In: Sherk HH, Dunn EJ, Eisomont FJ, et al (eds): The Cervical Spine, 2nd ed. Philadelphia: JB Lippincott Co, 1989, pp 693–722.

30. Hastings DE, Macnab I, Lawson V: Neoplasms of the atlas and axis. Can J Surg 11:290, 1968.

31. Fielding JW, Keim HA, Hawkins RJ, Kiem HA: Osteoid osteoma of the cervical spine. Clin Orthop 128:163, 1977.

32. Zwimpfer TJ, Tucker WS, Faulknes JF: Osteoid osteoma of the cervical spine: case reports and literature review. Can J Surg 25:637, 1982.

33. Camins MB, Rosenblum BR: Osseous lesions of the cervical spine. Clin Neurosurg 37:722, 1991.

34. Hershman E, Bjorkengren AJ, Fielding JW, Allen SC: Osteoid osteoma in a cervical pedicle: resection via transpillar approach. Clin Orthop 213:115, 1986.

35. Bohlman HH, Sachs BL, Carter JR, et al.: Primary neoplasms of the cervical spine: diagnosis and treatment of twenty-three patients. J Bone Joint Surg 68A:483, 1986.

36. Marsh HO, Choi CB: Primary osteogenic sarcoma of the cervical spine originally mistaken for benign osteoblastoma. J Bone Joint Surg 52A:1467, 1970.

37. Sundaresan N, Schiller AL, Rosenthal DI: Osteosarcoma of the spine. In: Sundaresan N, Schmidek HH, Schiller AL, Rosenthal DI (eds): Tumors of the Spine: Diagnosis and Clinical Management. Philadelphia: WB Saunders Co, 1990, pp 128–145.

38. Dorfman HD, Czerniack B: Bone cancers. Cancer 75:203, 1995.

39. Ghelman B: Radiology of bone tumors. Orthop Clin North Am 20:287, 1989.

40. Breton CL, Meziou M, Laredo JD, et al.: Sarcoma complicating Paget's disease of the spine. Rev Rhum (Engl ed) 60:17, 1993.

41. Fielding JW, Fietti VG, Hughes JO, et al.: Primary osteogenic sarcoma of the cervical spine. J Bone Joint Surg 58A:892, 1976.

42. Mnaymneh W, Brown M, Tejada F, et al.: Primary osteogenic sarcoma of the second cervical vertebra. J Bone Joint Surg 61A:460, 1979.

43. Dahlin DC, Unni KK: Bone Tumors: General Aspects and Data on 8,542 Cases, 4th ed. Springfield, Illinois: Charles C Thomas, Publisher, 1986, pp 269–307.

44. Siegel RD, Ryan LM, Antman KH: Osteosarcoma in adults: one institution's experience. Clin Orthop 240:263, 1989.

45. Lopez-Barea F, Rodriguez-Peralto JL, Hernandez-Moneo JL, et al.: Tumors of the atlas: three incidental cases of osteochondroma, benign osteoblastoma, and atypical Ewing's sarcoma. Clin Orthop 307:182, 1994.

46. Jaffe N: Chemotherapy for malignant bone tumors. Orthop Clin North Am 20:487, 1989.

47. Camitta B, Wells R, Segura A, et al.: Osteoblastoma response to chemotherapy. Cancer 68:999, 1991.

48. Lucas DR, Unni KK, McLeod RA, et al.: Osteo-

blastoma: clinicopathologic study of 306 cases. Hum Pathol 25:117, 1994.

49. Jackson RP: Recurrent osteoblastoma: a review. Clin Orthop 131:229, 1978.

50. Beauchamp CP, Duncan CP, Dzus AK, Morton KS: Osteoblastoma: experience with 23 patients. Can J Surg 35:199, 1992.

51. Schajowicz F, Lemos C: Malignant osteoblastoma. J Bone Joint Surg 58B:202, 1976.

OSTEOCHONDROMA

Capsule Summary

Frequency of neck pain—uncommon
Location of neck pain—cervical spine
Quality of neck pain—dull ache
Symptoms and signs—restricted motion
Laboratory and x-ray test—exostosis: single or multiple on plain roentgenogram
Treatment—en bloc excision for lesions that cause nerve impingement

Prevalence and Pathogenesis

Osteochondroma is a common benign tumor of bone that occurs in single or multiple locations in the skeleton. Osteochondroma represents up to 36% of all benign bone tumors and 8% to 11% of all primary tumors of bone.[1, 2] Approximately 60% of patients develop the lesion from the second to third decade of life. Patients with multiple osteochondromas develop lesions before they reach 20 years of age.[2] The male-to-female ratio is 2:1.[3]

The lesion was first described by Cooper in 1818.[4] Osteochondromas have been detected in skeletons dated from 3500 B.C. to 2000 B.C.[5] Exostosis and osteocartilaginous exostosis are two other names associated with this benign tumor. Mirra has proposed that the term exostosis be reserved for marginal osteophytes associated with osteoarthritis and that the term osteochondroma be reserved for the benign bone tumor because the two lesions occur in different areas of bone, occur at different ages of the skeleton, and have different pathogenetic mechanisms.[2]

The pathogenesis of osteochondroma is postulated to be related to an abnormality of cartilage growth. Keith thought that osteochondroma results from a defect in the periosteal cuff of bone that surrounds the lower end of the epiphyseal plate cartilage during embryogenesis.[6] The larger the defect, the larger the tumor. A single defect results in a solitary tumor, and multiple defects cause hereditary multiple osteochondromatosis. Nests of cartilage in a periosteal location grow out from the epiphyseal growth plate and result in a bony prominence capped by a layer of cartilage that is contiguous with the cortex of the underlying bone. They may be thought of as slow-growing developmental anomalies that cease to enlarge once growth has stopped. This progression correlates with the clinical history of recognition of the tumor during childhood and its cessation of growth once the epiphyses close.[2]

Osteochondroma occurs most commonly at the ends of tubular bones. Approximately 1% to 2% of osteochondromas are located in the spine.[7] Approximately 50% are found in the lumbosacral spine, 30% in the thoracic spine, and 20% in the cervical spine.[1] A review of 96 patients with solitary spinal osteochondromas reported the cervical spine to be the most commonly affected area, with a 50% frequency, with the lumbar spine being involved in 23% of cases.[8] In the cervical spine, C2 was the most frequently affected vertebra.

Clinical History

Osteochondroma is frequently asymptomatic and is discovered only as a painless prominence of bone or as a chance finding on a radiograph. If pain is present, it is mild, deep, and usually secondary to mechanical irritation of overlying soft tissue structures. Pain may increase with activity. Osteochondroma that continues to grow may cause loss of function and decreased motion. When attached to the spinal column, it has been associated with kyphosis and spondylolisthesis.[9] The lesion grows slowly over months to years. Most patients with osteochondroma of the spine have no compression of the spinal cord or nerve root. However, when neurologic symptoms occur, the location of the tumor corresponds to the area of compression. Compression of the spinal cord causes neurologic compromise, including quadriparesis. Myelopathy predominates to a greater extent in patients with multiple osteochondromas than in those with a solitary tumor in the spine. Sudden death, Brown-Séquard syndrome, and Horner's syndrome are among a variety of complications reported in patients with osteochondromas that have involved the axis and other portions of the cervical spine.[10–21] Intermittent episodes of C2 neuralgia, tinnitus, dizziness, and blurring of vision are associated with osteochondroma of the axis, which causes occlusion of the vertebral artery.[22] The onset of symptoms may be more acute when an individual has had a fall or hyperextension injury of the neck.[15, 23] Anterior spinal osteochondromas in the cervical spine may present with hoarseness, dysphagia, or a slowly growing mass.[24]

Physical Examination

Physical examination may be normal without any neurologic deficit; however, osteochondroma near facet joints of the spine may cause some restriction in motion. Osteochondroma that grows close to the body surface may cause a palpable mass that may be tender on palpation.[25] Neurologic findings, when present, correspond to the location of the lesion and related nerve root compression.

Laboratory Data

Screening laboratory tests are normal with this benign tumor of bone. Pathologically, a gross specimen of this lesion may take the form of a pedunculated stalk or a flat prominence. The tumor's cortex and its periosteal covering are continuous with those of the underlying bone. The cartilage cap may cover the entire lesion or the rounded end of a stalked exostosis. The cap's cartilage is smooth and 2 to 3 mm thick. An actively growing lesion may have cartilage 1 cm thick. As the lesion grows older, the cartilaginous cap disappears. The lesion may vary up to 10 cm in diameter and is well circumscribed. Histologic examination of the tumor shows benign chondrocytes with small nuclei. The islands of cartilage and cartilage cells are embedded in the underlying cancellous bone. As the bone matures, the amount of cartilage decreases. However, residual microscopic foci of cartilage may be identified well into adult life.

Radiographic Evaluation

The radiographic features of osteochondroma are diagnostic. The lesion protrudes from the underlying bone on a sessile or pedunculated bony stalk that is continuous with the cortex and spongiosa of the underlying bone. The outer surface of the lesion may be smooth or irregular, but it is almost always well demarcated (Fig. 13–4). If the cartilage cap is calcified, it may obscure the underlying stalk. Plain roentgenogram may not identify a significant number of lesions. Among 80 tumors

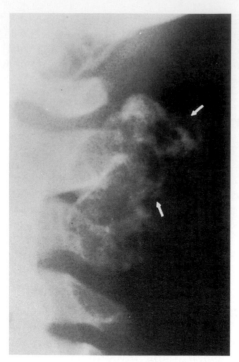

Figure 13–4. Solitary osteochondroma of the spine. This pedunculated osteochondroma *(arrows)* arises from the spinous process of the third cervical vertebra. It extends upward, behind the spinous process of the axis. (From Resnick D, Kyriakos M, Greenway GD: Tumors and tumor-like lesions of bone: Imaging and pathology of specific lesions. In: Resnick D [ed]: Diagnosis of Bone and Joint Disorders, 3rd ed. Philadelphia: WB Saunders Co, 1995, p 3729.)

studied by plain roentgenograms, 21% were diagnostic, 64% had nondiagnostic anomalies, and 15% were normal.[8] In the spine, osteochondromas are located close to centers of secondary ossification, including the spinous process, pedicle, and neural arch.[26] In the cervical spine, the axis and the lateral masses of the atlas may be involved.[13, 27]

Radionuclide bone scan reveals increased uptake at the site of the tumor. Malignant lesions may exhibit greater intensity of uptake, but this finding is not always a reliable distinguishing feature of malignant transformation.[28, 29] The increased activity of osteochondroma is related to endochondral ossification within the cartilaginous cap.

Computerized tomography (CT) and myelography are helpful in localizing the site of the lesion in the spinal column, its size, and its relationship to the nerve roots and spinal cord as well as differentiating it from malignant lesions.[30, 31] CT is the imaging modality of choice for identifying osteochondromas.[8] In the setting of neurologic abnormalities compatible with spinal cord compression, tumors may arise from the vertebral arch, or posterior aspect of the vertebral body.[32, 33] Magnetic resonance (MR) imaging is also a good technique for detecting spinal cord compression, but it does not image the bony architecture of the tumor as well as CT.[34] MR imaging is able to detect the thickness of the cartilaginous cap and the continuity of the bone marrow space between the original bone and new growth. Angiography may be helpful in detecting tumor occlusion of the vertebral artery in its location in the cervical spine.[22]

Differential Diagnosis

The diagnosis of an osteochondroma is based on its appearance on a radiograph and the lack of clinical and laboratory findings. Chondrosarcomatous degeneration of osteochondroma occurs in less than 1% of patients. Adult patients with multiple lesions are at greater risk in this respect. Malignant transformation is usually heralded by increasing pain, enlarging soft tissue mass, and loss of definition of the outer border of the lesion on radiograph. However, the onset of pain in a previously asymptomatic osteochondroma is not always associated with malignant degeneration, because infarction of the cartilage cap or fracture through the base of an osteochondroma may also cause pain and new bone growth.[2]

Other non-neoplastic lesions to be considered in the differential diagnosis are callus associated with fractures, chondroid metaplasia, and osteophytes associated with osteoarthritis. The size and location of the benign tumor should help differentiate these non-neoplastic entities with similar histologic features. Fibrocartilaginous nodules in the ligamentum nuchae may be confused with osteochondroma or a fracture of a spinous process. These painless nodules may be noted on physical examination.[35]

Treatment

Osteochondroma requires no therapy when it is asymptomatic.[36] Removal is indicated if the tumor is causing persistent pain or disability, has roentgenographic features suggestive of malignancy, or shows an abnormal increase in size. Patients with neurologic symptoms can be helped by removal of the lesion and decompression of the affected nerve root or spinal cord.[37] In the cervical spine, decompression, posterior stabilization, and facet fusion may be required for therapy for cord compression in patients with solitary or multiple osteochondromas (diaphyseal aclasis).[38]

Although chondrosarcoma is more common in patients with multiple osteochondromas, prophylactic removal of tumors in patients with multiple lesions is not practical. Patients must be followed closely for a change in symptoms or size of lesions. These lesions should be removed.

Prognosis

The course of the solitary osteochondroma is usually benign and asymptomatic and is not associated with any dysfunction or inability to work. In the rare patient who has a vertebral osteochondroma and neurologic dysfunction, surgical decompression of the site should result in a return of function and complete cure.[39] Resolution of neck pain and neurologic dysfunction affecting the arm after surgical excision has been reported.[40] There may be a recurrence if the tumor, particularly its cartilaginous cap and periosteum, are not completely removed. Continuous observation of patients with osteochondromas is important, particularly for patients with multiple lesions, because the lesions can occasionally become malignant.

References

OSTEOCHONDROMA

1. Dahlin DC, Unni KK: Bone Tumors: General Aspects and Data on 8,542 Cases, 4th ed. Springfield, Illinois: Charles C Thomas, 1986, pp 18–32.
2. Mirra JM: Bone Tumors: Clinical, Radiologic, and Pathologic Correlations. Philadelphia: Lea & Febiger, 1989, pp 1626–1659.
3. Huvos AG: Bone Tumors: Diagnosis, Treatment, and Prognosis, 2nd ed. Philadelphia: WB Saunders Co, 1991, pp 253–291.
4. Cooper A: Exostosis. In: Cooper A, Travers B (eds): Surgical Essays, 3rd ed. London: Cox and Son, 1818, pp 169–226.
5. Chamberlain AT, Rogers S, Romanowski CAJ: Osteochondroma in a British neolithic skeleton. Br J Hosp Med 47:51, 1992.
6. Keith A: Studies on the anatomical changes which accompany certain growth disorders of the human body. J Anat 54:101, 1920.
7. Resnick D, Kyriakos M, Greenway GD: Tumors and tumor-like lesions of bone: Imaging and pathology of specific lesions. In: Resnick D (ed): Diagnosis of Bone and Joint Disorders, 3rd ed. Philadelphia: WB Saunders Co, 1995, pp 3725–3746.
8. Albrecht S, Crutchfield S, Segall GK: On spinal osteochondromas. J Neurosurg 77:247, 1992.
9. Blaauw G: Osteocartilaginous exostosis of the spine.

In: Vinken PJ, Bruyn GW (eds): Handbook of Clinical Neurology Tumors of the Spine and Spinal Cord, Part I. New York: American Elsevier Publishing Co, 1975, pp 313–319.
10. Fielding JW, Ratzan S: Osteochondroma of the cervical spine. J Bone Joint Surg 55A:640, 1973.
11. Twersky J, Kassner EG, Tenner MS, et al.: Vertebral and costal osteochondromas causing spinal cord compression. AJR 124:124, 1975.
12. Inglis AE, Rubin RM, Lewis RJ, et al.: Osteochondroma of the cervical spine: case report. Clin Orthop 126:127, 1977.
13. Wu KK, Guise ER: Osteochondroma of the atlas: a case report. Clin Orthop 136:160, 1978.
14. Julien J, Riemens V, Vital C, et al.: Cervical cord compression by solitary osteochondroma of the atlas. J Neurol Neurosurg Psychiatry 41:479, 1978.
15. MacGee EE: Osteochondroma of the cervical spine: a cause of transient quadriplegia. Neurosurgery 4:259, 1979.
16. Palmer FJ, Blum PW: Osteochondroma with spinal cord compression: report of three cases. J Neurosurg 52:842, 1980.
17. Novick GS, Pavlov H, Bullough PG: Osteochondroma of the cervical spine: report of two cases in preadolescent males. Skeletal Radiol 8:13, 1982.
18. Karian JM, DeFilipp G, Buchheit WA, et al.: Vertebral osteochondroma causing spinal cord compression: case report. Neurosurgery 14:483, 1984.
19. Rose EF, Fekete A: Odontoid osteochondroma causing sudden death: report of a case and review of the literature. Am J Clin Pathol 42:606, 1964.
20. Linkowski GD, Tsai FY, Recher L, et al.: Solitary osteochondroma with spinal cord compression. Surg Neurol 23:388, 1985.
21. Calhoun JM, Chadduck WM, Smith JL: Single cervical exostosis: report of a case and review of the literature. Surg Neurol 37:26, 1992.
22. George B, Attallah A, Laurian C, et al.: Cervical osteochondroma (C2 level) with vertebral artery occlusion and second cervical nerve root irritation. Surg Neurol 31:459, 1989.
23. Wen DY, Bergman TA, Haines SJ: Acute cervical myelopathy from hereditary multiple exostoses: case report. Neurosurgery 25:472, 1989.
24. Peck JH: Dysphagia due to massive exostosis of the cervical spine. In: Proceedings of the Western Orthopaedic Association. J Bone Joint Surg 46A:1379, 1964.
25. Morard M, de Preux J: Solitary osteochondroma presenting as a neck mass with spinal cord compression syndrome. Surg Neurol 37:402, 1992.
26. Inglis AE, Rubin RM, Lewis RJ, Villacin A: Osteochondroma of the cervical spine: case report. Clin Orthop 126:127, 1977.
27. Lopez-Barea F, Rodriguez-Peralto JL, Hernandez-Moneo JL, et al.: Tumors of the atlas: three incidental cases of osteochondroma, benign osteoblastoma, and atypical Ewing's sarcoma. Clin Orthop 307:182, 1994.
28. Greenspan A: Tumors of cartilage origin. Orthop Clin North Am 20:347, 1989.
29. Edeling CJ: Bone scintigraphy in hereditary multiple exostoses. Eur J Nucl Med 14:207, 1988.
30. Kenney PJ, Gilula LA, Murphy WA: The use of computed tomography to distinguish osteochondroma and chondrosarcoma. Radiology 139:129, 1981.
31. Tigges S, Erb RE, Nance EP: Skeletal case of the day. AJR 158:1368, 1992.
32. Buckler RA, Chad DA, Smith TW, et al.: Sciatica: an early manifestation of thoracic vertebral osteochondroma. Neurosurgery 21:98, 1987.
33. Gottlieb A, Severi P, Ruelle A, et al.: Exostosis as a

cause of spinal cord compression. Surg Neurol 26:581, 1986.

34. Moriwaka F, Hozen H, Nakane K, et al.: Myelopathy due to osteochondroma: MR and CT studies. J Comput Assist Tomogr 14:128, 1990.

35. Lewinnek GE, Peterson SE: A calcified fibrocartilagenous nodule in the ligamentum nuchae: presenting as a tumor. Clin Orthop 136:163, 1978.

36. Chrisman OD, Goldenberg RR: Untreated solitary osteochondroma: report of two cases. J Bone Joint Surg 50A:508, 1968.

37. Gokay H, Bucy PC: Osteochondroma of the lumbar spine: report of a case. J Neurosurg 12:72, 1955.

38. Bhojraj SY, Panjwani JS: A new management approach to decompression, posterior stabilization, and fusion for cervical laminar exostosis with cord compression in a case of diaphyseal aclasis: case report and review of the literature. Spine 18:1376, 1993.

39. Esposito PW, Crawford AH, Vogler C: Solitary osteochondroma occurring on the transverse process of the lumbar spine. Spine 10:398, 1985.

40. Bohlman HH, Sachs BL, Carter JR, et al.: Primary neoplasms of the cervical spine: diagnosis and treatment of twenty-three patients. J Bone Joint Surg 68A:483, 1986.

GIANT CELL TUMOR

Capsule Summary

Frequency of neck pain—common
Location of neck pain—cervical spine
Quality of neck pain—intermittent ache
Symptoms and signs—localized mass, dysphagia
Laboratory and x-ray tests—anterior vertebral body involvement on plain roentgenogram
Treatment—en bloc excision

Prevalence and Pathogenesis

Giant cell tumor of bone is a common, locally aggressive lesion that may turn malignant. Giant cell tumor represents up to 21% of all benign tumors of bone and up to 5% of biopsied primary bone tumors.[1, 2] Approximately 70% of patients are diagnosed from the ages of 20 to 40 years. The average age of patients with malignant giant cell tumors is higher than that associated with benign tumors. Benign tumors predominate in women in a ratio of 3:2, and malignant tumors predominate in men in a ratio of 3:1.[3]

The first description of the benign characteristics was by Cooper in 1818.[4] Bloodgood in 1919 was the first to refer to this neoplasm as a benign giant cell tumor.[5] Other names that have been associated with this perplexing neoplasm include myeloid sarcoma, medullary sarcoma, and osteoclastoma.

The pathogenesis of giant cell tumor is not known. The tumor starts after the skeleton has ceased to grow and has matured. The tumor arises from non–bone-forming supporting connective tissue of the bone marrow space. The factors that make this tumor inherently invasive or potentially malignant are unknown.

Most giant cell tumor occurs at the ends of long bones, particularly around the knee. About 8% to 12% of giant cell tumor occur in the spine.[1, 6] The sacrum is the most frequently affected area in the spine. Approximately 68% occur in the sacrum, 11% in the lumbar and cervical spine, and 10% in the thoracic area. Other series have found lower frequencies of sacral involvement in the range of 3% to 8%.[7, 8] The ilium and ischium may also be involved in a small percentage of patients (.05%).[9]

Clinical History

Giant cell tumor of bone causes intermittent aching pain over the affected bone, which is almost always the predominant symptom. The duration of symptoms may vary from a few weeks to 6 months, but some patients have pain more than 2 years prior to diagnosis.[10] Patients with vertebral involvement may describe neurologic dysfunction, including paresthesias with radiation of pain into the upper extremities, and muscle weakness.[10] Expansion of the tumor anteriorly may be associated with the symptom of dysphagia.[11]

Physical Examination

Physical examination may demonstrate tenderness on palpation over the spine. Localized swelling may be noted if the location of the giant cell tumor is superficial, that is, in the spinous process. Muscle spasm and associated limitation of motion of the neck may also be noted. Neurologic findings may show sensory, motor, or reflex abnormalities, depending on the level of nerve root compression.[12]

Laboratory Data

Laboratory results are normal in patients with benign giant cell tumor, but serum calcium, phosphorus, and alkaline phosphatase tests should be obtained to differentiate giant cell tumor from hyperparathyroidism, Paget's disease, and malignant giant cell tumor. Patients with malignant giant cell tumor may show abnormalities such as anemia and elevated erythrocyte sedimentation rate.

On gross pathologic examination, the tumor is a soft, friable, gray-to-red mass. Areas of the tumor may be cystic or necrotic, filled with blood. This characteristic finding causes confusion with findings associated with aneurysmal bone cyst. The tumors cause expansion of host bone with cortical destruction. In most lesions, the periosteum is relatively spared, with the tumor contained by a shell of new bone.

The histologic appearance of giant cell tumor of bone is not distinctively characteristic because a number of other benign lesions may contain giant cells (Table 13–2). In general, giant cell tumor contains large numbers of osteoblast-like giant cells separated by inconspicuous mononuclear stromal cells. The proliferating giant cells have round to oval to spindle-shaped nuclei. Mitotic figures may be numerous. The nuclei lack the variation in size and shape that are characteristic of sarcoma. In a minority of lesions, small foci of osteoid and woven bone are seen. Thin-walled vessels with hemorrhages are also characteristic.

A debate exists over the histologic grading of giant cell tumor. Some pathologists believe that the histologic grade is predictive of subsequent tumor behavior.[6] Others do not believe that grading, particularly at the benign end of the scale (grades I and II), is predictive of any subsequent propensity to aggressive growth.[1, 2]

Cytogenic analysis of giant cell tumor reveals chromosomal abnormalities in tumor cells not detected in normal cells. Telomere-to-telomere chromosome translocations affecting the long arm of chromosomes 19 and 20 were noted in the tumors but were not predictive of the aggressiveness of the giant cell neoplasm.[13] The alteration in chromosome 19 may affect the function of transforming growth factor-beta (TGF-β) on osteoclasts. Giant cell tumor may consist of osteoclasts that have been affected by TGF-β activity. Researchers in another study used flow cytometric deoxyribonucleic acid (DNA) analysis of giant cell tumor in an attempt to predict the biologic behavior of this neoplasm. DNA analysis was unable to predict the likelihood of the tumor metastasizing.[14]

Radiographic Evaluation

The radiographic findings of giant cell tumor are characteristic but not pathogno-

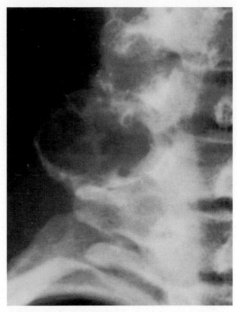

Figure 13–5. Giant cell tumor. A 21-year-old female with a radiolucent, well-marginated, expansile mass with a sclerotic rim that has been growing over a 7-year period in the lateral articular process of C7. (From Campanacci M, Boriani S, Giunti A: Giant cell tumors of the spine. In: Sundaresan N, Schmidek HH, Schiller AL, Rosenthal DI [eds]: Tumors of the Spine: Diagnosis and Clinical Management. Philadelphia: WB Saunders Co, 1990, p 169.)

monic. The lesion is expansile, with irregular thinning of the cortical margin. It is lytic but may contain a delicate trabecular meshwork. Little bony reaction occurs in response to this lesion. Extensive sclerotic borders or periosteal reaction are not seen. In the spine, the vertebral body is frequently affected, but the spinous and transverse processes may also be involved (Fig. 13–5).[15] The destruction of vertebral bone that is most commonly in the vertebral body, as opposed to the posterior elements in other benign tumors of the spine, results in lytic lesions without surrounding reactive sclerosis or matrix mineralization.[16]

If plain radiograph is unable to demonstrate abnormalities of the spine, a bone scan may be helpful in demonstrating abnormalities. However, radionuclide scintigraphy may exhibit increased tracer element in bone across the adjacent joint and in other joints in the same extremity not involved with the tumor.[17]

Computerized tomography (CT) is superior to plain roentgenogram in detecting the extent of tumor in the extraosseous space.[18] However, clear distinctions between tumor and muscle may be difficult to make with CT scan.

TABLE 13–2. DIFFERENTIAL DIAGNOSIS OF GIANT CELL LESIONS OF BONE

	MOST COMMON AGE GROUP	LOCATION IN BONE	RADIOLOGIC APPEARANCE	GROSS FEATURES	MICROSCOPIC FEATURES	
					Giant Cells	Stromal Cells
Giant cell tumor	Third and fourth decades	Epiphysis or metaphysis	Eccentric expanded radiolucent area	Fleshy soft tissue	Abundant number uniformly distributed	Plump and polyhedral cells with abundant cytoplasm
Nonossifying fibroma	First decade	Metaphysis	Eccentric oval defects	Fleshy soft tissue	Focal distribution, small and few nuclei	Slender and spindly cells with little cytoplasm; whorled pattern
Aneurysmal bone cyst	First and second decades	Vertebral column or metaphysis of long bone	Eccentric blow-out "soap bubble" appearance	Cavity filled with blood	Focal around vascular channels or hemorrhage	Large vascular channels; slender to plump cells with hemosiderin granules; metaplastic bone
Brown tumor of hyperparathyroidism	Any age	Anywhere in bone	Subperiosteal, subchondral, and subligamentous resorption of bone	Fleshy tissue or cystic spaces	Focal around hemosiderin pigment or hemorrhage	Fibrous stroma with slender spindle cells
Simple bone cyst	First and second decades	Metaphysis	Trabeculations in radiolucent area	Cyst filled with clear fluid	Focal around cholesterol clefts	Cyst wall of fibrous tissue; metaplastic bone
Chondroblastoma	Second decade	Epiphysis	Radiolucency in spotty opacities	Firm to fleshy tissue	Few and focal	Plump and round or ovoid cells with pericellular calcifications
Fibrous dysplasia	First and second decades	Metaphysis	Ground-glass appearance	Firm and gritty	Few and focal	Woven bone and whorled fibrous tissue; no osteoblasts
Giant cell reparative granuloma	Second and third decades	Maxilla and mandible	Radiolucent focus	Soft fleshy tissue	Focal around hemosiderin pigment or hemorrhage	Slender or plump spindle cells
Ossifying fibroma	Second and third decades	Maxilla and mandible	Radiopaque	Firm and gritty	Few and focal	Lamellar bony trabeculae in fibroma tissue; osteoblastic rimming
Osteosarcoma	Second and third decades	Metaphysis	Radiolucent	Soft, firm, or hard	Focal distribution	Malignant cells with direct osteoid formation
Chondromyxoid fibroma	Second and third decades	Metaphysis	Eccentric with expanded cortex	Soft to firm	Focal distribution	Chondroid, myxoid, and fibrous lobules
Osteoblastoma	Second and third decades	Vertebral column, diaphysis of long bone	Radiolucent or dense	Hemorrhagic, gritty	Focal distribution	Abundant osteoid trabeculae with osteoblasts

Modified from Ghandur-Mnaymneh L, Mnaymneh WA: Bone lesions with giant cells: problems in differential diagnosis. J Med Liban 25:91, 1972.

Magnetic resonance (MR) imaging is the best radiographic modality to study giant cell tumors and soft tissue extension because of superior contrast resolution. The tumor exhibits long T_1 and T_2 relaxation times that correspond to low intensity on T_1 images and high intensity on T_2 images. MR is better at determining the extraosseous extent of the tumor, and CT is better able to visualize mineralized structures, including subtle cortical breaks.[19]

Differential Diagnosis

A thorough review of the clinical laboratory, pathologic, and radiologic data is necessary to make the diagnosis of a giant cell tumor of bone. This evaluation is required because a number of benign and malignant lesions have pathologic findings that are similar. Table 13–2 has a list of benign and malignant lesions that contain giant cells that may mimic the findings of giant cell tumor of bone.[20] Not all of these neoplasms affect the cervical spine. Aneurysmal bone cyst, brown tumor of hyperparathyroidism, chondroblastoma, fibrous dysplasia, osteosarcoma, chondromyxoid fibroma, and osteoblastoma need to be included in the differential diagnosis of a giant cell–containing tumor located in the cervical spine.

Enchondroma. Enchondroma (EN) is a benign hyaline cartilage growth that develops within the medullary cavity of a single bone.[21] EN accounts for 1.4% of primary benign tumors. EN occurs most frequently in the small bones of the hands and feet; only 0.88% of EN occurs in the axial skeleton.[22] In the axial skeleton, the distribution of EN is 31% in the cervical spine, 32% in the thoracic spine, 23% in the lumbosacral spine, and 14% in the sacrum.[22] Most EN is asymptomatic and is identified as an incidental finding on roentgenographic examination. In the spinal column, EN may expand into the spinal canal or neural foramen to cause spinal cord or nerve root compression, respectively.[23–25] EN is a well-defined osteolytic lesion with sharp sclerotic margins. The lytic quality of this tumor may be confused with giant cell tumor. The lesion is radiolucent, although it may contain areas of cartilage matrix calcification. In vertebral bodies, the posterior elements are most frequently affected. The lesion may expand the surrounding bone. Pathologically, the lesion contains translucent hyaline cartilage with a varying amount of chondrocyte cellularity with little atypia. Most lesions do not require any

intervention. Curettage and filling the defect with bone chips is the usual treatment for symptomatic tumors.

Aneurysmal bone cyst is a fibrous-walled structure filled with blood that occurs in association with other neoplasms, including giant cell tumor. An aneurysmal bone cyst contains giant cells in its wall and may be confused with giant cell tumor.[26] Giant cell tumor with an aneurysmal bone cyst component should be treated as giant cell tumor.

Brown tumor of hyperparathyroidism contains cells that are similar histologically to those of giant cell tumor. The elevation of serum calcium level and decrease of serum phosphorus level along with multiple locations of lesions help differentiate this entity. In addition, the giant cells of hyperparathyroidism are arranged in a more nodular pattern and are surrounded by areas of active bone.

Chondroblastoma is a benign lesion that affects men younger than 30 years of age and is located near epiphyseal cartilage. The tumor is more commonly found in long bones and is only rarely located in the cervical spine.[27] In the thoracic spine, this tumor may expand into the spinal canal, causing spinal cord compression.[28] Radiographically, the lesion is a solitary lytic lesion with a surrounding sclerotic border and punctate calcifications that are difficult to visualize. Histologically, the tumor contains a variable number of giant cells containing multiple nuclei, polygonal to round stromal cells with distinct borders, "chicken-wire" calcification, and variable amounts of chondroid.[2]

Fibrous dysplasia is a benign process affecting either one bone or multiple bones in the skeleton. The disease is more common in women than men and becomes prominent before the second decade of life. Fibrous dysplasia rarely affects the cervical spine.[29–31] Cervical spine involvement occurs in 7% of patients with polyostotic fibrous dysplasia.[22] Radiologically, the medullary cavity of bone is replaced with fibrous tissue that appears as a predominantly radiolucent, albeit hazy, matrix, often described as "ground glass," that may contain focal calcific deposits. Lesions appear matted, loculated, or trabeculated with well-defined, sclerotic margins. The affected bone may be expanded, bowed, and deformed.[32] Histologically, the lesion contains a benign fibrous tissue matrix with variable quantities of woven bone, little to no cartilage, and only small foci of giant cells that are associated with areas of cystification or hemorrhage. The small number of these cells helps differentiate fibrous dysplasia from giant cell tumor.

Osteosarcoma is a rare tumor of the axial skeleton, occurring in about 1% to 3% of cases.[33–35] It most commonly affects men 10 to 30 years of age. The tumor may be osteoblastic or osteolytic. An osteoblastic lesion in a vertebral body affects one area of the body with dense sclerosis that may extend into the neural arch. Irregular areas of calcification or ossification in the paravertebral soft tissues are usual. Osteolytic lesion is also associated with soft tissue masses and collapse of the anterior portion of a vertebra. Giant cell tumor, when untreated, is a pure lytic lesion without any new bone formation. Histologic examination of osteosarcoma may demonstrate areas of osteoclast-like giant cells that superficially resemble giant cell tumor. However, close inspection of the specimen reveals frank anaplastic cells in areas away from bone-producing areas associated with dense sclerosis where nuclear anaplasia is absent.

Chondromyxoid fibroma is a rare benign tumor representing less than 1% of all primary bone neoplasms. The lesion occurs in men from the second to third decade of life. About 16% of these lesions occur in the cervical spine.[36] In the vertebral column, the lesion may affect the neural arch, vertebral body, or posterior elements.[37] Radiographically, the tumor causes an area of osteolysis with bone expansion and variable calcification that may be difficult to differentiate from other causes of bone damage.[38] On gross pathologic examination, this lesion is sharply delineated from surrounding bone. A thin sclerotic zone may be found in neighboring host bone. Histologically, the tumor has different zones containing myxomatous, fibrous, and chondroid tissue. Nuclei of cells may be round, oval, or spindle shaped. Giant cells, when present, are found in focal collections in fewer number than associated with giant cell tumor.

Osteoblastoma may be considered in the differential diagnosis because a giant cell tumor rich in osteoid and woven bone may be mistaken for osteoblastoma. However, concentrating on areas in giant cell tumor with no bone production shows masses of stromal and giant cells that are not seen in osteoblastoma.

Giant cell tumor may also be associated with Paget's disease.[39] This lesion is more common in the skull and facial bones than in the axial skeleton. Giant cell tumor may complicate extensive Paget's disease. Not every expansion of a pagetoid bone is sarcomatous degeneration. Lytic lesion with soft tissue extension in patients with Paget's disease does not necessarily imply a grave prognosis.[40, 41]

In rare circumstances, pigmented villonodular synovitis may be confused with giant cell tumor of bone. Villonodular synovitis may proliferate from the interior of the apophyseal joint and enter the spinal canal in the cervical spine. Patients with this lesion may demonstrate symptoms and signs of myelopathy.[42] The occasional multinucleated giant cells of this lesion should not be confused with giant cell tumor of bone or malignant processes.

Treatment

The lesion must be staged before therapy is instituted.[43] Staging of a giant cell tumor includes CT scanning to determine the exact extent of the tumor and MR imaging to determine the soft tissue distribution of the neoplasm in multiple planes. Angiography may be used to embolize the tumor prior to surgery.[8]

The therapy of choice for giant cell tumor is en bloc excision if the tumor is in an accessible location. Recurrence rates of 10% to 15% are reported in lesions that have been excised.[44] Curettage may control growth of the tumor, but the local recurrence rate is 50% within 5 years.[45] Radiation therapy is rarely curative, is associated with frequent recurrences, and may promote malignant transformation.[3] It is reserved for lesions that are inaccessible for surgical removal or curettage.[46] Lesions treated with radiation do not necessarily undergo malignant degeneration. Patients who were followed up to 35 years after receiving radiation therapy had remission of their tumor.[47–50]

The ideal treatment for giant cell tumor of the spine is complete removal of accessible lesions.[51] Decompression of the spine is necessary once neurologic symptoms appear. A delay of longer than 3 months after the onset of nerve root symptoms may result in irreversible nerve deficits.[12] However, complete resection is frequently impossible because of the location and size of the lesions and the potential for critical blood loss. Giant cell tumor of the upper cervical spine may be approached by splitting the mandible and tongue.[52] Posterior decompression and autograft to stabilize the spine have also been used for cervical lesions.[53] Chemotherapy is not effective in controlling growth of this benign tumor.[18] Embolization of tumors in the spine may be used for inaccessible tumors. A potential risk associated with embolization of spinal lesions is ischemic injury to peripheral nerves and the spinal cord.[18]

Prognosis

Giant cell tumor of bone is invasive and benign and has a high local recurrence rate. Malignant degeneration is associated with metastases that occur after a recurrence of the tumor and up to 10 years after diagnosis.[54] Regardless of treatment, the patients must continue to be examined for signs of recurrence. In some circumstances, up to five courses of therapy were needed to eradicate the disease successfully.[3]

References

GIANT CELL TUMOR

1. Dahlin DC, Unni KK: Bone Tumors: General Aspects and Data on 8,542 Cases, 4th ed. Springfield, Illinois: Charles C Thomas, Publisher, 1986, pp 119–140.
2. Mirra JM: Bone Tumors: Clinical, Radiologic, and Pathologic Correlations. Philadelphia: Lea & Febiger, 1989, pp 942–1020.
3. Hutter RVP, Worcester JW Jr, Francis KC, et al.: Benign and malignant giant cell tumors of bone: a clinicopathological analysis of the natural history of the disease. Cancer 15:653, 1962.
4. Cooper A, Travers B (eds): Surgical Essays, 3rd ed. London: Cox and Son, 1818.
5. Bloodgood JG: Bone tumors: central (medullary) giant cell tumor (sarcoma) of lower end of ulna, with evidence that complete destruction of the bony shell or perforation of the bony shell is not a sign of increased malignancy. Ann Surg 69:345, 1919.
6. Huvos AG: Bone Tumors: Diagnosis, Treatment, and Prognosis, 2nd ed. Philadelphia: WB Saunders Co, 1991, pp 429–467.
7. Schajowicz F, Granato DB, McDonald DJ, Sundaram M: Clinical and radiological features of atypical giant cell tumours of bone. Br J Radiol 64:877, 1991.
8. Campanacci M, Boriana S, Giunti A: Giant cell tumors of the spine. In: Sundaresan N, Schmidek HH, Schiller AL, Rosenthal DI (eds): Tumors of the Spine: Diagnosis and Clinical Management. Philadelphia: WB Saunders Co, 1990, pp 163–172.
9. Kuritzky AS, Joyce ST: Giant cell tumor in the ischium: a therapeutic dilemma. JAMA 238:2392–2394, 1977.
10. Dahlin DC: Giant cell tumor of vertebrae above the sacrum: a review of 31 cases. Cancer 39:1350–1356, 1977.
11. Regen EM, Haber A: Giant cell tumor of cervical vertebra with unusual symptoms. J Bone Joint Surg 39A:196, 1957.
12. Larrson SE, Lorentzon R, Boquist L: Giant cell tumors of the spine and sacrum causing neurological symptoms. Clin Orthop 111:201, 1975.
13. Schwartz HS, Jenkins RB, Dahl RJ, Dewald GW: Cytogenic analysis on giant cell tumors of bone. Clin Orthop 240:250, 1989.
14. Fukunaga M, Nikaido T, Shimoda T, et al: A flow cytometric DNA analysis of giant cell tumors of bone including two cases with malignant transformation. Cancer 70:1886, 1992.
15. DiLorenzo N, Spallone A, Nolletti A, Nardi P: Giant cell tumor of the spine: a clinical study of six cases, with emphasis on the radiological features, treatment, and follow-up. Neurosurgery 6:29, 1980.
16. Sim FJ, McDonald DJ, McLeod RA, Unni KK: Giant cell tumors: Mayo Clinic experience. In: Sundaresan N, Schmidek HH, Schiller AL, Rosenthal DI (eds): Tumors of the Spine: Diagnosis and Clinical Management. Philadelphia: WB Saunders Co, 1990, pp 173–180.
17. Van Nostrand D, Madewell JE, McNeish LM, et al: Radionuclide bone scanning in giant cell tumor. J Nucl Med 27:329, 1986.
18. Carrasco CH, Murray JA: Giant cell tumors. Orthop Clin North Am 20:395, 1989.
19. Masaryk TJ: Neoplastic disease of the spine. Radiol Clin North Am 29:829, 1991.
20. Ghandur-Mnaymneh L, Mnaymneh WA: Bone lesions with giant cells: problems in differential diagnosis. J Med Liban 24:91, 1972.
21. Huvos AG: Bone Tumors: Diagnosis, Treatment, and Prognosis, 2nd ed. Philadelphia: WB Saunders Co, 1991, pp 268–291.
22. Kricun ME: Tumors of the Spine. In: Kricun ME (ed): Imaging of Bone Tumors. Philadelphia: WB Saunders Co, 1993, p 262.
23. Lozes G, Fawaz A, Perper H, et al: Chondroma of the cervical spine: case report. J Neurosurg 66:128, 1987.
24. Slowik T, Bittner-Manioka M, Grochowski W: Chondroma of the cervical spine: case report. J Neurosurg 29:276, 1968.
25. Willis BK, Heilbrun MP: Enchondroma of the cervical spine. Neurosurgery 19:437, 1986.
26. Hess WE: Giant cell tumor of the cervical spine. J Bone Joint Surg 42A:480, 1960.
27. Wisniewski M, Toker C, Anderson PJ, et al: Chondroblastoma of the cervical spine: case report. J Neurosurg 38:763, 1973.
28. Buraczewski J, Lysakowska J, Rudowski W: Chondroblastoma (Codman's tumour) of the thoracic spine. J Bone Joint Surg 39B:705, 1957.
29. Harris WH, Dudley HR, Barry RJ: The natural history of fibrous dysplasia: an orthopaedic, pathological, and roentgenographic study. J Bone Joint Surg 44A:207, 1962.
30. Smith MD, Bohlman HH, Gidonse N: Fibrous dysplasia of the cervical spine: a fatal complication of treatment: a case report. J Bone Joint Surg 72A:1254, 1990.
31. Hu SS, Healey JH, Huvos AG: Fibrous dysplasia of the second cervical vertebra: a case report. J Bone Joint Surg 72A:781, 1990.
32. Resnick CS, Lininger JR: Monostatic fibrous dysplasia of the cervical spine: case report. Radiology 151:49, 1984.
33. Sundaresan N, Schiller AL, Rosenthal DI: Osteosarcoma of the spine. In: Sundaresan N, Schmidek HH, Schiller AL, Rosenthal DI (eds): Tumors of the Spine: Diagnosis and Clinical Management. Philadelphia: WB Saunders Co, 1990, pp 128–145.
34. Barwick KW, Huvos AG, Smith J: Primary osteogenic sarcoma of the column: a clinicopathologic correlation of ten patients. Cancer 46:595, 1980.
35. Dorfman HD, Czerniack B: Bone cancers. Cancer 75:203, 1995.
36. Dahlin DC, Unni KK: Bone Tumors: General Aspects and Data on 8,542 cases, 4th ed. Springfield, Illinois: Charles C Thomas, Publisher, 1986, pp 68–83.
37. Standefer M, Hardy RW Jr, Marks K, et al.: Chondromyxoid fibroma of the cervical spine: a case report with a review of the literature and a description of an operative approach to the lower anterior cervical spine. Neurosurgery 11:288, 1982.
38. Mayer BS: Chondromyxoid fibroma of the lumbar spine. J Can Assoc Radiol 29:271, 1978.
39. Hutter RVP, Foote FW, Frazell EL, Francis KC: Giant

cell tumors complicating Paget's disease of bone. Cancer 16:1044, 1963.

40. Potter HG, Schneider R, Ghelman B, et al.: Multiple giant cell tumors and Paget disease of bone: radiographic and clinical correlations. Radiology 180:261, 1991.

41. Bhambhani M, Lamberty BGH, Clements MR, et al.: Giant cell tumours in mandible and spine: a rare complication of Paget's disease of bone. Ann Rheum Dis 51:1335, 1992.

42. Kleinman GM, Dagi TF, Poletti CE: Villonodular synovitis in the spinal canal: case report. J Neurosurg 52:846, 1980.

43. Heare TC, Enneking WF, Heare MM: Staging techniques and biopsy of bone tumors. Orthop Clin North Am 20:273, 1989.

44. Parrish F: Treatment of bone tumors by total excision and replacement with massive autologous and homologous grafts. J Bone Joint Surg 48A:968, 1966.

45. Johnson EW Jr: Giant cell tumors of bone. J Bone Joint Surg 41A:895, 1959.

46. Dahlin DC, Cupps RE, Johnson EW: Giant cell tumor: a study of 195 cases. Cancer 25:106, 1970.

47. Seider MJ, Rich TA, Ayala AG, Murray JA: Giant cell tumors of bone: treatment with radiation therapy. Radiology 161:537, 1986.

48. Bennett CJ, Marcus RB Jr, Million RR, Enneking WF: Radiation therapy for giant cell tumor of bone. Int J Radiat Oncol Biol Phys 26:299, 1993.

49. Schwartz LH, Okunieff PG, Rosenberg A, Suit HD: Radiation therapy in the treatment of difficult giant cell tumors. Int J Radiat Oncol Biol Phys 17:1085, 1989.

50. DeGroof E, Verdonk R, Vercauteren M, et al.: Giant cell tumor involving a lumbar vertebra. Spine 15:835, 1990.

51. Savini R, Gherlinzoni F, Morandi M, et al.: Surgical treatment of giant cell tumor of the spine. J Bone Joint Surg 65A:1283, 1983.

52. Honma G, Murota K, Shiba R, Kondo H: Mandible and tongue-splitting approach to giant cell tumor of the axis. Spine 14:1204, 1989.

53. Shikata J, Yamamuro T, Shimizu K, et al.: Surgical treatment of giant cell tumors of the spine. Clin Orthop 278:29, 1992.

54. Tubbs WS, Brown LR, Beabout JW, et al.: Bening giant cell tumor of bone with pulmonary metastases: clinical findings and radiologic appearance of metastases in 13 cases. AJR 158:331, 1992.

ANEURYSMAL BONE CYST

Capsule Summary

Frequency of neck pain—common

Location of neck pain—cervical spine

Quality of neck pain—acute onset, increasing severity

Symptoms and signs—localized bone tenderness, overlying skin erythema

Laboratory and x-ray tests—expansile lesion of the posterior elements on plain roentgenograms

Therapy—en bloc excision

Prevalence and Pathogenesis

Aneurysmal bone cyst (ABC) is a benign, non-neoplastic, cystic vascular lesion of bone that occurs de novo or in the setting of another bone condition such as giant cell tumor, chondroblastoma, chondromyxoid fibroma, and fibrous dysplasia. ABC represents about 1% to 2% of primary bone lesions.[1, 2] Another review reports ABC to be 6% of primary bone lesions.[3] Schajowicz has reported on 217 ABCs, a number approximately 50% of the frequency of giant cell tumors.[4] The majority of adults who develop ABCs are younger than 30 years of age and, in contrast with other primary bone tumors, most series report a slight female predominance.[5, 6] A review of 238 patients with ABC also found a slight predominance of women at 54%.[7]

The first description of the distinctive characteristics of this lesion is attributed to Jaffe and Lichtenstein in 1950.[8, 9] Other names that have been associated with ABC include ossifying hematoma, plain bone cysts, and atypical giant cell tumor.

The etiology of ABC remains uncertain, although trauma may play a role in its initiation as injuries may induce the formation of arteriovenous malformations (AVMs). These malformations consist of abnormal vascular channels, and several reports have suggested that the trauma that initiated an AVM may have led to the development of an ABC.[10, 11]

In one third of the cases, ABC is superimposed on another pathologic process that may be either a benign or malignant bone tumor. Primary lesions that may be complicated by ABC include giant cell tumor, chondroblastoma, chondromyxoid fibroma, nonossifying fibroma, osteoblastoma, fibrosarcoma, fibrous histiocytoma, osteosarcoma, and fibrous dysplasia.[12] The basic abnormality in both circumstances is a local change in intraosseous blood flow. The blood pools in bone and results in increasing intraosseous pressure, followed by resorption, expansion, and cyst formation.[13] The recognition of an underlying causative process is important because the clinical course of the patient may more closely follow that of the primary lesion.

A majority of ABCs occur in the long bones of the extremities, and 15% to 25% of cases occur in the spine.[14, 15] The lumbosacral spine is affected in 36% of cases, the thoracic spine in 32%, and the cervical spine in 32%. In a review of 256 cases, the cervical spine was the location for 26% of ABCs affecting the axial skeleton.[16]

Clinical History

Patients with ABC usually present with symptoms of pain or swelling in the affected area. The pain is usually of acute onset that increases in severity for a short period. The duration of symptoms can range from months to several years. The patient may also experience limitation of motion.

The clinical manifestations of spinal ABC vary with the location and size of the lesion. A lesion of the spinous or transverse process may be entirely asymptomatic. Neurologic symptoms and signs include a range of abnormalities, from sensory changes to myelopathy, and these may occur if the expansion of the lesion results in nerve root or spinal cord compression.[17, 18] ABC tends to involve the posterior elements of the vertebra, and giant cell tumor affects the vertebral body. The posterior elements and the vertebral body may be affected simultaneously in large ABCs.[19]

Physical Examination

Physical examination may demonstrate tenderness on palpation at the site of involvement. The overlying skin may be erythematous and warm if the ABC is close to the surface. Patients demonstrate decreased range of motion with muscle spasm.[20] Slightly more than 10% of patients may have associated scoliosis or kyphosis.[21] Neurologic findings correlate with the location of nerve root or spinal cord compression.

Laboratory Data

Screening blood tests are normal in this benign, vascular lesion of bone. Patients with secondary cysts have abnormal tests that correspond with their underlying lesion (malignant tumor).

On gross inspection, ABC contains anastomosing, cavernous spaces that comprise the bulk of lesion. The blood is unclotted. The presence of unclotted blood indicates that the lesion is hemodynamically active with pools of blood filling and draining. The pressure in the tumor is arterial.[3] Subperiosteal new bone that is eggshell-thin in thickness separates the lesion from surrounding tissue.

Histologically, the cystic cavities are composed of vascular channels filled with fibrous connective tissue, osteoid, granulation tissue, and multinucleated giant cells.[4] The solid portions of ABC may be fibrous but may contain a lacework of osteoid trabeculae.

The solid variant of ABC occurs most commonly in long tubular bones but occasionally affects the axial skeleton. Histologically, the lesion is characterized by florid fibroblastic proliferation with osteoclast-like giant cell–rich areas, stromal hemorrhage, and newly formed osteoid. The histology is similar to that of ABC except for the presence of blood-filled spaces.[22]

Radiographic Evaluation

The radiographic features of ABC consist of a solitary, eccentrically located, osteolytic, expansile lesion that is sharply demarcated by a thin subperiosteal shell of bone. The cyst cavity is traversed by fine strands of bony cortex. A soft tissue mass may also be associated with the bony lesion. When in the spine, ABC occurs most commonly in the lumbar and thoracic area and affects the posterior elements of the vertebrae, including pedicles, laminae, and spinous and transverse processes in 60% of lesions (Fig. 13–6). About 30% to 40% of ABCs occur in vertebral bodies.[11] A lesion within the vertebral body may involve more than one vertebra by extension across the apophyseal joint or disc space.[23] The lesion may attain a considerable size. The lesion may also expand to encroach on the neural canal.[24]

Computerized tomography (CT) is useful in the diagnosis of ABC, especially for lesions in the axial skeleton. Multiple fluid levels (layering of solid blood components) on CT are suggestive but not diagnostic of ABC.[25] CT may show a thin rim of bone not evident on radiographs and helps exclude calcified tumor matrix.

Magnetic resonance (MR) imaging may be useful in identifying the extent of lesions in bone and soft tissues.[26] MR images have an expansile appearance of the lesion. The soft tissue extension of all cysts is well defined with a sharp interface. The fibrous tissue in the periphery of the tumor is highlighted by a low-intensity signal in the rim of the lesion on both T_1- and T_2-weighted sequences. Increasing the T_2 weighting of sequences, fluid levels are also detected by MR evaluation.[27] Fluid levels may also accompany telangiectatic osteosarcoma, giant cell tumor, and chondroblastoma.

Differential Diagnosis

The characteristic radiographic appearance of ABC helps differentiate it from other be-

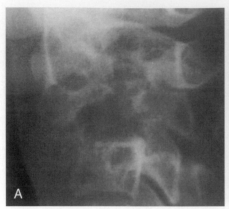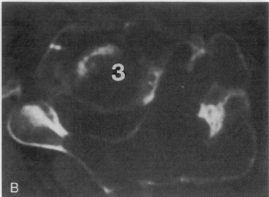

Figure 13–6. In this child, routine radiography, *A*, shows an expansile, osteolytic lesion of the body and posterior elements of the third cervical vertebra. Transaxial computerized tomography, *B*, confirms the extent of involvement and the expansile nature of the lesion. (Courtesy of L. Pinckney, M.D., San Diego, California.)

nign and malignant lesions. The posterior arch and the transverse or spinous process are the common locations of involvement in the spine. A solitary lytic lesion of the anterior body of a vertebra is more likely to be a metastasis, infection, or giant cell tumor. Some primary bone tumors, including chondroblastoma and giant cell tumor, may have areas that appear histologically like ABC. Careful evaluation of the entire specimen should alert the pathologist to the underlying lesion.

Treatment

ABC can be treated by surgery, radiation therapy, and cryotherapy. Although it is a benign lesion, it is highly prone to local recurrence after curettage. If the location of ABC allows for removal of a section of bone without loss of function, en bloc resection is the treatment of choice, and a lesion in the posterior elements of the spine may be treated with resection and bone grafting.[28–30] Excision of the tumor is associated with postoperative pain resolution.[31] Lesions that are too large or involve a vertebral body are treated with radiation therapy.[32] Radiation therapy is able to control the growth of lesions in inaccessible locations.[33] The benefit of radiation therapy must be weighed against the potential of radiation-induced sarcoma many years later. Cryosurgery, freezing the lesion, has also been reported to halt expansion of the cyst and prevent recurrence.[6, 34] Embolization of the tumor with polyvinyl alcohol particles may slow growth of tumors. Lesions may then calcify over months.[24] On occasion, spontaneous healing of a cyst may occur. Lesions may stabilize for extended periods. Older patients are more likely candidates for spontaneous tumor healing.[35]

Prognosis

ABC is a benign lesion but may cause severe dysfunction because of its expansile characteristics. If diagnosed early and treated appropriately, dysfunction may be kept to a minimum. However, if ABC is located in the spine and is allowed to expand unchecked, serious neurologic deficits may result. In addition, ABC weakens the bone and increases the risk of pathologic fracture. Lesions in the cervical spine may require excision with fusion with bone graft and wire.[36] In rare circumstances, the cyst may transform into a malignant tumor, particularly after irradiation.[37]

References

ANEURYSMAL BONE CYST

1. Mirra JM: Bone Tumors: Clinical, Radiologic, and Pathologic Correlations. Philadelphia: Lea & Febiger, 1989, pp 1267–1312.
2. Dahlin DC, Unni KK: Bone Tumors: General Aspects and Data on 8,542 cases, 4th ed. Springfield, Illinois: Charles C Thomas, Publisher, 1986, pp 420–430.
3. Huvos AG: Bone Tumors: Diagnosis, Treatment, and Prognosis, 2nd ed. Philadelphia: WB Saunders Co, 1991, pp 727–743.
4. Schajowicz F: Tumors and Tumorlike Lesions of Bone: Pathology, Radiology, and Treatment, 2nd ed. Berlin: Springer-Verlag, 1994, pp 514–531.
5. Dahlin DC, Besse BE, Pugh DG, Ghormley RK: Aneurysmal bone cysts. Radiology 64:56, 1955.
6. Biesecker JL, Marcove RC, Huvos AG, Mike V: Aneurysmal bone cyst: a clinicopathologic study of 66 cases. Cancer 26:615, 1970.

7. Vergel AM, Bond JR, Shives TC, et al.: Aneurysmal bone cyst: a clinicopathologic study of 238 cases. Cancer 69:2921, 1991.
8. Jaffe HL: Aneurysmal bone cyst. Bull Hosp Jt Dis 11:3, 1950.
9. Lichtenstein L: Aneurysmal bone cyst: a pathological entity commonly mistaken for a giant cell tumor and occasionally for hemangioma and osteogenic sarcoma. Cancer 3:279, 1950.
10. Barnes R: Aneurysmal bone cyst. J Bone Joint Surg 38B:301, 1956.
11. Donaldson WF: Aneurysmal bone cyst. J Bone Joint Surg 44A:25, 1962.
12. Martinez V, Sissons HA: Aneurysmal bone cyst: a review of 123 cases including primary lesions and those secondary to other bone pathology. Cancer 81:2291, 1988.
13. Clough JR, Price CHG: Aneurysmal bone cyst: pathogenesis and long-term results of treatment. Clin Orthop 97:52, 1973.
14. Lichtenstein L: Aneurysmal bone cyst: observations on fifty cases. J Bone Joint Surg 39A:873, 1957.
15. Dabska M, Buraczewski J: Aneurysmal bone cyst: pathology, clinical course and radiologic appearance. Cancer 23:371, 1969.
16. Kricun ME: Tumors of the Spine. In: Kricun ME (ed): Imaging of Bone Tumors. Philadelphia: WB Saunders Co, 1993, pp 260–262.
17. Hay MC, Patterson D, Taylor TKF: Aneurysmal bone cysts of the spine. J Bone Joint Surg 60B:406, 1978.
18. Dahlin DC, McLeod RA: Aneurysmal bone cyst and other non-neoplastic conditions. Skeletal Radiol 8:243, 1982.
19. Tillman BP, Dahlin DC, Lipscomb PR, et al.: Aneurysmal bone cyst: an analysis of ninety-five cases. Mayo Clin Proc 43:478, 1968.
20. Chakravarty K, Brett F, Merry P: Aneurysmal bone cyst: an unusual presentation of neck pain in a young adult. Br J Rheumatol 33:597, 1994.
21. Capanna R, Albisinni U, Picci P, et al.: Aneurysmal bone cyst of the spine. J Bone Joint Surg 67A:527, 1985.
22. Oda Y, Tsuneyoshi M, Shinohara N: Solid variant of aneurysmal bone cyst (extragnathic giant cell reparative granuloma) in the axial skeleton and long bones. Cancer 70:2642, 1992.
23. Banna M: Clinical Radiology of the Spine and the Spinal Cord. Rockville, Maryland: Aspen Systems Corp, 1985, pp 347–348.
24. Cory DA, Fritsch SA, Cohen MD, et al.: Aneurysmal bone cysts: imaging findings and embolotherapy. AJR 153:369, 1989.
25. Hudson TM: Fluid levels in aneurysmal bone cysts: a CT feature. AJR 141:1001, 1984.
26. Zimmer WD, Berquist TH, Sim FH, et al.: Magnetic resonance imaging of aneurysmal bone cysts. Mayo Clin Proc 59:633, 1984.
27. Munk PL, Helms CA, Holt RG, et al.: MR imaging of aneurysmal bone cysts. AJR 153:99, 1989.
28. Stillwell WT, Fielding JW: Aneurysmal bone cyst of the cervicodorsal spine. Clin Orthop 187:144, 1984.
29. Buck RE, Bailey RW: Replacement of a cervical vertebral body for aneurysmal bone cyst. J Bone Joint Surg 51A:1656, 1969.
30. Parrish FF, Pevey JK: Surgical management of aneurysmal bone cyst of the vertebral column. J Bone Joint Surg 49A:1597, 1967.
31. Bohlman HH, Sachs BL, Carter JR, et al.: Primary neoplasms of the cervical spine. J Bone Joint Surg 68A:483, 1986.
32. Slowick FA, Campbell CJ, Kettelkamp DB: Aneurysmal bone cyst. J Bone Joint Surg 50A:1142, 1968.
33. Maeda M, Tateishi H, Takaiwa H, et al.: High-energy, low-dose radiation therapy for aneurysmal bone cyst: report of a case. Clin Orthop 243:200, 1989.
34. Marcove RC, Miller TR: The treatment of primary and metastatic bone-localized tumors by cryosurgery. Surg Clin North Am 49:421, 1969.
35. Malghem J, Maldague B, Esselinckx W, et al.: Spontaneous healing of aneurysmal bone cysts: a report of three cases. J Bone Joint Surg 71B:645, 1989.
36. Gupta VK, Gupta SK, Khosla VK, et al.: Aneurysmal bone cysts of the spine. Surg Neurol 42:428, 1994.
37. Kyriakos M, Hardy D: Malignant transformation of aneurysmal bone cyst, with an analysis of the literature. Cancer 68:1770, 1991.

HEMANGIOMA

Capsule Summary

Frequency of neck pain—rare
Location of neck pain—cervical spine
Quality of neck pain—throbbing
Symptoms and signs—localized tenderness, decreased motion
Laboratory x-ray tests—prominent vertical vertebral body striations on plain roentgenogram
Treatment—radiation for symptomatic lesions

Prevalence and Pathogenesis

Hemangioma is a benign, vascular lesion, composed of cavernous, capillary, or venous blood vessels, that may affect soft tissues or bone. Hemangioma accounts for fewer than 1% of clinically symptomatic primary bone tumors.[1, 2] However, necropsy studies by a number of investigators have demonstrated that asymptomatic vertebral lesions are found in 12% of autopsies.[3, 4] The prevalence of hemangioma increases with age, affecting 25% of adults in the fifth decade of life. It is usually identified in patients in the fourth and fifth decades of life. When taking into account hemangiomas from all sites, women and men are affected equally.

The first reference to hemangioma was reported by Toynbee in 1845.[5] This vascular lesion has been known by many names, including capillary, cavernous, venous, hypertrophic, juvenile, arteriovenous, intramuscular, synovial, and histiocytic hemangioma.

The pathogenesis of hemangioma remains unknown. The lesion is considered a congenital vascular malformation by some and a benign neoplasm by others.

Approximately 50% of patients with hemangioma have the lesion in the spine or skull. The thoracic spine is the location for 65% of lesions, cervical spine for 25%, and lumbar spine for 10%.[2] In a review of 59 patients with vertebral hemangiomas, the distribution of lesions was thoracic spine 54%, lumbar spine 39%, and cervical spine 7%.[6]

Clinical History

The initial complaints of patients with symptomatic vertebral hemangioma are localized pain and tenderness over the involved vertebra along with associated muscle spasm.[7] The pain usually starts as a vague, nondescript ache that gradually increases in intensity and duration until it becomes constant and throbbing. Neurologic manifestations of cord compression by vertebral hemangiomas may include sensory changes, motor weakness, radiculitis, or transverse myelitis.[8, 9] In the study reported by Fox and Onofrio, 22% of vertebral hemangiomas presented with neck or back pain.[6]

Multiple hemangiomas may cause spinal cord compression resembling metastatic disease to the spine.[10] Neurologic symptoms tend to occur at time of expansion of the lesion in the vertebral body into the epidural space, pathological fracture, or extradural hematoma.[11] Neurologic symptoms may occur acutely and recurrently.[12] Many of the hemangiomas that cause neurologic symptoms are located in the thoracic spine, where the spinal canal is narrow. Most patients with neurologic dysfunction secondary to vertebral hemangioma have symptoms at the time of presentation. In the study by Fox and Onofrio, one of four cervical hemangiomas was associated with a neurologic deficit.[6]

Physical Examination

Physical examination may demonstrate tenderness on palpation over the affected vertebral body. Limitation of motion may be present if related muscle spasm is severe.

Hemangioma that expands bone may cause palpable swelling. Increased weakening of the vertebral body may result in fractures, which markedly increase tenderness, and muscle spasm.[13] Increased pain and spasm may also result in kyphoscoliosis.[14] Hemangioma may occur in the setting of systemic hemangiomatosis. In that circumstance, hemangiomas may be noted on the skin, mucous membranes, and other organs (multiple hemangiomatosis of bone or Osler-Weber-Rendu disease).[15, 16]

Laboratory Data

Screening blood tests are normal in this benign lesion of bone. Occasionally, the erythrocyte sedimentation rate (ESR) is elevated.[17] Rarely, a consumptive coagulopathy with thrombocytopenia has been reported in patients with multiple vertebral hemangiomas.[18] This syndrome, Kasabach-Merritt syndrome, occurs with multiple hemangiomas and hemangioendotheliomas.[19]

On gross examination, the well-demarcated lesion is reddish brown and is confined to the vertebral body or extends into the surrounding soft tissue. The vertebral body is the preferential location of primary involvement, with secondary extension into the arch or transverse process. Microscopically, hemangioma is composed of numerous capillary and larger vascular channels that are contained in a fibrous stroma. The trabeculae that are not affected by the tumor are thickened in comparison with the lesional, thinned osseous trabeculae.[6]

Radiographic Evaluation

Vertebral hemangioma primarily involves the vertebral bodies.[20] In an affected vertebral body, the vertical striations are prominent and horizontal striations are absent because of absorption. This gives rise to a "corduroy" appearance of the vertebral body. This is most prominent on the lateral projection (Fig. 13–7). The alteration of vertebral striations is diffuse, and vertebral body configuration is usually unchanged. Occasionally, vertebral body hemangioma may extend from the body to the laminae, pedicles, or transverse or spinous processes. Rarely does expansion or enlargement of a vertebra occur.[8]

Symptomatic vertebral hemangioma may have thinner and wider vertical striations. It may be associated with vertebral body collapse, hemorrhage, and soft tissue masses.[21] Hemangioma rarely causes compression fractures because of the buttressing of the weaker components by the coarse remaining trabeculations.[22] Radiologic study of 57 solitary vertebral hemangiomas identified six factors associated with a greater likelihood of compressing the spinal cord. These features were location in the tho-

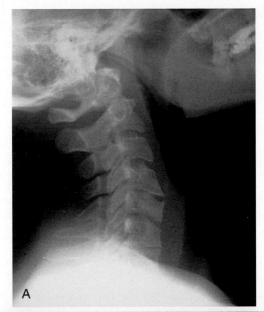

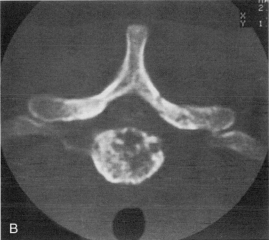

Figure 13–7. Hemangiomas. An 18-year-old female with cervical vertebral bodies (C4, C5, and C7) with hemangiomas. *A,* Lateral view of cervical spine shows prominence of vertical striations. *B,* Computerized tomography scan of cervical spine shows areas of osteolysis of the vertebral body and posterior lamina. (Courtesy of Anne Brower, M.D.)

racic spine, involvement of the entire vertebral body, extension into the neural arch, an expanded cortex with indistinct margins, an irregular honeycomb pattern, and soft tissue mass. Only one hemangioma at the L3 level was associated with compressive signs.[23]

Bone scintigraphy demonstrates increased tracer uptake at the site of vertebral hemangioma. The bone scan may demonstrate decreased uptake if the hemangioma has become thrombosed.[24]

Examination by computerized tomography

(CT) scan demonstrates the bony changes of hemangioma, including the expansion of the body and the involvement of the arch. Soft tissue extension is also noted by CT examination, with or without contrast agent.[25]

Magnetic resonance (MR) examination of hemangioma demonstrates increased signal intensity on both T_1- and T_2-weighted images. Increased signal intensity corresponds with fatty stroma (T_1) and vascularization (T_2). The aggressiveness of hemangioma associated with expansion has been related to the absence of fat and increased extent of vascularity as measured by MR.[26]

Angiography may help identify the blood vessels that are feeding the tumor. Occasionally, hemorrhage may impede the filling of the tumor during angiography.[25] Angiography does not distinguish hemangioma from other vascular tumors.

Differential Diagnosis

The diagnosis of vertebral hemangioma is uncomplicated when one vertebral body is affected with characteristic radiographic changes. It is more difficult when portions of a vertebra other than the body are affected. Bony resorption of a pedicle may mimic the destructive changes of metastatic cancer. A vertebral body fracture may occur with hemangioma but is more frequently seen in metastatic tumor.

Skeletal lymphangiomatosis may affect vertebral bodies, causing increased striation, bony lysis with bone compression, and spinal cord compression when affecting the cervical spine.[27] Lymphangiography may be required to confirm this diagnosis. Histologically, lymphoid tissue is present to an increased degree in the vascular channels of the bone.[28]

A closely related but rare cause of vertebral bone loss that may resemble hemangiomatosis is Gorham's disease (massive osteolysis).[2, 6] Multiple hemangiomas develop with total lysis of the affected bone and periosteum. The bone is replaced by fibrous tissue. The disease may be either self-limited or may progress to a fatal outcome.[29] Fatal outcome may occur despite therapy with radiation therapy.[30] Patients with structural instability of the cervical spine secondary to Gorham's disease have been reported.[31] Hemangiopericytoma is also a rare vascular tumor that may mimic hemangioma.[3] Angiolipoma, another tumor that affects vertebrae, may cause spinal cord compression and must be differentiated from a hemangioma.[32] Angiosarcoma is a rare malignant tumor that may affect areas of the vertebral column similar to those affected by hemangioma.[33]

Coarse trabeculation of a vertebral body may also be seen in Paget's disease. Abnormal laboratory tests (elevated ESR and serum alkaline phosphatase level) should differentiate tumor and Paget's disease from hemangioma.

Treatment

The treatment of choice for symptomatic vertebral hemangioma is irradiation because it is radiosensitive. Radiation therapy relieves symptoms effectively even though the appearance of the lesion remains unchanged.[34] Surgical intervention in the form of laminectomy has excessive morbidity and mortality due to profuse hemorrhage. Therefore, laminectomy should be reserved for those patients with neurologic deficits who require decompression of the spinal cord. Embolization of feeder vessels before surgery may render surgical decompression a safer procedure.[35] Embolization alone may be successful in controlling the growth of the tumor or may be used in combination with radiation therapy or surgery to reverse neurologic symptoms.[36-38] A new technique is the injection of methylmethacrylate under the guidance of CT and fluoroscopy into symptomatic vertebral bodies containing hemangiomas. Although the efficiency of this technique in preventing collapse cannot be evaluated, the injection is associated with pain resolution.[39]

Prognosis

Vertebral hemangioma is usually asymptomatic and has a benign course; however, when it becomes symptomatic, it requires therapy to prevent expansion of the lesion. The major complication of vertebral hemangioma is neural compression. Compression fractures may occur more easily in vertebrae affected by hemangioma. Hemangioma may cause neural compression by compression fracture, expansion of an involved vertebrae, direct extension of the hemangioma into the extradural space, or extradural hemorrhage. Appropriate diagnosis and treatment may help prevent this potentially disabling complication of this vascular neoplasm.

References

HEMANGIOMA

1. Mirra JM: Bone Tumors: Clinical, Radiologic, and Pathologic Correlations. Philadelphia: Lea & Febiger, 1989, pp 1338–1377.
2. Dahlin DC, Unni KK: Bone Tumors: General Aspects and Data on 8,542 Cases, 4th ed. Springfield, Illinois: Charles C Thomas, Publisher, 1986, pp 167–180.
3. Marcial-Rojas RA: Primary hemangiopericytoma of bone: review of the literature and report of the first case with metastasis. Cancer 13:308, 1960.
4. Schmorl G, Junghanns H: The Human Spine in Health and Disease, 2nd ed. New York: Grune & Stratton, 1971, p 325.
5. Toynbee J: An account of two vascular tumors developed in the substance of bone. Lancet 2:676, 1845.
6. Fox MW, Onofrio BM: The natural history and management of symptomatic and asymptomatic vertebral hemangiomas. J Neurosurg 78:36, 1993.
7. Huvos AG: Bone Tumors: Diagnosis, Treatment, and Prognosis, 2nd ed. Philadelphia: WB Saunders Co, 1991, pp 553–578.
8. Barnard L, Von Nuys RG: Primary hemangioma of the spine. Ann Surg 97:19, 1933.
9. McAllister VL, Kendall BE, Bull JWD: Symptomatic vertebral hemangiomas. Brain 98:71, 1975.
10. Zito G, Kadis GW: Multiple vertebral hemangiomas resembling metastases with spinal cord compression. Arch Neurol 37:247, 1980.
11. Mohan V, Gupta SK, Tuli SM, Sanyal B: Symptomatic vertebral hemangiomas. Clin Radiol 31:575, 1980.
12. Newmark J, Jones HR Jr, Thomas CB, et al.: Vertebral hemangioma causing acute recurrent spinal cord compression. J Neurol Neurosurg Psychiatry 54:471, 1991.
13. Bergstrand A, Hook O, Lidvall H: Vertebral hemangiomas compressing the spinal cord. Acta Neurol Scand 39:59, 1963.
14. Ghormley RK, Adson AW: Hemangioma of vertebrae. J Bone Joint Surg 23:887, 1941.
15. Gutierrez R, Spjut J: Skeletal angiomatosis: report of 3 cases and review of the literature. Clin Orthop 85:82, 1972.
16. Mirra JM, Arnold WD: Skeletal hemangiomatosis in association with hereditary hemorrhagic telangiectasia. J Bone Joint Surg 55A:850, 1973.
17. Govender S, Charles RW, Kelman IE: Vertebral haemangiomas: a report of 2 cases. S Afr Med J 72:640, 1987.
18. Lozman J, Holmblad J: Cavernous hemangiomas associated with scoliosis and a localized consumptive coagulopathy: a case report. J Bone Joint Surg 58A:1021, 1976.
19. Brower TD: Case records of the Massachusetts General Hospital. N Engl J Med 320:854, 1989.
20. Sherman RS, Wilner D: The roentgen diagnosis of hemangioma of bone. AJR 86:1146, 1961.
21. Banna M: Clinical Radiology of the Spine and the Spinal Cord. Rockville, Maryland: Aspen Systems Corp, 1985, pp 341–345.
22. McAllister VL, Kendall BE, Bull JW: Symptomatic vertebral hemangiomas. Brain 98:71, 1975.
23. Laredo J, Reizine D, Bard M, Merland J: Vertebral hemangiomas: radiologic evaluation. Radiology 161:183, 1986.
24. Gerard PS, Wilck E: Spinal hemangioma: an unusual photopenic presentation on bone scan. Spine 17:607, 1992.
25. Schnyder P, Frankhauser H, Mansouri B: Computed

tomography in spinal hemangioma with cord compression: report of two cases. Skeletal Radiol 15:372, 1986.

26. Laredo J, Assouline E, Gelbert F, et al.: Vertebral hemangiomas: fat content as a sign of aggressiveness. Radiology 177:467, 1990.

27. Edwards WH, Thompson RC, Varsa EW: Lymphangiomatosis and massive osteolysis of the cervical spine. Clin Orthop 177:222, 1983.

28. Reilly BJ, Davison JW, Bain H: Lymphangiectasis of the skeleton: a case report. Radiology 103:385, 1972.

29. Hambach R, Pujman J, Maly V: Massive osteolysis due to hemangiomatosis: report of a case of Gorham's disease with autopsy. Radiology 71:43, 1958.

30. Bohlman HH, Sachs BL, Carter JR, et al.: Primary neoplasms of the cervical spine. J Bone Joint Surg 68A:483, 1986.

31. Castleman B: Case records of the Massachusetts General Hospital. N Engl J Med 270:731, 1964.

32. Kuroda S, Abe H, Akino M, et al.: Infiltrating spinal angiolipoma causing myelopathy: case report. Neurosurgery 27:315, 1990.

33. Dagi TF, Schmidek HH: Vascular tumors of the spine. In: Sundaresan N, Schmidek HH, Schiller AL, Rosenthal DI (eds): Tumors of the Spine: Diagnosis and Clinical Management. Philadelphia: WB Saunders Co, 1990, pp 181–191.

34. Manning JH: Symptomatic hemangioma of the spine. Radiology 56:58, 1951.

35. Kapur P, Banna M: Spinous osseous angioma: Gelfoam embolization. J Can Assoc Radiol 31:271, 1980.

36. Raco A, Ciappetta P, Artico M, et al.: Vertebral hemangiomas with cord compression: the role of embolization in five cases. Surg Neurol 34:164, 1990.

37. Djindijian M, Nguyen J, Gaston A, et al.: Multiple vertebral hemangiomas with neurological signs: case report. J Neurosurg 76:1025, 1992.

38. Bednar DA, Esses SI: Double hemangioma of the spine with paraparesis: a case report. Spine 15:1377, 1990.

39. Gangi A, Kastler BA, Dietmann JL: Percutaneous vertebroplasty guided by a combination of CT and fluoroscopy. AJNR 15:83, 1994.

EOSINOPHILIC GRANULOMA

Capsule Summary

Frequency of neck pain—common
Location of neck pain—cervical spine
Quality of neck pain—localized aching
Symptoms and signs—nontender swelling
Laboratory and x-ray tests—occasional peripheral eosinophilia; osteolysis without sclerosis in a vertebral body on plain roentgenogram; epidural extension of granuloma on magnetic resonance image
Treatment—curettage

Prevalence and Pathogenesis

Eosinophilic granuloma occurs in solitary and multifocal forms and is characterized by the infiltration of bone with histiocytes, mononuclear phagocytic cells, and eosinophils. The cell of origin is the Langerhans's cell. Eosinophilic granuloma, Hand-Schüller-Christian disease, and Letterer-Siwe disease are thought to have the same pathogenesis and are referred to collectively as histiocytosis X. Eosinophilic granuloma is the mildest form, and Letterer-Siwe the most aggressive form, of histiocytosis X.

Eosinophilic granuloma is a rare lesion occurring in less than 1% of biopsied primary infiltrative lesions of bone.[1] It occurs most commonly in children and adolescents, with approximately 10% of patients being 20 years of age or older.[2] It has a higher incidence in males at a 2:1 ratio and is more frequent in whites than blacks. Approximately 1,200 new cases of eosinophilic granuloma are reported yearly in the United States.[3]

The first reference to the term eosinophilic granuloma was made by Jaffe and Lichtenstein in 1944.[4] This lesion has had many names, including pseudotuberculous granuloma, Taratynov's disease, traumatic myeloma, and histiocytic granuloma.

The pathogenesis of eosinophilic granuloma is not known. This disease belongs to the nonlipid histiocytoses, which are characterized by proliferation of histiocytes without a demonstrable disorder of lipid metabolism. These histiocytes accumulate cytoplasmic lipid but, unlike true lipid metabolic disorders (Gaucher's disease), these lipids develop as a consequence of the ingestion of necrotic debris rather than an inborn error of metabolism. The cause of this accumulation of these lipids is unknown. Some investigators have suggested that eosinophilic granuloma may be the result of a viral infection, but this hypothesis remains unproven.[5] Immunologic alterations have been demonstrated in association with eosinophilic granuloma. The immunologic changes are associated with abnormal histologic findings in the thymus.[6] Autoimmune complexes have also been implicated as a possible immunologic cause of this disorder.[7] Another suggested immunologic abnormality includes deficiency of suppressor T lymphocytes resulting in uncontrolled proliferation of monocytes and macrophages.[8]

Approximately 10% of patients with unifocal eosinophilic granuloma have lesions in the spine. Eosinophilic granuloma involving the spine was first recognized by Compere and colleagues in 1954.[9] It is dispersed equally through the lumbar, thoracic, and cervical spine.[1] Macnab first described eosinophilic granuloma in the cervical spine in 1955.[10] A review of 32 cases of eosinophilic granuloma affecting the cervical spine was reported by Dickson and Farhat.[11] Unifocal (solitary) bone presentation is twice as common as multifocal osseous involvement. Eosinophilic granuloma may affect multiple spinal levels.[12]

Clinical History

The symptoms of spinal eosinophilic granuloma vary with the location and severity of the lesion. Neck pain, which is constant, is the most common complaint in up to 87% of patients.[11] Pain is not relieved with rest or aspirin and may have a duration of weeks to months at presentation. The lesion may cause restricted motion and muscle spasm. A palpable mass may be noted if a lesion is close to the skin. Symptoms of spinal cord compression are uncommon but may occur secondary to vertebral body collapse or dislocation. These patients may have neurologic symptoms including radicular pain and paresthesias.[13] In the cervical spine, the extremities (arms and legs) and visceral functions may be affected in patients with cervical cord compression.[14–16]

Physical Examination

A palpable mass may be present over the affected bone, but it is neither tender nor associated with redness or heat in most circumstances. Tenderness on palpation has been noted in patients with cervical eosinophilic granuloma.[16] Pain may be provoked by neck movement and limited cervical range of motion may be noted. Torticollis has been reported.[11] A low-grade fever is present in few patients.[1] Spinal cord and nerve root compression secondary to vertebral body collapse result in corresponding abnormalities on neurologic examination.

Laboratory Data

Eosinophilic granuloma is associated with peripheral eosinophilia in 6% to 10% of patients. There is also an occasional patient with an elevated erythrocyte sedimentation rate. Bone marrow examination from an uninvolved area of bone yields increased numbers of eosinophils, even with normal differential counts.[17]

Gross pathologic specimens usually describe a soft reddish-brown tissue with hemorrhage and cysts. The histologic appearance of eosinophilic granuloma is characterized by collections of eosinophils and histiocytes without the formation of local, distinct granulomas. The characteristic cell of eosinophilic granuloma is similar to the Langerhans's cell of the epidermis. On electron microscopy, Langerhans's cells contain Birbeck granules. Birbeck granules are shaped like tennis rackets. These pentalaminar cytoplasmic inclusions are thought to be formed by the invagination of the cell membranes of Langerhans's cells. Birbeck granules are found in cells from eosinophilic granuloma lesions. Special stains may also be used to detect S-100 nuclear-positive dendritic-system histiocytes and lysozyme- and esterase-positive and S-100–negative macrophage-system histiocytes.[1] S-100 protein cells are ubiquitous and may be found in a variety of neoplastic and benign conditions. Peanut agglutinin (PNA) is a more specific histiocyte marker. The paranuclear and surface pattern of PNA binding helps define Langerhans's histiocytes.[18] The histiocytes have striking phagocytic activity. Some foci contain multinucleated giant cells with areas of hemorrhage and necroses. The cytoplasm of the phagocytic cells often exhibits double-refractile, neutral-fat deposition. In areas where eosinophilic leukocytes undergo fragmentation, Charcot-Leyden crystals are noted. As eosinophilic granuloma heals, eosinophils markedly diminish in number to be replaced by large histiocytes and fibrous tissue.[19, 20]

The pleomorphic appearance of the histiocytes may superficially resemble malignant cells of Hodgkin's disease. Histiocytes of eosinophilic granuloma are benign. With time, they may form giant cells and take on the appearance of foam cells after they have ingested necrotic tissue and convert it into cytoplasmic lipids. The presence of lipid in eosinophilic granuloma is a secondary phenomenon and is not of pathogenetic importance as it is in Gaucher's disease.

Radiographic Evaluation

Eosinophilic granuloma in the spine is associated with a range of radiographic abnormalities. The features of early lesions are a destructive, radiolucent oval area of bone lysis without peripheral sclerosis. Progressive destruction in a vertebral body results in a flattened vertebral body, termed vertebra plana, first described by Calvé.[21] The degree of compression may be symmetrical or asymmetrical with preservation of the intervertebral disc. Although the disc may be spared, the intervertebral disc space may be narrowed if the disc collapses into a weakened vertebral body.[22] The body of the vertebra is affected with sparing of the posterior elements.[23] The compressed vertebra may project anteriorly and, in extreme circumstances, cause spinal dislocation. The association of vertebra plana with eosinophilic granuloma has been verified by tissue biopsy.[24] Eosinophilic granuloma is the most common cause of vertebra plana in children (Fig. 13–8). It may erode the posterior elements of a vertebral body and spare the vertebral body. In the cervical spine, the vertebra may be involved without signs of vertebral body collapse.[25] One pedicle, one lamina, or one of the lateral masses may be affected. These lesions are not associated with vertebral collapse.[26] Rarely, eosinophilic granuloma can produce expansile lesions with extensive destruction of multiple vertebrae and paraspinal extension.[27] The vertebral height may be restored spontaneously or after treatment, with the affected vertebra

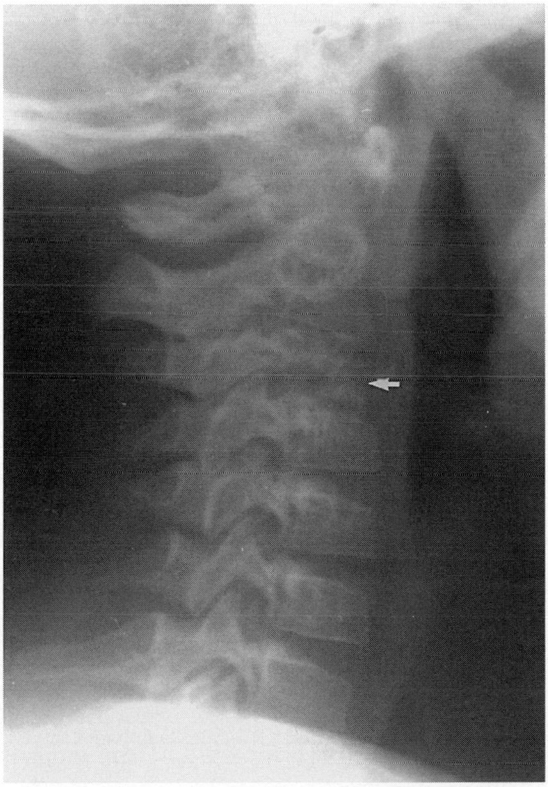

Figure 13–8. Eosinophilic granuloma. Lateral view of cervical spine shows some flattening of the C3 vertebral body (vertebra plana) *(arrow)* with preservation of disc spaces. (Courtesy of Anne Brower, M.D.)

reverting to an almost normal configuration.[28] Reconstitution of body height occurs more regularly in young children with continued vertebral growth.[29]

Other radiographic techniques may be useful in the determination of bone involvement and the extent of soft tissue extension of lesions in the spinal canal. Bone scintigraphy may detect lesions in complex bones, but roentgenogram may be superior in the detection of early lesions.[30] Computerized tomography is particularly helpful in confirming periosteal reaction and cortical invasion.[11] Magnetic resonance (MR) imaging is useful in the determination of epidural extension of extraosseous eosinophilic granulomas associated with neurologic compromise.[13] MR imaging is able to determine the level and extent of spinal cord compression.[15, 16]

Differential Diagnosis

The diagnosis of eosinophilic granuloma is made from the close inspection of biopsied material. Laboratory and radiographic features are too nonspecific to ensure an accurate diagnosis. The careful inspection of biopsied material is essential to making the correct diagnosis. There are many pitfalls that may cause misinterpretation of biopsy specimens. The characteristic cells associated with this tumor are eosinophils and monocytoid histiocytes. Improperly stained eosinophils may be mistaken for neutrophils. The large number of "neutrophils" might be mistaken for osteomyelitis caused by bacterial, tuberculous, or fungal organisms. Histiocytes associated with eosinophilic granuloma may have single or multiple nuclei that are round, oval, or lobulated. The pleomorphism of histiocytes can lead to the erroneous impression of a reticulum cell sarcoma or Hodgkin's disease. Histiocytes in these malignant diseases have greater nuclear pleomorphism and more irregular nucleoli.

During the healing phase of eosinophilic granuloma, masses of multinucleate giant cells are seen in areas of the tumor that are being revascularized. These giant cells may result in an inappropriate diagnosis of giant cell tumor. The clinical, radiologic, and histologic features should prevent an erroneous diagnosis being made.

Treatment

Spontaneous healing of eosinophilic granuloma is manifested by partial restoration of vertebral body height. Restoration of vertebral height occurs most commonly in younger patients.[12] Therefore surgery or radiation therapy may not be indicated unless specific indications such as neurologic complications are present. In patients with biopsy evidence of the neoplasm and intractable symptoms, the treatment of choice for eosinophilic granuloma is curettage, with or without packing of the lesion with bone chips. Patients with cervical lesions with neurologic impairment may require anterior or posterior exploration, vertebral body fusion, and halo traction.[11, 15] Inaccessible lesions in the spine that may lead to pathologic fractures are best treated with low-dosage radiation therapy of 300 to 600 rads. Healing may occur over months to years. Corticosteroids have been used in pediatric patients and have been effective in reversing bone lesions.[31] Steroids have been chosen for patients with lesions in a difficult operative location.[32] Bisphosphonates have been used in a small number of patients to decrease bone pain and prevent the progression of bone lesions. Clodronate given in a dose of 1.6 gm/day for 6 months allowed for healing of bone lesions in two adult patients. The remission lasted for 3 years in one patient and 5 years in another.[33]

Prognosis

Eosinophilic granuloma is a benign lesion and the prognosis is good. Patients with vertebra plana may heal in time with partial reconstitution of the affected vertebral body. The prognosis of patients with multifocal eosinophilic granuloma may not be as good if their disease progresses to the diffuse involvement associated with other components of histiocytosis X. This is more of a concern for younger patients than for adults. If a patient has only a single lesion for 6 months, the chances are that the lesion will remain unifocal.[1]

References

EOSINOPHILIC GRANULOMA

1. Mirra JM: Bone Tumors: Clinical, Radiologic, and Pathologic Correlations. Philadelphia: Lea & Febiger, 1989, pp 1023–1045.
2. Cheyne C: Histiocytosis X. J Bone Joint Surg 53B:366, 1971.
3. Lavin PT, Osband ME: Evaluating the role of therapy in histiocytosis X. Hematol Oncol Clin North Am 1:35, 1987.
4. Jaffe HL, Lichtenstein L: Eosinophilic granuloma of bone: a condition affecting one, several or many bones, but apparently limited to the skeleton and representing the mildest clinical expression of the peculiar inflammatory histiocytosis also underlying Letterer-Siwe disease and Schüller-Christian disease. Arch Pathol 37:99, 1944.
5. Schajowicz F, Slullitel J: Eosinophilic granuloma and its relationship to Hand-Schüller-Christian and Letterer-Siwe syndromes. J Bone Joint Surg 55B:545, 1973.
6. Sessa S, Sommelet D, Lascombes P, Prevot J: Treatment of Langerhans' cell histiocytosis in children: experience at the Children's Hospital of Nancy. J Bone Joint Surg 76A:1513, 1994.
7. Osband ME: Histiocytosis X: Langerhans' cell histiocytosis. Hematol Oncol Clin North Am 1:737, 1987.
8. Willman CL, Busque L, Griffith BB, et al.: Langerhans' cell histiocytosis (histiocytosis X): a clonal proliferative disease. N Engl J Med 331:154, 1994.
9. Compere EL, Johnson WE, Coventry MD: Vertebra plana (Calve's disease) due to eosinophilic granuloma. J Bone Joint Surg 36A:969, 1954.
10. Macnab GH: Discussion: eosinophilic granuloma, Letterer-Siwe disease, Hand-Schüller-Christian disease. Proc R Soc Med 48:711, 1955.
11. Dickson LD, Farhat SM: Eosinophilic granuloma of the cervical spine: a case report and review of the literature. Surg Neurol 35:57, 1991.
12. Tomita T: Special considerations in surgery of pediatric spine tumors. In: Sundaresan N, Schmidek HH, Schiller AL, Rosenthal DI (eds): Tumors of the Spine: Diagnosis and Clinical Management. Philadelphia: WB Saunders Co, 1990, pp 258–271.
13. Kantererewicz E, Condom E, Canete JD, Del Olmo JA: Spinal cord compression by a unifocal eosinophilic granuloma: a case report of an adult with unusual roentgenological features. Neurosurgery 23:666, 1988.
14. Alley RM, Sussman MD: Rapidly progressive eosinophilic granuloma: a case report. Spine 17:1517, 1992.
15. Sweasey TA, Dauser RC: Eosinophilic granuloma of the cervicothoracic junction: case report. J Neurosurg 71:942, 1989.
16. Acciarri N, Paganini M, Fonda C, et al.: Langerhans' cell histiocytosis of the spine causing cord compression: case report. Neurosurgery 31:965, 1992.
17. Marcove RC: Bone-marrow eosinophilia with solitary eosinophilic granuloma of bone: a report of two cases. J Bone Joint Surg 41A:1521, 1959.
18. Ree HJ, Kadin ME: Peanut agglutinin: a useful marker for histiocytosis X and interdigitating reticulum cells. Cancer 57:282, 1986.
19. Huvos AG: Bone Tumors: Diagnosis, Treatment, and Prognosis, 2nd ed. Philadelphia: WB Saunders Co, 1991, pp 695–711.
20. Green WT, Farber S: "Eosinophilic or solitary granuloma" of bone. J Bone Joint Surg 24:499, 1942.
21. Calvé JA: Localized affection of spine suggesting osteochondritis of vertebral body, with clinical aspects of Pott's disease. J Bone Joint Surg 7:41, 1925.
22. Sherk HH, Nicholson JT, Nixon JE: Vertebra plana and eosinophilic granuloma of the cervical spine in children. Spine 3:116, 1978.
23. David R, Oria RA, Kumar R, et al.: Radiologic features of eosinophilic granuloma of bone. AJR 153:1021, 1989.
24. Kieffer SA, Nesbit ME, D'Angio GJ: Vertebra plana due to histiocytosis X: serial studies. Acta Radiol [Diagn] (Stockh) 8:241, 1969.
25. Baber WW, Numaguchi Y, Nadell JM, et al.: Eosino-

philic granuloma of the cervical spine without vertebrae plana. J Comput Tomogr 11:346, 1987.
26. Kaye JJ, Freiberger RH: Eosinophilic granuloma of
the spine without vertebra plana: a report of two
unusual cases. Radiology 92:1188, 1969.
27. Ferris RA, Pettrone FA, McKelvie AM, et al.: Eosinophilic granuloma of the spine: an unusual radiographic presentation. Clin Orthop 99:57, 1974.
28. Nesbit ME, Kieffer S, D'Angio GJ: Reconstitution of
vertebral height in histiocytosis X: a long-term follow-
up. J Bone Joint Surg 51:1360, 1969.
29. Kricun ME: Tumors of the Spine. In: Kricun ME (ed):
Imaging of Bone Tumors. Philadelphia: WB Saunders
Co, 1993, pp 266–267.
30. Kumar R, Balachandran S: Relative roles of radionuclide scanning and radiographic imaging in eosinophilic granuloma. Clin Nucl Med 5:538, 1980.
31. Avioli LV, Lasersohn JT, Lopresti JM: Histiocytosis
X (Schüller-Christian disease): a clinico-pathological
survey, review of ten patients and the results of prednisone therapy. Medicine 42:119, 1963.
32. Carmago OPD, Oliveira NRBD, Andrade JS, et al.:
Eosinophilic granuloma of the ischium: long-term
evaluation of a patient treated with steroids. J Bone
Joint Surg 74A:445, 1992.
33. Elomaa I, Blomqvist C, Porkka L, Holmstrom T: Experiences of clodronate treatment of multifocal eosinophilic granuloma of bone. J Intern Med 225:59, 1989.

MALIGNANT TUMORS

MULTIPLE MYELOMA

Capsule Summary

Frequency of neck pain—common
Location of neck pain—cervical spine
Quality of neck pain—ache of increasing intensity
Symptoms and signs—generalized fatigue,
bone pain
Laboratory and x-ray tests—pancytopenia,
hypergammaglobulinemia; diffuse osteolysis without reactive sclerosis on plain
roentgenogram
Treatment—chemotherapy for general disease; radiation therapy and/or stabilization
for cord compression

Prevalence and Pathogenesis

Multiple myeloma is a malignant tumor of
plasma cells. Plasma cells are the cells that
produce immunoglobulins and antibodies,
and they are located throughout the bone
marrow. The multiplication of these cells in
the bone marrow is associated with diffuse
bone destruction characterized by bone pain,
pathologic fractures, and increases in serum
calcium level. Multiple myeloma is the most
common primary malignancy of bone in
adults, accounting for 27% of biopsied bone
tumors and 45% of all malignant bone
tumors.[1, 2] The incidence is 3 cases per 100,000
people in the United States.[3] The patients are
usually in an older age group, ranging from
50 to 70 years.[4] Multiple myeloma is rare in a
patient younger than the age of 40 years.[5]
There is a slight increase in the male-to-female
ratio, but the ratio may be increased further
for solitary plasmacytoma.[6]

Three physicians, Bence-Jones, Dalrymple,
and Macintyre, first identified the bone lesion
and urinary protein between 1845 and 1850.[7–9]
Von Rustizky in 1873 was the first to call the
disease multiple myeloma.[10]

The pathogenesis of this plasma cell tumor
is unknown. Viral infections, chronic inflammation, and myeloproliferative diseases have
been suggested as possible initiating factors.
Although the symptoms of a fracture associated with trauma are frequently the reason for
a patient's initial evaluation by a physician,
trauma is not a factor in the etiology of multiple myeloma. The lesions tend to occur in the
bones with the greatest hematopoietic activity,
such as the spine, pelvis, ribs, skull, and proximal ends of the femora and humeri. A
majority of patients with multiple myeloma
have lesions in the axial skeleton. The thoracic
spine is involved in 59% of patients, the lumbosacral spine in 31%, and the cervical spine
in 10%. A review by Clarke of medical literature prior to 1956 reported 33 of 193 (12%)
patients with multiple myeloma with cervical
spine lesions.[11] In Dahlin and Unni's series of
556 surgical cases of multiple myeloma, 6% of
patients with axial skeleton involvement had
cervical spine lesions.[2] The spine is affected in
30% to 50% of patients with solitary plasmacytomas.[1] Solitary plasmacytomas affect the cervical spine in 9% to 13% of patients with spinal
lesions. Most frequently, the thoracic and lumbar spine are affected with solitary plasmacytomas rather than the cervical spine.[12]

The term plasmacytoma is used when one
bone is involved by the disease. Multiple myeloma denotes the involvement of several
bones throughout the skeleton. Myelomatosis
refers to disseminated disease throughout the
hematopoietic system, including extraosseous
locations. Extramedullary plasmacytoma refers
to lesions in soft tissues independent of bone.[13]

Clinical History

Pain is the most common initial complaint
of patients with multiple myeloma and occurs

in 75% of patients.[3] Low back pain is the presenting symptom in 35% of patients. Localized neck pain is a symptom of individuals with cervical spine disease.[11] Neck pain is mild, aching, and intermittent at the onset. Pain on recumbency is one of the symptoms that should raise the possibility of a spinal tumor, including multiple myeloma.[14] The duration of pain prior to diagnosis may be 6 months or longer.[15] Some patients have radicular symptoms and are diagnosed as having herniated intervertebral discs, sciatica, and arthritis.[16–18] Approximately 20% of patients give a history of insignificant trauma that results in pathologic fractures of cervical vertebral bodies, which results in acute, severe localized pain. Paraplegia more often occurs with solitary plasmacytoma than with multiple myeloma.[19] Spinal cord compression or cauda equina compression also occurs in myeloma patients.[20, 21] Patients with multiple myeloma affecting the cervical spine may develop quadriplegia with minor trauma. Fracture with extrusion of bony fragments into the spinal canal, resulting in compression of the cervical spinal cord, has been reported in myeloma patients.[22] Approximately 10% of patients with multiple myeloma may first present with a solitary lesion.[23] Monoclonal antibodies develop as a sign of progression of isolated plasmacytoma to multiple myeloma.[24] Involvement of the ribs, sternum, and thoracic spine may result in kyphosis and loss in height. Pain is not confined to the neck in this disease, because bone pain may be found in any part of the skeleton and may be secondary to bone marrow expansion or to microfractures.[25]

As a consequence of widespread bone destruction, abnormal immunoglobulin production, and infiltration of bone marrow, patients with multiple myeloma develop a broad range of clinical symptoms. Hypercalcemia, due to bone destruction, is associated with bone weakness, easy fatigability, anorexia, nausea, vomiting, mental status changes including coma, and kidney stones. Increased abnormal immunoglobulin concentrations cause progressive renal insufficiency, increased susceptibility to infection, and amyloidosis. Amyloid is a protein that forms from portions of abnormal myeloma immunoglobulins. This protein infiltrates certain structures, including bone, muscle, perivascular connective tissue, kidney, and bladder.[26] Primary amyloidosis in the absence of multiple myeloma may infiltrate bone marrow and simulate radiographic changes in the vertebral column that are similar to those of multiple myeloma.[27] Infiltration of bone

marrow is associated with anemia, bleeding secondary to a deficiency of platelets, thrombocytopenia, and generalized weakness. Most patients have symptoms for less than 6 months before seeking medical attention. Patients who are subsequently diagnosed with solitary lesions may have had symptoms for several years.

Physical Examination

In the early stages of the disease, the physical examination may be unremarkable. As the duration of disease increases and bone marrow infiltration progresses, diffuse bone tenderness along with fever, pallor, and purpura become a prominent finding on examination. Fever is usually a manifestation of a complicating infection. Fever associated with myeloma alone is not common.[28] Rib cage and spine deformities are common in latter stages of the disease. Neurologic examination may demonstrate signs of compression of the spinal cord or nerve roots if vertebral collapse has progressed to a significant extent.[29] Neurologic signs of cervical spine nerve root compression include muscle weakness, sensory changes, and reflex asymmetry. Spinal cord compression is manifested by upper motor neuron signs, including spasticity, hyperreflexia, and positive Babinski's sign.

Laboratory Data

Laboratory examination may reveal many abnormalities, including normochromic normocytic anemia, rouleau formation on blood smear, elevated leukocyte count, thrombocytopenia, positive Coombs's test, and elevated erythrocyte sedimentation rate. Abnormal serum chemistries include hypercalcemia, hyperuricemia, and elevated creatinine levels.[30] Impaired coagulation is mediated through inhibitors of clotting factors, clearance of clotting factors, and platelet function abnormalities.[12]

Serum alkaline phosphatase level is normal in most patients with multiple myeloma. A normal leukocyte alkaline phosphatase level is associated with benign paraproteinemias, but an elevated level does not necessarily indicate a malignant condition.[31] Characteristic serum protein abnormalities occur in the majority of patients with multiple myeloma. The total serum protein concentrations are increased secondary to an increase in the globulin fraction. The increase in globulins is due to the presence of abnormal immunoglobulin (Ig) of the G, A, D, E, or M classes. Igs are composed of light and heavy chains. Multiple myeloma, instead of having a multitude of antibodies, has a single antibody, composed of a light and heavy chain, an M protein. It is produced to the exclusion of others. The balance between light and heavy chains may also be disturbed with excess light-chain production, resulting in Bence Jones protein in the urine, or excess heavy-chain production, resulting in heavy-chain disease. Serum protein electrophoresis demonstrates the elevation in globulin levels, and quantitative Ig determination detects the class of Ig that is present in increased concentration. Serum protein electrophoresis demonstrates a spike in 76% of patients, hypogammaglobulinemia in 9%, and no abnormality in 15%.[4] Urine protein electrophoresis detects the presence of Bence Jones proteinuria. Other tests associated with abnormal Igs include increased serum viscosity, which results in the blockage of blood vessels, and a positive test for rheumatoid factor.

Examination of a bone marrow aspirate and biopsy shows characteristic changes of multiple myeloma. Bone marrow aspirate demonstrates increased numbers of plasma cells, at levels greater than 30%. Bone marrow biopsy demonstrates diffuse infiltration of bone marrow with plasma cells. Plasma cells may be classified into three histologic grades: well differentiated, moderately differentiated, and poorly differentiated.[32] The well-differentiated plasma cells look much like normal plasma cells. Anaplastic myeloma cells may mimic undifferentiated carcinomas or small cell sarcomas. The differentiation of myeloma cells from non-neoplastic plasma cells is difficult. Subtle abnormalities in the size of the nucleus, nucleocytoplasmic disproportion, and the absence of inclusions are just a few of the many factors that may help with the differentiation of normal from malignant cells.[3]

Gross pathologic examination of bone shows a soft, gray, friable tumor in the bone. The tumor frequently expands beyond the confines of the bone into the soft tissue. In the spine, pathologic fractures are commonly identified.

Bone lesions are frequently associated with myeloma lesions. Most patients have lytic abnormalities associated with unbalanced bone remodeling, leading to reduced bone mass and bone destruction.[33] Patients with sclerotic bone lesions had increased osteoblastic activity in the setting of increased bone resorption. These patients had a lambda subtype IgG myeloma, an Ig subtype associated with sclerotic myeloma.[34] An early manifestation of myeloma is enhancement of osteoblastic recruitment with increased generation of new osteoclasts that cause increased bone resorption. The early stimulation of osteoblasts results in increased amounts of interleukin-6, a potent myeloma growth factor and a cytokine for the formation of osteoclasts in bone marrow.[35]

Radiographic Evaluation

The predominant radiographic abnormality of multiple myeloma is osteolysis (Fig. 13–9). Diffuse osteolysis of the axial skeleton resembles osteoporosis.[36] A characteristic finding is the absence of reactive sclerosis surrounding lytic lesions in the spine. Preferential destruction of vertebral bodies with sparing of posterior elements helps in differentiating multiple myeloma from osteolytic metastasis, which affects the vertebral pedicle and body (Fig. 13–10).[37] Paraspinous and extradural extensions of tumor are seen in patients with multiple myeloma.

Benign solitary plasmacytoma may occur almost anywhere in the body, including bone and kidney. Bone plasmacytoma is most common in the vertebral column, pelvis, and long bones, in that order of decreasing frequency.[38] Solitary plasmacytoma, when located in the spine, has variable radiographic features. A purely osteolytic area without expansion or an expansile lesion with thickened trabeculae may be observed. An involved vertebral body may fracture and disappear completely, or the lesion may extend across the intervertebral disc to invade an adjacent vertebral body, simulating the appearance of an infection.[19] The lesion may have coarse trabeculae with vertical striations simulating vertebral angioma or Paget's disease.[39] Occasionally, osteoblastic lesions have been reported in patients with multiple myeloma and plasmacytoma.[40, 41]

Although bone scans are used in the early detection of metastatic lesions, they are not helpful in multiple myeloma because the osteolytic lesions, which lack bone-forming (blastic) activity, are not abnormal.[42, 43] In the unusual patient with an abnormal scintiscan, regression of tumor activity may be characterized by the disappearance of scan abnormalities with treatment.[13]

Computerized tomography (CT) may demonstrate vertebral body involvement before plain radiograph. Radiography is able to detect abnormalities in bone only after 30% of

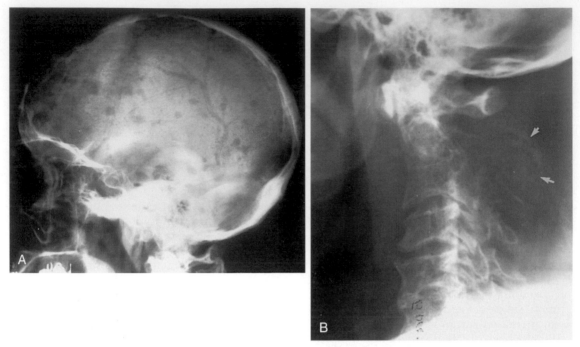

Figure 13–9. Multiple myeloma. A 62-year-old male with multiple myeloma and neck pain. *A*, Lateral view of skull reveals multiple osteolytic "punched out" lesions involving the entire calvarium. *B*, Lateral view of cervical spine shows generalized osteopenia and an expansile, osteolytic lesion of the posterior elements of C2 *(arrows)*. (Courtesy of Anne Brower, M.D.)

its calcium is lost.[44] CT is useful in demonstrating the extent of tumor, delineating the soft tissue component of an osseous lesion, or detecting extramedullary plasmacytoma. CT is a useful technique for detecting early bone or extraosseous lesions in areas of the spine that are difficult to image with simple radiographic techniques.[45]

Magnetic resonance (MR) imaging is able to detect abnormalities in bone marrow that are not readily visualized by other techniques. On T_1-weighted and T_2-weighted images, myeloma appears as decreased or increased signal intensity, respectively. Alterations in signal may occur with fatty infiltration of marrow. Foci of tumor are better visualized with T_2-weighted images. MR appearance does not correlate with laboratory or bone marrow findings.[46] The use of gadolinium as a contrast agent does not improve the ability of MR imaging to detect deposits of myeloma cells in the bone marrow of vertebral bodies.[47, 48]

Differential Diagnosis

The diagnosis of multiple myeloma requires the inclusion of clinical, radiographic, and laboratory data along with the presence of abnormal plasma cells on histologic examination. A combination of major and minor criteria for establishing the diagnosis of myeloma has been developed by the Southwest Oncology Group.[49] The major criteria include plasmacytoma demonstrated on biopsy; bone marrow plasmacytosis with more than a 30% content of plasma cells; and a monoclonal spike of more than 3.5 gm for IgG, 2.0 gm/100 mL for IgA, or 1.0 gm/24 hours for urinary light chains. Minor criteria include bone marrow plasmacytosis, a monoclonal spike with small globulin concentrations, a lytic bone lesion, and serum immunoglobulin values less than 50 mg for IgM, 100 mg for IgA, and 600 mg/ 100 mL for IgG. The presence of characteristic abnormalities, Bence Jones protein and M protein on electrophoresis, makes the diagnosis an easy one, but the diagnosis is more difficult in the patient who presents with diffuse osteoporosis and no detectable myeloma protein.[50] Neck pain in the middle-aged to elderly patient with osteoporosis of the cervical spine on roentgenogram must be evaluated thoroughly for possible myeloma.[28]

Solitary plasmacytoma is also difficult to diagnose. The diagnosis may be assumed if the character of the lesion is established by biopsy, if bone survey is negative, if the bone marrow specimen is free of plasma cells, if hypergammaglobulinemia and Bence Jones proteinuria

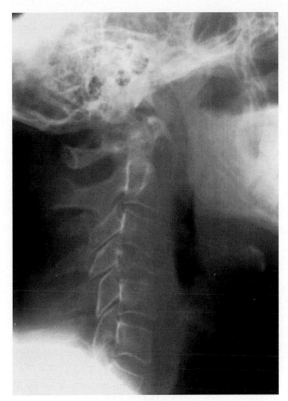

Figure 13–10. Multiple myeloma. Lateral view of cervical spine reveals generalized osteopenia and collapse of the vertebral body of C3 without any reactive sclerosis. (Courtesy of Anne Brower, M.D.)

are absent, and if the patient has been followed closely for years.

The list of other diseases that must be considered in the differential diagnosis of multiple myeloma is quite broad. Metastatic tumors and malignant lymphoma must be considered. Focal osteolysis on roentgenogram may be associated with a hemangioma. Infections, pyogenic and tuberculous, are associated with similar roentgenographic findings. Hyperparathyroidism may be associated with generalized bone lesions and hypercalcemia. Appropriate evaluation of blood tests and biopsy material should give the physician the data to make the appropriate diagnosis.

A differential diagnosis of monoclonal gammopathy must also be considered in the patient with elevated globulin levels.[51] Some of the gammopathies have elevated globulin levels but do not cause bone lesions to the same extent as multiple myeloma. Examples of these gammopathies include benign monoclonal gammopathy, Waldenström's macroglobulinemia, IgE myeloma, and alpha heavy-chain disease.[12]

Multiple myeloma is usually associated with osteolytic bone activity. In rare circumstances, osteoblastic activity has been associated with this neoplasm. Patients with IgG monoclonal proteins with lambda subtype are the ones with osteosclerotic bone lesions.[15]

Treatment

Clinically active multiple myeloma usually requires systemic therapy with melphalan and prednisone over an extended course.[52] Approximately 70% of patients respond to this therapy and have a reduction in bone destruction and pain; decreased concentration of abnormal proteins; and a normalization of hematocrit level, urea nitrogen, creatinine, and calcium. Some patients have responded well to high-dose dexamethasone treatment alone without the toxicities associated with other therapies.[53] Patients with more aggressive disease may benefit from the M-2 drug program, combining vincristine, melphalan, cyclophosphamide, prednisone, and bis-chloroethyl-nitrosourea.[54] Other therapies used for myeloma patients include high-dose melphalan, autologous bone marrow transplantation, interferon, and cytokines.[55] Response to therapy with changes in bone marrow cells can be seen on serial MR scans using contrast media.[56] The MR changes are important for documenting positive response to therapy in patients who may remain symptomatic from bony changes that are not related to the growth of plasma cells. In patients with cord compression secondary to multiple myeloma, decompressing laminectomy and local radiotherapy are indicated.[57] Radiotherapy is also indicated for solitary plasmacytoma. Patients with cervical spine instability secondary to compression fractures secondary to multiple myeloma or plasmacytoma should be considered for surgical stabilization. Instability at upper cervical levels may require occipitocervical fusion with bone graft and bone cement.[58] Stability may be maintained despite progression of the neoplastic lesion in the bone. Cervical lesions may invade the adventitia of the vertebral artery. Presurgical embolization of the lesion may be required to obliterate the tumor blood supply prior to surgery.[12]

Bisphosphonates inhibit calcium release from bone and prevent bone resorption through inhibition of osteoclastic activity. These drugs are most effective in patients with idiopathic osteoporosis. Daily etidronate is not effective in reversing the osteopenia associated with myeloma.[59]

Prognosis

The usual course of multiple myeloma is one of gradual progression. Therapy may have effects on clinical symptoms and amounts of myeloma protein, but the average survival remains about 5 years. Three patients with cervical spine disease with spinal cord compression were dead in 2 years in one study.[60] Patients with nerve compression secondary to myeloma may respond to chemotherapy with decreased paraproteinemia and tumor volume. However, the decrease in tumor size may be associated with increased instability of the spine requiring stabilization.[61] Patients with D and G myeloma have poorer prognoses than A myeloma patients.[62, 63] Many patients may have more extensive disease than is clinically apparent. More than 50% of patients may have compression fractures at autopsy.[64] In addition, the effects of myeloma may extend beyond the involvement of bone alone. Even in the absence of a marrow packed with plasma cells, erythropoiesis may be depressed by an effect of the disease on progenitor cells.[65] Male patients with plasmacytosis, hypoalbuminemia, elevated alkaline phosphatase, hyperuricemia, or renal insufficiency are predictors of poor outcome at 2 years.[66] In a study of 130 Japanese patients, only 6.9% of patients were alive at 10 years. Prognostic factors for survival included a younger age at diagnosis, low tumor mass, chemotherapy with cyclophosphamide, disappearance of myeloma protein, and a positive response to retreatment.[67]

Patients with solitary plasmacytoma have a better prognosis than those patients who initially have multiple lesions.[19] However, some patients with solitary lesions may develop disseminated disease 20 years or more after their initial diagnosis.[68]

References

MULTIPLE MYELOMA

1. Mirra JM: Bone Tumors: Diagnosis and Treatment. Philadelphia: JB Lippincott Co., 1980, pp 398–406.
2. Dahlin DC, Unni KK: Bone Tumors: General Aspects and Data on 8,542 Cases, 4th ed. Springfield, Illinois: Charles C Thomas, Publisher, 1986, pp 193–207.
3. Huvos AG: Bone Tumors: Diagnosis, Treatment, and Prognosis, 2nd ed. Philadelphia: WB Saunders Co, 1991, pp 653–676.
4. Kyle RA: Multiple myeloma: review of 869 cases. Mayo Clin Proc 50:29, 1975.
5. Hewell GM, Alexanian R: Multiple myeloma in young persons. Ann Intern Med 84:441, 1976.
6. Todd IDH: Treatment of solitary plasmacytoma. Clin Radiol 16:395, 1965.

7. Bence-Jones H: On a new substance occurring in the urine of a patient with mollities ossium. Philos Trans R Soc Lond (Biol) 1:55, 1848.
8. Dalrymple J: On the microscopical character of mollities ossium. Dublin Q J Med Sci 2:85, 1846.
9. Macintyre W: Case of mollities and fragilitas ossium accompanied with urine strongly charged with animal matter. Med Chir Soc Trans 33:211, 1850.
10. Von Rustizky J: Multiples myelom. Dtsch Z Chir 3:162, 1873.
11. Clarke E: Spinal cord involvement in multiple myelomatosis. Brain 79:332, 1956.
12. Kempin S, Sundaresan N: Disorders of the Spine Related to Plasma Cell Dyscrasias. In: Sundaresan N, Schmidek HH, Schiller AL, Rosenthal DI (eds): Tumors of the Spine: Diagnosis and Clinical Management. Philadelphia: WB Saunders Co, 1990, pp 214–225.
13. Bataille R, Chevalier J, Rossi M, Sany J: Bone scintigraphy in plasma cell myeloma: a prospective study of 70 patients. Radiology 145:801, 1982.
14. Nicholas JJ, Christy WC: Spinal pain made worse by recumbency: a clue to spinal cord tumors. Arch Phys Med Rehabil 67:598, 1986.
15. Bataille R, Delmas PD, Chappard D, Sany J: Abnormal serum bone Gla protein levels in multiple myeloma: crucial role of bone formation and prognostic implications. Cancer 66:167, 1990.
16. Lichtenstein L, Jaffee HL: Multiple myeloma: a survey based on 35 cases, 18 of which came to autopsy. Arch Pathol Lab Med 44:207, 1947.
17. Bayrd ED, Heck FJ: Multiple myeloma: a review of 83 proven cases. JAMA 133:147, 1947.
18. Lehmann O: Problems of pathological fractures. Bull Hosp Jt Dis 12:90, 1951.
19. Valderrama JAF, Bullough PG: Solitary myeloma of the spine. J Bone Joint Surg 50B:82, 1968.
20. Jacobs P, King HS, Le Roux I, Handler L: Extradural spinal myeloma and emergency neurosurgery. S Afr Med J 77:316, 1990.
21. Sinoff CL: Spinal cord compression due to myeloma. S Afr Med J 78:434, 1990.
22. Chan L, Snyder HS, Verdile VP: Cervical fracture as the initial presentation of multiple myeloma. Ann Emerg Med 24:1192, 1994.
23. Osserman EF: Plasma-cell myeloma II: clinical aspects. N Engl J Med 261:952, 1959.
24. Otto S, Vegh Z, Hindy I, Peter I: Multiple myeloma arising from solitary plasmacytoma of bone. Oncology 47:84, 1990.
25. Charkes ND, Durant J, Barry WE: Bone pain in multiple myeloma: studies with radioactive 87m SR. Arch Intern Med 130:53, 1972.
26. Klein LA: Case Record 7–1986. N Engl J Med 314:500, 1986.
27. Axelsson U, Hallen A, Rausing A: Amyloidosis of bone: report of two cases. J Bone Joint Surg 52B:717, 1970.
28. Duffy TP: The many pitfalls in the diagnosis of myeloma. N Engl J Med 326:394, 1992.
29. Davison C, Balser BH: Myeloma and its neural complications. Arch Surg 35:913, 1937.
30. Paredes JM, Mitchell BS: Multiple myeloma: current concepts in diagnosis and management. Med Clin North Am 64:729, 1980.
31. Majumdar G, Hunt M, Singh AK: Use of leukocyte alkaline phosphatase (LAP) score in differentiating malignant from benign paraproteinemias. J Clin Pathol 44:606, 1991.
32. Bayrd ED: The bone marrow on sternal aspiration in multiple myeloma. Blood 3:987, 1948.

33. Bataille R, Chappard D, Marcelli C, et al.: Mechanisms of bone destruction in multiple myeloma: the importance of an unbalanced process in determining the severity of lytic bone disease. J Clin Oncol 7:1909, 1989.
34. Bataille R, Chappard D, Marcelli C, et al.: Osteoblast stimulation in multiple myeloma lacking lytic bone lesions. Br J Haematol 76:484, 1990.
35. Bataille R, Chappard D, Marcelli C, et al.: Recruitment of new osteoblasts and osteoclasts is the earliest critical event in the pathogenesis of human multiple myeloma. J Clin Invest 88:62, 1991.
36. Carson CP, Ackerman LV, Maltby JD: Plasma cell myeloma: a clinical, pathologic and roentgenologic review of 90 cases. Am J Clin Pathol 25:849, 1955.
37. Jacobsen HG, Poppel MH, Shapiro JH, Grossberger S: The vertebral pedicle sign: a roentgen finding to differentiate metastatic carcinoma from multiple myeloma. AJR 80:817, 1958.
38. Eichner ER: The plasma cell dyscrasias: diverse presentations, pathophysiology and management. Postgrad Med 67:44, 1980.
39. Loftus CM, Micheisen CB, Rapoport F, Antunes JL: Management of plasmacytomas of the spine. Neurosurgery 13:30, 1983.
40. Brown TS, Paterson CR: Osteosclerosis in myeloma. J Bone Joint Surg 55B:621, 1973.
41. Roberts M, Rianudo PA, Vilinskas J, Owens G: Solitary sclerosing plasma-cell myeloma of the spine: case report. J Neurosurg 40:125, 1974.
42. Wooltenden JM, Pitt MJ, Durie BGM, Moon TE: Comparison of bone scintigraphy and radiography in multiple myeloma. Radiology 134:723, 1980.
43. Wahner HW, Kyle RA, Beabout JW: Scintigraphic evaluation of the skeleton in multiple myeloma. Mayo Clin Proc 55:739, 1980.
44. Helms CA, Genant HK: Computed tomography in the early detection of skeletal involvement with multiple myeloma. JAMA 248:2886, 1982.
45. Solomon A, Rahamani R, Seligsohn U, Ben-Artzi F: Multiple myeloma: early vertebral involvement assessed by computerized tomography. Skeletal Radiol 11:258, 1984.
46. Libshitz HI, Malthouse SR, Cunningham D, et al.: Multiple myeloma: appearance at MR imaging. Radiology 182:833, 1992.
47. Rahmouni A, Divine M, Mathieu D, et al.: Detection of multiple myeloma involving the spine: efficacy of fat-suppression and contrast-enhanced MR imaging. AJR 160:1049, 1993.
48. Avrahami E, Tadmor R, Kaplinsky N: The role of T2-weighted gradient echo in MRI demonstration of spinal multiple myeloma. Spine 18:1812, 1993.
49. Durie BGM, Salmon SE: A clinical staging system for multiple myeloma: correlation of measured myeloma cell mass with presenting clinical features response to treatment and survival. Cancer 36:842, 1975.
50. Arend WP, Adamson JW: Nonsecretory myeloma: immunofluorescent demonstration of paraprotein within bone marrow plasma cells. Cancer 33:721, 1974.
51. Gandara DR, Mackenzie MR: Differential diagnosis of monoclonal gammopathy. Med Clin North Am 72:1155, 1988.
52. Costa G, Engle RL Jr, Schilling A, et al.: Melphalan and prednisone: an effective combination for the treatment of multiple myeloma. Am J Med 54:589, 1973.
53. Alexanian R, Dimopoulos MA, Delasalle K, Barlogie B: Primary dexamethasone treatment of multiple myeloma. Blood 80:887, 1992.
54. Case DC Jr, Lee BJ III, Clarkson BD: Improved survival times in multiple myeloma treated with melphalan, prednisone, cyclophosphamide, vincristine and BCNU: M-2 protocol. Am J Med 63:897, 1977.
55. Camba L, Durie BGM: Multiple myeloma: new treatment options. Drugs 44:170, 1992.
56. Rahmouni A, Divine M, Mathieu D, et al.: MR appearance of multiple myeloma of the spine before and after treatment. AJR 160:1053, 1993.
57. Gilbert RW, Kim JH, Posner JB: Epidural spinal cord compression from metastatic tumor: diagnosis and treatment. Ann Neurol 3:40, 1978.
58. Lofvenberg R, Lofvenberg EB, Ahlgren O: A case of occipitocervical fusion in myeloma. Acta Orthop Scand 61:81, 1990.
59. Belch AR, Bergsagel DE, Wilson K, et al.: Effect of daily etidronate on the osteolysis of multiple myeloma. J Clin Oncol 9:1397, 1991.
60. Benson WJ, Scarffe JH, Todd IDH, et al.: Spinal cord compression in myeloma. Br Med J 1:1541, 1979.
61. Rapoport AP, Rowe JM: Plasma cell dyscrasia in a 15-year-old boy: case report and review of the literature. Am J Med 89:816, 1990.
62. Gompels BM, Votaw ML, Martel W: Correlation of radiological manifestations of multiple myeloma with immunoglobulin abnormalities and prognosis. Radiology 104:509, 1972.
63. Pruzanski W, Rother I: IgD plasma cell neoplasia: clinical manifestations and characteristic features. Can Med Assoc J 102:1061, 1970.
64. Kapadia SB: Multiple myeloma: a clinicopathologic study of 62 consecutively autopsied cases. Medicine 59:380, 1980.
65. Oken MM: Multiple myeloma: symposium on hematology and hematologic malignancies. Med Clin North Am 68:757, 1984.
66. Cherng NC, Asal NR, Kuebler JP, et al.: Prognostic factors in multiple myeloma. Cancer 67:3150, 1991.
67. Murakami H, Nemoto K, Miyawaki S, et al.: Ten-year survivors with multiple myeloma. J Intern Med 231:129, 1992.
68. Woodruff RK, Malpas JS, White FE: Solitary plasmacytoma II: solitary plasmacytoma of bone. Cancer 43:2344, 1979.

CHONDROSARCOMA

Capsule Summary

Frequency of neck pain—uncommon
Location of neck pain—cervical spine
Quality of neck pain—mild ache
Symptoms and signs—painless mass
Laboratory and x-ray tests—expansile, calcified mass on plain roentgenogram
Treatment—en bloc resection

Prevalence and Pathogenesis

Chondrosarcoma is a malignant tumor that forms cartilaginous tissue. It is rarely located in the cervical spine. Chondrosarcoma comprises 11% to 22% of biopsied primary tumors of bone.[1, 2] Among malignant tumors, chondrosarcoma is the third most common neoplasm, following multiple myeloma and osteosarcoma. In the cervical spine, chondrosarcoma occurs more commonly than osteosarcoma or Ewing's sarcoma.[3] The usual age of onset is 40 to 60 years, and the ratio of men to women is 3:2.[4] Another study of this tumor in the spine reported a ratio of men to women of 4:1.[3]

Chondrosarcoma has been known by many different names. These have included chondroblastic sarcoma, malignant chondroblastoma, myxoid chondrosarcoma, and clear cell chondrosarcoma.

The pathogenesis of chondrosarcoma is unknown. Primary chondrosarcoma arises de novo from previously normal bone, and secondary chondrosarcoma develops from other cartilaginous tumors, such as an osteochondroma and enchondroma. Chondrosarcoma may be induced by irradiation, accounting for 9% of radiation-induced bone sarcoma.[5] It also develops in a small number of patients with Paget's disease, fibrous dysplasia, and Maffucci's syndrome (enchondromas with soft tissue hemangiomas).[6–8]

Approximately 9% of patients with chondrosarcoma have lesions involving the spine. A review of 553 chondrosarcoma patients documented spinal involvement in 6% of them.[4] The cervical spine is the site of the tumor in 18% of patients, with 32% and 50% in the thoracic and lumbosacral spine, respectively.[2] In another review of 151 cases of spinal chondrosarcoma, the frequency of involvement was 28.5% lumbar spine, 28.5% sacrum, 23% thoracic spine, 12% cervical spine, and 8% of unspecified location.[9]

Clinical History

Chondrosarcoma may be asymptomatic or may present with only mild discomfort and palpable swelling. Tumors in the cervical spine are associated with neck pain. Pain is frequently worse at night. Pain, when it occurs, is strongly suggestive of actively growing tumor. This is particularly important in a patient who has had an osteochondroma for decades that suddenly becomes painful. This is a slow-growing tumor; therefore, a history of symptoms for several years before medical evaluation is sought is usual. Almost 50% of patients have neurologic symptoms at the time of diagnosis. Unilateral radicular pain is associated with chondrosarcoma of the cervical spine.[10] Referred arm pain may precede local neck pain,

delaying the discovery of the tumor. With increased tumor growth, the pain becomes more severe and persistent.[10]

Physical Examination

Physical examination may demonstrate a painless tumor mass or one that is mildly painful on palpation.[11] Range of motion of the spine is decreased secondary to pain and muscle spasm. Neurologic examination may be abnormal if neural elements are compressed by the tumor. With progression of compression, increasing weakness is noted. Lesions in the cervical spine produce sensory deficits in the corresponding nerve root distribution. Radicular involvement produces numbness, paresthesias, and dysesthesias in a dermatomal pattern in the arm. Myelopathic abnormalities, including paresis, have been reported in patients with tumors invading the spinal canal.[3] Compression of the spinal cord produces upper motor neuron weakness with spasticity, abnormal Babinski's sign, and increased reflexes. Spinal cord lesions produce a progression of sensory deficits from impaired vibratory sensation, joint position, temperature, and pain on light touch.[10]

Laboratory Data

Laboratory findings may not be abnormal until late in the course of the tumor. Abnormalities may correlate with tumor size and extent of metastasis. Useful tests to obtain include blood counts, serum chemistries, and erythrocyte sedimentation rates. As many as 75% of patients with chondrosarcoma demonstrate an abnormal glucose tolerance curve and high insulin levels. Insulin and insulin growth factor are documented stimulators of cartilage metabolism.[12] The relationship of insulin to the development of abnormal cartilage growth is unknown.[12]

Gross pathologic inspection of chondrosarcoma reveals a pearly, translucent tissue that is lobulated. Areas of calcification within the lesion are represented by yellow-white areas of speckling. The extent and exact boundaries of the lesion are hard to identify.[13] Slow-growing tumors elicit reactive new bone, and high-grade anaplastic chondrosarcomas exhibit less.[14]

The microscopic appearance of chondrosarcoma is graded by the extent of abnormality in the nuclei of the cells. Grade 1 is the most benign form of chondrosarcoma and does not have any associated cellular atypia. Some lesions have double nuclei and abundant hyalin matrix. Microscopically, a grade 1 chondrosarcoma differs only slightly from a benign enchondroma. The malignant lesion is more cellular, with larger cells that are binucleate. These changes may be present only in parts of the tumor, necessitating review of many sections of a biopsy specimen to confirm the diagnosis.[15] Grades 2 and 3 are increasingly malignant and are associated with greater amounts of cellularity, nuclear size, and mitoses.[16] Grade 2 lesions have increased atypia, are more densely cellular, and have multiple nuclei and foci of necrosis. Grade 3 lesions have marked atypia, mitotic figures, multinucleate cells, little matrix, and numerous areas of necrosis. Rare types of chondrosarcoma include clear cell, mesenchymal (characterized by a calcified soft tissue mass), myxoid, and periosteal. Dedifferentiation refers to the appearance of a more anaplastic connective tissue tumor in a grade 1 chondrosarcoma.[17]

Radiographic Evaluation

The characteristic radiographic findings of chondrosarcoma include a well-defined lesion with expansile contours (Fig. 13–11). The interior of the lesion may demonstrate lobular or fluffy calcification with scalloping of the interior cortex of bone. Periosteal and endosteal reactive bone formation leads to a thickened cortex of bone that is typical of a slow-growth tumor.[18] Cortical destruction and soft tissue invasion are indicative of more aggressive lesions. In the spine, the vertebral body or posterior elements may be the site of origin.[19] Plain radiograph is useful in detecting tumors that have calcified. However, soft tissue extension may not be appreciated on this radiograph. Chondrosarcoma may develop in the cartilaginous cap of an osteochondroma. The appearance of a malignant lesion should be suspected if the cap of the benign lesion becomes thicker than 1 cm, especially after skeletal maturity, and has the appearance of irregular calcification.[17] Plain roentgenogram is the single most effective means for establishing the diagnosis of a cartilaginous tumor. This technique detects calcifications, ossifications, and periosteal reaction more readily than computerized tomography (CT) or magnetic resonance (MR) imaging.[17]

For the evaluation of extraosseous extension of a tumor, CT and MR imaging are essential.

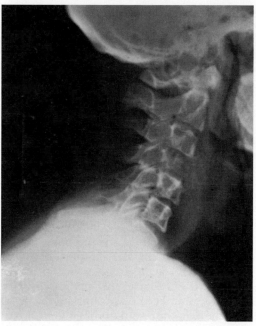

Figure 13–11. Chondrosarcoma of C4. Poorly marginated lytic destruction of vertebral body combined with anterior soft tissue mass indicates malignancy. (From Sim FH, Frassica FJ, Wold LE, McLeod RA: Chondrosarcoma of the spine: Mayo Clinic experience. In: Sundaresan N, Schmidek HH, Schiller AL, Rosenthal DI [eds]: Tumors of the Spine: Diagnosis and Clinical Management. Philadelphia: WB Saunders Co, 1990, p 157.)

CT and MR imaging can determine the presence or absence of soft tissue invasion by the tumor. CT depicts calcification in tumor matrix and cortical destruction that may be missed on MR imaging.[15] Recent studies with gadolinium contrast–enhanced MR imaging have detected scalloped margins and curvilinear septa of chondrosarcomas that correspond to fibrovascular bundles surrounding hyaline cartilage lobules.[20] Neither CT nor MR imaging is specific enough to establish a precise diagnosis before biopsy of the lesion. Particularly with MR imaging, benign and malignant chondrogenic lesions have similar MR characteristics that do not allow for accurate differentiation of tumors.

Arteriography may be useful in determining the extent of extraosseous involvement associated with a chondrosarcoma and defining the major feeding blood vessels to the tumor.[21] Bone scintigraphy is most helpful in detecting remote skeletal lesions and local intraosseous metastases.[15]

Differential Diagnosis

The diagnosis of grade 1 chondrosarcoma must be based on clinical, radiographic, and pathologic findings. Chondrosarcoma is the most difficult of the malignant tumors of bone for the histopathologist to diagnose. The histologic appearance of a low-grade chondrosarcoma may be similar to a cellular enchondroma, a benign lesion. Malignant tumors with similar histologic appearances may have different aggressive properties. The findings of pain, rapid growth, cortical destruction, soft tissue extension, and anaplastic cells on biopsy are characteristic of higher grade, more malignant chondrosarcoma.[4]

A wide range of benign and malignant processes may mimic the characteristics of chondrosarcoma. The processes that may cause lesions of the cervical spine include giant cell tumor, chordoma, and osteosarcoma. Careful attention to the clinical symptoms of the patient along with a thorough review of biopsy specimens should give the pathologist adequate data to make the appropriate diagnosis. The pathologic differentiation of chondrosarcoma and chordoma is a difficult one because of histologic similarities. Immunohistochemical evaluation of cartilaginous tumors with a panel of antibodies to cytokeratin, epithelial membrane antigen, vimentin, S-100 protein, carcinoembryonic antigen, and type II collagen is helpful in differentiating these tumors.[22]

Treatment

Surgery is the treatment of choice for chondrosarcoma. En bloc resection of the tumor with a margin of normal tissue so that malignant cells are not implanted in the surgical wound offers the best chance of long-term survival. Tumors that are partially resected frequently recur with increased cytologic malignancy.[23] Chondrosarcoma is radioresistant, and radiation therapy is reserved for tumors that are inaccessible to excision. Chemotherapy may play an adjunct role in these difficult situations. A combination of surgical removal, radiation, and chemotherapy has been associated with prolonged survival.[24]

Prognosis

The patients with chondrosarcoma who present with pain frequently have more malignant tumors.[25] Those with low-grade, well-differentiated chondrosarcoma have a longer survival rate and longer interval between treatment and recurrence than those with higher grade tumors. These facts hold true for chondrosarcoma of the cervical spine. Chondrosarcoma with low degree of malignancy grows slowly, recurs locally, and metastasizes late. High-grade tumors grow rapidly and metastasize early. The patients with the best outcome are those with low-grade tumors and successful en bloc excision. Patients without en bloc excision have progression of disease and are more likely to die from their tumor. In one study, 50% of patients with contaminated marginal excisions died after a local recurrence developed.[3] Patients with cervical spine lesions and larger tumors that limit the opportunity to remove the entire tumor have a higher risk of recurrence.[26] Patients with a cervical lesion may survive up to 20 years after a successful surgical excision.[3] In a study of 2,627 primary malignant bone tumors comparing chondrosarcoma, osteosarcoma, chordoma, and malignant fibrous histiocytoma, chondrosarcoma had the best 5-year survival rate (72.7%, 41.0%, 63.8%, and 42.9%, respectively), despite being the tumor, of this group, most commonly discovered in patients older than 50 years of age.[27]

New immunologic techniques are being developed to categorize the potential of bone tumors to respond to different types of therapy. A Ki-67 monoclonal antibody, specific for a nuclear antigen that is expressed throughout the cell cycle of an actively dividing cell, has been used to determine the proliferative activity of chondrosarcoma. The level of Ki-67 expression correlates with the level of malignancy of the tumor. In the future, this information may be useful for therapeutic decisions concerning specific grades of tumors, and it may have prognostic importance.[28]

References

CHONDROSARCOMA

1. Huvos AG: Bone Tumors: Diagnosis, Treatment, and Prognosis, 2nd ed. Philadelphia: WB Saunders Co, 1991, pp 343–381.
2. Dahlin DC, Unni KK: Bone Tumors: General Aspects and Data on 8,542 Cases, 4th ed. Springfield, Illinois: Charles C Thomas, Publisher, 1986, pp 227–259.
3. Shives TC, McLeod RA, Unni KK, Schray MF: Chondrosarcoma of the spine. J Bone J Surg 71A:1158, 1989.
4. Mirra JM: Bone Tumors: Diagnosis and Treatment. Philadelphia: JB Lippincott Co, 1980, pp 178–218.
5. Fitzwater JE, Caboud HE, Farr GH: Irradiation-induced chondrosarcoma: a case report. J Bone Joint Surg 58A:1037, 1976.
6. Feintuch TA: Chondrosarcoma arising in a cartilagi-

nous area of previously irradiated fibrous dysplasia. Cancer 31:877, 1973.

7. Lewis RJ, Ketcham AS: Maffucci's syndrome: functional and neoplastic significance: case report and review of the literature. J Bone Joint Surg 55A:1465, 1973.

8. Thomson AD, Turner-Warwick RT: Skeletal sarcomata and giant cell tumor. J Bone Joint Surg 37B:266, 1955.

9. Kricun ME: Imaging of Bone Tumors. Philadelphia: WB Saunders Co, 1993, p 263.

10. Sim FH, Frassica FJ, Wold LE, McLeod RA: Chondrosarcoma of the spine: Mayo Clinic experience. In: Sundaresan N, Schmidek HH, Schiller AL, Rosenthal DI (eds): Tumors of the Spine: Diagnosis and Clinical Management. Philadelphia: WB Saunders Co, 1990, pp 155–162.

11. Bohlman HH, Sachs BL, Carter JR, et al.: Primary neoplasms of the cervical spine: diagnosis and treatment of twenty-three patients. J Bone Joint Surg 68A:483, 1986.

12. Cammisa FP Jr, Glasser DB, Lane JM: Chondrosarcoma of the spine: Memorial Sloan-Kettering Cancer Center experience. In: Sundaresan N, Schmidek HH, Schiller AL, Rosenthal DI (eds): Tumors of the Spine: Diagnosis and Clinical Management. Philadelphia: WB Saunders Co, 1990, pp 149–154.

13. Goldenbeg RR: Chondrosarcoma. Bull Hosp Jt Dis 25:30, 1964.

14. Gilmer WS Jr, Kilgore W, Smith H: Central cartilage tumors of bone. Clin Orthop 26:81, 1963.

15. Greenspan A: Tumors of cartilage origin. Orthop Clin North Am 20:347, 1989.

16. Lichtenstein L, Jaffe HL: Chondrosarcoma of bone. Am J Pathol 19:553, 1943.

17. Ghelman B: Radiology of bone tumors. Orthop Clin North Am 20:287, 1989.

18. Barnes R, Catto M: Chondrosarcoma of bone. J Bone Joint Surg 48B:729, 1966.

19. Blaylock RL, Kempe LG. Chondrosarcoma of the cervical spine: case report. J Neurosurg 44:500, 1976.

20. Aoki J, Sone S, Fujioka F, et al.: MR of enchondroma and chondrosarcoma: rings and arcs of Gd-DTPA enhancement. J Comput Assist Tomogr 15:1011, 1991.

21. Kenncy PJ, Gilola LA, Murphy WA: The use of computed tomography to distinguish osteochondroma and chondrosarcoma. Radiology 139:129, 1981.

22. Wojno KJ, Hruban RH, Garin-Chesa P, Huvos AG: Chondroid chordomas and low-grade chondrosarcomas of the craniospinal axis: an immunohistochemical analysis of 17 cases. Am J Surg Pathol 16:1144, 1992.

23. Dahlin DC, Henderson ED: Chondrosarcoma: a surgical and pathological problem—review of 212 cases. J Bone Joint Surg 38B:1025, 1956.

24. Di Lorenzo N, Palatinsky E, Artico M, Palma L: Dural mesenchymal chondrosarcoma of the lumbar spine: case report. Surg Neurol 31:470, 1989.

25. Kaufman JH, Douglass HO Jr, Blake W, et al.: The importance of initial presentation and treatment upon the survival of patients with chondrosarcoma. Surg Gynecol Obstet 145:357, 1977.

26. Austin JP, Urie MM, Cardenosa G, Muzenrider JE: Probable cause of recurrence in patients with chordoma and chondrosarcoma of the base of skull and cervical spine. Int J Radiat Oncol Biol Phys 25:439, 1993.

27. Dorfman HD, Czerniak B: Bone cancers. Cancer 75:203, 1995.

28. Scotlandi K, Serra M, Manara C, et al.: Clinical relevance of Ki-67 expression in bone tumors. Cancer 75:806, 1995.

CHORDOMA

Capsule Summary

Frequency of neck pain—common

Location of neck pain—cervical spine

Quality of neck pain—ache

Symptoms and signs—painless mass, dysphagia

Laboratory and x-ray tests—anemia, vertebral osteolysis with calcific soft tissue mass on plain roentgenogram

Treatment—en bloc resection, radiation therapy

Prevalence and Pathogenesis

Chordoma is a malignant tumor that originates from the remnants of embryonic tissue, the notochord. The notochord is the structure that develops into a portion of the vertebral bodies of the spine in the embryo. Chordoma is located exclusively in the axial skeleton. This tumor is slow growing and may be present for an extended period before symptoms secondary to the compression of vital structures bring the patient to a physician.

Chordoma accounts for 3% of primary bone tumors.[1, 2] Another study found chordoma to be 1.3% of primary bone tumors.[3] The tumors usually become evident in people 40 to 70 years of age and are rarely reported in people 30 years of age or younger. The ratio of men to women with sacrococcygeal chordoma is 3:1; the ratio is 1:1 for chordoma in other locations in the spine.[4] A Mayo Clinic study of 40 patients with chordoma, exclusive of the sacrum, reported the ratio of men to women as 2:1.[5] A study of 88 chordoma patients, including those with sacral tumors, had a similar 2:1 ratio of men to women.[6] The mean age of sacral tumor patients was 56 years, and the mean age of those with tumors in the mobile spine was 47 years.

Virchow in 1857 was the first to suggest the persistence of cells from the notochord in skeletal structures. Horwitz in 1941 proposed that chordoma arose from abnormal chordal remnants in vertebral bones.[7]

The etiology of the factors that initiate the regrowth of notochordal vestigial cells in the spine is unknown, although trauma has been suggested.[8] Whether trauma is a causative factor or a chance event in the pathogenesis of the lesion in the cervical spine is currently conjectural.

All chordoma is located in the axial skeleton, ranging from the spheno-occipital area in the skull to the tip of the coccyx. The most common location for chordoma is the sacrum, which has 50% of the tumors. The skull is the location for 38% of the tumors. The cervical, lumbar, and thoracic spine are unusual locations for this neoplasm, accounting for 6%, 4%, and 2% of lesions, respectively, in one study.[9] The extent of involvement of the cervical spine with chordoma has ranged from 48% to 6% in a variety of studies of this tumor in the axial skeleton.[5, 10, 11] Chordoma has been reported affecting the axis and the atlas.[12] Occasionally, chordoma may be present in other areas of the spine, such as the transverse process, and extraosseous locations, including the epidural space.[13–15]

Clinical History

The symptoms depend on the location and extent of the tumor. Patients with cervical chordoma present with nondescript neck pain. Pain may be characterized as dull, sharp, intermittent, or constant and is localized in the neck. It may be of long duration because the patient may not have thought it to be a significant problem.[16] The mean duration of symptoms in the mobile spine between the onset of symptoms and time of diagnosis was 14 months.[5] The neurologic symptoms associated with the tumor depend on its location. Patients with cervical chordoma may complain of unilateral weakness and paresthesias.[10] Characteristically, pain is not relieved by recumbency and is greater at night.[13] Dysphagia is a symptom of patients with chordoma projecting anteriorly from the cervical spine.[11]

Physical Examination

Chordoma of the cervical spine may present anteriorly, laterally, or posteriorly. Physical and neurologic examination may demonstrate a wide variety of abnormalities corresponding to the location of the tumor. Anterior lesions, which may form a soft tissue mass, may cause a swelling in the retropharyngeal area. Lateral lesions may cause signs of radiculopathy. Posterior lesions may have symptoms consistent with myelopathy.

Laboratory Data

Laboratory findings may be unremarkable early in the course of this tumor. Abnormali-

ties in hematologic and chemical parameters may appear only late once the tumor has grown extensively or has metastasized.

Gross examination of the tumor reveals a soft, lobulated, grayish mass that is usually well encapsulated except in the region of bony invasion. In the vertebral column, it originates in the vertebral body and spreads either along the posterior longitudinal ligament or through the intervertebral disc.

Histologically, chordoma is characterized by cells of notochordal origin—physaliphorous cells. These cells contain a large, clear area of cytoplasm, with an eccentric, flattened nucleus, and form columns that are interspersed in fibrous tissue.[16] The tumor is also characterized by the production of large amounts of mucin, and this histologic appearance bears a close resemblance to that of an adenocarcinoma. The nuclear size of tumor cells may vary greatly. Mitotic figures are rare. The tumor may show a wide range in its histologic appearance, including physaliphorous cells along with cells in arrangements that mimic spindle cell sarcomas or epithelial tumors.[17] The differentiation of chordoma from cartilage tumor and adenocarcinoma may be made through the use of special stains. Chordoma is positive for keratin and S-100 protein; cartilage tumor is negative for keratin; and adenocarcinoma is negative for S-100 protein.[6, 18] Chondroid chordoma is a variant of chordoma, with histologic features that may mimic chondrosarcoma.[19] Chordoma that contains chondroid components is usually limited to the spheno-occipital region of the skull. However, chondroid chordoma of other regions of the spine has been reported. The distinction between conventional and chondroid chordoma is important because the latter has a longer endurance.[20]

Radiographic Evaluation

Vertebral chordoma produces lytic bone destruction with calcific foci and a soft tissue mass (Fig. 13–12).[21] The tumor originates in a single vertebral body in the mobile spine. The lesion is osteosclerotic in most circumstances.[11] The soft tissue may extend superiorly to the tumor, with amorphous, peripheral calcification. Calcification occurs more commonly in tumors of the sacrum than in tumors in the mobile spine.[12] The extent of soft tissue may be best determined by evaluation with computerized tomography (CT) (Fig. 13–12).[22, 23] Vertebral chordoma initially causes destruc-

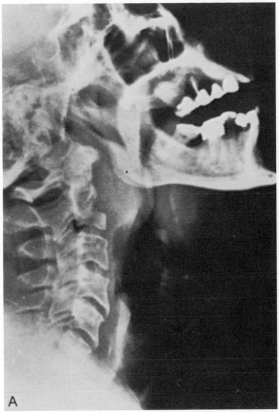
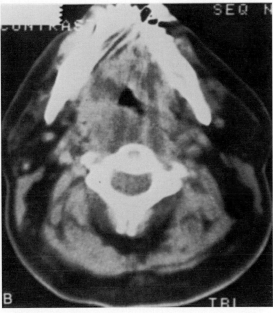

Figure 13–12. Chordoma. *A,* Lateral cervical spine. Note retropharyngeal soft tissue mass with minimal involvement of the C2 vertebra. *B,* Axial computerized tomography scan. Note parapharyngeal soft tissue extension of tumor. (From Sundaresan N, Rosenthal DI, Schiller AL, Krol G: Chordomas. In: Sundaresan N, Schmidek HH, Schiller AL, Rosenthal DI [eds]: Tumors of the Spine: Diagnosis and Clinical Management. Philadelphia: WB Saunders Co, 1990, p 200.)

tion of a vertebral body without intervertebral disc involvement. Subsequently, intervertebral discs become narrowed, and opposing vertebral end plates are eroded.[24] Myelography is helpful in determining extradural extension of the tumor even in the absence of neurologic symptoms.

Bone scintigraphy may be helpful in establishing the solitary nature of the tumor. Chordoma is a solitary mass, although extension to neighboring spinal bones occurs.[25]

CT scan is superior to plain roentgenogram for the evaluation of chordoma: it is able to determine the total extent of the tumor mass and soft tissue component without the need for angiography or myelography; it delineates bone destruction optimally; and it detects calcific debris not apparent on plain roentgenogram.[26]

Magnetic resonance (MR) imaging views the cervical region in three planes. MR imaging detects the presence of pathologic changes in bone and is particularly helpful in determining the extent of the soft tissue mass accompa-

nying the chordoma[27] (Fig. 13–13). MR charactcristics of chordoma include signal intensity similar to muscle on T_1-weighted images and increased intensity on T_2-weighted images.[28, 29] MR imaging is the best method for identifying local recurrence after patients have received therapy for their tumor.[13]

Differential Diagnosis

The diagnosis of chordoma is suggested by its location and radiographic features. Chordoma has been detected in all areas of the cervical spine, including the atlas.[30–32] However, the definitive diagnosis requires examination of a biopsy specimen. Fine-needle aspiration biopsy of chordomas produces adequate specimens for diagnosis. Specimens may be viewed by microscopic, histochemical, and immunocytochemical examination. The use of these methods, including tests for cytokeratin, epithelial membrane antigen, vimentin, carcinoembryonic antigen, and protein S-100,

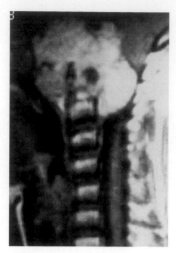

Figure 13–13. Chordoma: magnetic resonance (MR) imaging abnormalities. In a 12-year-old child, a sagittal T_1-weighted (TR/TE 600/20) spin echo MR image obtained after the intravenous injection of a gadolinium compound shows a large lesion in the base of the skull with inferior extension into the upper cervical vertebrae and spinal canal. The tumor is of high-signal intensity, representing enhancement related to the injected contrast agent. The tumor is lobulated, and there appear to be septations of low-signal intensity. (Courtesy of S.K. Brahme, M.D., La Jolla, California.)

allows for differentiation of chondrogenic and metastatic adenocarcinomas from chordomas.[9, 18, 19, 33]

A number of lesions need to be considered in the differential diagnosis of chordoma. Giant cell tumor of bone, osteochondroma, chondrosarcoma, metastases, multiple myeloma, osteosarcoma, osteoblastoma, and aneurysmal bone cyst may cause vertebral lesions that must be differentiated from chordoma. Tumor may cause intervertebral disc narrowing that may be confused with an inflammatory disorder, such as osteomyelitis.[25] Chordoma may cause widening of the cervical foramen, mimicking neurofibroma.[34]

Treatment

The definitive treatment for chordoma is en bloc excision. Unfortunately, because of tumor size at time of diagnosis and the approximation of the tumor to vital structures, partial resection may be the only surgical option. Staging of the tumor before surgery with radiographic techniques and percutaneous biopsy help determine the possible surgical options for removal.[35] Postoperative radiation therapy results in reasonable local control of tumor without significant toxicity.[36] Vertebral

chordoma is treated by decompression laminectomy, with excision of accessible tumor located in bone, soft tissues, and the extradural space. Aggressive surgical techniques have been developed that are able to remove an entire vertebra with little residual dysfunction.[35] Lesions in the upper cervical spine may be approached through a mandibular approach. Midcervical lesions may be approached from a lateral interscalene incision. Fusion with bone is preferable to methylmethacrylate for those with an unstable spine after removal of the tumor.[13] Chemotherapy is usually ineffective.[37] Improved long-term local control of axial skeleton chordoma has been reported with the combined use of high-dose proton and photon radiation therapy using three-dimensional planning to pinpoint the site of the radiation beam.[38]

Prognosis

Chordoma is a slowly growing tumor that metastasizes in 10% of patients late in the course of the disease.[39] The common locations for metastatic lesions are lung, bone, and lymph nodes.[40] Patients who undergo total resection of the tumor have a better survival than those with partial resection.[41, 42] The 5-year survival rate for sacrococcygeal tumors and vertebral tumors is 66% and 50%, respectively. The 10-year survival rate ranges from 10% to 40%.[22] A few patients have survived with chordoma for 20 years. These data support the impression that chordoma is a tumor with a wide range of behavior, from slow and indolent to rapidly progressive destructive growth. Cervical spine chordomas, particularly those that are larger, have a higher rate of recurrence than those at the base of the skull.[43] The prognosis of each patient must be determined by taking into account the location, pathologic characteristics, and invasiveness of the tumor. With the advent of more sensitive radiographic techniques, smaller tumors can be identified, which means improved opportunity for total removal of the tumor. This has resulted in a larger number of patients becoming disease-free.[44] In a large study of 2,627 primary malignant bone tumors comparing chordoma, chondrosarcoma, osteosarcoma, and malignant fibrous histiocytoma, chordoma had a 5-year survival rate of 63.8%, compared with 72.7%, 41.0%, and 42.9%, respectively.[45]

References

CHORDOMA

1. Mirra JM: Bone Tumors: Clinical, Radiologic, and Pathologic Correlation. Philadelphia: Lea & Febiger, 1989, pp 648–690.
2. Dahlin DC, Unni KK: Bone Tumors: General Aspects and Data on 8,542 Cases, 4th ed. Springfield, Illinois: Charles C Thomas, Publisher, 1986, pp 379–393.
3. Schajowicz F: Tumors and Tumorlike Lesions of Bone: Pathology, Radiology, and Treatment, 2nd ed. Berlin: Springer-Verlag, 1994, pp 459–468.
4. Mindell ER: Chordoma. J Bone Joint Surg 63A:501, 1981.
5. Bjornsson J, Wold LE, Ebersold MJ, Laws ER: Chordoma of the mobile spine: a clinicopathologic analysis of 40 patients. Cancer 71:735, 1993.
6. Sundaresan N, Rosenthal DI, Schiller AL, Krol G: Chordomas. In: Sundaresan N, Schmidek HH, Schiller AL, Rosenthal DI (eds): Tumors of the Spine: Diagnosis and Clinical Management. Philadelphia: WB Saunders Co, 1990, pp 192–213.
7. Horwitz T: Chordal ectopia and its possible relationship to chordoma. Arch Pathol 31:354, 1941.
8. Peyron A, Mellissinos J: Chordome, tumeur tramatique. Ann Med Legale 15:478, 1935.
9. Huvos AG: Bone Tumors: Diagnosis, Treatment, and Prognosis, 2nd ed. Philadelphia: WB Saunders Co, 1991, pp 599–624.
10. Chetty R, Levin CV, Kalan MR: Chordoma: a 20-year clinicopathologic review of the experience of Groote Schuur hospital, Cape Town. J Surg Oncol 46:261, 1991.
11. deBruine FT, Kroon HM: Spinal chordoma: radiologic features in 14 cases. AJR 150:861, 1988.
12. Kricun ME: Imaging of Bone Tumors. Philadelphia: WB Saunders Co, 1993, pp 263–265.
13. Healey JH, Lane JM: Chordoma: a critical review of diagnosis and treatment. Orthop Clin North Am 20:417, 1989.
14. Tomlinson FH, Scheithauer BW, Miller GM, Onofrio BM: Extraosseous spinal chordoma. J Neurosurg 75:980, 1991.
15. Sebag G, Dubois J, Benianinovitz A, et al.: Extraosseous spinal chordoma: radiographic appearance. AJNR 14:205, 1993.
16. Congdon CC: Benign and malignant chordomas: a clinico-anatomical study of twenty-two cases. Am J Pathol 28:793, 1952.
17. Volpe R, Mazabrund A: A clinicopathologic review of 25 cases of chordoma: a pleomorphic and metastatic neoplasm. Am J Surg Pathol 7:161, 1983.
18. Wojno KJ, Hruban RH, Garin-Chesa P, Huvos AG: Chondroid chordomas and low-grade chondrosarcomas of the craniospinal axis: an immunohistochemical analysis of 17 cases. Am J Surg Pathol 16:1144, 1992.
19. Jeffrey PB, Biava CG, Davis RL: Chondroid chordoma: a hyalinized chordoma without cartilaginous differentiation. Am J Clin Pathol 103:271, 1995.
20. Hruban RH, May M, Marcove RC, Huvos AG: Lumbosacral chordoma with high-grade malignant cartilaginous and spindle cell components. Am J Surg Pathol 14:384, 1990.
21. Higinbotham NL, Phillips RF, Farr HW, Husty HO: Chordoma: thirty-five-year study at Memorial Hospital. Cancer 20:1841, 1967.
22. Sundaresan N, Galicich JH, Chu FCH, Huvos AG: Spinal chordomas. J Neurosurg 50:312, 1979.
23. Krol G, Sundaresan N, Deck M: Computed tomography of axial chordomas. J Comput Assist Tomogr 7:286, 1983.
24. Pinto RS, Lin JP, Firooznia H, LeFleur RS: The osseous and angiographic manifestations of vertebral chordomas. Neuroradiology 9:231, 1975.
25. Meyer JE, Lepke RA, Lindfors KK, Pagani JJ, et al.: Chordomas: their CT appearance in the cervical, thoracic, and lumbar spine. Radiology 153:693, 1984.
26. Smith J, Ludwig RL, Marcove RC: Sacrococcygeal chordoma: a clinicoradiological study of 60 patients. Skeletal Radiol 16:37, 1987.
27. Wetzel LH, Levine E: MR imaging of sacral and presacral lesions. AJR 154:771, 1990.
28. Yuh WTC, Flickinger FW, Barloon TJ, Montgomery WJ: MR imaging of unusual chordomas. J Comput Assist Tomogr 12:30, 1988.
29. Yuh WTC, Lozano RL, Flickinger FW, et al.: Lumbar epidural chordoma: MR findings. J Comput Assist Tomogr 13:508, 1989.
30. Harwick RD, Miller AS: Craniocervical chordomas. Am J Surg 138:512, 1979.
31. Murali R, Rovit R, Benjamin MV: Chordoma of the cervical spine. Neurosurgery 9:253, 1981.
32. Wu KK, Mitchell DC, Guise ER: Chordoma of the atlas: a case report. J Bone Joint Surg 59A:140, 1979.
33. Walaas L, Kindblom L: Fine-needle aspiration biopsy in the preoperative diagnosis of chordoma: a study of 17 cases with application of electron microscopic, histochemical, and immunocytochemical examination. Hum Pathol 22:22, 1991.
34. Shallat RF, Taekman MS, Nagle RC: Unusual presentation of cervical chordoma with long-term survival: case report. J Neurosurg 57:716, 1982.
35. Stener B: Complete removal of vertebrae for extirpation of tumors: a 20-year experience. Clin Orthop 245:72:1989.
36. Schoenthaler R, Castro JR, Petti PL, et al.: Charged particle irradiation of sacral chordomas. Int J Radiat Oncol Biol Phys 26:291, 1993.
37. Kamrin RP, Potanos JN, Pool JL: An evaluation of the diagnosis and treatment of chordoma. J Neurol Neurosurg Psychiatry 27:157, 1964.
38. Hug EB, Fitzek MM, Liebsch NJ, Munzenrider JE: Locally challenging osteo- and chondrogenic tumors of the axial skeleton: results of combined proton and photon radiation therapy using three-dimensional treatment planning. Int J Radiat Oncol Biol Phys 31:467, 1995.
39. Wang CC, James AE Jr: Chordoma: brief review of the literature and report of a case with widespread metastases. Cancer 22:162, 1968.
40. Hertzanu Y, Glass RBJ, Mendelsohn DC: Sacrococcygeal chordoma in young adults. Clin Radiol 34:327, 1983.
41. Bethke KP, Neifeld JP, Lawrence W Jr: Diagnosis and management of sacrococcygeal chordoma. J Surg Oncol 48:232, 1991.
42. Bohlman HH, Sachs BL, Carter JR, et al.: Primary neoplasms of the cervical spine: diagnosis and treatment of twenty-three patients. J Bone Joint Surg 68A:483, 1986.
43. Austin JP, Urie MM, Cardenosa G, Muzenrider JE: Probable causes of recurrence in patients with chordoma and chondrosarcoma of the base of skull and cervical spine. Int J Radiat Oncol Biol Phys 25:439, 1993.
44. Sundaresan N, Huvos AG, Krol G, et al.: Surgical treatment of spinal chordomas. Arch Surg 122:1479, 1987.
45. Dorfman HD, Czerniack B: Bone cancers. Cancer 75:203, 1995.

LYMPHOMA

Capsule Summary

Frequency of neck pain—common
Location of neck pain—cervical spine
Quality of neck pain—persistent ache
Symptoms and signs—pain that increases on recumbency, generalized fatigue, localized tenderness
Laboratory and x-ray tests—anemia, osteolytic lesion with compression fracture on plain roentgenogram
Treatment—chemotherapy or radiation therapy or both

Prevalence and Pathogenesis

Lymphoma is a malignant disease of lymphoreticular origin. It usually arises in lymph nodes, rarely initially in bone, and is classified into two major groups: Hodgkin's and non-Hodgkin's lymphoma. Hodgkin's and non-Hodgkin's lymphoma are rare causes of neck pain in an adult patient.

The incidence of Hodgkin's and non-Hodgkin's lymphoma is approximately 40 to 60 cases per million persons per year. Primary Hodgkin's and non-Hodgkin's disease of bone unassociated with lymph node involvement are rare tumors occurring in 1% to 7% of biopsied tumors.[1, 2] Most bone involvement is secondary to hematogenous spread or direct extension of the tumor.[3] Approximately 30% of malignant lymphomas involve the skeletal system during the course of the disease.[4] A majority of the patients who develop lymphoma are 20 to 60 years of age. The male-to-female ratio is approximately 2:1. The disease occurs with increasing frequency from the second to the eighth decade, in which decade the frequency declines.[5]

The pathogenesis of lymphoma remains unknown. Although viral infections have been implicated as the etiologic agents that result in lymphoma, the exact pathogenetic factors causing lymphoreticular malignancy remain to be identified.

In a study of 25 patients with primary lymphoma of bone, 24% of lesions occurred in the axial skeleton.[6] About the same percentage was noted in a larger, retrospective study of 246 primary lymphoma of bone patients.[7] Another study found 14% of lymphomas in the axial skeleton. The cervical spine was the location of 11% of lesions, thoracic spine 34%, and lumbosacral spine 55%.[2] A study of 422 patients had 13% (66) with axial skeleton disease, with 3% (2) of the 66 with cervical spine lesions.[8] A study of non-Hodgkin's lymphoma also found only 8% (1 of 13) of lesions in the axial skeleton affecting the cervical spine.[9] Other studies have found lumbar, thoracic, and sacral lesions without cervical spine involvement.[10]

Clinical History

Patients with primary Hodgkin's or non-Hodgkin's lymphoma of bone develop persistent pain over the affected bone. Bone pain may increase when patients go to bed. A peculiar clinical finding relates to an increase of bone pain after the consumption of alcohol.[11] Pain duration is usually measured in months before patients seek medical evaluation. Most patients with solitary lesions have no constitutional symptoms. Constitutional symptoms are more closely associated with multiple lesions of bone. The diagnosis of lymphoma of bone should be considered in elderly patients with fever and compression fractures.[12] Patients with spinal epidural lymphoma may complain of symptoms compatible with spinal stenosis.[13] Lesions above the lumbar spine may be associated with acute onset of paraparesis.[14] Radicular pain in the upper or lower extremity may be caused not only by nerve compression due to an expanding mass in the spinal canal. Lymphoma may also infiltrate peripheral nerves, causing multifocal polyneuropathy and radicular pain.[15]

Physical Examination

The bone affected by primary lymphoma is tender on palpation. Soft tissue swelling may be associated with bony tenderness. Patients with axial skeleton disease may demonstrate neurologic deficits. Patients with primary disease of bone may have no peripheral signs of their tumor. Patients with generalized disease, of which bone infiltration is a part, may demonstrate lymphadenopathy and splenomegaly.

Laboratory Data

The patient with primary disease of bone does not demonstrate hematologic, chemical, and immunologic abnormalities associated with disseminated disease. The appearance of anemia, increased erythrocyte sedimentation rate, and increased serum protein levels in a patient with bone disease suggests that either the disease has extended to other tissue or that the bone lesion was secondary to disseminated disease and was late in its development.

Gross pathologic examination of affected bone reveals a main tumor mass in bone with variable amount of soft tissue extension.[16] The architecture of the bone is destroyed to a variable extent, and areas of necrosis are noted. The margins of the tumor and the involved bone are indistinct. The histologic picture of Hodgkin's disease includes typical Reed-Sternberg cells, atypical mononuclear cells, and an inflammatory component composed of lymphocytes, plasma cells, and scattered eosinophils. The reactive histiocytes and eosinophils look superficially like eosinophilic granuloma. In an older adult, a lesion that resembles eosinophilic granuloma may be Hodgkin's disease.[17] Non-Hodgkin's lymphomas may exhibit marked histologic variation.[18] These lesions lack Reed-Sternberg cells and demonstrate different combinations of abnormal lymphocytes and supporting cells. New staining techniques may help to improve the characterization of cells that cause the various kinds of lymphoma.[19] In a study of 34 Japanese patients with primary non-Hodgkin's lymphoma of bone, Ueda and colleagues identified T cell markers in 10% of tumors.[20] The frequency of T cell lymphoma may be related to the increased frequency of retroviral associated lymphoma that is common in Japan. In a series in the United States, a B-lineage, large-cell lymphoma was the cause of primary bone neoplasms.[21]

Radiographic Evaluation

Both primary Hodgkin's and non-Hodgkin's lymphoma involve the axial skeleton.[22] Neck pain often precedes the radiographic changes of lymphoma by months. The bone changes of Hodgkin's disease may include lytic (75%), sclerotic (15%), mixed (5%), or periosteal lesions (5%).[23] In the axial skeleton, Hodgkin's disease most frequently involves a vertebral body; involvement of posterior elements of a vertebral body is less common (Fig. 13–14). Occasionally, an osteoblastic lesion, an "ivory" vertebra, may be seen with Hodgkin's disease.[24] Hodgkin's involvement of the axial skeleton may result in compression fractures that spare the vertebral discs. Non-Hodgkin's lymphoma of bone has similar features charac-

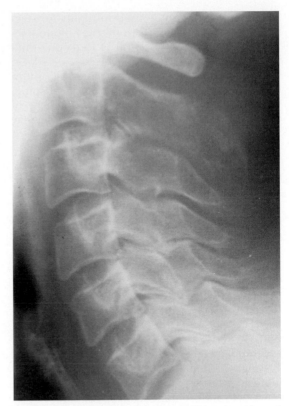

Figure 13–14. Lymphoma. A 32-year-old male with neck pain. Lateral view of the cervical spine reveals an expansile, lytic lesion of the posterior spine at C2. Lymphoma affects the vertebral body more commonly. (Courtesy of Anne Brower, M.D.)

terized by lytic and blastic areas, with cortical destruction and little reactive new bone.

The extent and type of bony lesions may vary with the histologic classification of lymphoma. In a study of 179 patients with primary lymphoma of bone, 33% (59) had two or more bones involved.[8] Skeletal lesions are more frequent and destructive in the more aggressive tumors. Sclerotic lesions are more common in less aggressive forms. Only 11% of patients with less aggressive tumor had bone lesions, in contrast with 64% who had more malignant disease.[25] The pathogenesis of extraosseous lesions without extensive osteolysis detected by roentgenograms of lymphoma of bone may be related to the production of cytokines with osteoclastic activity by the malignant cells. These cytokines include interleukin-1, interleukin-6, and tumor necrosis factor–alpha. The production of these factors allows for channels to form through the cortex of bone, allowing for the spread of tumor cells into surrounding soft tissues.[26]

Although computerized tomography (CT)

remains the commonly used modality for staging bone lymphoma before therapy, bone scintigraphy may also be helpful in detecting multiple lesions that may not be suspected on the initial presentation of the patient. Gallium scan may detect lesions in the cervical spine, including C2, that may be overlooked on a plain roentgenogram.[27] Bone scintigraphy may also be helpful in following the response of bone lesions to chemotherapy.[28]

CT and magnetic resonance (MR) imaging are helpful techniques for the determination of extraosseous, paravertebral extension of the neoplasm. CT reveals sequestra in 11% of patients with primary lymphoma of bone.[7] Sequestra are indicative of primary lymphoma and may also be associated with osteomyelitis, multiple myeloma, metastases, and bone sarcoma. CT scan is helpful in staging lymphomas to differentiate primary lymphoma of bone (stage I) from bone lesions associated with disease in other sites (stage IV).[29] MR evaluation demonstrates low-signal intensity on T_1-weighted images and high-intensity signal on T_2-weighted images. MR imaging is able to identify lymph gland enlargement, but it is unable to differentiate lymphadenopathy secondary to Hodgkin's disease, non-Hodgkin's disease, infection, and metastatic disease.[30] MR imaging may detect early changes in bones that may not be detected by plain bone scintigraphy or CT scan.[31]

Differential Diagnosis

The diagnosis of lymphoma is based on careful examination of adequate biopsy material. A CT-guided biopsy is able to obtain adequate material from the cervical spine without the need for an open surgical procedure.[32] Even with adequate histologic material, however, the diagnosis of specific lymphoma is difficult to make because of the pleomorphic forms of the disease. The differential diagnosis of a single osteoblastic vertebral body must include Paget's disease and carcinoma of the breast or prostate. In younger patients with vertebra plana, the possibility of eosinophilic granuloma must be investigated. Careful review of all the clinical and pathologic data should enable the physician to make the appropriate diagnosis.

Treatment

The treatment of lymphoma is based on the extent of the disease. All patients must be staged before treatment is initiated. Staging of lymphoma continues to be modified as additional information related to prognosis is gathered. A new, predictive model for aggressive non-Hodgkin's lymphoma includes extranodal sites as one of the factors determining outcome.[33] Once the stage of disease is known, the patient should receive appropriate therapy for that amount of involvement. Treatment may include radiation therapy or chemotherapy or both.[34–36]

Prognosis

Therapy for lymphoma has become more effective in the control of the disease. Patients have the potential for cure if the disease is not too extensive. In many circumstances, they are able to live productive lives for extended periods. Five-year survival rates of 40% to 50% have been reported. Recent studies report a 50% survival rate for patients with lymphoma of bone.[37] Patients with solitary bone lesions have a better prognosis when compared with the 42% 5-year survival rate for patients with multiple lesions.[5] Prognosis may also be related to the pattern of cell associated with the tumor. Favorable patterns include noncleaved and multilobated cells; unfavorable patterns include cleaved cells and immunoblasts. The 5-year survival rate is 67% for patients with cleaved cells and 21% for patients with uncleaved cells.[10] Young patients who develop neural compression should receive aggressive radiation therapy and chemotherapy. Decompression is reserved for young patients with rapidly progressive paralysis. The results of decompression in the elderly are poor.[9] Patients with primary epidural non-Hodgkin's lymphoma in the cervical spine may have a good response to medical and radiation therapy.[38]

References

LYMPHOMA

1. Mirra JM: Bone Tumors: Clinical, Radiologic, and Pathologic Correlation. Philadelphia: Lea & Febiger, 1989, pp 1119–1185.
2. Dahlin DC, Unni KK: Bone Tumors: General Aspects and Data on 8,542 Cases, 4th ed. Springfield, Illinois: Charles C Thomas, Publisher, 1986, pp 206–226.
3. Steiner PE: Hodgkin's disease: the incidence, distribution, nature and possible significance of lymphogranulomatous lesions in bone marrow; review with original data. Arch Pathol 36:627, 1943.
4. Coles WC, Schulz MD: Bone involvement in malignant lymphoma. Radiology 50:458, 1948.
5. Aisenberg AC: Malignant Lymphoma: Biology, Natu-

ral History, and Treatment. Philadelphia: Lea & Febiger, 1991, pp 288–290.

6. Desai S, Jambhekar NA, Soman CS, Advani SH: Primary lymphoma of bone: a clinicopathologic study of 25 cases reported over 10 years. J Surg Oncol 46:265, 1991.

7. Mulligan ME, Kransdorf MJ: Sequestra in primary lymphoma of bone: prevalence and radiologic features. AJR 160:1245, 1993.

8. Ostrowski ML, Unni KK, Banks PM, et al.: Malignant lymphoma of bone. Cancer 58:2646, 1986.

9. Laing RJ, Jakubowski J, Kunkler IH, Hancock BW: Primary spinal presentation of non-Hodgkin's lymphoma: a reappraisal of management and prognosis. Spine 17:117, 1992.

10. Clayton F, Butler JJ, Ayala AG, et al.: Non-Hodgkin's lymphoma of bone: pathologic and radiologic features with clinical correlates. Cancer 60:2492, 1987.

11. Conn HO: Alcohol-induced pain as a manifestation of Hodgkin's disease. Arch Intern Med 100:241, 1957.

12. Smith KY, Bradley SF, Kauffman CA: Fever of unknown origin in the elderly: lymphoma presenting as vertebral compression fractures. J Am Geriatr Soc 42:88, 1994.

13. Travlos J, du Toit G: Primary spinal epidural lymphoma mimicking lumbar spinal stenosis: a case report. Spine 16:377, 1991.

14. Moridaira K, Handa H, Murakami H, et al.: Primary Hodgkin's disease of the bone presenting with an extradural tumor. Acta Haematol 92:148, 1994.

15. Krendel DA, Stahl RL, Chan WC: Lymphomatous polyneuropathy: biopsy of clinically involved nerve and successful treatment. Arch Neurol 48:330, 1991.

16. Huvos AG: Bone Tumors: Diagnosis, Treatment, and Prognosis, 2nd ed. Philadelphia: WB Saunders Co, 1991, pp 625–637.

17. Jaffe HL: Metabolic, Degenerative and Inflammatory Diseases of Bones and Joints. Philadelphia: Lea and Febiger, 1972, p 887.

18. Reimer RR, Chabner BA, Young RC, et al.: Lymphoma presenting in bone: results of histopathology, staging, and therapy. Ann Intern Med 87:50, 1977.

19. Warnke RA, Gotter KC, Falini B, et al.: Diagnosis of human lymphoma with monoclonal antileukocyte antibodies. N Engl J Med 309:1275, 1983.

20. Ueda T, Aozasa K, Ohasawa M, et al.: Malignant lymphomas of bone in Japan. Cancer 64:2387, 1989.

21. Pettit CK, Zukerberg LR, Gray MH, et al.: Primary lymphoma of bone: a B-cell neoplasm with a high frequency of multilobated cells. Am J Surg Pathol 14:329, 1990.

22. Perttala Y, Kijanen I: Roentgenologic bone lesions in lymphogranulomatosis maligna: analysis of 453 cases. Ann Chir Gynaecol Fenn 54:414, 1965.

23. Granger W, Whitaker R: Hodgkin's disease in bone, with special reference to periosteal reaction. Br J Radiol 40:939, 1967.

24. Dennis JM: The solitary dense vertebral body. Radiology 77:618, 1961.

25. Braunstein EM: Hodgkin disease of bone: radiographic correlation with the histological classification. Radiology 137:643, 1980.

26. Hicks DG, Gokan T, O'Keefe RJ, et al.: Primary lymphoma of bone: correlation of magnetic resonance imaging features with cytokine production by tumor cells. Cancer 75:973, 1995.

27. Fertakos RJ, Swayne LC, Yablonsky TM: Gallium SPECT detection of lymphomatous involvement of the cervical dens. Clin Nucl Med 20:70, 1995.

28. White LM, Gray BG, Ichise M, et al.: Scintigraphic flare in skeletal lymphoma. Clin Nucl Med 19:661, 1994.

29. Malloy PC, Fishman EK, Magid D: Lymphoma of bone, muscle, and skin: CT findings. AJR 159:805, 1992.

30. Holtas SL, Kido DK, Simon JH: MR imaging of spinal lymphoma. J Comput Assist Tomogr 10:111, 1986.

31. Gaudin P, Juvin R, Rozand Y, et al.: Skeletal involvement as the initial disease manifestation in Hodgkin's disease: a review of 6 cases. J Rheumatol 19:146, 1992.

32. Babu NV, Titus VTK, Chittaranjan S, et al.: Computed tomographically guided biopsy of the spine. Spine 19:2436, 1994.

33. The International Non-Hodgkin's lymphoma prognostic factors project: a predictive model for aggressive non-Hodgkin's lymphoma. N Engl J Med 329:987, 1993.

34. Leslie NT, Mauch PM, Hellman S: Stage IA to IIB supradiaphragmatic Hodgkin's disease: long-term survival and relapse frequency. Cancer 55:2072, 1985.

35. Canellos GP, Come SE, Skarin AT: Chemotherapy in the treatment of Hodgkin's disease. Semin Hematol 20:1, 1983.

36. Dosoretz DE, Murphy GF, Raymond AK, et al.: Radiation therapy for primary lymphoma of bone. Cancer 51:44, 1983.

37. Edeiken-Monroe B, Ediken J, Kim EE: Radiologic concepts of lymphoma of bone. Radiol Clin North Am 28:841, 1990.

38. Lyons MK, O'Neill BP, Marsh WR, Kurtin PJ: Primary spinal epidural non-Hodgkin's lymphoma: report of eight patients and review of the literature. Neurosurgery 30:675, 1992.

SKELETAL METASTASES

Capsule Summary

Frequency of neck pain—very common

Location of neck pain—cervical spine

Quality of neck pain—ache of increasing intensity

Symptoms and signs—increased pain at night, prior malignancy

Laboratory and x-ray tests—anemia; bone biopsy may or may not show characteristics of primary tumor; bone scintigraphy most sensitive test

Treatment—palliative with radiation therapy, corticosteroids, decompressive laminectomy for spinal cord compression

Prevalence and Pathogenesis

A principal characteristic of malignant neoplastic lesions is the growth of tumor cells distant from the primary lesion. These distant lesions are referred to as metastases and are found commonly in the skeletal system. Skeletal lesions result from dissemination through the blood stream or by direct extension. The axial skeleton is a common site of metastatic disease.

Metastatic lesions in the skeleton are much more common than primary tumors of bone, with the overall ratio being 25:1.[1, 2] The prevalence of metastases increases with increasing age. This follows from the increasing numbers of tumors in a population as it grows older. Patients who are 50 years of age or older are at greatest risk of developing metastatic disease. The ratio of men to women who develop metastases varies for each type of malignancy. Men and women are equally at risk of developing metastatic lesions, when considering all neoplasms with the potential to metastasize.

Each tumor has a different propensity for metastasizing to bone. The true incidence of skeletal metastases from each tumor is difficult to ascertain. Complete examination of the skeleton cannot be done with the same amount of care as evaluating other body organs. Therefore, great variability may be reported for the incidence of metastases for the same tumor. Tumors that are frequently associated with skeletal metastasis include those of the prostate, breast, lung, kidney, thyroid, and colon (Table 13–3).[3] Metastases occur more commonly in the axial skeleton than in the appendicular skeleton. The axial skeleton is the third most common site of metastases after the lung and liver.[4]

Metastatic lesions affect the cervical spine less frequently than other portions of the axial skeleton. Many large studies of metastatic disease of the spine do not include the cervical spine either because of the extra dissection needed for autopsy evaluation or the notion that the cervical spine was less frequently involved.[5-7] A number of studies of the entire axial skeleton have identified cervical spine metastatic disease. The frequency of cervical spine involvement ranged from 6% to 19% in these studies.[8-13] A higher prevalence of 34% involvement of the cervical spine was reported with metastatic adenocarcinoma of unknown origin.[14] Metastases associated with breast cancer was reported in the cervical spine in 26% of individuals with that disease as detected by bone scintigraphy.[3] In general, the frequency of cervical spine metastases is less than that associated with the thoracic and lumbar spine.

The propensity of bone, and the axial skeleton in particular, to be the site of metastases may be explained in part by the presence of Batson's plexus around the vertebral column and bone marrow inside bone (Fig. 13–15). Batson's plexus is a network of veins located in the epidural space between the bony spinal column and the dura mater covering the spinal cord, and it is connected to the major veins that return blood to the heart, the inferior and superior venae cavae. This plexus of veins is unique in that there are no valves to control blood flow, and any increased pressure in the vena caval system results in increased flow into Batson's plexus. Metastatic cells may enter this plexus and be deposited in the venous and sinusoidal systems of bone that are connected to Batson's plexus.[15] Supporting data for the importance of Batson's plexus in the distribution of skeletal metastasis are the frequency of axial skeleton metastases and the predilection of metastasis of specific organs to travel to corresponding portions of the spine.[16, 17] Breast cancer tends to occur in the thoracic spine, and prostate cancer metastasizes to the lumbar spine. The red bone marrow, which is located inside vertebral bodies, long bones, and flat bones, has a rich sinusoidal system. Sinusoidal vessels are usually under low hemodynamic pressure, allowing for pooling of blood. The pooling of blood, along with other factors such as fibrin deposits and thrombosis, may encourage tumor growth.

The incidence of skeletal metastases may also be related to the ability of tumor cell emboli to develop into secondary tumors. This is a property of each form of tumor. The effects of tumor cells on bone also vary for each type of neoplasm. Tumor cells may cause bone destruction or formation. Osteoclasts may be stimulated by tumor cell products (myeloma and lymphoma, for example) that result in osteolysis.[18, 19] On the other hand, osteoblasts may also be directly stimulated by tumor cell factors (prostatic carcinoma) that stimulate

TABLE 13–3. INCIDENCE OF SKELETAL METASTASES

TUMOR ORIGIN	INCIDENCE (%)	
	High	*Low*
Breast	85	47
Prostate	85	33
Thyroid	60	28
Kidney	64	30
Esophagus	7	5
Intestine	11	3
Rectum	61	8
Bladder	42	
Uterine cervix	56	50
Ovary	9	
Liver	16	
Melanoma	7	

Modified from Galasko CSB: Skeletal Metastases. Boston: Butterworth, 1986.

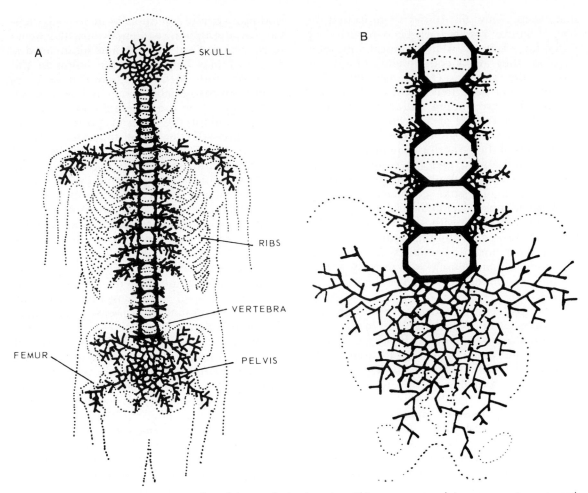

Figure 13–15. Diagrammatic representation of the vertebral vein system. This venous network is a common two-way path of the metastatic spread of pelvic, abdominal, and thoracic tumors. A large proportion of bony metastases results from dissemination of neoplastic cells through the vertebral vein system. (From del Regato JA: Pathways of metastatic spread of malignant tumors. Semin Oncol 4:33, 1977.)

bone formation or may produce bone in reaction to increased bone destruction.[20–24] The effects of these processes of tumor cells on bone result in osteolysis or osteosclerosis, which is discernible by radiographic techniques.

A number of chemical factors related to metastases have an effect on bone mineralization. These factors include parathyroid hormone, osteoclast-activating factor, prostaglandins (PGE_2), and transforming growth factor.[4, 25] Tumors associated with osteoblastic activity (prostate cancer) release factors that stimulate osteoblasts to produce bone.[26]

Clinical History

A high index of suspicion for the presence of metastasis is important in the evaluation of the patient with a history of malignancy or the adult older than 50 years of age with neck pain unassociated with trauma.[27] Neck pain has a gradual onset and increases in intensity. It tends to be localized initially and may radiate in a radicular pattern. Pain in the cervical spine is commonly increased with motion, cough, or strain. Radicular pain may increase at night as the spine lengthens on recumbency. Pain on recumbency is a symptom frequently associated with spinal tumors.[28] Patients with involvement of the atlas or axis may have decreased neck rotation.[29] In a study of 51 patients with metastatic disease to the cervical spine, 14 (27%) had cervical spine disease with pain as the initial manifestation of their illness.[30]

Not all patients with skeletal metastases have pain. In a review of 86 patients with breast cancer with radiographic evidence of skeletal metastases, only 56 (65%) complained of pain.[13] Similar results have been reported by other investigators.[23] When clinical symptoms develop, they are a consequence of one or more of the following: (1) an enlarging lesion in a vertebral body that fractures the cortex and invades surrounding soft tissues; (2) invasion or compression of adjacent nerve roots; (3) vertebral pathologic fractures; (4) destructive lesions of the posterior elements, resulting in spinal instability; and (5) compression of the spinal cord.[31] Patients with spinal cord or nerve root compression secondary to bony or epidural lesions develop neurologic dysfunction that correlates with the location of the lesion. Neurologic symptoms indicative of myelopathy may include numbness, tingling, unsteadiness of gait, muscle weakness, spasticity, bladder or bowel incontinence, and sexual dysfunction.[24, 32]

Three patterns of neurologic symptom progression may be noted. In 30% of patients, symptoms occur acutely, with progression to maximal neurologic deficit in 48 hours. Subacute deterioration from 7 to 10 days is noted in 60%. The remaining 10% develop symptoms from 4 to 6 months.[11]

Clinical symptoms of metastatic disease of the upper cervical spine (C1 and C2) are markedly different from those of the lower cervical spine.[33] Metastases tend to affect the anterior components of vertebrae. The anterior elements of C1 and C2 are different than those of the lower cervical vertebrae. The spinal canal is wide at the C1–C2 level, making neural impingement a late manifestation of metastatic disease in this location. Impingement occurs, not secondary to direct tumor growth, but from mechanical compression of the cord owing to gross instability.[34] The stability of the upper cervical spine depends on the lateral masses of C1 and C2. Destruction of the lateral masses results in rotatory instability and severe pain. Pathologic fracture of the dens leads to anterior or posterior instability.[35]

In the lower cervical spine, vertebral body disease results in kyphosis and direct tumor impingement on the anterior portion of the dural sac. Flexion instability and kyphosis may be the result of metastases of the lower portion of the cervical spine.[35]

Physical Examination

Physical examination may demonstrate pain on palpation over the affected bone. Muscle spasm and limitation of motion are associated findings. Careful attention to neurologic deficits (hyperesthesia, segmental muscular weakness, asymmetrical reflexes, and sphincter dysfunction) may help locate the lesion in the axial skeleton. Metastatic tumor masses expand from the vertebral body. Invasion of the spinal canal from the vertebral body results in compression of the anterior portion of the spinal cord, affecting motor functions. Sensory abnormalities follow as the cord is displaced posteriorly and impacts on the lamina. The thoracic spine is most commonly associated with neurologic compromise because the spinal cord is at its largest in comparison with the diameter of the spinal canal.[31] Upper motor neuron signs, including hyperreflexia, spasticity, and abnormal Babinski's signs, are present in patients with spinal cord compression of the cervical spine. Patients with lesions in the upper cervical spine have decreased rotation as a manifestation of disease of the atlantoaxial articulation.[29]

Also to be considered is the possibility of more than one level for extradural tumor compression. Lesions of the cauda equina cause lower motor neuron abnormalities, which are associated with motor and sensory loss and hyporeflexia.[36]

Frankel's classification is used to grade neurologic deficits.[4] Grade A is associated with complete motor and sensory loss, and grade E has normal motor and sensory function.

Laboratory Data

Early in the course of lesions, laboratory parameters may be unremarkable. However, subsequent evaluation may demonstrate anemia, increased erythrocyte sedimentation rate, abnormal urinalysis, or abnormal chemistries, including increased serum alkaline phosphatase concentrations. Therefore, initial negative laboratory data should not dissuade a physician from pursuing further diagnostic evaluation in an older patient with recent onset of neck pain.

Biochemical tests are not always positive in patients. In one study, only 30% of patients with positive scintiscan for metastatic disease had an elevated alkaline phosphatase level.[37]

In patients without a known primary tumor, bone biopsy may provide the first evidence of a malignancy. Occasionally, the histologic features of the biopsy specimen may suggest the source of the lesion, such as colloid material with thyroid adenocarcinoma, clear cells with renal cell carcinoma, and melanin with melanoma. On many occasions, the histologic features, squamous cells or mucin cells, may be associated with primary lesions in various organs. Some lesions may be so undifferentiated that the pathologic findings offer no clue to the possible source of the tumor.[2] Radiologic identification of lesions may help localize the area for biopsy.[38]

No consistent histologic abnormalities are described for compressive lesions of the spinal cord.[31] The gray matter is preserved; edema and cellular degeneration affect the white matter. Venous occlusion has been suggested as the most important factor leading to neuronal degeneration, although the distribution of pathologic changes does not conform to the arterial or venous drainage of the cord.[39]

Radiographic Evaluation

Radiographic abnormalities associated with the axial skeleton include osteolytic, osteoblastic, and mixed lytic and blastic lesions.[40] Osteolytic lesions, which affect a vertebral body or a posterior element such as a pedicle, are associated with carcinomas of the lung, kidney, breast, and thyroid. Multiple osteoblastic lesions are associated with prostatic, breast, and colon carcinoma and bronchial carcinoid. A single blastic vertebral body may be seen with prostatic carcinoma but is more closely associated with Hodgkin's disease or Paget's disease. Vertebral lesions that contain both lytic and blastic metastases are associated with carcinoma of the breast, lung, prostate, and bladder. Kidney and thyroid carcinoma, because of their usual slow growth, may cause an expansile lesion from periosteal growth without destruction. Osteolytic lesions are more frequently associated with vertebral body collapse than are osteoblastic lesions. Vertebral body destruction is not associated with changes in the intervertebral disc; therefore, the presence of vertebral body destruction and loss of intervertebral disc space suggest infection. However, radiographic and pathologic studies suggest that intervertebral discs may degenerate more rapidly, indent weakened vertebral bone, and form a Schmorl's node. Rarely, the vertebral body may be invaded by tumor and lose disc integrity.[41, 42]

A number of studies have investigated the initial location for metastases in individual vertebrae. The loss of a pedicle as the first roentgenographic finding of metastatic disease suggested that structure as the location for the initial nidus of cancerous cells. Studies by a variety of investigators have demonstrated the posterior vertebral body near the spinal venous plexus as the initial location for vertebral metastases. Computerized tomography (CT) studies have demonstrated vertebral body involvement without lesions of the pedicle.[43] Pedicle involvement has been documented by magnetic resonance (MR) imaging to be a direct extension from the vertebral body or the posterior elements.[44] The reason why the loss of the pedicle is the first abnormality noted despite earlier vertebral body disease is related to the loss of the cortical bone of the pedicle and the insensitivity of plain roentgenogram to detect loss of trabecular bone.

Lesions of the upper cervical spine may not be identified by plain roentgenographic evaluation. Overlapping of the dens and atlantoaxial joint may obscure early alterations in bony architecture. This may delay the timely diagnosis of a metastasis. In a study of 16 patients with upper cervical spine metastases, only 7 had identifiable diagnostic changes on plain roentgenogram of the cervical spine.[33] The open-mouth view may be helpful but is not routinely obtained (Fig. 13–16). In the lower cervical spine, alterations of the anterior vertebral body are easier to identify. However, the changes of degenerative disc disease seen frequently in elderly patients may draw attention away from the site of tumor involvement. Subsequently, progressive destruction may appear at a site distant from the location of degenerative disease.[33]

The involvement of the upper cervical spine as described by Phillips and Levine occurred in three patterns.[33] The most common pattern was disease in the anterior body of C2, including fracture of the dens. The second pattern was destruction of the lateral mass of C1. The third pattern had involvement of the posterior portion of C2. Patients with the third pattern are the most difficult for whom to make a definitive diagnosis. These patients have severe pain near the insertion of the ligamentum nuchae but do not exhibit instability.

Early in the course of a metastatic lesion, plain roentgenographic examination is unremarkable because 30% to 50% of bone must be destroyed before a lesion is evident on plain radiograph.[45] However, scintigraphic examination with bone scan makes it possible to detect areas of symptomatic and asymptomatic bone involvement in up to 85% of patients with metastases.[32, 46] A bone scan may also suggest the presence of tumor in patients with coincident degenerative disease or osteoporosis. In one study, bone scan was the single, most use-

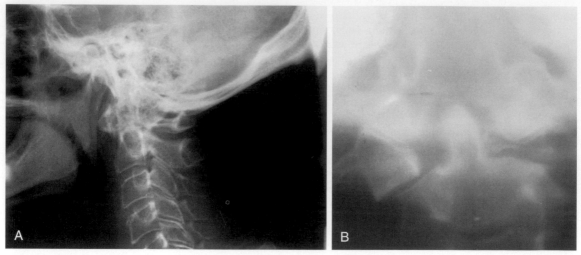

Figure 13–16. Metastatic tumor. A 64-year-old female with a history of breast cancer and neck pain. *A,* Lateral view of the cervical spine shows no detectable abnormality. *B,* Computerized tomographic open-mouth view shows loss of left portion of the C1 ring, compatible with metastatic breast cancer. (Courtesy of Anne Brower, M.D.)

ful diagnostic test in differentiating pain due to metastatic disease from pain due to a benign lesion.[47] There are reasons for false-negative and false-positive scintiscans[3] (Table 13–4). One of the most important is the "superscan." In this scan, marked increased, symmetrical, generalized uptake by diffuse metastases may be interpreted as normal. The reduction of a tracer agent in kidneys and urine should alert the radiologist to this possibility.[48] Bone marrow scintigraphy using ^{99m}Tc-labeled monoclonal antibodies is able to follow the extent and progression of metastases affecting bones containing bone marrow.[49] The bone scintiscan is the most sensitive and economical test for detecting bone metastases.[50]

CT may also be useful in localizing lesions that are difficult to identify on plain radiographs.[51, 52] CT is normally reserved for assessment of patients with positive isotope scans but with negative radiographs. CT may be particularly helpful in detecting upper cervical spine lesions that may be missed with plain roentgenograms.[33] CT is able to differentiate among bony metastases, benign lesions, and no abnormality.[53, 54] In one study, it was able to differentiate between metastases and degenerative joint disease when both existed in apophyseal articulations.[53] It is particularly useful in demonstrating small areas of bone destruction and bone and tumor impingement on the spinal canal.[55] CT should not be used as a screening technique because the exposure to radiation is great.

Myelography was the definitive diagnostic procedure for any patient with a metastatic lesion and spinal cord or nerve root compression. Injections of dye in two locations, lumbar and cisterna magna (cervical spine), were necessary to locate all potential areas of neural compression because lesions in the lumbar spine may be accompanied with "silent" lesions in the proximal spine.[56] Myelography may also identify the location of the lesion in the extradural or intradural space.

The role of MR imaging in the evaluation of patients with metastases continues to evolve as the technique becomes more sensitive in detecting neoplasms that replace normal tissues in the spine. MR imaging is an effective method for detecting upper spinal cord compression, particularly soft tissue lesions, that may not be adequately visualized by other radiographic techniques[57] (Fig. 13–17). Some studies have shown MR imaging to be better at showing the extent of tumor inside the

TABLE 13–4. BONE SCAN

FALSE-NEGATIVE	FALSE-POSITIVE
Tumor lacks osteoblastic response (myeloma)	Site of injection (elbow)
Small deposits	Urinary incontinence
Lesions of sacrum and ischium masked by bladder	Abnormal bladder collections (diverticulum)
Generalized increased uptake ("superscan")	Incomplete isotope Superimposition of uptake

Modified from Galasko CSB: Skeletal Metastases. Boston: Butterworth, 1986.

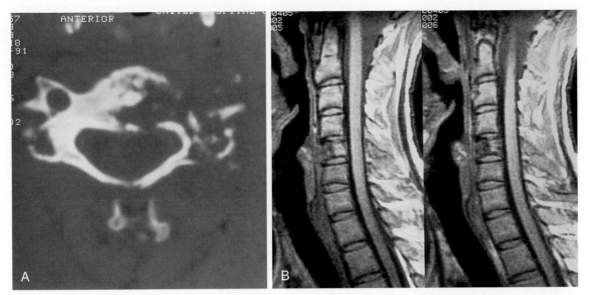

Figure 13–17. A 28-year-old male with a history of human immunodeficiency virus infection presented with increasing neck pain and swelling. *A,* Computerized tomography scan of C4 vertebral body shows osteolytic lesion of the vertebral body and transverse process. *B,* Magnetic resonance scan of a sagittal T₁-weighted image shows replacement of the anterior portion of C4 with anterior soft tissue extension. Biopsy of the lesion revealed metastatic follicular thyroid cancer. (Courtesy of Thomas Dina, M.D.)

cord, the size of extraosseous extension, and bone marrow invasion, and CT to be better at showing cortical bone destruction and extent of bone mineralization.[58, 59] MR imaging is able to differentiate compression fractures secondary to osteoporosis from replacement of bone marrow with malignant cells.[60] MR imaging detects lesions that are not identified by roentgenograms or scintiscan.[61] A study of 40 patients with metastatic disease revealed patients with breast, kidney, and prostate cancer and multiple myeloma who had abnormal MR imaging but normal findings with other radiographic techniques, including CT and scintiscan.[62] The importance of MR imaging as a diagnostic tool has been further advanced by the availability of gadolinium-diethylenetriamine penta-acetic acid as a paramagnetic contrast agent. MR imaging with contrast agent demonstrates the size, location, configuration, and characteristics of spinal tumors.[63] It is the first procedure to be used for patients with spinal cord compression. It is a noninvasive technique that is sensitive in detecting extradural masses.[64] Determination of the extent of lesions can be obtained without the need for lumbar puncture, which may lead to rapid neurologic deterioration.[65] MR imaging of the entire spinal cord should be obtained if compression is suspected because 10% of patients have multiple levels of impingement.[66] CT/myelogram should be reserved for patients for

whom MR imaging is not feasible or does not satisfactorily explain neurologic findings. CT may also prove to be more useful than MR imaging in upper cervical spine lesions at the C1–C2 level. In this location, neural impingement is a late consequence of metastasis. CT is more helpful in determining the status of bone architecture that has implications for surgical therapeutic intervention.[33]

Differential Diagnosis

In patients with a known primary tumor who develop neck pain, a destructive spinal lesion is associated with the primary neoplasm in the majority of cases. These patients may not require a biopsy of the spinal lesion for diagnosis. However, patients with no known primary neoplasm who develop destructive lesions of the spine require a biopsy for tissue diagnosis. Closed-needle biopsy of lesions in the cervical spine can safely yield useful information.[67, 68] CT-guided biopsy can obtain tissue from the cervical spine that is adequate to make the diagnosis of a metastatic lesion.[69]

Other conditions may cause bony changes on radiograph and "hot spots" on scintiscan. Elevated alkaline phosphatase levels may be seen in osteomalacia, Paget's disease, hyperparathyroidism, and sarcoidosis. Only with careful review of all the data can the various diagnosis be eliminated. In some circumstances, performing a tissue biopsy is the only sure way to obtain the data to make an accurate diagnosis.

Lesions in the superior sulcus (Pancoast's tumors) may invade the brachial plexus and extend into the epidural space through an intervertebral foramen.[70–72] These lesions cause radicular pain in the setting of normal plain roentgenograms and bone scintigraphy. MR imaging or CT/myelogram evaluation of the spinal column detects these lesions.

Treatment

Treatment of metastatic disease of the spine is directed toward palliation of pain. A cure is rarely possible because most solitary metastatic lesions are accompanied by a number of silent deposits that only become evident gradually. The pain of the metastatic lesion of the spine may be secondary to bony destruction or pathologic fracture.[73] The dependent weight of the head, the wide range of neck movements, and the lack of rib cage support combine to render the cervical spine vulnerable to pathologic fracture and dislocation.[27] Therapy directed specifically at vertebral and spinal cord lesions may include radiation therapy, corticosteroids, and decompressive laminectomy, along with stabilization of the spine. Radiation therapy may be used alone as primary treatment to decrease pain and slow growth or as adjunctive therapy after surgical decompression.[74, 75] Metastatic lesions from the breast, thyroid, and lymphomas are most sensitive to radiation therapy. Corticosteroids may help reduce edema and alleviate symptoms in patients with spinal cord compression.[76] Indications for surgical intervention in patients with symptomatic cervical spinal metastases include radiation failure, unknown tumor diagnosis, pathologic fracture or dislocation, and rapidly progressive neurologic dysfunction.[27, 77] Decompressive laminectomy is usually of no help in returning function to patients with long-standing paraplegia, but it is recommended for those who have recently developed neurologic symptoms.[78]

A number of new surgical procedures have been developed to offer spine stabilization to patients with an unstable vertebral column.[4] If instability develops, patients may require the placement of rods to control their pain.[79]

In the cervical spine, the extent and location of tumor, spinal level, bone integrity, and patient debility play a role in regard to choosing the appropriate surgical procedure.[27] Surgery should be considered before radiation if the cervical spine is unstable or has significant neurologic deficit secondary to compression.[12] A posterior approach to cervical metastatic lesions may decompress the spinal cord or root but may result in continued pain secondary to spinal instability. Attempts have been made to decrease the risk of instability by using methylmethacrylate—bone cement—for neck stabilization.[80] Subsequently, other investigators reported the failure of bone cement for cervical spine stabilization without the additional use of bone grafts and wire stabilization.[81] Anterior decompression allows for direct resection of the tumor but requires prolonged neck bracing for stabilization. In general, combined anterior and posterior stabilization may be required for cervical spine instability secondary to neoplastic destruction.

Prognosis

The course of each patient with skeletal metastasis depends on a number of factors: type of tumor, extent of involvement, sensitivity to therapy, and extent of neurologic symptoms; in general, the prognosis is poor. In one study, 20% of patients with vertebral metastases developed cord compression.[36] Unless decompression is accomplished quickly, the return of function is minimal, and the outcome is debilitating. Metastatic disease of an unknown primary tumor is an uncommon but a particularly aggressive form of neoplastic disease. The survival time of patients with this condition is extremely short, with a 6-month survival rate of only 6%.[14] Surgical intervention rarely extends the life of the patients. However, for patients with metastatic disease affecting the cervical spine, surgical treatment improves the quality of life.[82]

References

SKELETAL METASTASES

1. Francis KC, Hutter RV: Neoplasms of the spine in the aged. Clin Orthop 26:54, 1963.
2. Mirra JM: Bone Tumors: Clinical, Radiologic, and Pathologic Correlation. Philadelphia: Lea & Febiger, 1989, pp 1495–1517.
3. Galasko CSB: Skeletal Metastases. Boston: Butterworth, 1986.
4. Sundaresan N, Krol G, Digiacinto GV, Hughes JEO: Metastatic tumors of the spine. In: Sundaresan N, Schmidek HH, Schiller AL, Rosenthal DI (eds): Tumors of the Spine: Diagnosis and Clinical Manage-

ment. Philadelphia: WB Saunders Co, 1990, pp 279–304.

5. Wong DA, Fornasier VL, MacNab I: Spinal metastases: the obvious, the occult, and the impostors. Spine 15:1, 1990.

6. Fornasier VL, Horne JG: Metastases to the vertebral column. Cancer 36:590, 1975.

7. Fornasier VL, Czitrom AA: Collapsed vertebrae: review of 659 autopsies. Clin Orthop 131:261, 1978.

8. Barron KD, Hirano A, Araki S, Terry RD: Experiences with metastatic neoplasms involving the spinal cord. Neurology 9:91, 1959.

9. Kleinman WB, Kiernan HA, Michelsen WJ: Metastatic cancer of the spinal column. Clin Orthop 138:166, 1978.

10. Bernat JL, Greenberg ER, Barrett J: Suspected epidural compression of the spinal cord and cauda equina by metastatic carcinoma. Cancer 51:1953, 1983.

11. Constans JP, de Divitiis E, Donzelli R, et al.: Spinal metastases with neurological manifestations: review of 600 cases. J Neurosurg 59:111, 1983.

12. Onimus M, Schraub S, Bertin D, et al.: Surgical treatment of vertebral metastasis. Spine 11:883, 1986.

13. Schaberg J, Gainor BJ: A profile of metastatic carcinoma of the spine. Spine 10:19, 1985.

14. Saengnipanthkul S, Jirarattanaphochai K, Rojviroj S, et al.: Metastatic adenocarcinoma of the spine. Spine 17:427, 1992.

15. Batson OV: The function of the vertebral veins and their role in the spread of metastasis. Ann Surg 112:138, 1940.

16. Galasko CSB, Doyle FH: The detection of skeletal metastases from mammary cancer: a regional comparison between radiology and scintigraphy. Clin Radiol 23:295, 1972.

17. Lenz M, Fried JR: Metastasis to skeleton, brain, and spinal cord from cancer of the breast and effects of radiotherapy. Ann Surg 93:278, 1931.

18. Mundy GR, Raisz LG, Cooper RA, et al.: Evidence for the secretion of an osteoclast activating factor in myeloma. N Engl J Med 291:1041, 1974.

19. Hicks DG, Gokan T, O'Keefe RJ, et al.: Primary lymphoma of bone: correlation of magnetic resonance imaging features with cytokine production by tumor cells. Cancer 75:973, 1995.

20. Jacobs SC, Pikna D, Lawson RK: Prostate osteoblastic factor. Invest Urol 17:195, 1979.

21. Galasko CSB: The pathological basis for skeletal scintigraphy. J Bone Joint Surg 57B:353, 1975.

22. Galasko CSB: Skeletal metastases and mammary cancer. Ann R Coll Surg Engl 50:3, 1972.

23. Front D, Schenck SO, Frankel A, Robinson E: Bone metastases and bone pain in breast cancer: are they closely associated? JAMA 242:1747, 1979.

24. Rodriguez M, Dinapoli RP: Spinal cord compression with special reference to metastatic epidural tumors. Mayo Clin Proc 55:442, 1980.

25. Frassica FJ, Sim FH: Pathophysiology. In: Sim FH (ed): Diagnosis and Management of Metastatic Bone Disease: A Multidisciplinary Approach. New York: Raven Press, 1988, pp 7–14.

26. Rubens RD, Fogelman I: Bone Metastases: Diagnosis and Treatment. London: Springer-Verlag, 1991, pp 1–247.

27. Perrin RG, McBroom RJ, Perrin RG: Metastatic tumors of the cervical spine. Clin Neurosurg 37:740, 1991.

28. Nicholas JJ, Christy WC: Spinal pain made worse by recumbency: a clue to spinal cord tumors. Arch Phys Med Rehabil 67:598, 1986.

29. Hastings DE, Macnab I, Lawson V: Neoplasms of the atlas and axis. Can J Surg 11:290, 1968.

30. Jonsson B, Jonsson H Jr, Karlstom G, Sjostrom L: Surgery of cervical spine metastases: a retrospective study. Eur Spine J 3:76–83, 1994.

31. Harrington KD: Metastatic disease of the spine. J Bone Joint Surg 68A:1110, 1986.

32. Fager CA: Management of malignant intraspinal disease. Surg Clin North Am 47:743, 1967.

33. Phillips E, Levine AM: Metastatic lesions of the upper cervical spine. Spine 14:1071, 1989.

34. Sherk HH: Lesions of the atlas and axis. Clin Orthop 109:33, 1975.

35. Sundaresan N, Galcich JH, Lane JM, Greenberg HS: Treatment of odontoid fractures in cancer patients. J Neurosurg 54:187, 1981.

36. Emsellem HA: Metastatic disease of the spine: diagnosis and management. South Med J 76:1405, 1986.

37. Cowan RJ, Young KA: Evaluation of serum alkaline phosphatase determination in patients with positive bone scans. Cancer 32:887, 1973.

38. Gatenby RA, Mulhearn CB Jr, Moldofsky PJ: Computed tomography guided thin needle biopsy of small lytic bone lesions. Skeletal Radiol 11:289, 1984.

39. Boland PJ, Lane JM, Sundaresan N: Metastatic disease of the spine. Clin Orthop 169:95, 1982.

40. Young JM, Fung FJ Jr: Incidence of tumor metastasis to the lumbar spine: a comparative study or roentgenographic changes and gross lesions. J Bone Joint Surg 35A:55, 1953.

41. Hubbard DD, Gunn DR: Secondary carcinoma of the spine with destruction of the intervertebral disc. Clin Orthop 88:86, 1972.

42. Resnick D, Niwayama G: Intervertebral disc abnormalities associated with vertebral metastasis: observations in patients and cadavers with prostatic cancer. Invest Radiol 13:182, 1978.

43. Algra PR, Heimans JJ, Valk J, et al.: Do metastases in vertebrae begin in the body or the pedicles? Imaging in 45 patients. AJR 158:1275, 1992.

44. Asdourian PL, Weidenbaum M, DeWald RL, et al.: The pattern of vertebral involvement in metastatic vertebral breast cancer. Clin Orthop 250:164, 1990.

45. Edelstyn GA, Gillespie PG, Grebbel FS: The radiological demonstration of skeletal metastases: experimental observations. Clin Radiol 18:158, 1967.

46. Craig FS: Metastatic and primary lesions of bone. Clin Orthop 73:33, 1970.

47. Galasko CSB, Sylvester BS: Backpain in patients treated for malignant tumors. Clin Oncol 4:273, 1978.

48. Sy WM, Patel D, Faunce H: Significance of absent or faint kidney sign on bone scan. J Nucl Med 16:454, 1975.

49. Rieker O, Grunwald F, Layer G, et al.: Disseminated bone marrow metastases from primary breast cancer: detection and follow-up by radioimmune bone marrow scintigraphy. J Nucl Med 35:1485, 1994.

50. McNeil BJ: Value of bone scanning in neoplastic disease. Semin Nucl Med 4:277, 1984.

51. Wilson JS, Korobkin M, Genant HK, Bovill EG: Computed tomography of musculoskeletal disorders. AJR 13:55, 1978.

52. Patten RM, Shuman WP, Teefey S: Metastases from malignant melanoma to the axial skeleton: a CT study of frequency and appearance. AJR 155:109, 1990.

53. Redmond J, Spring DB, Munderloh SH, et al.: Spinal computed tomography scanning in the evaluation of metastatic disease. Cancer 54:253, 1984.

54. Muindi J, Coombes RC, Golding S, et al.: The role of computed tomography in the detection of bone

metastases in breast cancer patients. Br J Radiol 56:233, 1983.

55. Weissman DE, Gilbert M, Wang H, Grossman SA: The use of computed tomography of the spine to identify patients at high risk for epidural metastases. J Clin Oncol 3:1541, 1985.

56. Gilbert RW, Kim JH, Posner JB: Epidural spinal cord compression from metastatic tumor: diagnosis and treatment. Ann Neurol 3:340, 1978.

57. McAfee PC, Bohlman HH, Han JS, Salvagno RT: Comparison of nuclear magnetic resonance imaging and computed tomography in the diagnosis of upper cervical spinal cord compression. Spine 11:295, 1986.

58. Zimmer WD, Berquist TH, McLeod RA, et al.: Bone tumors: magnetic resonance imaging versus computed tomography. Radiology 155:709, 1985.

59. Maravilla KR, Lesh P, Weinre JC, et al.: Magnetic resonance imaging of the lumbar spine with CT correlation. AJNR 6:237, 1985.

60. Yuh WT, Zachar CK, Barloon TJ, et al.: Vertebral compression fractures: distinction between benign and malignant causes with MR imaging. Radiology 172:215, 1989.

61. Khurana JS, Rosenthal DI, Rosenberg A, Mankin HJ: Skeletal metastases in liposarcoma detectable only by magnetic resonance imaging. Clin Orthop 243:204, 1989.

62. Avrahami E, Tadmor R, Dally O, Hadar H: Early MR demonstration of spinal metastases in patients with normal radiographs and CT and radionuclide bone scans. J Comput Assist Tomgr 13:598, 1989.

63. Sze G, Stimac GK, Bartlett C, et al.: Multicenter study of gadopentetate dimeglumine as an MR contrast agent: evaluation in patients with spinal tumors. AJNR 11:967, 1990.

64. Carmody RF, Yang PJ, Seeley GW, et al.: Spinal cord compression due to metastatic disease: diagnosis with MR imaging versus myelography. Radiology 173:225, 1989.

65. Masaryk TJ: Neoplastic disease of the spine. Radiol Clin North Am 29:829, 1991.

66. Bonner JA, Lichter AS: A caution about the use of MRI to diagnose spinal cord compression. N Engl J Med 322:556, 1990.

67. Craig FS: Vertebral body biopsy. J Bone Joint Surg 38A:93, 1956.

68. Camins MB, Rosenblum BR: Osseous lesions of the cervical spine. Clin Neurosurg 37:722, 1991.

69. Babu NV, Titus VTK, Chittaranjan S, et al.: Computed tomographically guided biopsy of the spine. Spine 19:2436, 1994.

70. Pancoast HK: Superior pulmonary sulcus tumor: tumor characterized by pain, Horner's syndrome, destruction of bone and atrophy of hand muscles. JAMA 99:1391, 1932.

71. Cascino TL, Kori S, Krol G, Foley KM: CT of the brachial plexus in patients with cancer. Neurology 33:1553, 1983.

72. Kori SH, Foley KM, Posner JB: Brachial plexus lesions in patients with cancer: 100 cases. Neurology 31:45, 1981.

73. Bhalla SK: Metastatic disease of the spine. Clin Orthop 73:52, 1970.

74. Bruckman JE, Bloomer WD: Management of spinal cord compression. Semin Oncol 5:135, 1978.

75. Khan FR, Glickman AS, Chu FCH, Nickson JJ: Treatment by radiotherapy of spinal cord compression due to extradural metastases. Radiology 89:495, 1967.

76. Clark PRR, Saunders M: Steroid-induced remission in spinal canal reticulum cell sarcoma: report of two cases. J Neurosurg 42:346–348, 1975.

77. Byrne TN: Spinal cord compression from epidural metastases. N Engl J Med 327:614, 1992.

78. Vieth RG, Odom GL: Extradural spinal metastases and their neurosurgical treatment. J Neurosurg 23:501, 1965.

79. Dewald RL, Bridwell KH, Prodromas C, Rodts MF: Reconstructive spinal surgery as palliation for metastatic malignancies of the spine. Spine 10:21, 1985.

80. Harrington KD: The use of methylmethacrylate for vertebral-body replacement and anterior stabilization of pathological fracture-dislocations of the spine due to metastatic malignant disease. J Bone Joint Surg 63A:36, 1981.

81. McAfee PC, Bohlman HH, Ducker T, Eismont FJ: Failure of stabilization of the spine with methylmethacrylate. J Bone Joint Surg 68A:1145, 1986.

82. Raycroft JF, Hockman RP, Southwick WO: Metastatic tumors involving the cervical vertebrae: surgical palliation. J Bone Joint Surg 60A:763, 1978.

INTRASPINAL NEOPLASMS

Capsule Summary

E = extradural
IE = intradural-extramedullary
I = intramedullary

Frequency of neck pain
    E: very common
    IE: common
    I: rare
Location of neck pain
    E: cervical spine
    IE: neck and arm
    I: neck and arm
Quality of neck pain
    E: increasing local ache
    IE: referred pain
    I: radicular
Laboratory and x-ray tests
    E: magnetic resonance imaging
    IE: magnetic resonance imaging
    I: magnetic resonance imaging
Treatment
    E: radiation therapy, corticosteroids, laminectomy
    IE: surgical excision
    I: surgical excision

Prevalence and Pathogenesis

Whereas bone is the tissue in the axial skeleton most frequently affected by primary and metastatic tumors, less commonly tissues inside the spinal column may also be affected by neoplastic processes. These intraspinal neoplasms may be extradural—between the bone and the covering of the spinal cord, the dura;

intradural-extramedullary—between the dura and the spinal cord; and intramedullary—in the spinal cord (Fig. 13–18). Extradural tumors are most commonly metastatic in origin. Intradural-extramedullary tumors are predominantly meningioma, neurofibroma, and lipoma. Intramedullary tumors are ependymoma and glioma (Table 13–5).

Intraspinal tumors occur less frequently than tumors of the brain.[1] Tumors of the spinal cord and its coverings are uncommon, constituting 10% to 15% of primary central nervous system neoplasms, with an incidence of 1.3 per 100,000 per year.[1] A study in Norway revealed the annual incidence of primary intraspinal neoplasms as 5 per million for females and 3 per million for males.[2] They occur, most commonly, from 20 to 60 years of age.[3]

Extradural tumors are usually metastatic lesions that have invaded the intraspinal space from contiguous structures. These are the most common tumors of the spinal canal. Of the intradural lesions, extramedullary neo-

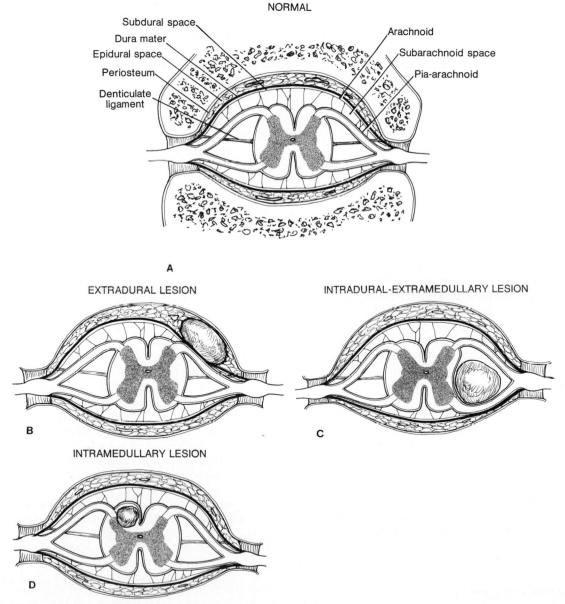

Figure 13–18. The location of intraspinal tumors. *A*, Normal anatomy. *B*, Extradural lesion (metastases). *C*, Intradural-extramedullary lesion (neurofibroma). *D*, Intramedullary lesion (glioma).

TABLE 13–5. INTRASPINAL MASSES

EXTRADURAL (50%–60%)

Metastases
  Lung
  Prostate
  Breast
Lymphoma
Chordoma
Meningioma
Fibroma
Lipoma/Lipomatosis
Vascular malformation with bleeding
Abscess

INTRADURAL—EXTRAMEDULLARY (30%–35%)

Neurofibroma
Neurilemoma
Meningioma
Neurinoma
Lipoma
Arachnoid cyst
Leptomeningeal metastases
Vascular abnormalities

INTRAMEDULLARY (10%–20%)

Glioma
  Ependymoma
  Astrocytoma
Arteriovenous malformation
Syringomyelia

plasms occur more commonly than intramedullary neoplasms.

The extradural, or epidural, space is the predominant site for intraspinal malignant tumors. Metastatic tumors in the spinal canal are extradural in location because the dura is resistant to invasion from lesions that extend from foci in vertebral bone. The extradural space is also the location of Batson's plexus, which is a site for hematogenous spread of tumor.[4] Major structures in the intradural-extramedullary space are meninges and spinal nerve roots. Meningioma and neurofibroma arise from these structures. Depending on the population of patients being studied, meningioma may cause 25% of intraspinal neoplasms. Intramedullary tumors arise in the spinal cord itself and are composed of cells that make up the support structure of the cord, ependymal and glial cells. Metastatic lesions of the spinal cord are extremely rare.[5] Glioma of the spinal cord occurs less frequently than neurofibroma or meningioma. Glioma affects men more commonly than women.

Clinical History

Intraspinal tumors may demonstrate a wide variety of clinical symptoms. Clinical symptoms associated with spinal cord disease may include a combination of pain, motor weakness, sensory changes, reflex alterations, and bladder incontinence.[6] Pain, which may be local, radicular, or causalgic, may develop in minutes, days, months, or years. Specific clinical disorders are associated with patterns of onset and location of pain. Acute local pain may be related to trauma, spinal hemorrhage, cord infarction, or disc herniation. Subacute pain may develop as the result of tumor growth or infection. Chronic pain may be related to syringomyelia or spondylosis.

Acute paralysis is a manifestation of acute trauma or cord infarction. Weakness occurring in a subacute period is frequently secondary to epidural tumor, epidural abscess, or transverse myelitis. Slowly progressive weakness is associated with multiple sclerosis, spondylosis, vitamin B_{12} deficiency, and amyotrophic lateral sclerosis. Muscle weakness may be associated with muscle atrophy and fasciculations affecting hand muscles when cervical myelopathy affects anterior horn cells.[7]

Sensory symptoms may help define the spinal cord tracts affected by a disorder. Symptoms of tingling, buzzing, or pins and needles sensations are a manifestation of dorsal column disease. Complaints of warmth, cold, or itching are more closely associated with lesions of the dorsal horn and spinothalamic tract, which mediates temperature sensation. Brown-Séquard syndrome is associated with loss of pinprick sensation on one side of the body, with loss of position and vibratory sensation on the contralateral side.

Reflex changes are dependent on the time course and location of the lesions. Spinal shock secondary to severe trauma to the cord is associated with areflexia, atonia, and nonresponsiveness to plantar stimulation. More slowly progressive lesions may be associated with hyperreflexia. Hyperactivity of all lower and upper extremity reflexes with a normal jaw jerk is indicative of a high cervical spine lesion. Hyperactive lower extremity and finger reflexes with normal biceps reflex suggest a lower cervical cord lesion.

Bladder incontinence is not an early symptom of spinal cord disease. Urinary incontinence is the hallmark of bladder involvement. Flaccid bladder paralysis is associated with overflow incontinence. More slowly progressive abnormalities result in a spastic bladder with the features of frequency and urgency.

Patients with extradural metastatic disease have pain as their initial complaint. Pain may localize to the affected area in the spine or may radiate to the upper or lower extremities if neural elements are compressed. Pain characteristically increases in intensity and is unrelenting. It increases at night on recumbency due to lengthening of the spine. Pain on recumbency may occur with extradural or intradural-extramedullary lesions such as multiple myeloma, meningioma, and neurilemoma.[8] Activity may also exacerbate the discomfort. The pain is unresponsive to mild analgesics and requires narcotics for control. Not uncommonly, neurologic dysfunction rapidly follows axial pain. Neurologic symptoms include weakness, loss of sensation, and incontinence. The symptomatic course of a cervical spine extradural lesion may be precipitous if blockage of the spinal canal occurs. Respiratory distress and diaphragmatic paralysis may occur with high cervical cord lesions.

Intradural-extramedullary tumors grow in proximity to nerve roots and are associated with radicular pain or axial skeletal pain. Meningioma and neurofibroma are slow-growing tumors, which corresponds with the slow evolution of symptoms. Nocturnal symptoms are increased; activity during the day may not be associated with symptoms. Neurologic symptoms are slower to develop than in metastatic disease.

Symptoms may persist and increase to the point that complaints associated with a herniated lumbar disc are reproduced. The slow, insidious onset of pain, without intermittency, may be helpful in identifying these patients, but in one study was not of great enough specificity to distinguish the neurofibroma patients from those with disc disease.[9] These tumors affect the nerves that travel to the upper extremities. Patients may present with dysesthesias in the shoulder and arm, without neck pain. This circumstance may occur with generalized neurofibromatosis (Recklinghausen's disease), solitary neurofibroma, or other intramedullary-extradural neoplasms (lipoma).[10]

Intramedullary tumors are frequently painless owing to their location within the spinal cord proper, which disrupts the normal transmission of pain impulses. However, not all these neoplasms are painless. Some patients may develop radicular or girdle-type pain as an early and persistent symptom. The onset may be insidious and the progression unrelenting. Frequently, weakness, spasticity, and sensory deficits below the level of the lesion develop. Some authors have described dysesthesias and "electricity-like" sensations in patients with intramedullary tumors.[11]

The pain associated with intraspinal tumors is different from the pain associated with mechanical disease of the spine. Patients with intraspinal tumors often tell of sleeping sitting up in a chair because of marked increase in severity of pain when trying to sleep in a normal position. The presence of this one part of the history should lead to a thorough evaluation for an intraspinal tumor.[12]

The motor and sensory features of compression depend on the extent and pattern of cord distribution. Pure intramedullary tumors do not disturb nerve roots. Therefore, pain is common at the level of the lesion but is not radicular. Sensory and motor loss are routinely worse at the level of the lesion and less severe distally. This pattern is in contradistinction to that of nerve root lesion or extramedullary tumor.[1] Corticospinal tract involvement with quadriparesis and spasticity is late in onset. Incontinence also occurs later in the course of the tumor. Cerebrospinal fluid blockage occurs only when the tumor is extensive throughout the cord.

Physical Examination

The physical examination is helpful in identifying patients with neurologic abnormalities by suggesting a location of a lesion affecting the spinal cord. Lesions at the level of the foramen magnum, upper cervical spine, and lower cervical spine are associated with different neurologic signs characteristic of compression of components of the spinal cord[13] (Table 13–6). Clinical findings may correspond to damage of the specific level of the spinal cord or may have effects that are proximal, secondary to descending fibers from cranial nerve V, or distal to that level, secondary to compromise of the vascular system supplying the cord, including the anterior spinal artery. In addition, extradural, intradural-extramedullary, and intramedullary tumors have distinct clinical signs that help the clinician determine the site of the tumor.

Examination of patients with extradural tumors may demonstrate pain on palpation, with associated muscle spasm and limitation of motion. Neurologic findings correspond to the level and extent of compression of the spinal roots and cord. Patients with intradural-extramedullary tumors demonstrate slowly changing neurologic abnormalities, including arm weakness or sensory changes. They may also demonstrate upper extremity muscle atrophy. Patients with multiple neurofibromas may demonstrate spinal angulation, scoliosis, and

TABLE 13–6. CLINICAL SYMPTOMS AND SIGNS OF LESIONS AT DIFFERENT CERVICAL SPINAL CORD LEVELS

	FORAMEN MAGNUM	UPPER CERVICAL SPINE	LOWER CERVICAL SPINE
Pain	Occipital/neck	Neck/shoulder	Shoulder
Pain Radiation	Shoulder/ipsilateral arm	Posterior scalp	Lower arm/hand
Sensory Loss Location	Face	Scalp	Arm/hand
Type	Decreased pin/temperature Intact tactile	Astereognosis	Paresthesias
Motor	Spastic weakness	Ipsilateral upper motor neuron	Ipsilateral arm/leg (extradural) Bilateral upper arm (intramedullary)
Reflex	Depressed arms/hands (decreased cord blood flow)	Increased or decreased	C5—biceps; C6—brachioradialis; C7—triceps; C8—Hoffman's syndrome
Other	Cranial nerves dysarthria, dysphonia, dysphagia	Diaphragmatic weakness	Horner's syndrome

kyphosis.[14] Others with Recklinghausen's disease develop paraplegia.[15] Patients with intramedullary tumors may have specific sensory changes that correlate with the location of these tumors in the center of the cord. Light touch and position sensation are normal, but pain and temperature sensation are lost. Hyperreflexia is a result of pressure on the pyramidal tracts. Hyperreflexia may also be associated with spasticity.

In addition to the neurologic examination, careful inspection of other organ systems may discover abnormalities that suggest possible diagnoses. Examination of skin may reveal café au lait patches or axillary freckles associated with neurofibromatosis. The presence of a tuft of hair, pigmented nevus, or skin dimple indicates the presence of spina bifida or tumor such as lipoma, dermoid, and epidermoid cyst.

Laboratory Data

Abnormal laboratory values are most closely associated with extradural metastatic lesions. The location, extent of spread, and histologic type of tumor have an effect on the pattern of laboratory abnormalities. Intradural tumors do not metastasize outside the spinal canal and are not associated with abnormal hematologic or chemical factors. Evaluation of cerebrospinal fluid obtained by cisternal or lumbar puncture may demonstrate marked elevation in spinal fluid protein in all of these tumors. The fluid is usually obtained during myelographic

study in a patient with suspected intraspinal tumor.

Histologic findings depend on the cell of origin of the tumor. The most common primary tumor causing extradural metastases in women is carcinoma of the breast and, in men, carcinoma of the lung.[16–18]

Intradural tumors are meningioma and neurofibroma. Meningioma is an encapsulated, nodular soft tumor with a wide range of histologic patterns, including meningothelial, fibroblastic, and psammomatous types.[19] The most common forms of cord meningioma, in order of decreasing incidence, are psammomatous, angioblastic, fibrous, and anaplastic. Neurofibroma may form fusiform swelling of a nerve root or a pedunculated mass. Intraspinal neurofibroma may take on a dumbbell form, with a central mass inside the vertebral canal connected by a shaft of tumor passing through the intervertebral foramen forming a peripheral mass.[20] Histologic patterns of neurofibroma may vary but usually contain fibrous tissue in an interlacing configuration.

Intramedullary tumors are most frequently gliomas, including ependymoma and astrocytoma. Ependymoma arises from cells that line the central ventricular system of the spinal cord. Glioma arises from glial cells, which are the supporting cells for the nerve cells of the nervous system. Glioma may be located peripherally or centrally in the spinal cord. Ependymoma and glioma are associated with a variety of histologic forms. In adults, the gliomas most often encountered are ependymoma (60%), astrocytoma (20%), glioblastoma (7%), and oligodendroglioma (4%).[12, 21]

Radiographic Evaluation

Radiographic evaluation of the patient with an intraspinal tumor can be helpful in determining the exact location of the tumor in the caudal-rostral orientation and its position in the extradural, intradural-extramedullary, or intramedullary space. Abnormalities noted on plain roentgenogram, computerized tomography (CT), or magnetic resonance (MR) imaging can pinpoint the location of lesions and help determine their potential source.

Radiographic abnormalities on plain roentgenogram of extradural tumors are characterized by destruction of bone in proximity to the growing lesion. Malignant tumors are associated with rapid destruction of bone, with loss of posterior elements of vertebral body or vertebral body collapse. On lateral roentgenogram, intraspinal lesions may be associated with posterior scalloping of the vertebral bodies, a consequence of their location and slow growth occurring more commonly in the lumbar spine than the cervical spine (Table 13–7).[22] Plain radiograph is insensitive to the presence of metastatic disease because at least 30% to 50% of bone must be destroyed before a lesion is identified.[23] In those patients with identifiable lesions in the spine, cervical spine

TABLE 13–7. POSTERIOR VERTEBRAL SCALLOPING

INCREASED INTRASPINAL PRESSURE

Generalized: communicating hydrocephalus
Localized: syringomyelia, intraspinal cysts, intradural neoplasms

BONE RESORPTION

Acromegaly

CONGENITAL DISORDERS

Idiopathic
Neurofibromatosis
Marfan's syndrome
Ehlers-Danlos syndrome
Mucopolysaccharidosis IV (Morquio's disease)
Dysostosis multiplex (Hurler's syndrome)
Osteogenesis imperfecta

SMALL SPINAL CANAL

Achondroplasia

NORMAL VARIANT

Physiologic scalloping

Modified from Mitchell GE, Lourie H, Berne AS: The various causes of scalloped vertebrae with notes on their pathogenesis. Radiology 89:67–74, 1967.

involvement occurs less frequently than other portions of the axial spine.[24] Neurofibroma may grow through intervertebral foramina, which results in uniform dilatation when compared with adjacent foramina (Fig. 13–19). Intramedullary tumors rarely cause anatomic alterations that are discernible on plain roentgenogram. Changes on plain roentgenogram are seen in 10% or less of patients with spinal meningioma.[25]

Myelographic studies are useful in determining the exact location of an intraspinal tumor.[26–28] Extradural tumor frequently causes a complete block of the myelographic dye at the point of spinal cord compression. The block has irregular edges, varies radiographic densities, and displaces the spinal contents. In a study of patients with metastatic cancer of the spine, 15% of 130 cases had a complete block or high-grade partial block on myelogram in the absence of bony abnormalities on plain roentgenogram.[29]

The myelographic features may be divided into the following four basic forms: (1) a lesion may be situated peripherally, displacing the dura and cord, resulting in a widening of the space between the dye column and pedicle on the side with the tumor and narrowing contralaterally; (2) an anterior or posterior tumor may cause flattening of the cord. This finding may simulate that associated with intramedullary tumors; (3) a shallow filling defect without cord displacement may be seen; and (4) a lesion that encircles the cord causes constriction of the subarachnoid space without cord displacement.

An intradural-extramedullary lesion produces a sharp, smooth concave outline because the tumor is in direct contact with the dye. The spinal cord may be displaced to one side, and spinal nerve roots may be stretched over the lesion.

Intramedullary tumor arises in the spinal cord. The myelogram demonstrates fusiform enlargement of the spinal cord, with tapering of the column of dye superiorly and inferiorly. Not all fusiform swelling of the cord is secondary to intramedullary tumor. Extradural tumor may flatten the contralateral aspect of the cord. Therefore, films must be taken at 90° angles so that an intramedullary lesion is not confused with an extradural lesion.

CT may be used after placement of myelographic dye to better delineate the status of the spinal cord. CT/myelogram is helpful in locating an extension of tumor from vertebrae and paravertebral structures to the epidural space.[30] For example, lesions in the superior

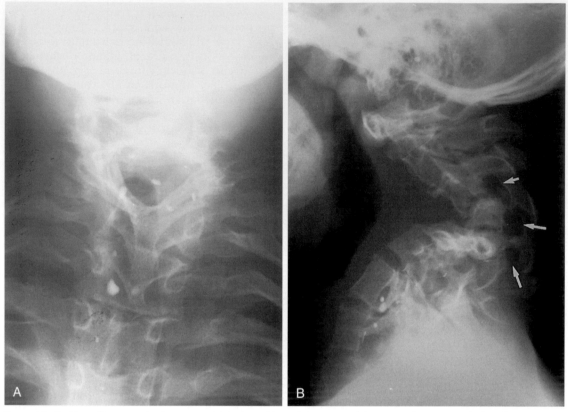

Figure 13–19. Neurofibromatosis. Anteroposterior, *A*, and lateral, *B*, views of the cervical spine. Marked scoliotic curve of cervical spine with reversal of normal lordotic curve. The neural foramina are expanded, corresponding to the growth of neurofibroma *(arrows).* (Courtesy of Anne Brower, M.D.)

pulmonary sulcus (Pancoast's tumors) may invade the brachial plexus and extend into the epidural space through an intervertebral foramen.[31–33] These lesions cause radicular pain in the setting of normal plain roentgenogram and bone scintigraphy. CT/myelogram evaluation of the spinal column detects these lesions missed by other radiographic techniques. CT techniques are useful in detecting alterations in bone architecture in those individuals unable to undergo MR imaging studies (Fig. 13–20). CT technology has progressed to the development of three-dimensional imaging of the bony architecture of the spine.[34] The technique has been used in the lumbar spine for the detection of foraminal stenosis and the status of postoperative fusions. In anticipation of stabilization surgery, the same technology may also be applied to the cervical spine to determine the extent of damage to structures from extradural tumors.

MR imaging has revolutionized the visualization of intraspinal lesions.[35] MR is the single best modality for imaging spinal tumor. It is the best technique for distinguishing soft tissue densities (normal versus neoplastic) inside bony structures.[36] Extradural, intradural-extramedullary, and intramedullary tumors can be clearly depicted by MR imaging in multiple planes and can be distinguished from cerebrospinal fluid without the need for contrast media (Figs. 13–21 and 13–22).

The addition of gadolinium contrast agent to the technique of MR imaging has helped increase the sensitivity of this method in the detection of intraspinal tumors. In one study of intraspinal tumor, gadolinium enhancement detected ependymoma (intense, homogeneous, sharply margined lesions) and astrocytoma (patchy, ill-defined lesions).[37] The differences in appearance of these two lesions were not adequate to allow MR imaging to be useful in differentiating the histology of these intraspinal tumors. However, enhancement with gadolinium helps better define the locations, size, configuration, and character of the lesion.[38] Intradural-extramedullary tumor is also enhanced by MR imaging with gadolinium contrast agent. The mechanism of enhancement is not breakdown of the blood-

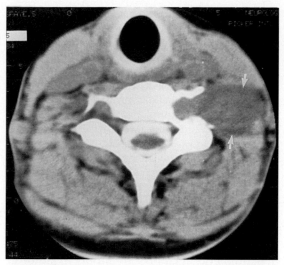

Figure 13–20. Neurofibromatosis. Computerized tomography scan of C6 vertebral body with soft tissue mass growing from the neural foramen, compatible with neurofibroma *(arrows)*. (Courtesy of Thomas Dina, M.D.)

brain barrier but the highly vascular character of tumors such as meningioma and neurinoma. Gadolinium is also helpful in detecting leptomeningeal spread of metastatic tumor and in differentiating cystic lesion (syringomyelia) from intramedullary tumor that has similar radiographic characteristics on unenhanced MR images. In patients with unexpected neurologic signs, contrast-enhanced MR imaging may detect metastases to the pial membrane secondary to lymphoma, leukemia, adenocarcinoma of the lung, prostate carci-

noma, and malignant melanoma, allowing for better resolution of lesions with shorter imaging times.[39] However, the changes in MR parameters have significant effects on the resulting images. For example, on T_1-weighted images, gadolinium enhancement results in marrow metastases becoming isointense with normal bone marrow, obscuring their presence. Therefore, discussion with neuroradiologists concerning the techniques used in obtaining the MR images is essential in determining the images' clinical significance.

Differential Diagnosis

The diagnosis of intraspinal tumor is suggested by the presence of persistent neck pain, neurologic dysfunction, and radiographic abnormalities. The definitive diagnosis requires histologic confirmation. A high level of suspicion is necessary to make this diagnosis. Patients with intradural tumor, such as neurofibroma, may present with upper extremity symptoms of long duration. This association must be kept in mind or the correct diagnosis may be missed.[40]

EXTRADURAL LESIONS

The differential diagnosis of extradural lesions includes neoplastic and non-neoplastic lesions. Metastatic lesions from the lung, prostate, and breast are the most frequent cause of

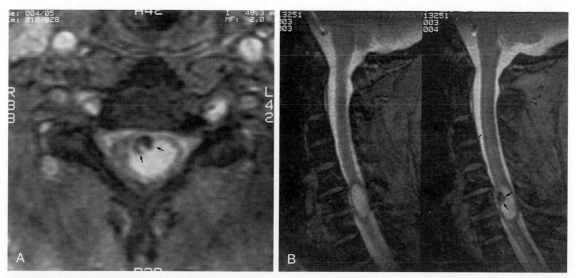

Figure 13–21. Intramedullary tumor. Magnetic resonance scan of T_1-weighted axial, *A*, and sagittal, *B*, views of cervical spinal cord. A large intramedullary tumor (glioma) with possible area of hemorrhage *(arrows)* is noted. (Courtesy of Thomas Dina, M.D.)

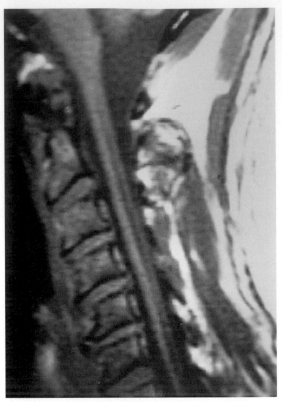

Figure 13–22. Syringomyelia. Magnetic resonance T_1-weighted sagittal image of the cervical spine with an enlarged central cavity that is isodense with cerebrospinal fluid. (Courtesy of Thomas Dina, M.D.)

epidural lesions. Primary tumors—lymphoma, chordoma, meningiomas, fibroma, and lipoma—also may cause epidural lesions. Fibrosarcoma is a rare extradural tumor of the cervical spine.[41, 42] This tumor may need to be differentiated from benign lesions, such as giant cell, and malignant lesions, such as osteosarcoma.

Epidural Abscess. This is a potential, disastrous non-neoplastic epidural lesion associated with delayed diagnosis. These patients present with acute-onset, severe neck pain and progressive neurologic dysfunction that can progress to quadriparesis within hours.[43] In a study of 43 spinal epidural abscesses, 7 (15%) were in the cervical spine and 14 (30%) were in the lumbar spine.[44] These patients, who are predominantly men, usually have evidence of a bacterial infection elsewhere, are acutely ill with fever and disoriented, and exhibit signs of a parameningeal infection on cerebrospinal fluid examination. On myelogram, the extradural defect may extend over several vertebral levels.[45] MR imaging has increased the opportunity to make the correct diagnosis of extra-

dural abscess without the need for invasive procedures, such as myelogram (see the section on epidural abscess in Chapter 12). MR evaluation of the cervical spine is able to determine the extent of the abscess and differentiate it from spinal cord, vertebral bodies, intervertebral discs, and paraspinal soft tissues.[46]

Epidural Hematoma. Spontaneous epidural hematoma may mimic the course of time and symptoms of epidural abscess.[47] The bleeding may be associated with a small extradural vascular malformation or occur spontaneously without any specific anatomic abnormality. Most reported epidural hematoma is spontaneous and acute. The decreasing order of frequency of axial involvement is cervical, thoracic, and lumbar spine.[48] Cervical epidural hematoma occurs more commonly in children and young adults.[49] Most hematomas extend two or more segments and are located in a posterolateral position.[50] Chronic epidural hematoma is rare but does occur in the cervical spine.[51]

A variety of structural and physiologic abnormalities have been associated with development of spontaneous hematoma. Patients with extradural cavernous hemangioma and bleeding have developed symptoms of neck pain and stiffness as well as radicular arm pain secondary to nerve root compression.[52, 53] Epidural hematoma has been reported as complications of invasive procedures, including surgery and myelograms, and may occur in patients who are normotensive with normal blood coagulability.[54–56] Bleeding may also occur in a patient on anticoagulants.[57] Hematoma may also be a complication of patients with axial arthritis, including ankylosing spondylitis.[58]

Most patients with spinal epidural hematoma have axial pain that may radiate in a radicular pattern.[59] The motor, sensory, and sphincter function abnormalities correspond to the level of the spinal axis damaged. Dysfunction usually has onset from minutes to hours. The diagnosis is corroborated by a mass with a T_1-weighted increased signal intensity and T_2-weighted decreased signal intensity on MR image.[60] Surgical intervention is required in the setting of neurologic dysfunction. Fresh frozen plasma and vitamin K may be given to patients with anticoagulation. Platelet transfusions may be tried in patients with thrombocytopenia. Prompt surgical decompression is required because the prognosis for neurologic recovery depends on the extent of damage and the duration of neurologic dysfunction. Patients with the best chance of recovery have surgical decompression rapidly and have incomplete sensorimotor deficits. Cervical and thoracic hematomas have a poorer prognosis compared with that for lumbar hematomas.[59]

Epidural Lipomatosis. High-dose corticosteroid therapy may cause the accumulation of fat in an epidural location. Patients who have renal transplants, asthma, rheumatoid arthritis, radiation pneumonitis, polyarteritis nodosa, Cushing's disease, or morbid obesity have developed epidural lipomatosis.[61] Corticosteroids in doses ranging from 5 to 180 mg/day have been associated with lipomatosis. The onset of lipomatosis may occur in 6 months to 13 years after starting therapy. Cervical spine involvement is rare compared with disease located in the thoracic and lumbar areas.[62] Transaxial CT scan reveals abundant soft tissue surrounding the thecal sac. T_1-weighted MR imaging reveals increased signal intensity in the lipid mass. Fat has an almost pathognomonic appearance on MR images (increased T_1-weighted signal and intermediate T_2-weighted signal intensity). MR imaging is ideal for identifying extradural fat.[63] The treatment for this condition may be surgical or medical. Multilevel laminectomy may improve symptoms and signs but is also associated with significant mortality in patients requiring high-dose steroid treatment.[61] With cessation of steroid therapy, however, epidural fat deposits may disappear with resolution of symptoms.[64]

Spinal Synovial Cyst. Intraspinal synovial cyst arises from the joint lining of the apophyseal joint and occurs on rare occasions in the cervical spine.[65] The cyst occurs most frequently in the lumbar spine at the L4–L5 level.[66] This lesion is associated with degenerative joint disease and trauma. Cervical spine cyst may occur in individuals whose occupations have considerable neck movement, including assembly-line workers, dentists, and salespeople.[65] These extradural lesions may be asymptomatic or may cause myelopathic symptoms and signs associated with sensory and motor dysfunction, including paraparesis.[67] Spinal synovial cyst may appear and cause symptoms acutely with a traumatic event or slowly throughout a number of years.[68, 69] CT appearance of intraspinal synovial cyst is characterized by a cystic mass with a broad base extending from the apophyseal joint. Calcification of the cyst may occur in a chronic stage after hemorrhage.[68] The presence of an attachment between the apophyseal joint and the synovial cyst can be proven by injection of contrast material into the joint and its subsequent dispersal throughout the cyst.[70] MR imaging allows for the evaluation of synovial cyst at the C1–C2 level.[71] Cysts that cause nerve root compression or neurogenic claudication require surgical decompression.[65] Ganglion cysts arising from the ligamentum flavum in the cervical spine, independent of the neighboring apophyseal joint, have been described causing myelopathic signs secondary to cervical spinal cord compression. These lesions also require surgical removal.[72]

INTRADURAL-EXTRAMEDULLARY LESIONS

Intradural-extramedullary lesions in adults are predominantly primary tumors of the neural tissues, including neurofibroma, neurilemoma (schwannoma), meningioma, and vascular malformation. Neurofibroma arises from proliferating nerve fibers, fibroblasts, and Schwann cells. Neurilemoma consists of Schwann's cells and collagen fibers. Meningioma arises from the meninges, which support the spinal cord. The arachnoid may also be a source of lesions as well as vessel abnormalities.[13]

Neurofibroma. Recclinghausen's neurofibromatosis type-1 (peripheral neurofibromatosis) is the most common hereditary syndrome, predisposing to neoplasm at a rate of 1 in 3,000 live births in the United States.[73] Neurofibromatosis type-2 is associated with bilateral acoustic neuroma. These entities are genetically separate, type-1 associated with a locus on chromosome 17 and type-2 associated with a deletion on the long arm of chromosome 22.[74] Neurofibroma, like neurilemoma, contains Schwann's cells but can be differentiated by histologic examination because the former has a more disorganized, plexiform appearance. Among 322 patients with nerve sheath tumors, the cervical spine was affected in 26% of cases, the thoracic spine in 41%, the lumbar spine in 31%, and the sacrum in 2%.[75–77] The tumor may involve sensory or motor roots or the entire nerve. Neurofibroma may occur singly or multiply (Recclinghausen's disease). The autosomal dominant disease with variable penetrance may be easily recognized when the cutaneous manifestations (café au lait spots, axillary freckling, and cutaneous neurofibroma) are present. The disease may become manifest when the patient is a child or is an adult with kyphoscoliosis, vertebral scalloping, and intervertebral foramen widening.[78] Malignant deterioration of neurofibroma occurs in 3% of cases and is more likely to occur in patients with multiple tumors as opposed to solitary lesion.[79]

Neurofibroma occurs in adults 30 to 60 years of age.[76] The primary symptom is pain that may be axial, radicular, or referred. Pain is exacerbated at night on recumbency, Valsalva's maneuver, or sneezing. Abnormalities, including loss of reflexes, motor function (muscle atrophy), and sensory function (loss of touch), are present at the time of diagnosis. Spinal cord compression signs are asymmetrical. Motor function is impaired on the side of the tumor, and pain and temperature loss are experienced on the opposite side. Motor loss is usually spastic, with involvement of flexor muscles rather than extensor muscles. The time from the onset of symptoms to diagnosis may average 1 to 4 years. The shortest period before diagnosis is associated with cervical lesions.[76]

Plain roentgenogram demonstrates intervertebral foramen widening, erosion of a pedicle, or widening of the interpedicular distance with tumors that extend into the extradural area. A normal roentgenogram is associated with a completely intradural tumor.[80] MR findings in patients with type-1 and type-2 neurofibromatosis include multiple masses in both extramedullary and intradural locations.[81] Skeletal abnormalities include dural ectasias and posterior scalloping. In a study of 47 neurofibromatosis patients, scoliosis occurred in 17% of the cases.[82] The primary location for spinal deformation secondary to neurofibromatosis is the thoracic spine.[83] Neurofibroma in the cervical spine vertebrae may be associated with abnormalities affecting the vertebral arteries.[84] Arterial disease may cause symptoms that may be attributed to neurofibroma. Evaluation with angiography identifies those patients with both anomalies. Surgical removal of tumors is the preferred therapy if spinal cord or nerve root compression is present. The opportunity for tumor removal is diminished in the setting of multiple lesions.

Neurilemoma. Neurilemoma (schwannoma) is also a common cord tumor, constituting 30% to 35% of all primary intraspinal neoplasms, occurring most often in adults 30 to 40 years of age. Neurilemoma is a solitary tumor consisting of Schwann's cells and is more frequently found on sensory nerve roots than on motor roots.[40] This tumor is considered benign. It grows slowly, causing symptoms by exerting pressure on adjacent structures.[12] In keeping with lesions exerting pressure on adjacent structures, neurilemoma is one of the extraosseous spinal lesions mimicking disc dis-

ease.[85] Patients with intraspinal tumors have painless neurologic deficits, pain on recumbency, pain disproportionate to that expected with disc disease, no improvement with disc surgery, and elevated spinal fluid protein. Neurilemoma is not limited to the cervical spine but may also affect the cervical sympathetic plexus, brachial plexus, and spinal accessory nerve.[86] MR evaluation of the cervical spine is a noninvasive means of scanning the cervical spine and surrounding soft tissues for this tumor. This tumor is encapsulated and is amenable to surgical removal without loss of neurologic function.[86]

Meningioma. Meningioma is a benign, well-circumscribed tumor that constitutes about 25% of all primary intraspinal neoplasms.[13] This tumor affects adults older than 50 years of age. Approximately 80% of patients are women.[87] As opposed to neurofibroma, meningioma tends to remain intradural. Only 10% of meningiomas are extradural.[87] In two studies of 705 and 97 spinal meningiomas, the cervical spine was the site of involvement in 17% of patients.[25, 87] They are most common in the thoracic spine. Meningioma differs from neurofibroma by occurring in adults 50 to 70 years of age, being located commonly in a lateral position, having a dumbbell shape only on occasion, calcifying more often, and producing sensory abnormalities more prominently than motor symptoms. Pain is the most common early complaint with spinal meningioma. The pain is axial or radicular in radiation. Sensory disturbances include paresthesias and numbness. Motor weakness in the form of hemiplegia has been reported in patients with meningiomas affecting the upper cervical spine near the craniocervical junction.[88] The average duration of symptoms before diagnosis is 2 years, but about 50% of patients come to surgery within a year of onset. Plain roentgenogram is not helpful in identifying the location of intradural tumor. The ideal treatment is surgical excision of the tumor and its dural attachment. CT scan may be helpful if the location of the lesion has been identified by another radiographic technique. MR imaging with contrast agent is the most sensitive technique for identifying the location of the tumor.[89] Extensive tumors may be successfully removed with the appropriate surgical approach and technique.[90, 91]

Intradural Lipoma. Intradural lipoma may occur in the presence or absence of a spinal malformation. The prevalence of spinal lipoma with spinal dysraphism is 90%. This form of lesion is associated with pediatric patients with congenital abnormalities. In adults, spinal lipoma may be present without evidence of other structural abnormalities. However, about one third of intradural lesions in adults is associated with some malformation. Therefore, a distinction may not truly exist between the childhood and adult lesions. The cervicothoracic region is the most common location for the adult lesion.[92] The duration of symptoms before diagnosis is usually measured in years. Numbness and ataxia rather than pain may be the initial symptoms.[92] In time, the symptoms of cord compression become more obvious. MR imaging is the best radiographic technique for identifying the location of lipoma.[93] Surgical excision of the lesion is the most effective therapy.[10, 94]

Arachnoid Cyst. Cysts may arise from the arachnoid of the spinal cord. They are known by the terms arachnoid cyst or diverticulum.[95] These lesions occur in young adults, most commonly in the thoracic spine and less commonly in the cervical area. Most cysts are asymptomatic. Patients with this lesion may have fluctuating neck and arm pain that is made worse by physical activity. Pain is relieved on recumbency. The presence of posterior scalloping of a vertebral body helps raise the possibility of this lesion in a patient with neurologic symptoms. The lesion is identified with MR imaging or myelogram. Surgical removal is usually effective in relieving symptoms.[96]

Arachnoiditis. Arachnoiditis is a nonspecific inflammatory process causing fibrosis of arachnoid membrane. The pathogenesis of arachnoiditis involves the development of a mild inflammatory cellular exudate similar to the inflammatory response necessary to repair serous membranes like the peritoneum.[97] A fibrous exudate covers the nerve roots and causes them to adhere to one another and the thecal sac. Proliferating fibrocytes form dense collagenous adhesions around the spinal cord or nerve roots. Arachnoiditis evolves from a stage of inflammation of the pia-arachnoid, with hyperemia and swelling of the nerve tissue followed by arachnoiditis and fibroblast proliferation and adhesion. The final stage of arachnoiditis causes complete encapsulation of the structure, with hypoxia and atrophy of the nerve tissue.[78, 98]

Causes of arachnoiditis are listed in Table 13–8.[99–101] Frequently implicated in the development of arachnoiditis are oily contrast agents (such as iophendylate) when they are not removed from the spinal canal after myelography. In any event, oily contrast agents have been replaced with water-soluble contrast

TABLE 13–8. CAUSES OF ARACHNOIDITIS

Surgery
  Extradural
    Discectomy
    Laminectomy
    Lumbar spine fusion
  Intradural
    Closure of spinal fistula
    Nerve root severed
Injected agents
  Contrast media
  Anesthetic agents
  Intradural steroids
Space-occupying lesion
  Neurofibroma
Infection
Intrathecal hemorrhage

agents that are unassociated with the development of arachnoiditis. Other exogenous agents associated with arachnoiditis include infection (tuberculosis)[102] and intrathecal medications, including anesthetics such as bupivacaine.[103, 104] Arachnoiditis may be the cause of unsuccessful spine surgery, with scar formation affecting the spinal cord at the surgical level.[105] Retained swab debris may be one potential source of the inflammatory response.[106]

The clinical symptoms associated with arachnoiditis include diffuse constant neck pain, radicular pain, paresthesias, dysesthesias, causalgia, motor weakness, and sphincter dysfunction. Physical signs may include neck tenderness, muscular spasm, atrophy, hyporeflexia in the upper extremities, and hyperreflexia in the lower extremities.

Inflammatory changes of the arachnoid space (arachnoiditis) may cause changes on myelogram that should not be confused with an arachnoid cyst. Cysts cause localized lesions. Arachnoiditis causes loculations of contrast dye, partial or complete obstruction of dye flow, and obliteration of nerve root sleeves. MR scan is the best radiographic technique for evaluating arachnoiditis. In the upper spinal cord, arachnoiditis may be visualized as thickening of the leptomeninges. If the cord is involved with the inflammation, it lies eccentrically within the canal.[107] Arachnoiditis that fills the subarachnoid space may have MR characteristics that mirror those of a spinal cord tumor.[108] Gadolinium-enhanced MR imaging does not increase the signal intensity of arachnoiditis.[109] The absence of gadolinium enhancement helps differentiate neoplastic lesions from arachnoiditis.

The disability of arachnoiditis patients is related to the severe pain they experience. The physical impairments change relatively little during the course of the disease. Urinary symptoms characterized by urgency, frequency, and incontinence develop late in its course. These patients have a poor prognosis because no therapy has been developed that consistently decreases inflammation or diminishes the symptoms.

Another disorder associated with thickening of the dura is pachymeningitis hypertrophica.[110] This disorder may affect the dura in the cervical spinal cord. The natural history is one of progression from local pain to radiculopathy and spinal cord compression. Surgical removal of the thickened dura is associated with resolution of neurologic symptoms. The response to surgical therapy is in clear distinction from the lack of improvement with surgery for arachnoiditis.

Arteriovenous Malformation (AVM). Vascular malformations may be located in the cervical spinal column. Lesions may be arterial, capillary, cavernous, or arteriovenous (Table 13–9). Vascular malformations and neoplasms account for 5% to 10% of space-occupying lesions of the spine.[13] Malformations are more common than tumors. Vascular lesions affect the thoracic spinal cord more commonly than the other portions. About 20% of AVMs are located in the cervical segments.[49] Increased pressure in vessels causes structural alterations that result in vessel enlargement. Dysfunction of the spinal cord may occur secondary to impingement by the vessel mass or impairment of normal venous drainage may occur secondary to abnormally high pressure in spinal cord capillaries. The majority of adults with AVMs are older than 30 years of age and are men.[111]

The clinical course is one of progressive symptoms of neck and radicular pain, dysesthesias, and painful claudication. Episodes of vessel thrombosis may accentuate the symptoms and signs. The symptom course of these patients may be hours to weeks. The symptom of exercise claudication with gradual onset of neurologic symptoms, including quadriparesis, helps distinguish vascular abnormalities from other tumors.[112] Patients with cervical AVM and other vascular tumors are at risk of developing subarachnoid hemorrhages.[113] Some of these vascular lesions causing hemorrhages may be extramedullary or intramedullary.[114–116] Cervical subarachnoid bleeds may be difficult to differentiate from intracranial bleeds. This may include photophobia, change in mentation, and meningismus as well as signs of cord compression. Physical examination of patients with a bleed should include inspection for cutaneous angioma and auscultation over the spine for bruits associated with vascular malformations.[49]

Vascular lesions, including feeding vessels, draining veins, and vascular nidus, are best localized by spinal angiography.[117, 118] AVMs may not always be visualized by MR evaluation.[119] However, MR imaging is a useful technique for the study of AVMs and is able to detect myelomalacia, edema, and reversible scalloping of the spinal cord; thrombosis and thickening of blood vessels; new bleeding versus old hematoma; and the alterations associated with angiographic or surgical correction of the lesion.[120, 121] Cerebrospinal fluid evaluation may demonstrate elevated protein level and red blood cell count in the setting of a recent bleed. Normal cerebrospinal fluid does not eliminate the possibility of AVM. Indications for therapy is for prevention of recurrent bleeding and progressive neurologic dysfunction. Asymptomatic lesions are left undisturbed. Therapy for AVMs and vascular tumors includes the use of embolization, alone or preoperatively.[122, 123] Embolization or surgery may decrease the risk of bleeding but at the risk of increased neurologic dysfunction.

Vascular malformations may also be identified in an intramedullary location. These intramedullary vascular lesions are located in the cervical and thoracic spine. Lesions in the cervical spine are associated with arm and leg dysfunction, and thoracic cord lesions are associated with lower extremity motor and sensory abnormalities.[124, 125] Once identified, these lesions may be left alone, embolized, or treated surgically.[126] Clinical improvement is common in patients who have operative resection or angiographic ablation.[127, 128]

Leptomeningeal Metastases. Leptomenin-

TABLE 13–9. SPINAL CORD VASCULAR TUMORS AND MALFORMATIONS

Vascular tumors
  Capillary hemangioblastoma
Vascular tumors of the meninges
  Hemangioblastoma
  Hemangiopericytoma
Vascular malformations
  Capillary telangiectasia
  Cavernous angioma
  Arteriovenous malformation
    Dural
    Intradural
  Venous malformation

Modified from Byrne TN, Waxman SG: Spinal Cord Compression: Diagnosis and Principles of Management. Philadelphia: FA Davis Co, 1990, pp. 1–278.

geal spread of tumor is relatively rare because the dura is a barrier to the spread of malignant tumors. In adults, this form of metastasis occurs with breast cancer, lung or oat cell carcinoma, melanoma, non-Hodgkin's lymphoma, and leukemia.[129] In one study, 5% of patients with breast cancer had leptomeningeal involvement.[130] Patients may also have concomitant intraparenchymal brain metastases or epidural lesions.

The hallmark of leptomeningeal metastases is the multifocal nature of the neurologic deficits. The symptom of neck or back pain, as part of the list of multiple abnormalities, occurs in 25% of patients with widespread leptomeningeal disease.[129] This list may include extremity weakness, paresthesias, radicular pain, causalgia, sphincter dysfunction, and all the symptoms of cauda equina compression. On physical examination, patients have focal weakness, asymmetrical reflexes, and spotty sensory loss. The diagnosis is confirmed by cerebrospinal fluid cytologic examination.[131] A variety of biochemical markers may be obtained from cerebrospinal fluid to better determine the source of cancerous cells and the response to therapy.[13] MR scan, with or with-

out contrast agent, is able to identify leptomeningeal metastases in a minority of patients[132] (Fig. 13–23). Patients may be treated with irradiation or intrathecal therapy. The prognosis is usually poor. The median survival rate of patients with leptomeningeal tumors is 4 to 6 months.[133]

INTRAMEDULLARY LESIONS

Intramedullary lesions are primarily glioma, vascular malformation, syringomyelia, lipoma, lymphoma, and melanoma. Other lesions that may cause intramedullary cord lesions include multiple sclerosis, sarcoidosis, abscess, myelitis, radiation exposure, nutritional deficiency, cord infarction, and vasculitis. These lesions may occur with neurologic dysfunction without neck pain.

Syringomyelia. Syringomyelia is a fluid-filled cyst lined with benign glial cells that is located in the central portion of the spinal cord. Syringomyelia may be classified into communicating and noncommunicating types (Table 13–10). Communicating types are associated with obstructive lesions at the foramen magnum,

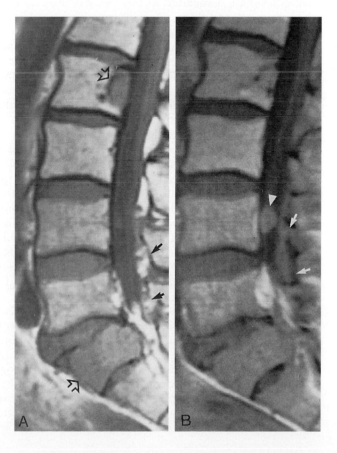

Figure 13–23. Intradural metastasis: magnetic resonance (MR) imaging. Spin echo MR imaging technique with and without gadolinium enhancement. In this 72-year-old female with metastatic breast carcinoma, precontrast, *A* and postcontrast, *B*, sagittal T_1-weighted (TR/TE 400/20) spin echo MR images are shown. The linear streak of enhancement agent along the dorsal surface of the spinal cord *(arrows)* represents the site of pial metastasis. (From Lim V, Sobel DF, Zyroff J: Spinal cord pial metastases: MR imaging with gadopentetate dimeglumine. AJNR 11(5):975–982, 1990. © by American Society of Neuroradiology.)

TABLE 13–10. CLASSIFICATION OF SYRINGOMYELIA

COMMUNICATING (SYRINGOHYDROMYELIA)

Associated with developmental abnormalities of the cranial-cervical junction and posterior fossa (e.g., Arnold-Chiari malformation)

Associated with acquired obstructive lesions of the foramen magnum (basilar meningitis)

NONCOMMUNICATING

Traumatic myelopathy
Spinal arachnoiditis
Spinal cord tumors
Idiopathic

Modified from Byrne TN, Waxman SG: Spinal Cord Compression: Diagnosis and Principles of Management. Philadelphia: FA Davis Co, 1990, pp 1–278.

resulting in alterations in cerebrospinal fluid flow. These cysts, attached to the central canal, are lined with glial cells. Noncommunicating types are a consequence of lesions of the spinal cord. For example, arachnoiditis may cause syrinx formation by obliterating the spinal vasculature supplying the center of the cord, thereby causing ischemia. These cysts are lined with cells associated with the pathologic process that caused the lesion (tumor cells). Syringomyelia is associated with congenital abnormalities (Arnold-Chiari malformations—cerebellar tissue extending through the foramen magnum; and downward displacement of the medulla), trauma, infections (meningitis), or inflammatory abnormalities (arachnoiditis).[134]

This lesion is found most commonly in the cervical spine.[135] The cyst frequently extends from below the first cervical segment to the thoracic spinal cord. Cysts frequently span seven or more cord levels.[136] The cavity is located within the gray matter of the cord, posterior to the central canal. The cyst contains fluid with the composition of cerebrospinal fluid but may not always be connected to the central canal. The lesion most commonly occurs in men 25 to 40 years of age.

Syringomyelia, by its growth laterally and longitudinally through the spinal cord, first causes loss of pain sensation, then abnormalities of motor function, with weakness in the extremities and scoliosis in the axial skeleton, long tract signs (Babinski's reflex), and autonomic dysfunction of the bladder and rectum. The sensory loss is bilateral, over the shoulders secondary to the loss of decussating pain and temperature fibers with preservation of posterior column fibers. The onset or exacerbation of symptoms may be marked by a minor trauma, a sneeze, or cough. Pain in the neck is a symptom in 24% of patients.[134] If pain is exacerbated by Valsalva's maneuver or minor strain, the cyst may be associated with a compressive lesion, such as an Arnold-Chiari malformation.[137] This lesion may be associated with brain stem and cerebellar signs. Muscle weakness is associated with atrophy and loss of reflexes. Neuropathic joint disease, particularly of the shoulder, is a recognized complication of a cervical syringomyelia.[138] Lesions of the cervicothoracic junction affect the intermediolateral column and result in Horner's syndrome.

Plain roentgenogram of the cervical spine may demonstrate a variety of abnormalities, including canal widening, basilar impression, atlantoaxial dislocation, and occipitalization of the atlas, that are associated with congenital lesion and syringomyelia.[139] Diagnosis in the past was made by myelography or CT.[140] MR imaging has become the technique of choice for localizing syringomyelia.[141] MR is able to differentiate intramedullary neoplasms from cysts[142] (Fig. 13–24).

The treatment of syringomyelia is guided by the progression of the symptoms and signs associated with the lesion. Approximately 22% of patients may have no progression of symptoms over a 20 year period.[13] Patients with progressive symptoms require therapy that includes surgical removal of the fluid in the cystic cavity by needle aspiration or myelotomy.[143] The surgical therapy for syringomyelia must be approached with consideration of the pathogenesis of the specific lesion. Different shunting procedures are required depending on the location of the lesion.[144] Without effective therapeutic intervention to halt the progressive growth of the lesion, patients with syringomyelia experience marked disability, with spastic paraplegia, arthropathy, and infectious complications. Syringomyelia may develop years after the surgical removal of lesions from the spinal cord.[145]

Neoplasms. Intramedullary tumors, mostly ependymoma and astrocytoma, grow slowly and insidiously in adults with few symptoms for many years. In adults, ependymoma comprises the majority of intramedullary tumors, accounting for nearly 65% of lesions.[40] Astrocytoma causes 20% to 25% of primary intraspinal neoplasms. Glioblastoma and oligodendroglioma occur much less frequently.

Ependymoma occurs most commonly in the caudal portion of the spinal canal. The cervical spinal cord is the location of ependymoma in 20% of patients.[146] Men are more frequently

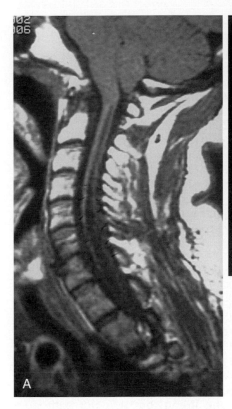

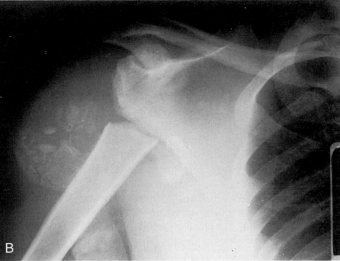

Figure 13–24. Syringomyelia. A 52-year-old female developed a neuropathic shoulder joint over a 6-week period. *A*, magnetic resonance scan of T_1-weighted sagittal image of cervical spinal cord shows isodense area in central cord extending from the level of C1 to the thoracic spine. *B*, Anteroposterior view of the right shoulder shows disorganization, destruction, and decidua characteristic of a neuropathic joint. (Courtesy of Anne Brower, M.D.)

affected than women, 63% and 57%, respectively.[147] The clinical symptoms associated with ependymomas may include local, radicular, or funicular (ascending spinal tract involvement) pain. Neck pain is a symptom in a minority of patients. Astrocytoma occurs more commonly in the medullary portion of the spinal cord than ependymoma. The cervical spinal cord is affected in 33% of patients with astrocytoma.[40] Astrocytoma most commonly affects men 34 to 40 years of age. Clinical symptoms and signs are similar to those of cervical ependymoma. When the lesion is in the cervical spine, upper extremity atrophy may be associated with lower extremity spasticity. Benign astrocytoma is a slow-growing tumor associated with slowly progressive clinical symptoms. Cerebrospinal fluid evaluation of both types of tumors demonstrates elevated protein concentration with a minimal increase in cerebrospinal leukocytes.

Radiographic evaluation with myelogram demonstrates a fusiform expansion of the spinal cord. Contrast-enhanced MR imaging is particularly effective at identifying the presence of intramedullary tumors. In one study of 32 spinal tumors, 30 intramedullary neoplasms were enhanced. Ependymomas and astrocytomas were located and differentiated.[37] Enhanced MR imaging has advantages over other radiographic techniques in differentiating

solid tumor from syrinx and cysts. MR imaging is also able to detect hemorrhage within tumor masses.[148] Also, recurrent or residual tumor can be differentiated from scar tissue in postoperative patients. The diagnosis of lesions in the spinal cord requires biopsy of the lesion. MR imaging is unable to differentiate neoplastic from benign lesions in all cases.[149]

The treatment of these lesions is microsurgical removal of the accessible ones. Resection is completed to the extent consistent with preservation of neurologic function. Ependymomas are more readily removed in their entirety compared with astrocytomas.[150] Postoperative irradiation is helpful for those patients who have not had complete resection of the lesion but does not result in as good a clinical outcome.[151] The 10-year survival rate of patients with ependymoma is 80%.[152–154] Only a minority of these patients have experienced neurologic deterioration during the follow-up period. Crisante and Herrmann described the functional outcome of 69 patients with intramedullary tumors, including ependymoma, astrocytoma, lipoma, neurofibroma, and oligodendroglioma.[155] Surgery on lesions in the lower cervical spinal cord had a greater morbidity rate than those in other locations in the cord. Patients with ependymoma had a better recovery rate than those with astrocytomas.

Primary tumors such as lipoma, lymphoma, and melanoma are very rare causes of intramedullary tumor. For example, lipomas are 2% of intramedullary tumors.[40] Compared with extradural metastases, intramedullary metastatic lesions are uncommon.[5] Some patients with intramedullary metastases may develop symptoms over 6 months. The common sources for metastases to the cord are, in descending order, lung, breast, lymphoma, colorectal, head and neck, and renal cell. The prognosis is poor, with a 20% survival rate at 3 months in one study.[156] Angioma may also be an intramedullary lesion. The cervical spinal cord is affected less frequently than the thoracic cord. This lesion may be confused with syringomyelia.[157] Surgical removal is possible without significant neurologic deficit.[158]

Vasculitis/Infarction. In the region below T8, the spinal cord is supplied anteriorly by the anterior spinal artery that arises from a single large vessel, the artery of Adamkiewicz, that arises from a segmental vessel between T9 and L2 on the left side. This artery is the largest vessel to reach the spinal cord and supplies 25% of the cord in 50% of individuals.[159] Branches of the anterior and posterior spinal arteries form a plexus around the cord that supplies the white matter and posterior horns of gray matter. The largest branches of the anterior spinal artery form a central artery that supplies the anterior gray matter and the innermost white matter.[49] Radicular arteries supply individual nerve roots. In the cervical spine, the anterior spinal artery receives branches from three or more segmental arteries, including one from the costocervical trunk.

In rare circumstances, connective tissue disorders that cause vasculitis may affect blood vessels that supply blood to the spinal cord. Isolated granulomatous angiitis of the central nervous system is a form of vasculitis more commonly associated with cerebral vasculitis. Patients with isolated angiitis may develop spinal cord symptoms with or without cerebral involvement.[160, 161] In a study of 40 patients with isolated angiitis, 23% had spinal cord disease.[162] Acute onset of neurologic symptoms may be secondary to hemorrhage from a ruptured inflammatory aneurysm.[163] These patients describe lower extremity weakness accompanied by sensory abnormalities including loss of pain, proprioception, and vibratory sense. Patients also develop incontinence. The prognosis for return of function is poor, although patients may survive for a number of years after therapy with corticosteroids and radiation. Polyarteritis nodosa may cause neurologic dysfunction by affecting spinal cord arteries or by compression secondary to subarachnoid hemorrhage.[164, 165]

Infarction of the spinal cord may occur by mechanisms other than inflammation of blood vessels. Occlusion of the artery of Adamkiewicz results in paraplegia with relative sparing of the sacral roots. Blockage of this artery usually leads to watershed ischemia in its peripheral extension. Patients with severe atherosclerosis, emboli, and sustained hypotension all may be associated with cord infarction.[166] Spinal cord infarction may also occur in the cervical spinal cord after exposure to radiation therapy.[166]

Miscellaneous Lesions

Intramedullary spinal cord abscess is a rare but overwhelming infection.[167] This cord infection occurs in the setting of a systemic infection. The onset of symptoms is rapid. Local pain with neurologic dysfunction is found in most patients with this acute infection. MR evaluation is able to identify the location and extent of the lesion, but it is not pathognomonic.[168] In a study of 93 patients with intramedullary abscesses, 32% of the abscesses occurred in the cervical spine.[169] The prognosis for these patients is poor.

Sarcoidosis affects the central nervous system in 5% of patients.[170] Involvement of the spinal cord is rare. Granuloma affecting the spinal cord causes expansion of the cord. Granuloma may also cause vascular compression with ischemic changes in the cord. Patients may develop signs of myelopathy.[171] MR scan is able to determine the location of granuloma in the spinal cord.[172] Biopsy of the lesion is necessary. This lesion requires decompression and corticosteroid therapy.

Multiple sclerosis (MS) is a demyelinating disease that affects the white matter of the nervous system, including the spinal cord. Although involvement of the cerebrum is more common, spinal cord disease occurs in 9% of patients.[173] Another study reported involvement in 25% of patients.[174] The signs and symptoms of the disease, which develop over weeks, include muscle weakness, decreased light touch and temperature sensation, and sphincter dysfunction. MR imaging demonstrates "plaque" lesions in the spinal cord.[175] MR imaging is positive in 86% of patients with clinically suspected spinal cord MS[176] (Fig. 13–25). In the cervical spine, 48% of patients, with or without myelopathic symptoms, have

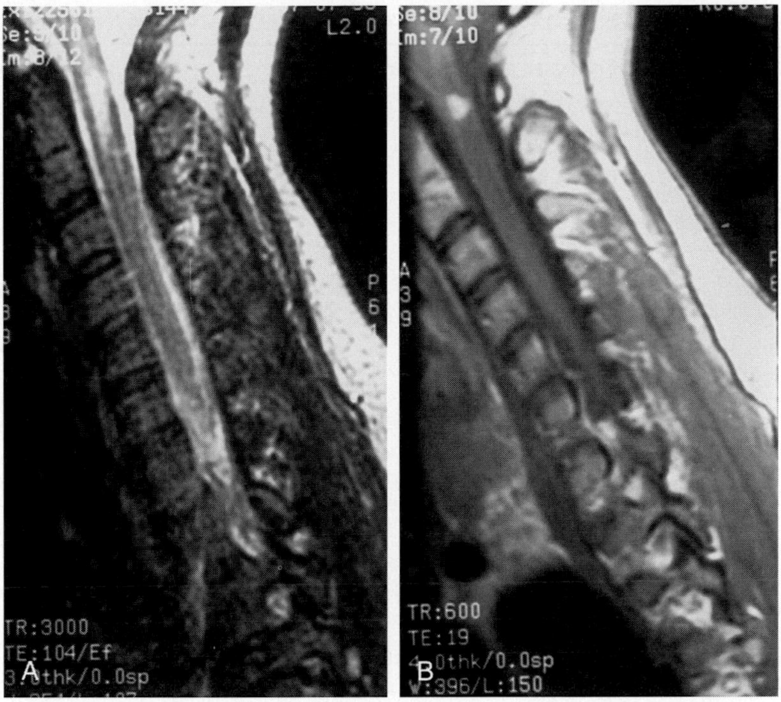

Figure 13–25. Multiple sclerosis. A 26-year-old female with a history of facial and right-arm numbness. She developed pain and paresthesias in her legs when she bent her neck. She had a positive Lhermitte's sign and a positive Babinski's sign. Magnetic resonance scan of T_2-weighted sagittal image of the cervical spinal cord, A, reveals an area of increased signal approximately one vertebral body in length. Abnormal enhancement is visible with gadolinium in T_1-weighted sagittal image, B. This appearance is compatible with demyelinating plaque in the cord substance.

MR findings. In addition to MR imaging, visual, auditory, and somatosensory evoked potentials are helpful diagnostic tests.[177] Cerebrospinal fluid evaluation for oligoclonal bands or immunoglobulin G synthesis rates may be helpful when the diagnosis is in doubt. There are no pathognomonic tests for the diagnosis of MS.[178] Therapy for MS includes immunosuppressive drugs.[179]

Myelitis, in its various forms, may also cause lesions in the cervical spinal cord (Table 13–11). The categories of myelitis include postinfectious (postvaccinal), primary infectious (viral, bacterial and spirochetal), primary intraspinal infectious (meningitis), toxic (drugs), physical agent (radiation), metabolic (B12 deficiency), blood vessel (connective tissue disease and systemic lupus erythematosus), and paraneoplastic.[40] Parainfectious myelitis may be differentiated from MS by the presence of spinal shock, MR evidence of cord swelling, and absence of oligoclonal bands.[180] Connective tissue disease may also cause transverse myelitis that may mimic MS. For example, in a study of 31 patients with central nervous system systemic lupus erythematosus, 16% had symptoms and signs of transverse myelitis.[181] Patients with Behçet's syndrome may develop neurologic involvement that may also include myelitis.[182] MR evaluation of the cerebral cortex may be a useful additional test for the patient with myelitis if the diagnosis is not evident with spinal cord tests. Plaques compatible with MS may be noted in the cortex.[183] Myelitis usually occurs in a single episode. Repeated episodes of myelitis may occur, associated with no specific diagnostic group.[184] The differential diagnosis of myelitis should be considered when other causes of spinal cord dysfunction have been eliminated as possibilities.[185]

Treatment

Therapy directed at extradural metastatic lesions may include radiation therapy, corticosteroids, and decompressive laminectomy.[186, 187] The treatment of intradural-extramedullary tumors is complete surgical removal. Intramedullary tumors accessible to surgical excision should be removed.[188] Some physicians suggest postsurgical radiation therapy of the spinal cord.

Prognosis

In general, extradural and intramedullary tumors are malignant, and intradural-extramedullary tumors are benign. The course and prognosis of these tumors correspond to their invasiveness, rapidity of growth, and location. Extradural and intramedullary tumors have

TABLE 13–11.   CAUSES OF MYELITIS AND NONCOMPRESSIVE MYELOPATHY

POSTINFECTIOUS/PARAINFECTIOUS	**PHYSICAL AGENTS**
Postvaccinal	Irradiation
Postviral infection	Electrical injury
Spontaneous	**METABOLIC/NUTRITIONAL**
DEMYELINATING	Diabetes mellitus
Multiple sclerosis	Cyanocobalamin deficiency
Neuromyelitis optica	Pellagra
Acute necrotizing	Chronic liver disease
PRIMARY INFECTIOUS	**BLOOD VESSELS**
Viral	Arteriosclerosis
Poliomyelitis/Postsyndrome	Dissecting aortic aneurysm
Acute encephalomyelitis	Coarctation of the aorta
Herpes zoster	Vascular malformations
Rabies	**CONNECTIVE TISSUE DISEASE**
Subacute myoclonic spinal neuritis	Polyarteritis nodosa
Human T-cell lymphotrophic virus type	Systemic lupus erythematosus
Acquired immunodeficiency syndrome	Sjögren's syndrome
Bacterial/Spirochetal	Behçet's syndrome
Spinal abscess	**TOXIC**
Tuberculoma	Organic iodide contrast media
Syphilis	Penicillin
Lyme disease	Spinal anesthetics
Rickettsial/fungal/parasitic	Arsenic
INTRASPINAL INFECTIONS	Lathyrism
Bacterial meningitis	Orthocresyl phosphate
Tuberculous meningitis	**PARANEOPLASTIC**

Modified from Byrne TN, Waxman SG: Spinal Cord Compression: Diagnosis and Principles of Management. Philadelphia: FA Davis Co, 1990.

poor prognoses, and intradural-extramedullary tumors may be cured with surgical removal.

References

INTRASPINAL NEOPLASMS

1. Long DM: Cervical cord tumors. In: Sherk HH, Dunn EJ, Eismont FJ, et al. (eds): The Cervical Spine, 2nd ed. Philadelphia: JB Lippincott Co, 1989, pp 526–543.
2. Helseth A, Mork SJ: Primary intraspinal neoplasms in Norway 1955 to 1986: a population based survey of 467 patients. J Neurosurg 71:842, 1989.
3. Elsberg CA: Diagnosis and Treatment of Surgical Diseases of the Spinal Cord and its Membranes, 2nd ed. Philadelphia: WB Saunders Co, 1941.
4. Batson OV: The function of vertebral veins and their role in the spread of metastases. Ann Surg 112:138, 1940.
5. Edelson RN, Deck MDF, Posner JB: Intramedullary spinal cord metastases: clinical and radiographic findings in nine cases. Neurology 22:1222, 1972.
6. Woolsey RM, Young RR: The clinical diagnosis of disorders of the spinal cord. Neurol Clin 9:573, 1991.
7. Goodridge AE, Feasby TE, Ebers GC, et al: Hand wasting due to mid-cervical spinal cord compression. Can J Neurol Sci 14:309, 1987.
8. Nicholas JJ, Christy WC: Spinal pain made worse by recumbency: a clue to spinal cord tumors. Arch Phys Med Rehabil 67:598, 1986.
9. Wiesel SW, Ignatius P, Marvel JP, Rothman RH: In-

tradural neurofibroma simulating lumbar disc disease. J Bone Joint Surg 58A:1040, 1976.
10. Crols R, Appel B, Klaes R: Extensive cervical intradural and intramedullary lipoma and spina bifida occulta of C1: a case report. Clin Neurol Neurosurg 95:39, 1993.
11. Austin GM: The significance and nature of pain in tumors of the spinal cord. Surg Forum 10:782, 1960.
12. Davidoff RA: Handbook of the Spinal Cord, vols 4 and 5. Congenital Disorders, Trauma, Infections, and Cancer. New York: Marcel Dekker, 1987.
13. Byrne TN, Waxman SG: Spinal Cord Compression: Diagnosis and Principles of Management. Philadelphia: FA Davis Co, 1990, pp 1–278.
14. Winter RB, Moe JH, Bradford DS, et al.: Spine deformity in neurofibromatosis: a review of 102 patients. J Bone Joint Surg 61A:677, 1979.
15. Curtis BH, Fisher RL, Butterfield WL, Sauders FP: Neurofibromatosis in paraplegia. J Bone Joint Surg 51A:843, 1969.
16. Barron KD, Hirano A, Araki S, Terry RD: Experiences with metastatic neoplasms involving the spinal cord. Neurology 9:91, 1959.
17. Vieth RG, Odom GL: Extradural spinal metastases and their neurosurgical treatment. J Neurosurg 23:501, 1965.
18. Schaberg J, Gainor BJ: A profile of metastatic carcinoma of the spine. Spine 10:19, 1985.
19. Love JG, Dodge HW: Dumbbell (hourglass) neurofibromas affecting the spinal cord. Surg Obstet Gynecol 94:161, 1952.
20. Levy WJ, Bay J, Dohn D: Spinal cord meningioma. J Neurosurg 57:804, 1982.
21. Heshmat MY, Kovi J, Simpson C, et al.: Neoplasms of the central nervous system. Cancer 38:2135, 1976.

22. Mitchell GE, Lourie H, Berne AS: The various causes of scalloped vertebrae with notes on their pathogenesis. Radiology 89:67, 1967.

23. Edelstyn GA, Gillespie PJ, Grebbell FS: The radiological demonstration of skeletal metastases. Clin Radiol 18:158, 1967.

24. Stark RJ, Henson RA, Evans SJW: Spinal metastases: a retrospective survey from a general hospital. Brain 105:189, 1982.

25. Nittner K: Spinal meningiomas, neurinomas, and neurofibromas and hourglass tumors. In: Vinken PJ, Bruyn GW (eds): Handbook of Clinical Neurology, vol 20. Amsterdam: North Holland Publishing, 1976, pp 177–322.

26. Alazraki N: Radionuclide Techniques. In: Resnick D, Niwayama G (eds): Diagnosis of Bone and Joint Disorders. Philadelphia: WB Saunders Co, 1981, pp 432–445.

27. Banna M: Clinical Radiology of the Spine and the Spinal Cord. Rockville, Maryland: Aspen Systems Corporation, 1985.

28. Resnick D, Niwayama G: Soft Tissues. In: Resnick D (ed): Diagnosis of Bone and Joint Disorders, 3rd ed. Philadelphia: WB Saunders Co, 1995, p 4555.

29. Gilbert RW, Kim JH, Posner JB: Epidural spinal cord compression from metastatic tumor: diagnosis and treatment. Ann Neurol 3:40, 1978.

30. Weissman DE, Gilberg M, Wang H, et al.: The use of computed tomography of the spine to identify patients at high risk for epidural metastases. J Clin Oncol 3:1541, 1985.

31. Pancoast HK: Superior pulmonary sulcus tumor: tumor characterized by pain, Horner's syndrome, destruction of bone and atrophy of hand muscles. JAMA 99:1391, 1932.

32. Cascino TL, Kori S, Krol G, Foley KM: CT of the brachial plexus in patients with cancer. Neurology 33:1553, 1983.

33. Kori SH, Foley KM, Posner JB: Brachial plexus lesions in patients with cancer: 100 cases. Neurology 31:45, 1981.

34. Zinreich SJ: Three-dimensional computed tomography of the spine: evaluation of failed back surgery syndrome and spinal stenosis. Spine 9:287, 1995.

35. Modic MT, Masaryk T, Paushter D: Magnetic resonance imaging of the spine. Radiol Clin North Am 24:229, 1986.

36. Lee RR: Spinal tumors. Spine 9:261, 1995.

37. Parizel PM, Baleriaux D, Rodesch G, et al.: Gd-DTPA–enhanced MR imaging of spinal tumors. AJR 152:1087, 1989.

38. Sze G, Stimac GK, Bartlett C, et al.: Multicenter study of gadopentetate dimeglumine as a MR contrast agent: evaluation in patients with spinal tumors. AJNR 11:967, 1990.

39. Lim V, Sobel DF, Zyroff J: Spinal cord pial metastases: MR imaging with gadopentetate dimeglumine. AJNR 11:975, 1990.

40. Gurusinghe NT: Spinal cord compression and spinal cord tumours. In: Critchley E, Eisen A (eds): Diseases of the Spinal Cord. London: Springer-Verlag, 1992, pp 351–408.

41. Huvos AG: Bone Tumors: Diagnosis, Treatment, and Prognosis, 2nd ed. Philadelphia: WB Saunders Co, 1991, pp 413–427.

42. Schierholz U: Fibrosarcoma of the cervical spine. Arch Orthop Trauma Surg 93:145, 1979.

43. Levy ML, Wieder BH, Schneider J, et al.: Subdural empyema of the cervical spine: clinicopathological correlates and magnetic resonance imaging. J Neurosurg 79:929, 1993.

44. Darouiche RO, Hamill RJ, Greenberg SB, et al.: Bacterial spinal epidural abscess: review of 43 cases and literature survey. Medicine 71:369, 1992.

45. Baker AS, Ojemann RG, Swartz MN, Richardson EP Jr: Spinal epidural abscess. N Engl J Med 293:463, 1975.

46. Kricun R, Shoemaker EI, Chovanes GI, Stephens HW: Epidural abscess of the cervical spine: MR findings in five cases. AJR 158:1145, 1992.

47. Markham JW, Lynge HN, Stahlman GEB: The syndrome of spontaneous spinal epidural hematoma: report of three cases. J Neurosurg 26:334, 1967.

48. Levitan LH, Wiens CW: Chronic lumbar extradural haematoma: CT findings. Radiology 148:707, 1983.

49. Aminoff MJ: Spinal vascular disease. In: Critchley E, Eisen A (eds): Diseases of the Spinal Cord. London: Springer-Verlag, 1992, pp 281–299.

50. Beatty RM, Winston KR: Spontaneous cervical epidural hematoma: consideration of etiology. J Neurosurg 61:143, 1984.

51. Morio Y, Kuranobu K, Yamamoto K: Chronic spontaneous cervical epidural hematoma. Spine 18:405, 1993.

52. Acciarri N, Padovani R, Pozzati E, et al.: Spinal cavernous angioma: a rare cause of subarachnoid hemorrhage. Surg Neurol 37:453, 1992.

53. Hillman J, Bynke O: Solitary extradural cavernous hemangiomas in the spinal canal: report of five cases. Surg Neurol 36:19, 1991.

54. Stevens JM, Kendall BE, Gedroyc W: Acute epidural haematoma complicating myelography in a normotensive patient with normal blood coagulability. Br J Radiol 64:860, 1991.

55. DiLauro L, Poli R, Bortoluzzi M: Paresthesiae after lumbar disc removal and their relationship to epidural haematoma. J Neurosurg 57:135, 1982.

56. Gustafson H, Rutberg H, Bengtsson M: Spinal haematoma following epidural analgesia: report of a patient with ankylosing spondylitis and a bleeding diathesis. Anesthesia 43:220, 1988.

57. Vinters HV, Barnett HJM, Kaufmann JCE: Subdural hematoma of the spinal cord and widespread subarachnoid hemorrhage complicating anticoagulant therapy. Stroke 11:459, 1980.

58. Hissa E, Boumphrey F, Bay J: Spinal epidural hematoma and ankylosing spondylitis. Clin Orthop 208:225, 1986.

59. Mattle H, Sieb JP, Rohner M, Mumenthaler M: Nontraumatic spinal epidural and subdural hematomas. Neurology 37:1351, 1987.

60. Crisi G, Sorgato P, Colombo A, et al.: Gadolinium-DTPA-enhanced MR imaging in the diagnosis of spinal epidural haematoma: report of a case. Neuroradiology 32:64, 1990.

61. Fessler RG, Johnson DL, Brown FD, et al.: Epidural lipomatosis in steroid-treated patients. Spine 17:183, 1992.

62. Roy-Camille R, Mazel C, Husson JL, Saillant G: Symptomatic spinal epidural lipomatosis induced by a long-term steroid treatment: review of the literature and report of two additional cases. Spine 16:1365, 1991.

63. Quint DJ, Boulos RS, Sanders WP, et al.: Epidural lipomatosis. Radiology 169:485, 1988.

64. Butcher DL, Sahn SA: Epidural lipomatosis: a complication of corticosteroid therapy. Ann Intern Med 90:60, 1979.

65. Choe W, Walot I, Schlesinger C, et al.: Synovial cyst of dens causing spinal cord compression: case report. Paraplegia 31:803, 1993.

66. Lemish W, Apsimon T, Chakera T: Lumbar intra-

spinal synovial cysts: recognition and CT diagnosis. Spine 14:1378, 1989.

67. Quaghebeur G, Jeffree M: Synovial cyst of the high cervical spine causing myelopathy. AJNR 13:981, 1992.

68. Nijensohn E, Russell EJ, Milan M, Brown T: Calcified synovial cyst of the cervical spine: CT and MR evaluation. J Comput Assist Tomogr 14:473, 1990.

69. Weymann CA, Capone P, Kinkel PR, Kinkel WR: Synovial cyst of the upper cervical spine: MRI with gadolinium. Neurology 43:2151, 1993.

70. Bjokengren AG, Kurz LT, Resnick D, et al.: Symptomatic intraspinal synovial cysts: opacification and treatment by percutaneous injection. AJR 149:105, 1987.

71. Goffin J, Wilms G, Plets C, et al.: Synovial cyst at the C1–C2 junction. Neurosurgery 30:914, 1992.

72. Takano Y, Homma T, Okumura H, Takahashi HE: Ganglion cyst occurring in the ligamentum flavum of the cervical spine: a case report. Spine 17:1531, 1992.

73. Skuse GR, Kosciolek BA, Rowley PT: The neurofibroma in von Recklinghausen neurofibromatosis has a unicellular origin. Am J Hum Genet 49:600, 1991.

74. Wertelecki W, Rouleau G, Superneau D, et al.: Neurofibromatosis: clinical and DNA linkage studies of a large kindred. N Engl J Med 319:278, 1988.

75. Broager B: Spinal neurinoma. Acta Psychiatr Scand (Suppl) 85:1, 1953.

76. Gautier-Smith PC: Clinical aspects of spinal neurofibromas. Brain 90:359, 1970.

77. Rasmussen TB, Kernohan JW, Adson AW: Pathologic classification with surgical consideration of intraspinal tumors. Ann Surg 111:513, 1940.

78. Wander JV, Das Gupta TK: Neurofibromatosis. Curr Probl Surg 14:1, 1977.

79. Thomeer RT, Bots GT, Van Dulken H, et al.: Neurofibrosarcoma of the cauda equina: case report. J Neurosurg 54:409, 1981.

80. Bull JWD: Spinal meningiomas and neurofibromas. Acta Radiol 40:283, 1953.

81. Egelhoff JC, Bates DJ, Ross JS, et al.: Spinal MR findings in neurofibromatosis types 1 and 2. AJNR 13:1071, 1992.

82. Disimone RE, Berman AT, Schwentker EP: The orthopedic manifestation of neurofibromatosis: a clinical experience and review of the literature. Clin Orthop 230:277, 1988.

83. Funasaki H, Winter RB, Lonstein JB, Denis F: Pathophysiology of spinal deformities in neurofibromatosis: an analysis of seventy-one patients who had curves associated with dystrophic changes. J Bone Joint Surg 76A:692, 1994.

84. Schievink WI, Piepgras DG: Cervical vertebral artery aneurysms and arteriovenous fistulae in neurofibromatosis type 1: case reports. Neurosurgery 29:760, 1991.

85. Guyer RD, Collier RR, Ohnmeiss DD, et al.: Extraosseous spinal lesions mimicking disc disease. Spine 13:328, 1988.

86. Katz AD, McAlpin C: Face and neck neurogenic neoplasms. Am J Surg 166:421, 1993.

87. Levy WJ, Bay J, Dohn D: Spinal cord meningioma. J Neurosurg 57:804, 1982.

88. Weil SM, Gewirtz RJ, Tew JM Jr: Concurrent intradural and extradural meningiomas of the cervical spine. Neurosurgery 27:629, 1990.

89. Sze G, Abramson A, Krol G, et al: Gadolinium-DTPA in the evaluation of intradural extramedullary spinal disease. AJNR 9:153, 1988.

90. Sen CN, Sekhar LN: An extreme lateral approach to intradural lesions of the cervical spine and foramen magnum. Neurosurgery 27:197, 1990.

91. Sawa H, Tamaki N, Kurata H, Nagashima T: Complete resection of a spinal meningioma extending from the foramen magnum to the second thoracic vertebral body via the anterior approach: case report. Neurosurgery 33:1095, 1993.

92. Giuffre R: Spinal lipomas. In: Vinken PJ, Bruyn GW (eds): Handbook of Clinical Neurology, vol 20. Amsterdam: North Holland Publishing, 1976, pp 389–414.

93. Lantos G, Epstein F, Kory L: Magnetic resonance imaging of intradural spinal lipoma. Neurosurgery 20:469, 1987.

94. Bertalanffy H, Mitani S, Otani M, et al.: Usefulness of hemilaminectomy for microsurgical management of intraspinal lesions. Keio J Med 41:76, 1992.

95. Adams RD, Wegner W: Congenital cyst of the spinal meninges as cause of intermittent compression of the spinal cord. Arch Neurol Psychiatry 58:57, 1947.

96. Cillufo JM, Gomez MR, Reese DF, et al.: Idiopathic ("congenital") spinal arachnoid diverticula: clinical diagnosis and surgical results. Mayo Clin Proc 56:93, 1981.

97. Delamarter RB, Ross JS, Masaryk TJ, et al.: Diagnosis of lumbar arachnoiditis by magnetic resonance imaging. Spine 15:304, 1990.

98. Burton CV: Lumbosacral arachnoiditis. Spine 3:24, 1978.

99. Shaw MDM, Russel JA, Grossart KW: The changing pattern of spinal arachnoiditis. J Neurol Neurosurg Psychiatry 41:97, 1978.

100. Bourne IHJ: Lumbo-sacral adhesive arachnoiditis: a review. J R Soc Med 83:262, 1990.

101. Quiles M, Marchisello PJ, Tsairis P: Lumbar adhesive arachnoiditis: etiologic and pathologic aspects. Spine 3:45, 1978.

102. Freilick D, Swash M: Diagnosis and management of tuberculosis paraplegia with special reference to tuberculosis radiculomyelitis. J Neurol Neurosurg Psychiatry 42:12, 1979.

103. Sghirlanzoni A, Marazzi R, Pareyson D, et al.: Epidural anaesthesia and spinal arachnoiditis. Anaesthesia 44:317, 1989.

104. Sklar EML, Quencer RM, Green BA, et al.: Complications of epidural anesthesia: MR appearance of abnormalities. Radiology 181:549, 1991.

105. Caplan LR, Norohna AB, Amico LL: Syringomyelia and arachnoiditis. J Neurol Neurosurg Psychiatry 53:106, 1990.

106. Hoyland JA, Freemont AJ, Denton J, et al.: Retained surgical swab debris in post-laminectomy arachnoiditis and peridural fibrosis. J Bone Joint Surg 70B:659, 1988.

107. Ross JS: Inflammatory Disease. In: Modic MT, Masaryk TJ, Ross JS: Magnetic Resonance Imaging of the Spine. Chicago: Year Book Medical Publishers, 1989, pp 167–182.

108. Vloeberghs M, Herregodts P, Stadnik T, et al.: Spinal arachnoiditis mimicking a spinal cord tumor: a case report and review of the literature. Surg Neurol 37:211, 1992.

109. Johnson CE, Sze G: Benign lumbar arachnoiditis: MR imaging with gadopentetate dimeglumine. AJR 155:873, 1990.

110. Rosenfeld JV, Kaye AH, David S, Gonzales M: Pachymeningitis cervicalis hypertrophica: case report. J Neurosurg 66:137, 1987.

111. Rosenblum B, Oldfield EH, Doppman JL, DiChiro G: Spinal arteriovenous malformations: a comparison of

dural arteriovenous fistulas and intradural AVM's in 81 patients. J Neurosurg 67:795, 1987.

112. Madsen JR, Heros RC: Spinal arteriovenous malformations and neurogenic claudication: report of two cases. J Neurosurg 68:793, 1988.

113. Aminoff MJ, Logue V: Clinical features of spinal vascular malformation. Brain 97:197, 1974.

114. Acciarri N, Padovani R, Pozzati E, et al.: Spinal cavernous angioma: a rare cause of subarachnoid hemorrhage. Surg Neurol 37:453, 1992.

115. Biondi A, Merland JJ, Hodes JE, et al.: Aneurysms of spinal arteries associated with intramedullary arteriovenous malformations I: angiographic and clinical aspects. AJNR 13:913, 1992.

116. Chalif DJ, Black K, Rosenstein D: Intradural spinal cord tumor presenting as a subarachnoid hemorrhage: magnetic resonance imaging diagnosis. Neurosurgery 27:631, 1990.

117. Djindjian R: Arteriography of the spinal cord. AJR 107:461, 1969.

118. Choi IS, Berenstein A: Surgical neuroangiography of the spine and spinal cord. Radiol Clin North Am 26:1131, 1988.

119. Rosenblum DS, Myers SJ: Dural spinal cord arteriovenous malformation. Arch Phys Med Rehabil 72:233, 1991.

120. Minami S, Sagoh T, Nishimura K, et al.: Spinal arteriovenous malformations: MR imaging. Radiology 169:109, 1988.

121. Isu T, Iwasaki Y, Akino M, et al.: Magnetic resonance imaging in cases of spinal dural arteriovenous malformation. Neurosurgery 24:919, 1989.

122. Nichols DA, Rufenacht DA, Jack CR Jr, Forbes GS: Embolization of spinal dural arteriovenous fistula with polyvinyl alcohol particles: experience with 14 patients. AJNR 13:933, 1992.

123. Glasser R, Masson R, Mickle P, Peters KR: Embolization of a dural arteriovenous fistula of the ventral cervical spinal canal in a nine-year-old boy. Neurosurgery 33:1089, 1993.

124. Ogilvy CS, Louis DN, Ojemann RG: Intramedullary cavernous angiomas of the spinal cord: clinical presentation, pathological features, and surgical management. Neurosurgery 31:219, 1992.

125. Fontaine S, Melanson D, Cosgrove R, Bertrand G: Cavernous hemangiomas of the spinal cord: MR imaging. Radiology 166:839, 1988.

126. Logue V: Angiomas of the spinal cord: review of the pathogenesis, clinical features, and results of surgery. J Neurol Neurosurg Psychiatry 42:1, 1979.

127. McCormick PC, Michelsen WJ, Post KD, et al.: Cavernous malformations of the spinal cord. Neurosurgery 23:459, 1988.

128. Lundqvist C, Berthelsen B, Sullivan M, et al.: Spinal arteriovenous malformations: neurological aspects and results of embolization. Acta Neurol Scand 82:51, 1990.

129. Wasserstrom WR, Glass JP, Posner JB: Diagnosis and treatment of leptomeningeal metastases from solid tumors: experience with 90 patients. Cancer 49:759, 1982.

130. Yap HY, Yap BS, Tashima CK, et al.: Meningeal carcinomatosis in breast cancer. Cancer 42:283, 1978.

131. Murray JJ, Greco FA, Wolff SN, Hainsworth JD: Neoplastic meningitis: marked variations of cerebrospinal fluid composition in the absence of extradural block. Am J Med 75:289, 1983.

132. Yousem DM, Patrone PM, Grossman RI: Leptomeningeal metastases: MR evaluation. J Comput Assist Tomogr 14:255, 1990.

133. Bleyer WA, Byrne TN: Leptomeningeal cancer in leukemia and solid tumors. Curr Probl Cancer 12:185, 1988.

134. Batzdorf U (ed): Syringomyelia: Current Concepts in Diagnosis and Treatment. Baltimore: Williams & Wilkins, 1991.

135. McIlory WJ, Richardson JC: Syringomyelia: a clinical review of 75 cases. Can Med Assoc J 93:731, 1965.

136. Sherman JL, Barkovich AJ, Citrin CM: The MR appearance of syringomyelia: new observations. AJR 148:381, 1987.

137. Zager EL, Ojemann RG, Poletti CE: Acute presentations of syringomyelia: Report of three cases. J Neurosurg 72:133, 1990.

138. Singer GL, Brust JCM, Challenor YB: Syringomyelia presenting as shoulder dysfunction. Arch Phys Med Rehabil 73:285, 1992.

139. Spillane JD, Pallis C, Jones AM: Developmental abnormalities in the region of the foramen magnum. Brain 80:11, 1957.

140. Aubin ML, Vignaud J, Jardin C, Bar D: Computed tomography in 75 clinical cases of syringomyelia. AJNR 2:199, 1981.

141. Yeates A, Brant-Zowadzki M, Norman D, et al.: Nuclear magnetic resonance of syringomyelia. AJNR 4:234, 1983.

142. Shen W, Lee S: MRI of concurrent spinal meningioma, ependymoma, and syringomyelia. J Comput Assist Tomogr 16:665, 1992.

143. Gardner WJ, Bell HS, Poolos PN, et al.: Terminal ventriculostomy for syringomyelia. J Neurosurg 46:609, 1977.

144. Milhorat TH, Johnson WD, Miller JI, et al.: Surgical treatment of syringomyelia based on magnetic resonance imaging criteria. Neurosurgery 31:231, 1992.

145. Cusick JF, Bernardi R: Syringomyelia after the removal of benign spinal extramedullary neoplasms. Spine 20:1289, 1995.

146. Fischer G, Tommasi M: Spinal ependymomas. In: Vinken PJ, Bruyn GW (eds): Handbook of Clinical Neurology, vol 20. Amsterdam: North Holland Publishing, 1976, pp 759–780.

147. Barone BM, Elvidge AR: Ependymomas: a clinical survey. J Neurosurg 33:428, 1970.

148. Nemoto Y, Inoue Y, Tahiro T, et al: Intramedullary spinal cord tumors: significance of associated hemorrhage at MR imaging. Radiology 182:793, 1992.

149. Brotchi J, DeWitte O, Levivier M, et al.: A survey of 65 tumors within the spinal cord: surgical results and the importance of preoperative magnetic resonance imaging. Neurosurgery 29:651, 1991.

150. Guidetti B, Mercuri S, Vagnozzi R: Long-term results of the surgical treatment of 129 intramedullary spinal gliomas. J Neurosurg 54:323, 1981.

151. Whitaker SJ, Bessell EM, Ashley SE, et al.: Postoperative radiotherapy in the management of spinal ependymoma. J Neurosurg 74:720, 1991.

152. Clover LL, Hazuke MB, Kinzie JJ: Spinal cord ependymomas treated with surgery and radiation therapy: a review of 11 cases. Am J Clin Oncol 16:350, 1993.

153. Ferrante L, Mastronardi L, Celli P, et al.: Intramedullary spinal cord ependymomas: a study of 45 cases with long-term follow-up. Acta Neurochir (Wien) 119:74, 1992.

154. McCormack PC, Torres R, Post K, Stein BM: Intramedullary ependymoma of the spinal cord. J Neurosurg 72:523, 1990.

155. Crisante L, Herrmann H: Surgical management of intramedullary spinal cord tumors: functional outcome and sources of morbidity. Neurosurgery 35:69, 1994.

156. Grem JL, Burgess J, Trump DL: Clinical features

and natural history of intramedullary spinal cord metastasis. Cancer 56:2305, 1985.

157. Hida K, Tada M, Iwasaki Y, Abe H: Intramedullary disseminated capillary hemangioma with localized spinal cord swelling: case report. Neurosurgery 33:1099, 1993.

158. Oglivy CS, Louis DN, Ojemann RG: Intramedullary cavernous angiomas of the spinal cord: clinical presentation, pathological features, and surgical management. Neurosurgery 31:219, 1992.

159. Sliwa JA, Maclean IC: Ischemic myelopathy: a review of spinal vasculature and related clinical syndromes. Arch Phys Med Rehabil 73:365, 1992.

160. Caccamo DV, Garcia JH, Ho K: Isolated granulomatous angiitis of the spinal cord. Ann Neurol 32:580, 1992.

161. Inwards DJ, Piepgras DG, Lie JT, et al.: Granulomatous angiitis of the spinal cord associated with Hodgkin's disease. Cancer 68:1318, 1991.

162. Vollmer TL, Guarnaccia J, Harrington W, et al.: Idiopathic granulomatous angiitis of the central nervous system. Arch Neurol 50:925, 1993.

163. Yoong MF, Blumberg PC, North JB: Primary (granulomatous) angiitis of the central nervous system with multiple aneurysms of spinal arteries: case report. J Neurosurg 79:603, 1993.

164. Ojeda VJ: Polyarteritis affecting the spinal cord arteries. Aust N Z J Med 13:287, 1983.

165. Rodgers H, Veale D, Smith P, Corris P: Spinal cord compression in polyarteritis nodosa. Ann Neurol 32:580, 1992.

166. Sandson TA, Friedman JH: Spinal cord infarction: report of 8 cases and review of the literature. Medicine 68:282, 1989.

167. Ditulio MV: Intramedullary spinal abscess: a case report with a review of 53 previously described cases. Surg Neurol 7:351, 1977.

168. Babu R, Jafar JJ, Huang PP, et al.: Intramedullary abscess associated with a spinal cord ependymoma: case report. Neurosurgery 30:121, 1992.

169. Bartels RH, Gonera EG, van der Spek JAN, et al.: Intramedullary spinal cord abscess: a case report. Spine 20:1199, 1995.

170. Delaney P: Neurologic manifestations in sarcoidosis: review of the literature with a report of 23 cases. Ann Intern Med 87:336, 1977.

171. Tuel SM, Meythaler JM, Cross LL: Rehabilitation of quadriparesis secondary to spinal cord sarcoidosis. Am J Phys Med Rehabil 70:63, 1991.

172. Clifton AG, Stevens JM, Kapoor R, Rudge P: Spinal cord sarcoidosis with intramedullary cyst formation. Br J Radiol 63:805, 1990.

173. Poser S, Hermann-Gremmeis I, Wikstrom J, Poser W: Clinical features of the spinal form of multiple sclerosis. Acta Neurol Scand 57:151, 1978.

174. Leibowitz U, Halpern L, Alter M: Clinical studies of multiple sclerosis in Israel: progressive spinal syndromes and multiple sclerosis. Neurology 17:988, 1967.

175. Sze G: Gadolinium-DTPA in spinal disease. Radiol Clin North Am 26:1009, 1988.

176. Greenberg JO: Neuroimaging of the spinal cord. Neurol Clin 9:679, 1991.

177. Adams RD, Salam-Adams M: Chronic nontraumatic disease of the spinal cord. Neurol Clin 9:605, 1991.

178. Paty DW, McFarlin DE, McDonald WI: Magnetic resonance imaging and laboratory aids in the diagnosis of multiple sclerosis. Ann Neurol 29:3, 1991.

179. Carter JL, Hafler DA, Dawson DM, et al.: Immunosuppressive with high-dose IV cyclophosphamide and ACTH in progressive multiple sclerosis: cumulative 6-year experience in 164 patients. Neurology (suppl 2)38:9, 1988.

180. Jeffrey DR, Mandler RN, David LE: Transverse myelitis: retrospective analysis of 33 cases, with differentiation of cases associated with multiple sclerosis and parainfectious events. Arch Neurol 50:532, 1993.

181. Neuwelt CM, Lacks S, Kaye BR, et al.: Role of intravenous cyclophosphamide (IV-CYC) in the treatment of severe neuropsychiatric lupus erythematosus (NOSLE). Am J Med 98:32, 1995.

182. Shakir RA, Sulaiman K, Rudman M: Neurological presentation of Behçet's syndrome: clinical categories. Eur Neurol 30:249, 1990.

183. Arlien-Soborg P, Kjaer L, Praestholm J: Myelography, CT and MRI of the spinal canal in patients with myelopathy: a prospective study. Acta Neurol Scand 87:95, 1993.

184. Tippett DS, Fishman PS, Panitch HS: Relapsing transverse myelitis. Neurology 41:703, 1991.

185. Dawson DM, Potts F: Acute nontraumatic myelopathies. Neurol Clin 9:585, 1991.

186. Bruckmas JE, Bloomer WD: Management of spinal cord compression. Semin Oncol 5:135, 1978.

187. Clark PRR, Saunders M: Steroid-induced remission in spinal canal reticulum cell sarcoma: report of two cases. J Neurosurg 42:346, 1975.

188. Khan FR, Glickman AS, Chu FCH, Nickson JJ: Treatment by radiotherapy of spinal cord compression due to extradural metastases. Radiology 89:495, 1967.

14

Endocrinologic and Heritable Disorders of the Cervical Spine

Endocrinologic and heritable disorders are systemic diseases that can affect components of the musculoskeletal system throughout the body. Those diseases that produce symptoms of neck pain are less numerous than those that cause lumbosacral disorders. For example, idiopathic osteoporosis occurs commonly in the lumbar spine but rarely in the cervical spine. The diseases that affect the cervical spine are microcrystalline disorders. Patients with these systemic diseases may present to a physician with neck pain in the setting of joint disease in other locations in the skeleton. The endocrinologic and heritable disorders are not limited to the axial skeleton. These diseases cause bone changes in many locations. The bone abnormalities may be subtle but can be discovered if sought carefully.

The history of neck pain in patients with endocrinologic and heritable diseases is usually nonspecific. Neck pain is located predominantly in the cervical spine with occasional radiation into the arms. Pain is acute in onset when gout or pseudogout is present. Patients frequently have symptoms of bone or joint pain in other locations. In addition, the systemic manifestations of the endocrinologic or heritable disorder may include symptoms of muscle weakness, renal stones, or gastrointestinal malabsorption. Patients with abnormalities associated with the deposition of mucopolysaccharide in soft tissues or laxity of ligamentous structures are at risk of developing myelopathic symptoms. Physical examination may demonstrate the systemic quality of the under-

lying disorder. Patients have neck pain on percussion and may also have muscle weakness, peripheral joint inflammation, or tophaceous deposits. Neurologic examination may demonstrate spasticity, hyperflexia, and positive Babinski's sign, indicative of spinal cord compression. Laboratory evaluation may be helpful in making a specific diagnosis of the underlying disorder.

Detection of urate and calcium pyrophosphate dihydrate crystals is essential for the diagnosis of gout and pseudogout, respectively. Radiographic findings, such as disc calcification, bone erosions, and atlantoaxial subluxation, may be prominent, but they are nonspecific. Although radiologic evaluation is not diagnostic, it is important in documenting the global involvement of the skeletal system with these diseases.

Therapy is tailored for each endocrinologic or heritable disease. Episodes of acute microcrystalline arthritis are benefited by courses of nonsteroidal anti-inflammatory drugs. Patients with myelopathy benefit from spinal decompression and stabilization.

MICROCRYSTALLINE DISEASE

Capsule Summary

Frequency of neck pain—rare
Location of neck pain—cervical spine
Quality of neck pain—acute and sharp, chronic ache

Symptoms and signs—generalized micro-crystalline disease, straightened cervical spine

Laboratory and x-ray tests—monosodium urate or calcium pyrophosphate dihydrate crystals; joint erosions, disc calcification on plain roentgenogram

Therapy—nonsteroidal anti-inflammatory drugs, colchicine

Prevalence and Pathogenesis

Microcrystalline disease, gout, and calcium pyrophosphate dihydrate disease (CPPD) are commonly associated with peripheral joint arthritis. Rarely, patients with gouty axial skeletal disease may develop episodes of acute neck pain secondary to spinal involvement. CPPD is associated with radiographic findings of disc calcification and degenerative changes of the discs and vertebral bodies. Symptoms of neck pain may develop secondary to these degenerative changes. Calcification of the ligamentum flavum or atlantoaxial ligaments within the cervical canal may cause compression of the spinal cord, resulting in symptoms and signs of myelopathy.

The actual prevalence of gout and CPPD is not known. In one report, approximately 5% of a large adult population had hyperuricemia[1]; in another report 6% of an elderly population had CPPD in a joint.[2] Men develop gout during the fourth or fifth decade; women develop it after menopause. In a study of 37 women with gout, 86% developed gout after menopause.[3] The premenopausal women developed gout secondary to renal insufficiency or increased activity of phosphoribosylpyrophosphate synthetase. Prevalence increases with age in both sexes and is higher among males at all ages.[4] In North America, gout develops at rates of 1.7 and 0.2 cases per 1,000 person-years among men and women, respectively, 30 years of age and older.[5] A similar rate was found in a cohort of male physicians who were enrolled in a study at Johns Hopkins.[6] The majority of people with primary gout are men, with a 20:1 ratio to women. In secondary gout, approximately 30% of patients are women.[7] The etiology is related to the inability of the body to eliminate uric acid. This may occur secondary to underexcretion of uric acid through the kidney or to overproduction during protein metabolism. Uric acid accumulates in tissues throughout the body. The presence of crystals in joints, soft tissues, and other areas may initiate the inflammatory response that results in acute symptoms. Uric acid may accumulate into large collections, called tophi, that may be located in superficial structures, such as the olecranon bursae, as well as in deep areas, such as the kidney, heart, and cervical spine.[8] Risk factors for the development of acute gout include, primarily, hyperuricemia, along with obesity, hypertension, alcohol consumption, lead exposure, and renal insufficiency.[9]

High concentrations of uric acid alone are not adequate for the formation of crystals in synovial fluid. Gouty synovial fluids promote urate crystal formation significantly better than fluids from rheumatoid arthritis and osteoarthritis. A heat-sensitive macromolecule in gout fluid may promote the formation of crystals.[10] Crystals may act as antigens that induce immunoglobulin G antibodies. These antibodies may act as a nucleating matrix for new uric acid crystallization.[11] The ability of crystals to trigger attacks of acute inflammation is linked to their capacity to induce the release of a plethora of inflammatory mediators from phagocytes, serum proteins, and synovial lining cells into the synovial space.[12–14] The ingress of polymorphonuclear leukocytes supplies the soluble inflammatory mediators that initiate and perpetuate the acute attack.

CPPD causes symptomatic disease in about half the number of patients affected by gouty arthritis.[15] CPPD occurs in 5% to 10% of all adults. CPPD shows a marked increase with age, with a prevalence as high as 30% in those older than 75 years of age.[16] As with gout, men are more commonly affected than women. The disease becomes symptomatic in people from the sixth to seventh decade. Calcium pyrophosphate dihydrate is the crystal in CPPD that initiates the inflammatory response, but the factors that facilitate the deposition of this crystal in cartilage and surrounding articular structures are poorly understood. Inorganic pyrophosphate (PP) is a byproduct in the formation of cyclic adenosine monophosphate. PP is normally hydrolyzed by an inorganic pyrophosphatase, resulting in very low tissue concentrations of PP. Elevated levels of PP are noted in individuals who develop CPPD.[17] PP levels are increased five to eight times, compared with individuals who develop other arthropathies. Pyrophosphatase is inhibited by the presence of divalent cations including iron, calcium, and copper. This may be reflected in the diseases that are associated with CPPD. CPPD may be associated with a number of metabolic conditions, including hyperparathyroidism, hemochromatosis, hypothyroidism, Wilson's disease, and ochronosis. The disorders that are currently believed to be associated with chondrocalcinosis and pseudogout include hypophosphatasia, hypomagnesemia, hyperparathyroidism, and hypothyroidism. Chronic arthropathy of CPPD is associated with hemochromatosis, acromegaly, and ochronosis.[18]

Clinical History

Neck pain secondary to gout is a rare occurrence. Those patients who present with neck pain secondary to gout have a long history of peripheral gouty arthritis and are usually older than 50 years of age.[19] Most patients are men and have nonradiating neck pain due to chronic gouty arthritis. Occasionally they may have a sudden onset of severe neck pain associated with an acute gouty attack in peripheral joints.[20] Patients may experience severe pain, limiting spinal motion greatly.[21] Tophaceous deposits may affect the spine and spinal cord to the point of development of radicular symptoms, paraparesis, or quadriparesis.[22–25] Patients with spinal cord compression from tophi frequently have chronic polyarthritis.[23]

Patients with CPPD of the spine may also have symptoms of axial skeleton pain associated with straightening and stiffening of the spine.[8, 26] Neurologic symptoms compatible with myelopathy occur in the occasional patient with CPPD involvement of the ligamentum flavum in the foramen magnum and cervical spine.[27] Involvement of the cervical spine may occur independent of CPPD in other areas of the skeleton.[28] CPPD deposits may be found throughout the cervical, thoracic, and lumbar spine.[29] Pseudogout may cause an acute attack that causes spasm of the cervical spine that mimics the symptoms and signs associated with meningitis.[30]

Physical Examination

Physical findings in the cervical spine in the patient with gout may include spinal stiffness, loss of motion, and muscle spasm with pain on motion. A patient with acute gout of the axial skeleton may be febrile on initial presentation.[21] Examination of extensor surfaces (elbows and Achilles tendons) and ears may reveal tophaceous deposits. Peripheral joints may be affected with an acute attack at the same time as the cervical spine. However, even

in patients with polyarticular gout, involvement of the cervical spine is unusual.[31]

Patients with CPPD may have restricted motion from associated degenerative disease of the spine. Neurologic signs with CPPD are rare.[32] Patients with CPPD may also develop prolonged fever (50%) and an increased erythrocyte sedimentation rate.[33, 34]

Laboratory Data

Hyperuricemia is a prerequisite for the diagnosis of gout, and many patients have an elevated level of uric acid during an acute attack; however, a normal level does not eliminate the possibility of gout because uric acid concentrations fluctuate, particularly with anti-inflammatory medications. The presence of arthritis and elevated uric acid concentration does not equate with a diagnosis of gout. Hyperuricemia may occur without acute gout. The diagnosis of gout is established definitively by the demonstration of characteristic crystals of monosodium urate monohydrate in synovial fluid or from aspirates of tophaceous deposits. These crystals are negatively birefringent. Other synovial fluid characteristics of gout include fair mucin clot, elevated white blood cell count, and increased protein concentration. In a patient with gouty nephropathy, renal function as measured by blood urea nitrogen and creatinine may be impaired, and red blood cells may be present in the urine of the patient with uric acid renal stones. Components of the acute phase response, including serum leukocytes, platelet count, erythrocyte sedimentation rate, and C-reactive protein, are elevated in patients with acute gout.[35]

Blood studies in CPPD are of no use except to detect associated diseases, such as hemochromatosis and hyperparathyroidism. Synovial fluid aspiration of acute effusions demonstrates calcium pyrophosphate dihydrate crystals in the majority of patients. A careful examination for these crystals is necessary because they are less numerous than uric acid crystals in an inflamed joint and they polarize light weakly in contrast with urate crystals. White blood cell count and protein concentration in synovial fluid are elevated in a fashion similar to that of gout.

Radiographic Evaluation

Radiographic abnormalities in the axial skeleton are unusual in gout, but gout may cause

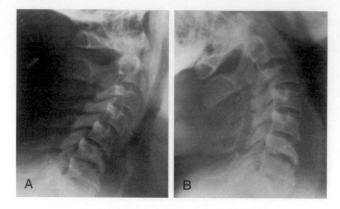

Figure 14–1. Gout. Flexion, *A*, and extension, *B*, cervical spine roentgenograms demonstrate endplate erosive changes in C6–C7. (Alarcón G, Reveille J: Gouty arthritis of the axial skeleton including the sacroiliac joints. Arch Intern Med 147:2018–2019, 1987. Copyright 1987, American Medical Association.)

joint margin sclerosis with cystic areas of erosion in the vertebral bodies.[19] Gout may also cause erosions of end plates, disc space narrowing, and vertebral subluxation[36–38] (Fig. 14–1). The changes associated with gout in the intervertebral disc may be confused with infectious discitis. Biopsy material from suspected areas should be placed in absolute alcohol, not formalin, so that crystals are not leached out from the specimen.[39] Occasionally, extradural deposits of urate may cause nerve compression and can be detected by myelographic examination.[40] Pathologic fractures in posterior elements of vertebral bodies are also found in patients with extensive gouty involve-

ment.[41] Indium-111 leukocyte scintigraphy identifies accumulation of tracer in involved joints during an acute attack. This type of scan has been used in patients with appendicular arthritis. The usefulness of this scan with axial involvement with gout is not known.[42] Repeat scan demonstrates decreased uptake after therapy corresponding to the patient's course.

Radiographic manifestations of CPPD in the spine include intervertebral disc calcifications, primarily in the annulus fibrosus. The nucleus pulposus is not involved.[43, 44] Calcification may occur throughout the cervical spine, most commonly at the C5–C6 interspace.[45] Calcifications of the ligamentum flavum and other

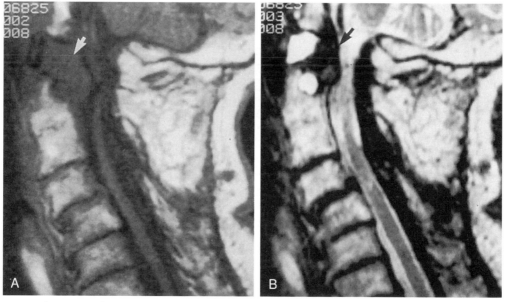

Figure 14–2. Calcium pyrophosphate dihydrate disease (CPPD). In this 70-year-old man, sagittal T_1-weighted (TR/TE 500/12), *A*, and T_2-weighted (TR/TE 3400/96), *B*, spin echo magnetic resonance images show a mass *(arrows)* about the eroded odontoid process. Note adjacent areas of high-signal intensity in *B*. The spinal cord is displaced. On computerized tomography scans, the mass was found to be calcified. CPPD crystal deposition was documented when the mass was surgically removed. (Resnick D, Niwayama G: Calcium pyrophosphate dihydrate (CPPD) crystal deposition disease. In: Resnick D [ed]: Diagnosis of Bone and Joint Disorders, 3rd ed. Philadelphia: WB Saunders Co, 1995, p 1598.)

spinous structures may be better visualized by computerized tomography (CT) or magnetic resonance (MR) imaging (Fig. 14–2). On CT, the calcifications are contiguous to the laminae but not continuous with the spinal cord. Disc space narrowing associated with vertebral osteophyte formation may also occur and is a common finding in the spine.[46] Vertebral body destruction may become severe enough to cause degenerative spondylolisthesis.[47, 48] Subluxation of the atlantoaxial joint has been reported with CPPD.[49] Ninety to 100 patients with CPPD of the spine have been reported in the medical literature.[45]

Differential Diagnosis

The diagnosis of microcrystalline disease is confirmed by the detection of the specific crystal in a clinical specimen. Patients with neck pain secondary to microcrystalline disease usually have extensive disease in other locations so that aspiration of facet joints is not necessary. Careful monitoring of response to therapy should show rapid improvement if the diagnosis is correct.

Infection must always be considered if the patient has extreme pain, fever, and an elevated peripheral white blood count. Patients with osteomyelitis do not improve with antigout therapy, and they require further evaluation with blood cultures and joint aspiration to rule out infection.

Cervical spine subluxation in the upper cervical spine in CPPD disease resembles the findings of rheumatoid arthritis. The absence of diffuse osteopenia, apophyseal erosions, and rheumatoid factor helps distinguish the diseases.

Acute calcific retropharyngeal tendinitis is a rare form of calcific periarthritis and is associated with acute upper neck pain and transient calcification of the tendon of the longus colli muscle, the principal flexor of the neck.[50] Middle-aged persons of both sexes are affected. These patients develop painful restriction of motion and pain on swallowing. Tenderness may occur over the C2 and C3 spinous processes. Lateral roentgenogram of the cervical spine reveals a calcific deposit anterior to the atlantoaxial junction and below the anterior arch of C1 (Fig. 14–3). Resorption of the deposit may occur throughout a 14-day period. Therapy is a cervical collar and nonsteroidal anti-inflammatory drugs. This form of calcific tendinitis is one of the forms of hydroxyapatite calcification that may cause calcification in

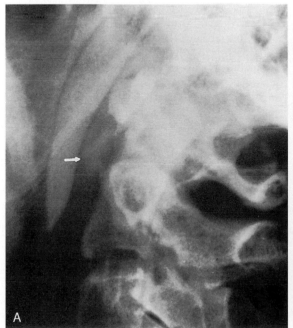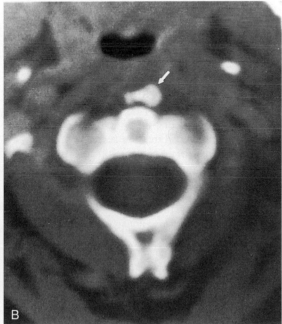

Figure 14–3. Longus colli calcification. A 46-year-old woman developed neck pain, fever, and decreased range of motion over a 2-week period. A lateral radiograph, *A*, and transaxial computerized tomography scan, *B*, at the level of the base of the odontoid process document calcification *(arrows)* within the longus colli muscle. The symptoms and imaging abnormalities disappeared over a period of weeks. (Courtesy of G. Greenway, M.D., Dallas, Texas.)

and around structures of the cervical spine and spinal canal. These calcifications look similar to those of CPPD and may be associated with radiculopathy and myelopathy.[51]

Hyperparathyroidism. Parathyroid hormone is the dominant factor in the maintenance of serum calcium level in a normal range. Hyperparathyroidism results in excess concentrations of parathyroid hormone in the blood stream and in elevated serum calcium level. Primary hyperparathyroidism is caused by abnormal growth of the parathyroid glands. Secondary hyperparathyroidism results from the secretion of parathyroid hormone in response to persistently low serum concentrations of calcium as associated with chronic renal failure. Hyperparathyroidism, regardless of type, leads to bone disease and abnormal physiology in a number of organ systems dependent on calcium for normal function (nervous, genitourinary, and gastrointestinal). The loss of calcium from bone results in pain, weakening, and fracture. Untreated disease causes marked osteopenia of the vertebral column, with progressive vertebral body fractures and spinal deformity. Hyperparathyroidism is associated with CPPD. Primary hyperparathyroidism is a disease process within the parathyroid glands and, in approximately 90% of cases, the abnormality is a neoplasm, usually the overgrowth of one gland forming an adenoma; less often, the abnormality is multiple adenomas (2%), diffuse hyperplasia (6%), or a carcinoma of the parathyroids (2%).[52] Secondary hyperparathyroidism is the increased secretion of parathormone in response to low scrum calcium level caused by abnormalities in other organ systems, such as the kidney, or when there is inadequate vitamin D metabolism. Alterations in calcium metabolism and relevant hormones occur with aging. The mean serum parathormone level is 20% to 40% higher in persons older than 70 years of age.[53] Calcitriol, the active form of vitamin D, is lower in older persons.[54] Calcitonin levels are lower in older women. Tertiary hyperparathyroidism occurs when parathormone is irrepressible in patients with normal or low serum calcium levels.[55] Acute pseudogout occurs in about 3.8% of patients with hyperparathyroidism.[56] Serum calcium level is elevated in more than 96% of patients with primary hyperparathyroidism.[57] Tests to determine parathormone levels have been improving. In a study of 101 patients with a variety of disorders of calcium homeostasis, including hyperparathyroidism, hypoparathyroidism, hypercalcemia of malignancy, and chronic renal failure, intact parathormone assay was superior to midregion/c-terminal parathormone assay in reflecting parathyroid function.[58] Roentgenographic abnormalities associated with hyperparathyroidism in the axial skeleton include pseudowidening of the sacroiliac joints and osteopenia with wedging of vertebral bodies.[59] Marked kyphosis may also be present. Sclerosis may develop at the superior and inferior margins of vertebral bodies, resulting in a "rugger-jersey" spine. This form of vertebral bony sclerosis may be associated with vertebrae of normal configuration of those who have undergone fracture and collapse. Subchondral resorption at the discovertebral junction results in bone weakening and Schmorl's nodes. Other axial skeleton and joint manifestations of hyperparathyroidism include calcium pyrophosphate dihydrate deposition disease and gout.[60, 61] Hyperparathyroidism secondary to renal failure causes renal osteodystrophy and has radiologic similarities with primary hyperparathyroidism. Osteosclerosis with soft tissue and arterial calcification occurs more commonly with secondary hyperparathyroidism than with the primary disease.[62] Most patients have a single parathyroid adenoma; its removal brings the hyperparathyroidism under control without recurrence.[63] In a smaller group of patients with diffuse hyperplasia of all the glands, total removal of all but a small portion of a single parathyroid gland is required.[64]

Destructive Spondyloarthropathy Associated with Hemodialysis. Patients who have chronic renal failure on dialysis and those with chronic renal failure alone may develop a destructive lesion of the cervical spine.[65] The prevalence of destructive lesions in the cervical spine in patients with chronic hemodialysis is 15%.[66] The mean period on dialysis before the development of spondyloarthropathy is 34 months.[67] Symptoms associated with this disorder include neck pain and radiculopathy.[68] The mechanism by which destructive spondyloarthropathy occurs is not clear. Some investigators have suggested that the destructive lesions are related to hyperparathyroidism.[69] This fact correlates with the presence of the syndrome in patients who have chronic renal failure who have not received dialysis. Other investigators have reported beta$_2$-microglobulin amyloid deposits in the destructive lesions in the spine.[70, 71] Amyloid deposits in the ligaments of the spine cause laxity, resulting in excess motion and eventual bony destruction. Although CPPD crystals are not frequently detected in these lesions, calcium hydroxyapatite crystals have been recovered from involved

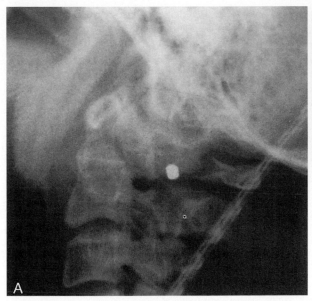

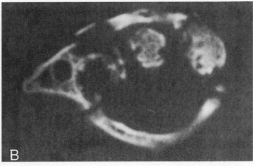

Figure 14–4. Spondyloarthropathy during hemodialysis, *A* and *B*. In this patient on long-term hemodialysis, findings included bone destruction of the atlas, odontoid erosions, a pathologic fracture at the base of the dens, fractures of the ring of the atlas, and posterior atlantoaxial subluxation. (Courtesy of S. Moreland, M.D., San Diego, California.)

joints. Amyloid deposits may reach adequate size in the cervical spine to cause spinal cord impingement and signs of myelopathy.[72] Radiographic abnormalities of disc space narrowing may simulate changes of osteomyelitis. The use of MR and CT to exclude the presence of soft tissue alterations helps exclude the possibility of infection[73] (Fig. 14–4). Patients may require surgical stabilization if subluxation occurs. Most patients with destructive spondyloarthropathy improve with stabilization.[67]

Treatment

Therapy for gout requires the immediate control of inflammation during the acute attack and the chronic control of hyperuricemia to prevent tophaceous deposits.[74] An acute gouty attack may be controlled with colchicine or nonsteroidal anti-inflammatory drugs, particularly indomethacin. The medication is continued for 7 to 10 days or until the attack is alleviated. In patients for whom nonsteroidal drugs or colchicine are contraindicated, corticotropin in the form of an intramuscular injection of 40 to 80 IU is used. Corticosteroids given by either oral or intravenous route may also be effective. The corticosteroids are gradually tapered during 2 to 3 weeks as the attack subsides. A maximum dose of intravenous colchicine for the treatment of an acute attack of gout should not exceed 2 mg. The use of a maximum dose of 2 mg per attack may prevent potential toxicities of cytopenias and renal fail-

ure.[75] The dose of colchicine should be reduced in the setting of renal or hepatic failure. Once the acute inflammation has subsided, uric acid concentrations may be controlled by increasing uric acid excretion with probenecid or sulfinpyrazone or by inhibiting uric acid production with the xanthine oxidase inhibitor, allopurinol, along with colchicine prophylaxis.[76]

Therapy for CPPD is primarily directed toward control of inflammation with nonsteroidal anti-inflammatory drugs. Occasionally, aspiration of a joint to remove crystals is helpful in controlling joint symptoms, but this is not practical for axial skeleton involvement. Oral colchicine is not as effective in preventing attacks in CPPD as it is in gout. Controlling diseases associated with CPPD may help to arrest their progression, but the calcium pyrophosphate deposits are not resorbed.[77]

Prognosis

Acute attacks of gout and CPPD do not occur with any specific intervals between episodes. Some patients have only one attack; others have frequent, painful bouts of inflammatory arthritis. Both the acute and chronic manifestations of gout can be well controlled with available therapy and, if diagnosed early enough, patients should have limited dysfunction from the disease. Those with CPPD also have a variable period between attacks, but anti-inflammatory drug therapy is usually effective at controlling the associated inflammation. There is, however, no effective therapy to either control or reverse the calcification of tissues or the secondary degenerative changes associated with crystal deposition. Patients with severe disease may develop progressive axial skeletal involvement with limited function. However, these circumstances are rare.

References

MICROCRYSTALLINE DISEASE

1. Hall AP, Barry PE, Dawber TR, McNamara PM: Epidemiology of gout and hyperuricemia: a long-term population study. Am J Med 42:27, 1967.
2. McCarty DJ, Hogan JM, Gatter RA, Grossman M: Studies on pathological calcifications in human cartilage, part I: prevalence and types of crystal deposits in the menisci of 215 cadavers. J Bone Joint Surg 48A:309, 1966.
3. Puig JG, Michan AD, Jimenez ML, et al.: Female gout: clinical spectrum and uric acid metabolism. Arch Intern Med 151:726, 1991.
4. Star VL, Hochberg MC: Prevention and management of gout. Drugs 45:212, 1993.
5. Abbott RD, Brand FN, Kannel WB, Castelli WP: Gout and coronary heart disease: the Framingham study. J Clin Epidemiol 41:237, 1988.
6. Roubenoff R, Klag MJ, Mead LA, et al.: Incidence and risk factors for gout in white men. JAMA 266:3004, 1991.
7. Cornelius R, Schneider HJ: Gouty arthritis in the adult. Radiol Clin North Am 26:1267, 1988.
8. Lichtenstein L, Scott HW, Levin MH: Pathologic changes in gout: survey of eleven necropsied cases. Am J Pathol 32:871, 1956.
9. Campion EW, Glynn RJ, DeLabry LO: Asymptomatic hyperuricemia: risks and consequences in the Normative Aging Study. Am J Med 82:421, 1987.
10. McGill NW, Dieppe PA: Evidence for a promotor of urate crystal formation in gouty synovial fluid. Ann Rheum Dis 50:558, 1991.
11. Kam M, Perl-Treves D, Caspi D, Addadi L: Antibodies against crystals. FASEB J 6:2608, 1992.
12. Terkeltaub R: Pathogenesis and treatment of crystal-induced inflammation. In: McCarty DJ, Koopman WJ (eds): Arthritis and Allied Conditions, 12th ed. Philadelphia: Lea & Febiger, 1993, pp 1819–1833.
13. Terkeltaub RA, Zachariae C, Santoro D, et al.: Monocyte-derived neutrophil chemotactic factor/IL-8 is a potential mediator of crystal-induced inflammation. Arthritis Rheum 34:894, 1991.
14. Terkeltaub RA: What stops a gouty attack? J Rheumatol 19:8, 1992.
15. O'Duffy JD: Clinical studies of acute pseudogout attacks: comments on prevalence, predispositions and treatment. Arthritis Rheum 19:349, 1976.
16. Felson DT, Anderson JJ, Naimark A, et al.: The prevalence of chondrocalcinosis in the elderly and its association with knee osteoarthritis: the Framingham study. J Rheumatol 16:1241, 1989.
17. Jensen PS: Chondrocalcinosis and other calcifications. Radiol Clin North Am 26:1315, 1988.
18. Jones AC, Chuck AJ, Arie EA, et al.: Diseases associated with calcium pyrophosphate deposition disease. Semin Arthritis Rheum 22:188, 1992.
19. Alarcon GS, Reveille JD: Gouty arthritis of the axial skeleton including the sacroiliac joints. Arch Intern Med 147:2018, 1987.
20. Sabharwal S, Gibson T: Cervical gout. Br J Rheumatol 27:413, 1988.
21. Leventhal LJ, Levin RW, Bomalaski JS: Peripheral arthrocentesis in the work-up of acute low back pain. Arch Phys Med Rehabil 71:253, 1990.
22. Reynolds AF, Wyler AR, Norris HT: Paraparesis secondary to sodium urate deposits in the ligamentous flavum. Arch Neurol 33:795, 1976.
23. Varga J, Giampaolo C, Goldenberg DL: Tophaceous gout of the spine in a patient with no peripheral tophi: case report and review of the literature. Arthritis Rheum 28:1312, 1985.
24. Magid SK, Gray GE, Anand A: Spinal cord compression by tophi in a patient with chronic polyarthritis: case report and literature review. Arthritis Rheum 24:1431, 1981.
25. Sequeira W, Bouffard A, Salgia K, Skoskey J: Quadriparesis in tophaceous gout. Arthritis Rheum 24:1428, 1981.
26. Reginato A, Valenzuela F, Martinez V, et al.: Polyarticular and familial chondrocalcinosis. Arthritis Rheum 13:197, 1970.
27. Circillo SF, Weinstein PR: Foramen magnum syndrome from pseudogout of the atlanto-occipital ligament: case report. J Neurosurg 71:141, 1989.
28. Brown TR, Quinn SF, D'Agostino AN: Deposition of calcium pyrophosphate dihydrate crystals in the ligamentum flavum: evaluation with MR imaging and CT. Radiology 178:871, 1991.
29. Resnick D, Pineda C: Vertebral involvement in calcium pyrophosphate dihydrate crystal deposition disease. Radiology 153:55, 1984.
30. Hammoudeh M, Siam AR: Pseudogout mimicking meningitis. Br J Rheumatol 32:351, 1993.
31. Lawry GV, Fan PT, Bluestone R: Polyarticular versus monoarticular gout: a prospective, comparative analysis of clinical features. Medicine 67:335, 1988.
32. Ellman MH, Vazquez T, Ferguson L, Mandel N: Calcium pyrophosphate deposition in ligamentum flavum. Arthritis Rheum 21:611, 1978.
33. Berger RG, Levitin PM: Febrile presentation of calcium pyrophosphate dihydrate deposition disease. J Rheumatol 15:642, 1988.
34. Masuda I, Ishikawa K: Clinical features of pseudogout attack: a survey of 50 cases. Clin Orthop 229:173, 1988.
35. Roseff R, Wohlgethan JR, Sipe JD, Canoso JJ: The acute phase response in gout. J Rheumatol 14:974, 1987.
36. Hall MC, Selin G: Spinal involvement in gout. J Bone Joint Surg 42A:341, 1960.
37. Kersley GD, Mandel L, Jeffrey MR: Gout: an unusual case with softening and subluxation of the first cervical vertebra and splenomegaly. Ann Rheum Dis 9:282, 1950.
38. Aaron SL, Miller JDR, Percy JS: Tophaceous gout in the cervical spine. J Rheumatol 11:862, 1984.
39. De AD: Intervertebral disc involvement in gout: brief report. J Bone Joint Surg 70B:671, 1988.
40. Litvak J, Briney W: Extradural spinal depositions of urates producing paraplegia: case report. J Neurosurg 39:656, 1973.
41. Burnham J, Fraker J, Steinbach H: Pathologic fracture in an unusual case of gout. AJR 129:116, 1977.
42. Palestro CJ, Vega A, Kim CK, et al.: Appearance of acute gouty arthritis on indium-111-labeled leukocyte scintigraphy. J Nucl Med 31:682, 1990.
43. McCarty DJ Jr, Haskin ME: The roentgenographic

aspects of pseudogout (articular chondrocalcinosis): an analysis of 20 cases. AJR 90:1248, 1963.

44. Bundens WD Jr, Brighton CT, Weitzman G: Primary articular cartilage calcification with arthritis (pseudogout syndrome). J Bone Joint Surg 47A:111, 1965.

45. Baba H, Maezawa Y, Kawahara N, et al.: Calcium crystal deposition in the ligamentum flavum of the cervical spine. Spine 18:2174, 1993.

46. Webb J, Deodhar S, Lee P: Chronic destructive polyarthritis due to pyrophosphate crystal arthritis ("pseudogout" syndrome). Med J Aust 2:206, 1974.

47. Resnick D, Niwayama G, Goergen TG, et al.: Clinical, radiographic, and pathologic abnormalities in calcium pyrophosphate dihydrate deposition disease (CPPD): pseudogout. Radiology 122:1, 1977.

48. Richards AJ, Hamilton EBD: Spinal changes in idiopathic chondrocalcinosis articularis. Rheumatol Rehabil 15:138, 1976.

49. Resnick D, Niwayama G: Calcium pyrophosphate dihydrate (CPPD) crystal deposition disease. In: Resnick D (ed): Diagnosis of Bone and Joint Disorders, 3rd ed. Philadelphia: WB Saunders Co, 1995, pp 1556–1614.

50. Saskozi J, Fam AG: Acute calcific retropharyngeal tendinitis: an unusual cause of neck pain. Arthritis Rheum 27:708, 1984.

51. Nakajima K, Miyaoka M, Sumie H, et al.: Cervical radiculomyelopathy due to calcification of the ligamenta flava. Surg Neurol 21:479, 1984.

52. Pyrah LN, Hodgkinson A, Anderson CK: Primary hyperparathyroidism. Br J Surg 53:245, 1966.

53. Endres DB, Morgan CH, Garry PJ et al.: Age-related changes in serum immunoreactive parathyroid hormone and its biological action in healthy men and women. J Clin Endocrinol Metab 65:724, 1987.

54. Clemens TL, Zhou XY, Myles M, et al.: Serum vitamin D$_2$ and vitamin D$_3$ metabolite concentrations and absorption of vitamin D$_2$ in elderly subjects. J Clin Endocrinol Metab 63:656, 1986.

55. Voorman GS, Petti GH Jr, Chankich GD, et al.: The pitfalls of technetium Tc-99mm–thallium-201 parathyroid scanning. Arch Otolaryngol Head Neck Surg 114:993, 1988.

56. Potts JT Jr: Management of asymptomatic hyperparathyroidism. J Clin Endocrinol Metab 70:1489, 1990.

57. Hect A, Gershberg H, St Paul H: Primary hyperparathyroidism: laboratory and clinical data in 73 cases. JAMA 233:519, 1975.

58. Rudnicki M, McNair P, Transbol I, Lindgren P: Diagnostic applicability of intact and midregion/C-terminal parathyroid hormone assays in calcium metabolic disorders. J Intern Med 228:465, 1990.

59. Genant HK, Heck LL, Lanzi LH, et al.: Primary hyperparathyroidism: a comprehensive study of clinical, biochemical, and radiographic manifestations. Radiology 109:513, 1973.

60. Resnick D, Niwayama G: Subchondral resorption of bone in renal osteodystrophy. Radiology 118:315, 1976.

61. Pritchard MH, Jessop JD: Chondrocalcinoisis in primary hyperparathyroidism: influence of age, metabolic bone disease, and parathyroidectomy. Ann Rheum Dis 36:146, 1977.

62. Greenfield GB: Roentgen appearance of bone and soft tissue changes in chronic renal diseases. AJR 116:749, 1972.

63. Attie JN, Wise L, Mir R, Ackerman LV: The rationale against routine subtotal parathyroidectomy for primary hyperparathyroidism. Am J Surg 136:437, 1978.

64. Block MA, Frame B, Jackson CE, Horn RC Jr: The extent of operation for primary hyperaparathyroidism. Arch Surg 109:798, 1974.

65. Kuntz D, Bertrand N, Bardin T, et al.: Destructive spondyloarthropathy in the hemodialyzed patients: a new syndrome. Arthritis Rheum 27:369, 1984.

66. Kerr R, Bjorkengren A, Bielecki DK, et al.: Destructive spondyloarthropathy in hemodialysis patients. Skeletal Radiol 17:176, 1988.

67. Cuffe MJ, Hadley MN, Herrera GA, Morawetz RA: Dialysis-associated spondyloarthropathy: report of 10 cases. J Neurosurg 80:694, 1994.

68. Westmark KD, Weissman BN: Complications of axial arthropathies. Orthop Clin North Am 21:423, 1990.

69. McCarthy JT, Dahlberg PJ, Kriegshauser JS, et al.: Erosive spondyloarthropathy in long-term dialysis patients: relationship to severe hyperparathyroidism. Mayo Clin Proc 63:446, 1988.

70. Moriniere P, Marie A, el Esper N, et al.: Destructive spondyloarthropathy with beta$_2$-microglobulin amyloid deposits in a uremic patient before chronic hemodialysis. Nephron 59:654, 1991.

71. Welk LA, Quint DJ: Amyloidosis of the spine in a patient on long-term hemodialysis. Neuroradiology 32:334, 1990.

72. Allain TJ, Stevens PE, Bridges LR, et al.: Dialysis myelopathy: quadriparesis due to extradural amyloid of beta$_2$-microglobulin origin. Br Med J 296:752, 1988.

73. Rafto SE, Dalinka MK, Schiebler ML, et al.: Spondyloarthropathy of the cervical spine in long-term hemodialysis. Radiology 166:201, 1988.

74. Yu TF, Gutman AB: Principles of current management of primary gout. Am J Med Sci 254:893, 1967.

75. Roberts WN, Liang MH, Stern SH: Colchicine in acute gout: reassessment of risks and benefits. JAMA 257:1920, 1987.

76. Klinenberg JR, Goldfinger S, Seegmiller JE: The effectiveness of the xanthine oxidase inhibitor allopurinol in the treatment of gout. Ann Intern Med 62:639, 1965.

77. McCarty DJ: Calcium pyrophosphate dihydrate crystal deposition disease (pseudogout syndrome): clinical aspects. Clin Rheum Dis 3:61, 1977.

HERITABLE GENETIC DISORDERS

Capsule Summary

Frequency of neck pain—common
Location of neck pain—cervical spine
Quality of neck pain—chronic ache
Symptoms and signs—abnormalities noticeable early in life; structural alterations: kyphoscoliosis, short stature
Laboratory and x-ray tests—specific for each disease
Therapy—surgical decompression of stenosis

This section reviews a number of heritable disorders of connective tissue that are associated with neck pain and cervical spinal cord compression. For the most part, these disorders are rare. Many of the patients with these disorders are not evaluated by internists because these patients do not live to adulthood.

Within the major categories of heritable disorders of connective tissue, impairment of the neck and spine is common. However, not all of the entities included in a single disorder (mucopolysaccharidoses, for example) have associated neck pain. Those subclasses of these disorders associated with neck pain are identified and the clinical characteristics are listed. The disorders of connective tissue may involve fibrous connective tissue elements (collagen and elastin), ground substance (mucopolysaccharide), cartilage, or bone.[1]

Achondroplasia

Achondroplasia is a skeletal defect associated with a quantitative decrease in endochondral bone growth and is the most frequent cause of dwarfism.[1-3] The etiology of the disease is unknown, and no biochemical abnormality has been identified. The disease is transmitted as an autosomal dominant trait, but only 20% of individuals have an affected parent. Spontaneous mutations occur in 90%.[4]

The diagnosis of achondroplasia is made at birth. Patients have short limbs, prominent forehead, kyphoscoliosis, and prominent buttocks associated with accentuated lumbar lordosis. Patients have normal intelligence and no visceral lesions.

Achondroplasts have abnormalities affecting the entire axial skeleton. The vertebral bodies of the spine have normal width, are slightly elongated, but have diminished diameter in the spinal canal. The space for the spinal cord is narrowed throughout the length of the spine.[5] Patients may also have critical narrowing at the level of the foramen magnum.

Cerebrospinal fluid may accumulate in the brain secondary to narrowing of all the foramina and venous channels exiting the skull.[6] Infants may have respiratory difficulties secondary to both central (cervical medullary compression) and peripheral (small chest) causes.[7] Sudden death may occur when the child stands upright, with the increased weight of the head increasing cord compression.[2] Quadriplegia may occur at any age.[8] Achondroplasts also have severe and persistent sciatica secondary to disc disease and stenosis in the lower lumbar canal.[9] These patients also develop cord or cauda equina compression at the thoracic or upper lumbar level.[10]

Radiographically, the height of vertebral bodies is reduced, with flaring of the upper and lower end plates resulting in posterior scalloping. The pedicles are short and thick. The interpediculate distances become progressively smaller from L1 to L5[11] (Fig. 14–5). Increased disc spaces are also noted. The spinal canal is very narrow throughout its length.[12, 13] Reconstructed sagittal computerized tomography (CT) may be the most sensitive radiographic technique for detecting craniocervical stenosis with medullary compression.[7] Somatosensory evoked potential (SEP) is a specific but not a sensitive test for documenting cervical cord compression. SEP may be a confirmatory test of compression in patients with signs of compression on CT evaluation.[7]

Treatment for neurologic complications is surgical. As the achondroplastic dwarf ages, stenosis is increased with hypertrophy of the ligamentum flavum and degenerative spondylosis.[14] Repetitive compression injuries to

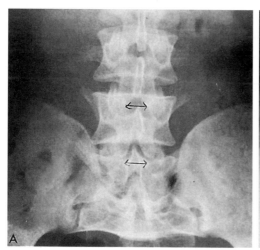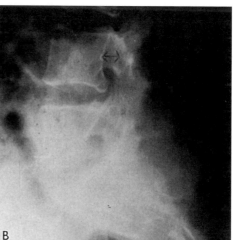

Figure 14–5. Anteroposterior, *A*, and lateral, *B*, views of an achondroplast show decreased spinal canal size and posterior scalloping of the vertebral bodies. (Wiesel SW, Bernini P, Rothman RH [eds]: The Aging Lumbar Spine. Philadelphia: WB Saunders Co, 1982, p 12.)

the cord and spinal nerves lead to irreversible atrophy. Patients with signs of myelopathy require surgical decompression. Patients with severe stenosis of the spinal canal may require surgical decompression from the foramen magnum to the sacrum.[15]

Mucopolysaccharidoses

The diseases in the mucopolysaccharidosis class of inborn errors of metabolism result in deposition of mucopolysaccharides in various tissues. The distinct types of mucopolysaccharidoses are distinguished on the basis of combined clinical, genetic, biochemical, and allelic subtypes.[16] Many of the patients with mucopolysaccharidoses do not live into adulthood. Forms of mucopolysaccharidoses that may be seen by an internist include Hunter's syndrome (type II), Morquio's syndrome (type IV), and Maroteaux-Lamy syndrome (type VI).

Hunter's syndrome (type II) is an X-linked syndrome with a deficiency of iduronate sulfatase, which results in accumulation of dermatan sulfate and heparan sulfate. Patients are men with mild mental retardation and mild hearing loss. The roentgenographic abnormalities include ovoid vertebral bodies with hypoplasia of vertebrae near the thoracolumbar junction, resulting in kyphosis and osteoporosis.[17] Hunter's syndrome is considered a milder form of Hurler's syndrome (type I), a disorder associated with severe deficiency of iduronate sulfatase and death before the age of 10 years. In Hurler's syndrome, cervical spine laxity with subluxation occurs in patients with hypoplasia of the odontoid process.[18] In Hunter's syndrome, compressive myelopathy is a complication of the illness. A combination of progressive thickening of the dura with glycosaminoglycan deposition (pachymeningitis cervicalis) and stenosis of the cervical canal results in myelopathy.[19]

Morquio's syndrome (type IV) is an autosomal recessive disorder with abnormalities in galactosamine-6-sulfate sulfatase (type A) or beta-galactosidase (type B), resulting in ineffective keratan sulfate catabolism and keratan sulfaturia. Clinical manifestations of Morquio's syndrome include dwarfism, facial deformity, short neck, corneal opacification, deafness, pectus carinatum, ligamentous laxity, hepatomegaly, and normal intelligence. The spinal roentgenogram of patients with Morquio's syndrome reveals platyspondylia, with central beaking of vertebral bodies, atlantoaxial subluxation, and kyphoscoliosis.[20] High spinal cord compression related to ligamentous laxity and hypoplasia of the odontoid is a frequent complication of Morquio's syndrome (Fig. 14–6). These individuals have myelopathic signs, spastic paraplegia, and decreased physical endurance secondary to repeated trauma and atrophy of the cervical spinal cord.[21–23] Compression of the spinal cord is a major cause of death in these individuals. Surgical fusion of the cervical spine is indicated in the majority of these patients.[16]

Maroteaux-Lamy syndrome (type VI) is an autosomal recessive syndrome with arylsulfatase B deficiency, which results in accumulation of dermatan sulfate. Clinical manifestations of the syndrome include kyphoscoliosis, pectus carinatum, genu valgum, hepatosplenomegaly, and joint contractures.[24] Variations in the severity of clinical manifestations of the disorder may be related to the heterogeneity of genetic mutations that result in corresponding alterations in the activity or amounts of the arylsulfatase B enzyme. Roentgenogram of the spine may demonstrate beaked vertebral bodies, hypoplasia of vertebral bodies, abnormal ossification of ring epiphyses, and atlantoaxial subluxation with hypoplasia of the odontoid process. Compressive myelopathy may be the result of chronic spinal cord com-

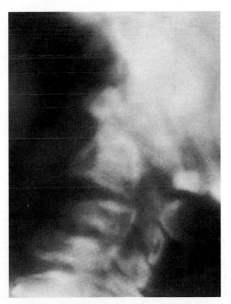

Figure 14–6. Mucopolysaccharidoses IV (Morquio's syndrome). A lateral computerized tomogram of the cervical spine shows odontoid hypoplasia and narrowing of the spinal canal. (McAlister WH, Herman TE: Osteochondrodysplasias, dysostoses, chromosomal aberrations, mucopolysaccharidoses, and mucolipidoses. In: Resnick D [ed]: Diagnosis of Bone and Joint Disorders, 3rd ed. Philadelphia: WB Saunders Co, 1995, p 4233.)

pression secondary to cervical spine instability.[25-27] Patients with this syndrome require surgical decompression of the cervical spinal cord. Bone marrow transplant may be used early in the course of the disorder to prevent harmful deposition of mucopolysaccharide systemically.[28]

Spondyloepiphyseal Dysplasia

The epiphyseal dysplasias have been defined by Spranger as a group of heterogeneous disorders characterized by defective or excessive bone formation in the secondary ossification centers of tubular bones and vertebrae.[29] Because there is no known biochemical abnormality to differentiate these disorders, they have been divided into two large categories based on skeletal disease: (1) spondyloepiphyseal dysplasia (SD) with vertebral beaking and (2) multiple epiphyseal dysplasia without spinal involvement.[30] Abnormalities in type II collagen have been identified in some forms of SD.[31] One abnormality is associated with a higher ratio of hydroxylysine to lysine than in normal collagen.[32] The spectrum of clinical severity of SD may be related to the extent and proximity of defects to the carboxyl terminus of the collagen molecule.

The disorder has an autosomal dominant inheritance. Spinal involvement in multiple epiphyseal dysplasia, if it occurs, is mild compared with the marked alterations that occur in the appendicular skeleton. Most forms of the disorder affect the phalanges, shoulders, and hips, or elbow and knee joints. The vertebral changes mimic those of Scheuermann's disease. The vertebral bodies are wedge-shaped, with mild platyspondylia and scoliosis. The spine is also osteoporotic.[33] This disorder is occasionally confused with Morquio's syndrome. Patients with SD of Maroteaux also mimic Morquio's syndrome but have no abnormality at birth and no biochemical abnormality.[34] Morquio's syndrome is not manifest at birth and has increased mucopolysaccharide in the urine.[35]

SD is recognized to have two primary forms, congenita and tarda. In the congenita form, the spine and some appendicular bones are involved. The vertebrae are flattened, with an irregular aspect to the superior and inferior end plates along with a bulging configuration to the posterior portion of the vertebral body.[36] People with this disorder have a short neck and odontoid hypoplasia and are at risk

for C1–C2 subluxation and myelopathy.[31] They may require cervical stabilization with fusion.[37]

The tarda form is a male sex-linked recessive disorder that becomes manifest in late childhood as short stature with spinal abnormalities, pectus carinatum, and a broad thorax.[38] Roentgenogram of these patients reveals generalized flattening of vertebral bodies, with irregular end plates, intervertebral disc space narrowing, and small iliac bones. The appendicular skeleton is minimally affected.

Down's Syndrome

Patients with Down's syndrome have a trisomy of chromosome 21. These people are recognized at birth with certain phenotypic characteristics, including epicanthal folds, hypotonia, brachycephaly, and large tongue. At any age, they are at risk of developing atlantoaxial subluxation (Fig. 14–7). A prevalence of 15% has been reported in these patients.[39, 40] Although the transverse ligaments are attenuated, the alar ligaments remain intact and protect the spinal cord from compression. Therefore, although excess motion may be measured, few individuals are symptomatic from this abnormality.[41] Patients with Down's syndrome may also develop lower cervical spondylosis and myelopathy below C1–C2.[42] No single assessment technique is available to determine those patients with increased risk for neurologic compromise.[43] In general, routine clinical and radiographic evaluation is indicated for Down's patients, particularly those

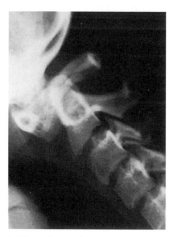

Figure 14–7. Down's syndrome. Note the considerable atlantoaxial subluxation. (McAlister WH, Herman TE: Osteochondrodysplasias, dysostoses, chromosomal aberrations, mucopolysaccharidoses, and mucolipidoses. In: Resnick D [ed]: Diagnosis of Bone and Joint Disorders, 3rd ed. Philadelphia: WB Saunders Co, 1995, p 4227.)

involved in athletics, including the Special Olympics. Patients with atlantoaxial subluxation should not engage in contact sports or those activities associated with flexion of the neck.[44]

References

HERITABLE GENETIC DISORDERS

1. Pyeritz RE: Heritable and development disorders of connective tissue and bone. In: McCarty DJ, Koopman WJ (eds): Arthritis and Allied Conditions, 12th ed. Philadelphia: Lea & Febiger, 1993, pp 1483–1509.
2. Beighton P (ed): McKusick's Heritable Disorders of Connective Tissue, 5th ed. St. Louis: CV Mosby, 1993, p 748.
3. Kahn MF, De Sese S: Rheumatic manifestations of heritable disorders of connective tissue. Clin Rheum Dis 1:3, 1975.
4. Horton WA, Hecht JT: The chondrodysplasias. In: Royce PM, Steinmann B (eds): Connective Tissue and Its Heritable Disorders: Molecular, Genetic, and Medical Aspects. New York: Wiley-Liss, 1993, pp 641–675.
5. Lutter LD, Langer LO: Neurological symptoms in achondroplastic dwarfs: surgical treatment. J Bone Joint Surg 59A:87, 1977.
6. Hecht JT, Butler IJ: Neurologic morbidity associated with achondroplasia. J Child Neurol 5:84, 1990.
7. Reid CS, Pyeritz RE, Kopits SE, et al.: Cervicomedullary compression in young patients with achondroplasia: value of comprehensive neurologic and respiratory evaluation. J Pediatr 110:522, 1987.
8. Yang SS, Corbett DP, Bough AJ, et al.: Upper cervical myelopathy in achondroplasia. Am J Clin Pathol 68:68, 1977.
9. Bailey JA: Orthopaedic aspects of achondroplasia. J Bone Joint Surg 52A:1285, 1970.
10. Epstein JA, Malis LI: Compression of spinal cord and cauda equina in achondroplastic dwarfs. Neurology 5:875, 1955.
11. Alexander E Jr: Significance of the small lumbar spinal canal: cauda equina compression syndromes due to spondylosis, part 5: achondroplasia. J Neurosurg 31:513, 1969.
12. Caffey J: Achondroplasia of pelvis and lumbosacral spine: some roentgenographic features. AJR 80:449, 1958.
13. Suss RA, Udvarhelyi GB, Wang H, et al.: Myelography in achondroplasia: value of a lateral C1–C2 puncture and non-ionic, water-soluble contrast medium. Radiology 149:159, 1983.
14. Hancock DO, Phillips DG: Spinal compression in achondroplasia. Paraplegia 3:23, 1965.
15. Uematsu S, Wang H, Kopits SE, Hurko O: Total craniospinal decompression in achondroplastic stenosis. Neurosurgery 35:250, 1994.
16. Whitley CB: The mucopolysaccharidoses. In: Beighton P (ed): McKusick's Heritable Disorders of Connective Tissue, 5th ed. St. Louis: CV Mosby, 1993, pp 367–499.
17. Hunter C: A rare disease in two brothers. Proc R Soc Med 10:104, 1971.
18. Thomas SL, Childress MH, Quinton B: Hypoplasia of the odontoid with atlanto-axial subluxation in Hurler's syndrome. Pediatr Radiol 15:353, 1985.
19. Kaendler S, Bockenheimer S, Grafin VIH, et al.: Cervical myelopathy in mucopolysaccharidosis type II

(Hunter's syndrome): neuroradiologic, clinical and histopathologic findings. Dtsch Med Wochenschr 115:1348, 1990.
20. McAlister WH, Herman TE: Osteochondrodysplasias, dysostoses, chromosomal aberrations, mucopolysaccharidoses, and mucolipidoses. In: Resnick D (ed): Diagnosis of Bone and Joint Disorders, 3rd ed. Philadelphia: WB Saunders Co, 1995, pp 4163–4244.
21. Blaw ME, Langer LO: Spinal cord compression in Morquio-Brailsford's disease. J Pediatr 74:593, 1969.
22. Lipson SJ: Dysplasia of the odontoid process in Morquio's syndrome causing quadriparesis. J Bone Joint Surg 59A:340, 1977.
23. Trojak JE, Ho C, Roesel RA, et al.: Morquio-like syndrome (MPS IV B) associated with deficiency of a beta-galactosidase. Johns Hopkins Med J 146:75, 1980.
24. Jin W, Jackson CE, Desnick RJ, Schuchman EH: Mucopolysaccharidosis type IV: identification of patients with the severe and mild phenotypes provides molecular evidence for genetic heterogeneity. Am J Hum Genet 50:795, 1992.
25. Wald SL, Schmidek HH: Compressive myelopathy associated with type IV mucopolysaccharidosis (Maroteaux-Lamy syndrome). Neurosurgery 14:83, 1984.
26. Banna M, Hollenberg R: Compressive meningeal hypertrophy in mucopolysaccharidosis. AJNR 8:385, 1987.
27. Tamaki N, Kojima N, Tanimoto M, et al.: Myelopathy due to diffuse thickening of the cervical dura mater in Maroteaux-Lamy syndrome. Neurosurgery 21:416, 1987.
28. Krivit W, Pierpont ME, Ayaz KL, et al.: Bone-marrow transplant in Maroteaux-Lamy syndrome (mucopolysaccharidoses type VI biochemical and clinical status 24 months after transplantation). N Engl J Med 311:1606, 1984.
29. Spranger J: The epiphyseal dysplasias. Clin Orthop 114:46, 1976.
30. Rubin P: Dynamic Classification of Bone Dysplasias. Chicago, Year Book Medical Publishers, 1964, p 120.
31. Rimoin DL, Lachman RS: Genetic disorders of the osseous skeleton. In: Beighton P (ed): McKusick's Heritable Disorders of Connective Tissue, 5th ed. St. Louis: CV Mosby, 1993, pp 557–689.
32. Murray LW, Bautista J, James PL, Rimoin DL: Type II collagen defects in chondrodysplasias, 1: spondyloepiphyseal dysplasias. Am J Hum Genet 45:5, 1989.
33. Hulvey JT, Keats T: Multiple epiphyseal dysplasia: a contribution to the problem of spinal involvement. AJR 106:170, 1969.
34. Doman AN, Maroteaux P, Lyne ED: Spondyloepiphyseal dysplasia of Maroteaux. J Bone Joint Surg 72A:1364, 1990.
35. Saldino RM: Radiographic diagnosis of neonatal short-linked dwarfism. Med Radiogr Photogr 49:61, 1973.
36. Spranger JW, Langer LO Jr: Spondyloepiphyseal dysplasia congenita. Radiology 94:313, 1970.
37. Kopits S: Orthopedic complications of dwarfism. Clin Orthop 114:153, 1976.
38. Langer LO Jr: Spondyloepiphyseal dysplasia tarda: hereditary chondrodysplasia with characteristic vertebral configuration in the adult. Radiology 82:833, 1964.
39. Burke SW, French HG, Roberts JM et al: Chronic atlanto-axial instability in Down's syndrome. J Bone Joint Surg 67A:1356, 1985.
40. Pueschel SM, Scola FH: Atlantoaxial instability in individuals with Down's syndrome: epidemiologic, radiographic, and clinical studies. Pediatrics 80:555, 1987.

41. Davidson RG: Atlantoaxial instability in individuals with Down's syndrome. A fresh look at the evidence. Pediatrics 81:857, 1988.

42. Olive PM, Whitecloud TS III, Bennett JT: Lower cervical spondylosis and myelopathy in adults with Down's syndrome. Spine 13:781, 1988.

43. Pueschel SM, Findley TW, Furia J, et al.: Atlantoaxial instability in Down syndrome: roentgenographic, neurologic, and somatosensory evoked potential studies. J Pediatr 110:515, 1987.

44. Hensinger RN: Congenital anomalies of the cervical spine. Clin Orthop 264:16, 1991.

15

Neurologic and Psychiatric Disorders of the Cervical Spine

Disorders of the neurologic system may be associated with systemic illnesses that alter nerve function or with local compression that causes isolated neurologic abnormalities.

In addition to systemic disorders, such as vasculitis, peripheral neuropathy may affect nerves that course through the cervical spine and arm. Abnormalities of these nerves may superficially resemble impingement of a nerve root by a herniated nucleus pulposus or spinal stenosis. However, careful history and physical examination should localize the lesion outside the central nervous system and should raise the possibility of nerve compression.

The diagnosis of neurologic disorders is made by careful review of findings discovered during the physical examination and of data obtained from a limited number of electrophysiologic and radiographic tests.

Therapy for neurologic disorders associated with neck pain must be directed at the underlying disorder causing nerve dysfunction. Most commonly, control of vessel inflammation is necessary to decrease nerve dysfunction. When nerve compression is relieved, total return of function is possible in a peripheral nerve.

Psychiatric disorders are also associated with neck pain. A minority of patients with psychiatric illness actually complain of neck pain. The hallucinations and other psychotic thoughts of these patients do not usually involve pain.

In contrast, those patients with chronic neck pain frequently develop neurotic behavior. Neurosis increases with the duration of pain. Patients with chronic pain lose control of their lives and become depressed. The initial injury that caused their pain may heal entirely, but the patient continues to exhibit pain behavior. The diagnosis of chronic pain syndrome is made in a patient who has no new organic disease, who has pain for 6 months or longer, and who has experienced progressive, physical, and emotional deterioration. In patients with chronic pain, therapy must take a multidisciplinary form, including drugs, physical therapy, psychiatric therapy, and vocational rehabilitation.

Malingerers are individuals who feign their symptoms and signs willfully to gain some advantage. The number of patients with neck pain who malinger is small. A careful history and physical examination frequently reveal the inconsistencies between malingerers' symptoms and signs and those of patients who have organic disease. If a patient is thought to be malingering, that suspicion should be corroborated by another physician. Extensive evaluation and prolonged treatment are counterproductive for patients with feigned illness.

NEUROLOGIC DISORDERS

Capsule Summary

Frequency of neck pain—rare
Location of neck pain—radicular distribution: shoulder, arm
Quality of neck pain—stinging, radiating
Symptoms and signs—tingling pain or numb-

ness, loss of sensation, local muscle wasting

Laboratory and x-ray tests—electromyogram (EMG) nerve compression; x-ray for Pancoast's tumor

Treatment—nonsteroidal anti-inflammatory drugs (NSAIDs), surgical decompression

NEUROPATHIES

Neurologic disorders most commonly involved with the cervical spine are radiculopathies associated with alterations of cervical intervertebral discs (herniation) and the spinal canal (spinal stenosis with myelopathy). These entities are discussed in Chapter 10. Patients with a herniated disc or myelopathy may have neck pain as part of their symptom complex, but more prominently, they have symptoms that affect the upper extremities. The involvement of the arms follows a specific pattern that correlates with motor and sensory abnormalities associated with dysfunction of a specific nerve root.

Distal to the neural foramen, spinal nerve roots from multiple levels form trunks that are incorporated into the cervical and brachial plexi (see Fig. 5–5). Pathologic processes that affect nerves distal to the spinal cord have a distribution, not as a single root, but as a peripheral nerve with abnormalities in cutaneous or muscular structures innervated by multiple nerve root segments.

Spinal Nerves

Spinal nerve roots become spinal nerves as they leave the spinal canal and lose their dural covering. Spinal nerves may continue as individual nerves or coalesce to form plexi. Different clinical syndromes are produced by problems affecting different segments of the spinal nerves. In the cervical area, paravertebral tumors may damage spinal nerves before they form the brachial plexus.

Pancoast's Tumor. Pancoast's tumor (superior sulcus tumor) arises near the pleural surface at the apex of the lung. This tumor may grow outward and posteriorly into the paravertebral space and posterior chest wall.[1] Pancoast's syndrome occurs as the tumor extends posteriorly toward the costovertebral joints, invading the sympathetic nerve chain (stellate ganglion) and the spinal roots proximal to the brachial plexus from C8 to T3.[2] Because Pancoast's tumor involves extraspinal nerve roots in the paravertebral gutter proxi-

mal to the brachial plexus, clinical syndromes associated with individual cervical nerve root dysfunction are compatible with Pancoast's tumor.[3] Other structures that may be involved less frequently include the lower trunk of the brachial plexus, subclavian artery and vein, internal jugular vein, phrenic nerve, vagus nerve, common carotid artery, and recurrent laryngeal nerve. Tumors may also invade the first three ribs, the transverse processes of C7 through T3. Further invasion results in compromise of the bone surrounding the spinal canal and eventual compression of the spinal cord.[4] Pancoast's tumor comprises 3% of all lung cancers.[5] This tumor is the most common malignancy to invade the brachial plexus.[3] The condition occurs most commonly in smokers. In one study, 49 of 51 patients with Pancoast's tumor were smokers.[6]

The clinical syndrome associated with this tumor includes aching pain in the shoulder of 90% of patients, followed by upper anterior chest wall pain and medial scapular pain posteriorly.[3] Subsequently, pain and numbness develop down the medial aspect of the lower arm and hand (C8 and T1). The arm may become discolored or edematous.[7] Motor weakness and wasting of intrinsic hand muscles occur with further compression. Invasion of the sympathetic ganglia results in decreased autonomic function, with increased warmth of the appendage (without perspiration) and Horner's syndrome. The presence of Horner's syndrome associated with dysfunction of the entire plexus and a primary lung tumor suggests epidural involvement.[8] Movement of the arm may cause muscle spasm and radiating arm pain with lower arm paresthesias. Reflex sympathetic dystrophy of the upper extremity has been associated with Pancoast's tumor.[9]

Radiographic evaluation of the apex of the lung with plain roentgenogram, apical lordotic view, or computerized tomography (CT) is able to detect the presence of a lung lesion once the diagnosis is suspected. Plain roentgenograms in 40% of instances may show only apical thickening. The tumor may grow from areas of old subpleural scarring.[2] Magnetic resonance (MR) imaging is useful for assessing the local extent of the tumor and predicting the possibility of resection of the tumor.[10] Bronchoscopy is not helpful because the lesion is peripheral in the lung. EMG is able to determine the presence of a radiculopathy and the location of the lesion proximal to the brachial plexus.[3] The diagnosis of Pancoast's tumor is frequently delayed. The onset of symptoms and the determination of the correct diagnosis may take more than 7 months.[11] Other disorders confused with Pancoast's tumor include shoulder bursitis, cervical osteoarthritis, and thoracic outlet syndrome.

The treatment of Pancoast's tumor requires a combination of preoperative irradiation, pulmonary wedge resection of the lung, and excision of the involved chest wall and rib.[12] Mediastinoscopy should be accomplished prior to surgery to determine the extent of involvement of mediastinal lymph nodes.[13] The best outcome is found in those patients with complete resection of the tumor. Different median survival rates are associated with involvement of various chest structures. A survival of 4 months is associated with brachial plexus disease, and 7 months is associated with vertebral body invasion. Early diagnosis is essential for the best outcome. Patients with bilateral Pancoast's tumors may survive 6 years or longer with complete resection and radiation.[14]

Cervical Plexus

The cervical plexus is composed of the anterior primary rami of the upper four cervical nerves, the superior cervical sympathetic ganglia, the spinal accessory nerve, and the hypoglossal nerve. The plexus supplies cutaneous nerves to the lateral occipital portion of the scalp, the pinna, the angle of the jaw, the neck, the supraclavicular area, and the upper thorax. The motor branches supply the scalene, levator, sternocleidomastoid, trapezius, infrahyoid, diaphragm, and posterior vertebral muscles. The plexus forms the greater and lesser occipital, greater auricular, and supraclavicular nerves. The plexus is located behind the sternocleidomastoid and anterior to the levator muscle.

Brachial Plexus

Tumors. The brachial plexus is composed of the anterior primary rami of the lower four cervical nerves and the first thoracic nerve. The upper portion supplies the supraclavicular nerve, innervating the supraspinatus and infraspinatus muscles. The lateral cord forms the anterior thoracic nerve supplying the pectoralis muscle. The medial cord supplies the medial brachiocutaneous nerves. The posterior cord forms the subscapular nerve supplying the subscapular muscle, teres major, and the latissimus dorsi. The brachial plexus also receives sympathetic nerves from the lower cervical ganglia.

Metastatic lesions of the axillary or cervical lymph nodes, causing compression or direct invasion of nerves in the neck, axilla, or upper arm, are the most common cause of neoplasms affecting the brachial plexus.[2] The pattern of involvement corresponds to the location of the nodes or the primary source of the tumor. Breast cancer causes compression of the medial cord and medial cutaneous nerves of the arm and forearm (median and ulnar) secondary to involvement of axillary nodes that compress the anteromedial aspect of the plexus. Metastatic cancer of the deep cervical nodes at the base of the neck involves the upper portion of the brachial plexus and the cervical sympathetic chain.

The clinical symptom commonly associated with tumors affecting the brachial plexus is constant, deep, boring pain with dysesthesias. The pain is predominantly in the medial aspect of the arm, forearm, and hand. Weakness in the hand, in a distribution similar to that of Pancoast's lesions, occurs with motor involvement. These lesions may be differentiated from Pancoast's tumors by the absence of paravertebral and subscapular pain and ocular sympathetic nerve abnormalities.

In a study of 100 patients with brachial plexus cancer lesions, Kori and colleagues reported 78 with metastatic disease and 22 with radiation therapy lesions.[15] Lung and breast cancer were the most frequent causing diseases in 32 and 38 individuals, respectively. Other tumors included lymphoma, melanoma, and sarcoma. Pain was the most constant symptom in individuals with metastatic disease. Physical examination demonstrates dysesthesias in the arm and intrinsic hand muscle atrophy with lower brachial plexus lesions. MR imaging is a useful radiographic technique for identifying mass lesions adjacent to the brachial plexus.[16] MR imaging detects tumor infiltration, which helps to distinguish lesions from damage associated with exposure to radiation. MR imaging also identifies the presence of anatomic abnormalities that may cause brachial plexus dysfunction (cervical rib).[17] A latent period of 16 years has been reported in individuals who have developed brachial plexus metastatic lesions after treatment for primary breast cancer.[18] Radiation treatment is used in the area to decrease pain, but there may not be improvement in arm or hand weakness.[15]

Vasculitis. Systemic vasculitis can affect the blood vessels supplying nerves. When blood flow to a nerve is compromised, neurologic dysfunction in the form of motor or sensory loss, or both, occurs. Most often, mononeuritis multiplex is associated with this pathologic process.[19] Medium-sized arteries are most frequently associated with mononeuritis. Mononeuritis multiplex is associated with a variety of connective tissue disorders, including polyarteritis nodosa, systemic lupus erythematosus (SLE), and rheumatoid arthritis.[20] In Wegener's granulomatosis, mononeuritis multiplex affects 12% of patients.[21] The most frequently involved nerves include the median, ulnar, peroneal, and tibial.[22] Mononeuritis multiplex may affect as many as 75% of individuals with Churg-Strauss allergic granulomatosis.[23] However, in a review of 35 patients with mononeuritis, 15 had no identifiable rheumatic disease.[19] Of the 14 patients with mononeuritis multiplex and a connective tissue disease, five had SLE.[19] In general, mononeuritis multiplex occurs less commonly in SLE than isolated sensory neuropathy.[24] A significant number of individuals may develop mononeuritis without an identifiable, associated connective tissue disorder. Dyck and colleagues reported that ischemic nerve lesions are located in the proximal nerve trunks of the upper arms in patients with necrotizing arteritis associated with rheumatoid arthritis.[25] The extent of lesions is throughout the length of the nerve. The areas of nerve ischemic degeneration are watershed zones of poor perfusion. Because peripheral nerves have extensive collateral circulations, vasculitis must be extensive to cause dysfunction.

Upper extremities are less frequently affected than lower extremities. Sensory abnormalities affected 5 of 35 mononeuritis patients with upper extremity symptoms versus 15 of 35 patients with lower extremity symptoms.[19] Eleven patients had both upper and lower extremities. In the upper extremities, the median (9 of 35 patients) and ulnar (9 of 35 patients) nerves were affected. Weakness in a nerve distribution occurred in the setting of a corresponding sensory loss. Motor loss affected the same number of patients with median and ulnar nerve weakness.

The clinical symptoms associated with vasculitis of a plexus or major nerve branch is sudden onset of profound weakness or paralysis of a group of muscles supplied by a major nerve and radiating, burning, aching, or shooting pain associated with dysesthesias or numbness in a matching cutaneous distribution.[26] The onset may take hours to days, but the condition is maximal at the beginning of the insult to the nerve. The damage to the nerve can be profound so that function does not return. If the damage is not complete, return of function may occur from months to a year or longer. Laboratory evaluation reveals systemic factors associated with the specific form of vasculitis (rheumatoid factor—rheumatoid vasculitis; eosinophils—allergic granulomatosis) and nonspecific signs of generalized vessel inflammation (elevated erythrocyte sedimentation rate, thrombocytosis). Antineutrophil cytoplasmic autoantibody (ANCA) is useful in the diagnosis of some forms of vasculitis. Antibodies directed against proteinase 3, a granular cytoplasmic pattern (cANCA), are most closely associated with Wegener's granulomatosis. Antibodies directed against myeloperoxidase, a perinuclear pattern (pANCA), are associated with microscopic polyangiitis.[27] Cerebrospinal fluid remains normal in most cases because the nerve lesions are extraspinal. Electromyogram reveals denervation in the affected muscle along with slowed conduction in the corresponding nerve on nerve conduction studies. Nerve biopsies are most commonly limited to the lower extremities, primarily the sural nerve. Upper extremity biopsies result in neurologic deficits and are not done. The appearance of neurologic abnormalities in the setting of vasculitis is indicative of more aggressive, potentially life-threatening disease. Patients with this condition usually require large doses of corticosteroids and immunosuppressive drugs such as cyclophosphamide.[28, 29]

Radiation Therapy. Radiation therapy to the apex of the lung or neck has been reported to cause damage to the brachial plexus.[15] Patients receiving greater than 6,000 rads to the brachial plexus developed signs of neurologic injury about a year after exposure. The major difficulty for the clinician in this circumstance is to distinguish plexus abnormalities from recurrent tumor. Patients with radiation damage develop neurologic dysfunction primarily in the upper portion of the brachial plexus, involving the C5, C6, or C7 roots. Radiation damage is usually painless, associated with lymphedema of the treated arm, and is not associated with Horner's syndrome. Patients with neoplastic invasion of the brachial plexus have lower branch involvement, with arm pain, and Horner's syndrome.

Brachial Neuritis. Neuralgic amyotrophy, or Parsonage-Turner syndrome, is a viral infection of motor nerves solely with acute onset of pain and weakness of the shoulder and arm.[30] Multiple nerve roots are affected without any sensory deficit, and it occurs most commonly in middle-aged men. The relative absence of sensory abnormalities helps differentiate this disorder from root or plexus abnormalities. Pain is exacerbated by arm movement but is relatively unaffected by neck motion or maneuvers that increase intervertebral disc pressure. The absence of exacerbation of symptoms with mechanical stresses helps differentiate this disorder from radiculopathy secondary to an osteophyte or herniated disc. No specific therapy is effective for this disorder.

Erb's Palsy. Injury to the upper and middle trunk of the brachial plexus, affecting C5 and C6 cervical roots, causes paralysis to the deltoid, biceps, brachial, and brachioradial muscles and less often to the supraspinatus, infraspinatus, and rhomboid muscles. The arm hangs down and cannot be abducted or externally rotated; the forearm cannot be flexed or supinated. The sensory changes are more variable because of overlapping distribution. This disorder occurs secondary to excessive traction on the arm.

Dejerine-Klumpke Palsy. Injury to the lower trunk of the brachial plexus affecting the C8 and T1 roots causes paralysis to the flexors of the wrist, fingers, adductor thumb muscles, interossei, and hypothenar muscles, and, to a lesser extent, to the thumb flexors. Sensory abnormalities correspond to the distribution of the ulnar and median nerves. Causes of this syndrome are apical tumors, aneurysm of the aortic arch, fracture of the clavicle or humerus, and sudden upward traction on the arm.

PERIPHERAL NERVE SYNDROMES

Peripheral nerves are the extension of the spinal nerve roots that comprise the brachial plexus. These nerves supply sensory function alone or a combination of sensory and motor function. Pathologic processes that compress (tunnel syndromes) or decrease blood flow (diabetes) to peripheral nerves are associated with neurologic symptoms of dysesthesias and muscular weakness in the distribution of the corresponding nerve. In diabetes, mononeuropathies of acute onset are located almost exclusively in the lower extremities.[31] Diabetes may increase the sensitivity of peripheral nerves to compression syndromes. Many of the rheumatic diseases that cause mononeuritis multiplex may also be associated with a peripheral polyneuropathy or a multifocal mononeuropathy. A number of nerves are affected in different locations in the upper extremity. Careful physical examination allows for the

differentiation of spinal root from peripheral nerve lesions. Specific areas of sensory loss are characteristic of individual peripheral nerve lesions, such as carpal tunnel syndrome (CTS). A complete listing of upper extremity tunnel syndromes is shown in Table 15–1.

Upper Extremity Compression Neuropathies

Thoracic Outlet Syndrome. This syndrome is caused by compression of the brachial plexus and subclavian vessels as they course from the neck into the arm. The area before the division of the plexus into its component parts is called the thoracic outlet. Compression of structures in this area is called thoracic outlet syndrome and was named by Peet and colleagues in 1956.[32] Depending on the location of compression, thoracic outlet syndrome patients may have symptoms associated with anterior scalene syndrome, costoclavicular syndrome, or hyperabduction syndrome[33] (Fig. 15–1).

Anterior Scalene Syndrome. The brachial plexus and subclavian artery may be compressed between the anterior and medial scalene muscles and the first rib, causing the anterior scalene syndrome. A cervical rib was thought to be the most common cause of this syndrome.[34] However, only 10% of patients who underwent surgery for thoracic outlet syndrome had a cervical rib.[35] Hypertrophy of the scalene muscles, fibrous bands, and vibration injuries are a few of the alternative reasons for this syndrome.[36–38]

The symptoms of this syndrome are related to compression of the lower roots of the brachial plexus on the first rib. Symptoms include pain in the shoulder, arm, forearm, hand, and fingers in a C8 and T1 distribution. The neck and shoulders are in a forward flexed position. Overhead activity stretches the plexus and causes compression by the scalene muscles. Tightness of the scalene muscles may produce occipital headaches.[39] Distal structures are more consistently affected with numbness in the fingers. The degree of arterial compression corresponds to the extent of ischemic changes in the hand, including mottled skin color, swelling, and ulcerations. Motor abnormalities include weakness and atrophy of the hypothenar eminence and interossei. The diagnosis is best determined by reproduction of symptoms with compression and positional provocative testing. Examples of provocative tests include Adson's test and Phalen's maneu-

TABLE 15–1. COMPRESSION NEUROPATHIES OF THE UPPER EXTREMITY

SYNDROME	NERVE	LOCATION	CLINICAL MANIFESTATIONS
Thoracic outlet	C8–T1 nerve roots	Anterior scalene muscle, first rib	Hand dysesthesias
Suprascapular	Suprascapular (C5, C6)	Scapular notch	Abduction, external humeral rotation, shoulder joint capsule
Quadrilateral tunnel	Axillary (C5, C6)	Lateral axillary hiatus	Dysesthesias: shoulder joint, upper arm; deltoid weakness
Supracondylar process	Median (C6, C7, C8)	Supracondylar process (elbow)	Dysesthesias: palmar, dorsal hand; wrist, finger flexor weakness
Pronator teres tunnel	Median (C6, C7)	Pronator teres (anterior lower arm near elbow)	Dysesthesias: palmar, dorsal hand; wrist, finger flexor weakness
Radial tunnel	Radial (C5, C6, C7) (motor branch) (posterior interosseus)	Supinator (lateral elbow)	Weakness of extensors, wrist, fingers
Anterior interosseus	Median (C7, C8)	Medial forearm	Weakness of thumb, index finger flexors (motor only)
Ulnar (ulnar sulcus)	Ulnar (C7, C8)	Medial epicondyle (elbow)	Dysesthesias: ring, little fingers; weakness of finger flexors
Cubital	Ulnar (C7, C8)	Distal to epicondyle (between heads of flexor carpi ulnaris)	Dysesthesias: ring, little fingers; weakness of finger flexors
Carpal	Median (C8, T1)	Wrist	Dysesthesias: palmar surface fingers; weakness of thumb
Guyon's	Ulnar (C8, T1)	Lateral wrist, hypothenar	Dysesthesias: ring, little fingers; weakness of hypothenar eminence
Cheiralgia paresthetica	Radial (C7, C8) (superficial)	Medial thumb, forearm	Dysesthesias: dorsal wrist, thumb, web space
Collateral digital nerve	Median, ulnar (C8, T1)	Fingers	Dysesthesias: neighboring fingers

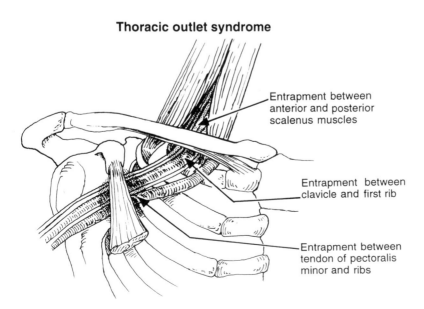

Thoracic outlet syndrome

Entrapment between anterior and posterior scalenus muscles

Entrapment between clavicle and first rib

Entrapment between tendon of pectoralis minor and ribs

Figure 15–1. Compression of the brachial plexus and subclavian artery may occur near the anterior scalenus muscle or the costoclavicular area or under the pectoralis minor muscle.

ver.[40] Adson's test stretches the scalene muscles to create neurovascular compression in the region of the first rib. Loss of pulse volume is not pathognomonic of the syndrome as 15% of normal individuals have similar findings.[41] Electrodiagnostic testing is usually normal because compression changes are reversible with alteration of position. Arteriography may be considered for those patients with signs of vascular compression. Poststenotic dilatation may be found in these patients.[33] No individual test is adequate to determine the presence of this syndrome.

Primary treatment of anterior scalene syndrome is physical therapy with exercises to increase the range of motion of the neck and shoulders, strengthen the trapezius and rhomboid muscles, and improve posture. Increased tone in the shoulder muscles has the potential to reduce tension in the cervical muscles. Conservative therapy, including exercises, can be successful in the majority of patients.[42] If conservative therapy is ineffective, surgical intervention in the form of scalenotomy or rib resection may be considered. The success rate for these operations is 50% or less and is associated with risk of damage to the brachial plexus.[33, 43] In a study of 45 thoracic outlet syndrome patients treated with surgery and followed for a mean of 8 years, successful outcome was reported in 43%.[44]

Costoclavicular Syndrome. Compression of the subclavian artery and vein and brachial plexus between the clavicle and the first rib causes symptoms of vascular insufficiency. The costoclavicular space is bordered by the medial third of the clavicle, the anterior third of the first rib, and insertions of the scalene muscles. The brachial plexus and subclavian artery run through this triangle, with the subclavian vein medial to the insertion of the anterior scalene muscle. Arm raising, posterior movement of the shoulder, or deep inhalation move the clavicle posteriorly in the first two instances or raise the first rib to narrow the costoclavicular space.[45]

Vascular symptoms, as opposed to neurogenic symptoms with the anterior scalene syndrome, tend to predominate and are characterized by claudication or edema. Symptoms may be exacerbated by carrying weight on the back, as in backpacking. The costoclavicular maneuver, rotating shoulders backward and downward, increases symptoms and causes a decrease in pulse volume. Control individuals may also have diminution in pulse volume.[46] Arteriography with movement of the affected shoulder may be required to determine the location of the vascular compression.[47]

Conservative therapy with isometric shoulder girdle exercises, improved posture, and avoidance of movements of the arm above the head are useful means of decreasing symptoms. Conservative therapy should be tried for a minimum of 6 months before surgical intervention is considered. Patients with evidence of vascular insufficiency with digital ischemia may require more immediate surgical intervention.[48]

Hyperabduction Syndrome. The neurovascular bundle continues to the axilla, passing under the attachment of the pectoralis minor muscle tendon to the coracoid process. With abduction of the arm to 180°, the neurovascular bundle is stretched around the tendon and humeral head.[49]

Symptoms of pain, paresthesias, and numbness develop in the fingers and then the hand. Vascular changes may resemble Raynaud's phenomenon, which has been reported in 38% of individuals with the syndrome.[50] Neurologic symptoms tend to be temporary because returning the arm to normal position resolves the pain. Hyperabduction of the arm during physical examination initiates symptoms in most patients.

Treatment consists of avoiding hyperabduction of the arm. This may be difficult for individuals who work overhead, such as painters, bricklayers, or electricians. Operative intervention consists of dividing the pectoralis minor tendon.

Carpal Tunnel Syndrome. Compression of the wrist-to-palm segment of the median nerve under the flexor retinaculum causes the clinical condition known as CTS.[51] CTS patients have numbness in the palmar side of the thumb and the three medial fingers, excluding the lateral half of the ring finger and the little finger (Fig. 15–2). Pain may spread proximally from the hand to the level of the shoulder. The symptoms increase at night and with movement during the day. Motor weakness occurs in the thenar eminence with more severe compression. The usual pressure in the tunnel is 7 or 8 mm Hg. In CTS, the resting pressure is 30 mm Hg, a pressure associated with nerve dysfunction.[52] Pressure may increase to 90 mm Hg with extremes of wrist motion.[41]

CTS is the most common entrapment neuropathy.[53] In a national health survey in 1988, 2.65 million of 170 million adults (1.55%) reported CTS.[54] White women were most frequently affected. In another study, an inci-

MEDIAN NERVE

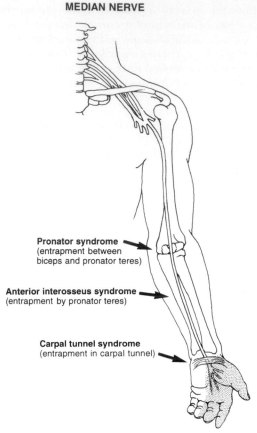

Pronator syndrome
(entrapment between
biceps and pronator teres)

Anterior interosseus syndrome
(entrapment by pronator teres)

Carpal tunnel syndrome
(entrapment in carpal tunnel)

Figure 15–2. Median nerve distribution in the upper extremity. Shaded area in the hand corresponds to the area of numbness with carpal tunnel syndrome.

group remains the most common cause of CTS (Table 15–2).[62]

Electrodiagnostic studies in the form of median sensory and motor nerve conduction studies provide the greatest diagnostic accuracy for CTS.[63] These tests are able to differentiate upper-limb numbness caused by cervical radiculopathy, peripheral neuropathy, and entrapment syndromes. Of the electrodiagnostic tests, the predictive value of sensory conduction is greatest with the maximum latency difference.[64] Uncini and colleagues reported the difference between median and ulnar sensory latencies at digit-four stimulation being the most sensitive test for mild CTS.[65] Distal motor latency determinations are the most helpful tests for detecting severe CTS.[66] Nerve conduction and EMGs are required to determine the extent of nerve compression.[67] The sensitivity of these tests is not total. Normal studies may be found in up to 8% of patients with CTS.[68] Electrophysiologic studies are most abnormal when large myelinated fibers are damaged. Symptoms of CTS may be related to damage of smaller-diameter myelinated and nonmyelinated fibers or to a small number of large fibers to be detected by conduction tests.

Double-crush syndrome refers to the coexistence of CTS and cervical spondylosis causing a C6 radiculopathy.[69] Patients with cervical radiculopathy have pain in the neck, shoulder,

dence of 125 per 100,000 general population was reported.[55] The incidence of CTS in workers covered by workers' compensation is 15 times that in the general population, with a greater proportion of men (60% versus 25%) and a younger peak age at onset (37.4 years versus 51 years).[56] Occupations with awkward wrist positions, increased force across the wrist, and repetitive hand motions have been proposed as causes of this compression syndrome. Musician, assembly line worker, and dental hygienist are a few of the occupations associated with CTS.[57, 58] Overuse or repetitive motion syndromes, including CTS, account for 50% of occupational illnesses in the United States.[59] However, continued debate exists concerning the specific criteria for diagnosis of CTS and the importance of nonergonomic factors (age and obesity) on the development of symptoms.[60, 61] CTS is also associated with a wide variety of medical conditions that cause swelling of the contents of the carpal tunnel, resulting in nerve compression. The idiopathic

TABLE 15–2. CAUSES OF CARPAL TUNNEL SYNDROME

CONDITION	PATIENTS (n = 1,016)	
	Number	Percentage
IDIOPATHIC	439	43.2
ASSOCIATED CONDITIONS	577	56.8
Trauma	136	13.4
Collagen vascular (rheumatoid arthritis, subacute lupus erythematosus)	66	6.5
Hormone replacement	65	6.4
Diabetes mellitus	62	6.1
Excessive hand use	60	5.9
Wrist osteoarthritis	54	5.3
Pregnancy	47	4.6
Tenosynovitis	31	3.1
Miscellaneous (tumors, amyloidosis)	25	2.5
Myxedema	14	1.4
Other (acromegaly, tuberculosis)	17	1.7

Modified from Stevens JC, Beard CM, O'Fallon WM, et al.: Conditions associated with carpal tunnel syndrome. Mayo Clin Proc 67:541, 1992. By permission.

arm, and hand, whereas the pain of CTS is primarily in the hand, with radiation to the shoulder but not to the neck. Pain radiating to the chest wall or the scapula suggests radiculopathy. When both lesions are present, the neurologic examination may demonstrate findings beyond those expected with pure median nerve compression, such as decrease of biceps (C6) or triceps (C7) reflexes.

Radiographic evaluation of the carpal tunnel is not necessary for diagnosis of CTS. MR imaging is able to determine a causative lesion in a minority of CTS patients.[70] MR imaging detects tenosynovitis, cysts, and aberrant muscles. Edema or enlargement of the nerve may also be detected, which may be unrecognized at time of surgery. However, MR imaging does not have greater diagnostic accuracy than electrodiagnostic tests and should be reserved for the patient who does not respond to usual treatment.

Conservative treatment with wrist splints, patient education, NSAIDs, and occasional carpal tunnel corticosteroid injection is effective therapy for the majority of patients with CTS. In a study of 265 patients, 188 (71%) improved without the need for carpal tunnel release surgery.[71] Follow-up electrodiagnostic studies obtained normal results in 72 (27%) and improvement in 106 (40%).[71] Potential indicators of poor response to conservative therapy include age greater than 50 years, duration of disease of more than 10 months, and constant paresthesias.[72] Patients who have a poor response to conservative therapy and demonstrate motor weakness confirmed with electrodiagnostic tests are candidates for sectioning of the volar carpal tunnel ligament. This outpatient procedure has good to excellent improvement of symptoms in 80% to 86% of patients, with 40% regaining normal function.[73, 74] Patients with a poor result from surgery may have had only partial sectioning of the retinaculum or they develop neural fibrosis. Reexploration of the tunnel, with internal neurolysis of the median nerve, may be required to relieve symptoms in these patients.[75, 76] Patients with occupations that do not require excessive use of the hands may return to work in 7 to 14 days. Patients whose occupations involve exposure of the hands to repeated trauma (such as carpenters) may not return for months. Some people may need to change jobs because of stress to the hands.[41]

Other conditions associated with compression of the median nerve in the upper extremity include supracondylar process syndrome, pronator syndrome, and anterior interosseous syndrome.[77] The supracondylar process is an atavistic bone connected to the anteromedial surface of the distal humerus. A fibrous band (ligament of Struthers) attaches this bone to the median epicondyle. The median nerve can be compressed under this band, causing pain and paresthesias in the median nerve distribution in the hand, motor signs of decreased thumb opposition, and flexion of the first three fingers. Nerve conduction (NC) tests document slowing across the supracondylar tunnel. Pronator syndrome occurs as the median nerve leaves the cubital fossa at the elbow, passing between the heads of the pronator teres and the tendinous arch of the flexor digitorum superficialis. The test on physical examination that helps differentiate this syndrome from CTS is the absence of Phalen's sign at the wrist, Tinel's sign in the forearm, pain on resistance to pronation, and pain in the forearm on resistance to isolated flexion of the proximal joints of the long and ring fingers.[77] Anterior interosseous syndrome affects the anterior interosseous nerve, which is a pure motor branch of the median nerve that supplies the flexor pollicis longus (thumb) and flexor digitorum profundus (index finger). The nerve appears from the posterior portion of the median nerve distal to the medial humeral epicondyle and travels to the deep fascial layer to run with the interosseous membrane, ending under the pronator quadratus. Individuals are unable to pinch the thumb and index finger and are usually unable to write.[78]

Ulnar Nerve Entrapments

The ulnar nerve entrapment syndromes occur less commonly than median nerve syndromes. Ulnar nerve syndromes include ulnar nerve sulcus syndrome, cubital tunnel syndrome, and ulnar tunnel (Guyon's canal) syndrome (Fig. 15–3).

Ulnar Nerve Sulcus Syndrome. The ulnar nerve is compressed in the sulcus at the medial side of the distal humerus. The sulcus is covered by the epicondylo-olecranon ligament to prevent subluxation with forearm movement. Swelling of or trauma to the sulcus may result in ulnar nerve dysfunction. Pain and dysesthesias appear in the lateral aspect of the hand. Pain may also radiate to the shoulder. Further compression results in atrophy of intrinsic hand muscles, including hypothenar wasting.

Cubital Tunnel Syndrome. Cubital tunnel syndrome occurs as the ulnar nerve passes un-

ULNAR NERVE

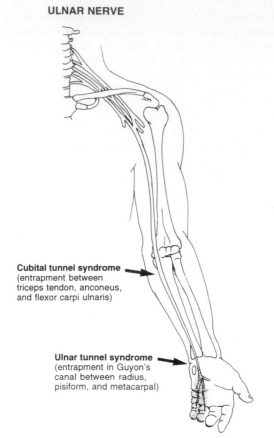

Cubital tunnel syndrome
(entrapment between
triceps tendon, anconeus,
and flexor carpi ulnaris)

Ulnar tunnel syndrome
(entrapment in Guyon's
canal between radius,
pisiform, and metacarpal)

Figure 15–3. Ulnar nerve distribution in the upper extremity. Shaded area in the hand corresponds to the area of numbness with ulnar tunnel syndrome.

der the aponeurosis of the flexor carpi ulnaris 1.5 to 3.5 cm distal to the humeral sulcus. When the elbow is flexed, the aponeurosis becomes taut, compressing the ulnar nerve, increasing symptoms. External compression results from resting the elbow on a flat surface and may occur in anesthetized patients.[79] Patients develop pain, paresthesias, and weakness in the hand in an ulnar nerve distribution. The location of a Tinel's sign helps differentiate this syndrome from the sulcus syndrome. NC tests detect pathologic conditions near the elbow. Intrinsic hand muscles are used to determine motor velocity and the little finger for sensory abnormalities. Despite careful examination, the exact location of the lesion may not be found in up to 50% of patients.[41] The differential diagnosis for cubital tunnel syndrome includes C8–T1 radiculopathy, compression of the medial cord of the brachial plexus with Pancoast's tumor, or thoracic outlet syndrome. Conservative therapy with decreased elbow flexion and NSAIDs is only partially effective. Surgical therapy is not nec-

essarily a preferred option because the exact location of impingement may not be identified. Surgical decompression should be reserved for individuals with disability associated with muscle weakness. Surgical intervention may include transposition of the nerve with protective muscle flap or removal of the epicondyle.[80, 81]

Ulnar Tunnel Syndrome. Ulnar tunnel syndrome occurs on compression of the nerve in Guyon's canal in the hand. The tunnel's floor is formed by the transverse carpal ligament and its roof by the insertion of the flexor carpi ulnaris muscle. Only the superficial and deep palmar branches of the nerve run in the ulnar tunnel. The superficial portion of the palmar branch supplies the palmaris brevis muscle, the palmar skin of the little finger, and the ulnar skin of the ring finger. The deep branch supplies the hypothenar muscles, the two lateral lumbrical muscles, the interossei muscles, the adductor pollicis, and the flexor pollicis brevis. Depending on the location of nerve injury, ulnar nerve symptoms may be mixed or purely motor in origin. The differential diagnosis between compression at the wrist or elbow of the ulnar nerve may be made by involvement of the flexor to the little finger, as this muscle is only affected by ulnar nerve compression at the elbow. Conservative therapy may be used for a 6-month trial. If symptoms persist, surgical decompression of the canal with release of sensory and motor branches is indicated.[33]

Radial Nerve Entrapments

The radial nerve may be involved in radial tunnel syndrome, posterior interosseous syndrome, and compression of the superficial branch of the radial nerve (cheiralgia paresthetica) (Fig. 15–4). The terminal motor branch of the radial nerve passes under the tendinous arch (Frohse's arcade, present in only 30% of adults) of the supinator muscle at the elbow, with the superficial sensory nerve branching proximal to the muscle.[82] The component of the radial nerve supplying the extensors of the elbow and wrist also branches before the supinator muscle so motion of these joints remains unaffected by radial tunnel syndrome.

Radial Tunnel Syndrome. The radial nerve may be compressed by fibrous bands in the region of the radiocapitellar joint, the radial recurrent vessels, the tendinous origin of the extensor carpi radialis brevis, the tendon of

RADIAL NERVE

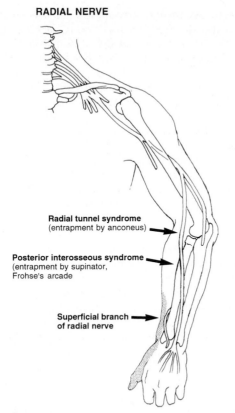

Radial tunnel syndrome
(entrapment by anconeus)

Posterior interosseous syndrome
(entrapment by supinator,
Frohse's arcade

Superficial branch
of radial nerve

Figure 15–4. Radial nerve distribution in the upper extremity. Shaded area in the hand corresponds to the area of numbness with cheiralgia paresthetica.

the supinator, and the distal edge of the supinator muscle. Finger weakness in association with pain over the lateral epicondyle is a finding associated with this nerve entrapment. Pain may be elicited with forced resistance to middle finger extension with the wrist and elbow extended.[83] Approximately 10% of patients with radial tunnel syndrome may also have lateral epicondylitis.[84] Treatment of the entrapment includes avoidance of repetitive trauma to the nerve in the tunnel. Physical therapy, splinting, and local injections may be helpful. Surgical decompression of the radial tunnel along with decompression of the epicondyle are frequently done as these areas of inflammation coexist.

Posterior Interosseous Syndrome. Posterior interosseous syndrome occurs with compression of the deep branch of the radial nerve at the distal end of the supinator muscle. Patients with this entrapment have transient pain and weakness of thumb extension. Electrodiagnostic tests are able to differentiate this nerve compression from those affecting the brachial plexus or more proximal lesions of the radial

nerve. This syndrome is treated in a fashion similar to that for radial tunnel syndrome.

Cheiralgia Paresthetica. Cheiralgia paresthetica is caused by damage to the superficial cutaneous portion of the radial nerve supplying the dorsal skin over the wrist and the thumb and index and middle fingers to the base of the second phalanx. The superficial branch of the radial nerve passes over the supinator muscle, dips under the brachioradialis muscle, and emerges in the skin near the radial styloid. Any trauma to the radial side of the hand results in a burning sensation in the wrist, thumb, and first two fingers. A variety of traumas, including those resulting from plaster casts, watchbands, handcuffs, and intravenous infusions, may irritate the nerve. Patients present with paresthesias without motor signs. Trophic changes in the skin appendages occur if the damage is chronic and extensive. The symptoms may respond to conservative therapy, including topical agents. If scar tissue develops, reduction of tissue with neurolysis is indicated.

OTHER PERIPHERAL NEUROPATHIES

Greater Occipital Nerve (C2). The greater occipital nerve ascends through the semispinalis capitis and trapezius muscles close to their attachments to the occipital bone and travels with the occipital artery over the medial portion of the scalp to the vertex of the skull. Entrapment of this nerve causes pain over the occiput without lower neck or shoulder pain. Increased pain with flexion or extension may suggest C1–C2 joint disease as a cause of nerve irritation. Palpation over the occipital prominence frequently increases scalp pain. Conservative management in the form of exercises and oral anti-inflammatory medications may be helpful. Injection over the maximum point of tenderness near the occiput with a local anesthetic may offer temporary relief of pain.

Dorsal Scapular Nerve (C5). The dorsal scapular nerve arises from the upper trunk of the brachial plexus, primarily from C5. The nerve passes through the body of the scalenus medius muscle. The nerve approaches the levator at its anterior border, passing under the muscle and the rhomboids adjacent to the medial border of the scapula. The nerve is the sole nerve supply to the rhomboids, and it supplies the lower portion of the levator scapulae. Pain is located over the rhomboid muscle and may be associated with muscular spasm. Subjective weakness may also be noted by the patient. On examination, pain is aggravated by turning the head towards the affected extremity and by lateral flexion to the opposite side. Physical therapy for strengthening the shoulder girdle muscles is helpful in decreasing compression of the nerve. Surgical decompression is limited to those with EMG evidence of denervation of the appropriate muscles.

Long Thoracic Nerve (Bell's Nerve). The long thoracic nerve arises from roots from C5, C6, and C7 and supplies the serratus anterior muscle. The nerve passes through the scalenus medius muscle. Loss of function results in winging of the scapula. The nerve may be injured by continuous heavy effort with the arm above the shoulder or by heavy objects being carried on the shoulder.

Suprascapular Nerve. The suprascapular nerve is derived from the upper trunk of the brachial plexus (C5, C6). The nerve passes behind the brachial plexus to enter the suprascapular notch under the transverse ligament. This pure motor nerve supplies the supraspinous and infraspinous muscles. Stretching of the arm causes a deep pain that is poorly localized. The pain results in decreased motion of the shoulder. In a patient with adhesive capsulitis with decreased motion of the humerus, forward flexion of the arm causes increased stretch of the nerve under the transverse ligament, resulting in pain. Persistent injury results in weakness in abduction and external rotation of the arm, tenderness on palpation, and atrophy of the muscles. Injection in the suprascapular notch may decrease pain. Division of the transverse ligament is indicated if conservative therapy is ineffective and muscle weakness is persistent.

MISCELLANEOUS DISORDERS

Other conditions that may, on occasion, be associated with neck pain or cause symptoms that may be confused with radicular arm pain include reflex sympathetic dystrophy and shoulder arthritis. These disorders cause radiating pain into the arm, to the trapezius and, on occasion, pain up to the base of the neck.

Reflex Sympathetic Dystrophy (RSD)

RSD is a syndrome associated with causalgia, extremity swelling, and vascular instability.

The International Association for the Study of Pain has defined RSD as "continuous pain in a portion of an extremity after trauma which may include fracture but does not involve a major nerve, associated with sympathetic hyperactivity."[85] Kozin has suggested that a patient may experience pain as the sole manifestation of RSD and other patients may have only vasomotor or sudomotor changes without pain or tenderness.[86] The American Association for Hand Surgery considered RSD to be a pain syndrome in which pain is accompanied by loss of function and evidence of autonomic dysfunction.[87] Not only is there debate about the components of RSD, but the syndrome has also had a number of different names, including Sudeck's atrophy, algodystrophy, and shoulder-hand syndrome.

The pathogenesis of the syndrome is a matter of debate in the medical literature. Some reports have suggested that peripheral sensory nerve increases afferent input to the internuncial nerve in the spinal cord, which results in continuous stimulation of the sympathetic system. Others have suggested vasomotor reflex spasm resulting in loss of vascular tone. Abnormalities in blood flow control result in atrophy of affected tissues.[85] Recent experiments suggest that alterations in blood flow are related to supersensitivity to sympathetic neurotransmitters rather than overactivity of the sympathetic system because levels of adrenaline and noradrenaline are lower in affected limbs compared with the unaffected limb. This finding suggests that the manifestations of RSD are a result of disruption of efferent sympathetic modulation of pain.[88] Hannington-Kiff suggested that failure of natural opioid modulation of pain mediated by regional sympathetic ganglia after injury results in dystrophic alterations of a limb.[89] Others believe that RSD is a disorder of the psyche associated with personality traits of rigidity and somatization.[90] Others promote the idea that the sympathetic system plays little role in RSD and consider neuropsychiatric mechanisms the cause of the syndrome.[91]

RSD is usually incited after a trauma (fracture), central or peripheral nerve injuries (stroke and shingles), cardiovascular events (myocardial infarction), drugs (barbiturates), pulmonary disease (tuberculosis), and immobilization. The clinical symptoms and signs of RSD include severe, burning pain; vasomotor instability; diffuse swelling of the appendage; and dystrophic skin changes. Most patients do not demonstrate all the manifestations of the syndrome. Many patients do not recall a traumatic event. Bonica defined three stages of RSD, starting with dysesthesias, swelling, increased blood flow, and increased skin temperature; followed by burning pain, decreased blood flow, decreased skin temperature, and decreased limb motion; and concluding with subcutaneous tissue atrophy and contractures.[92] A study of 829 patients did not find a chronologic progression in this syndrome.[93] Patients could be divided according to warm and cold appendages. Individuals with a longer duration of RSD were in the cold group. RSD may spread to affect other limbs without additional trauma,[94] or it may affect only part of a limb, such as a single digit.[95]

Routine laboratory test results are normal or reflect abnormalities with associated conditions. Plain roentgenograms of the affected limb may demonstrate diffuse osteopenia, which is greater than what would be expected from disuse alone.[96] Three-phase technetium 99m methylene diphosphonate bone scintiscans are useful in identifying individuals with RSD. The delayed images are better than blood flow or pool phase images to determine the presence of RSD.[97]

Treatment of RSD should be initiated as soon as the diagnosis is suspected. Physiotherapy for mobilization of the limb is essential to avoid progression of the syndrome. Patients should receive analgesics, NSAIDs, temperature modalities, and exercises to increase range of motion. Systemic corticosteroids in the range of 20 to 40 mg should be added if symptoms persist. Sympathetic blocks may be used to decrease pain in order to increase movement of the affected limb.[98] Surgical sympathectomy may be considered for those patients who have responded to injections. Some individuals have a sustained response to surgical sympathectomy.[99] Others have suggested that sympathectomy is not helpful and that symptoms return after operation.[91] Other therapies that have been used include calcitonin, guanethidine, and nifedipine.[85, 100] Intrathecal morphine has been used for RSD patients whose intractable pain is resistant to all other therapies.[101] This technique has been used for only a few patients and requires additional study with prolonged follow-up to determine its efficacy.

Shoulder Arthritis

Shoulder abnormalities cause pain primarily over the joint itself.[102] Instability, trauma, arthritis, bursitis, rotator cuff lesions, and bicipi-

tal tendinitis are a partial list of the lesions that affect the shoulder.[103] Referred pain from the shoulder may radiate proximally towards the base and lateral aspect of the neck. This radiation of pain may be mediated through tension in the trapezius muscle. Patients complain of pain in both locations. Acromioclavicular joint disease may also refer pain toward the base of the neck. C5 radiculopathy is associated with pain over the deltoid area that coincides with the location of pain associated with shoulder problems. Careful examination of the shoulder joint and cervical spine, including careful palpation of the structures, can help differentiate the primary focus of pain. Cervical spine disorders frequently refer pain to both shoulders. The absence of any tenderness in the neck or exacerbation of symptoms on manipulation of the cervical spine is important evidence that another musculoskeletal structure is the source of pain. The shoulder is usually more sensitive to mechanical enhancement of symptoms. Pain is more acute with movement and may remain more persistent. Shoulder disorders are also accompanied with stiffness or instability that would not be expected with primary cervical spine disease.

References

NEUROLOGIC DISORDERS

1. Pancoast HK: Superior pulmonary sulcus tumor: tumor characterized by pain, Horner's syndrome, destruction of bone and atrophy of hand muscles. JAMA 99:1391, 1932.
2. Layzer RB: Neuromuscular Manifestations of Systemic Disease. Philadelphia: FA Davis Co, 1985.
3. Vargo MM, Flood KM: Pancoast tumor presenting as cervical radiculopathy. Arch Phys Med Rehabil 71:606, 1990.
4. Batzdorf U, Brechner V: Management of pain associated with the Pancoast syndrome. Am J Surg 137:638, 1979.
5. Ziporyn T: Upper body pain: possible tipoff to Pancoast tumor. JAMA 246:1759, 1981.
6. Spengler DM, Kirsh MM, Kaufer H: Orthopaedic aspects and early diagnosis of superior sulcus tumor of the lung (Pancoast). J Bone Joint Surg 55A:1645, 1973.
7. Miller JI, Mansour KA, Hatcher CR: Carcinoma of the superior pulmonary sulcus. Ann Thorac Surg 28:44, 1975.
8. Stubgen J: Neuromuscular disorders in systemic malignancy and its treatment. Muscle Nerve 18:636, 1995.
9. Derbekyan V, Novales-Diaz J, Lisbona R: Pancoast tumor as a cause of reflex sympathetic dystrophy. J Nucl Med 34:1992, 1993.
10. Beale R, Siater R, Hennington M, et al.: Pancoast tumor: use of MRI for tumor staging. South Med J 85:1260, 1992.
11. Hepper NGG, Herskovic T, Witten DM, et al.: Thoracic inlet tumors. Ann Intern Med 64:979, 1966.

12. Maggi G, Casadio C, Pischedda F, et al.: Combined radiosurgical treatment of Pancoast tumor. Ann Thorac Surg 57:198, 1994.

13. Remmen HJ, Lacquet LK, Van Son JA, et al.: Surgical treatment of Pancoast tumor. J Cardiovasc Surg 34:157, 1993.

14. Rea F, Mazzucco C, Breda C, et al.: Bilateral Pancoast syndrome in a patient with metachronous primary lung cancer. Ann Thorac Surg 58:550, 1994.

15. Kori SH, Foley KM, Posner JB: Brachial plexus lesions in patients with cancer: 100 cases. Neurology 31:45, 1981.

16. Thyagarajan D, Cascino T, Harms G: Magnetic resonance imaging in brachial plexopathy of cancer. Neurology 45:421, 1995.

17. Collins JD, Shaver ML, Disher AC, et al.: Compromising abnormalities of the brachial plexus as displayed by magnetic resonance imaging. Clin Anat 8:1, 1995.

18. Thomas JE, Colby MY Jr: Radiation-induced or metastatic brachial plexopathy: a diagnostic dilemma. JAMA 222:1392, 1972.

19. Hellmann DB, Laing TJ, Petri M, et al.: Mononeuritis multiplex: the yield of evaluations for occult rheumatic diseases. Medicine 67:145, 1988.

20. Scott DGI, Bacon PA, Tribe CR: Systemic rheumatoid vasculitis: a clinical and laboratory study of 50 cases. Medicine 60:288, 1981.

21. Duna GF, Galperin C, Hoffman GS: Wegener's granulomatosis. Rheum Dis Clin North Am 21:949, 1995.

22. Nishino H, Rubino FA, DeRemee RA, et al.: Neurological involvement in Wegener's granulomatosis: an analysis of 324 consecutive patients at the Mayo Clinic. Ann Neurol 33:4, 1993.

23. Lhote F, Guillevin L: Polyarteritis nodosa, microscopic polyangiitis, and Churg-Strauss syndrome: clinical aspects and treatment. Rheum Dis Clin North Am 21:911, 1995.

24. Bacon PA, Carruthers DM: Vasculitis associated with connective tissue disorders. Rheum Dis Clin North Am 21:1077, 1995.

25. Dyck PJ, Conn DL, Okazaki H: Necrotizing angiopathic neuropathy: three-dimensional morphology of fiber degeneration related to sites of occluded vessels. Mayo Clin Proc 47:461, 1972.

26. Olney RK: AAEM minimonograph #38: neuropathies in connective tissue disease. Muscle Nerve 15:531, 1992.

27. Gross WL: Antineutrophil cytoplasmic autoantibody testing in vasculitides. Rheum Dis Clin North Am 21:987, 1995.

28. Guillevin L, Du LTH, Godeau P, et al.: Clinical findings and prognosis of polyarteritis nodosa and Churg-Strauss angiitis: a study in 165 patients. Br J Rheumatol 27:258, 1988.

29. Moore PM, Fauci AS: Neurologic manifestations of systemic vasculitis: a retrospective and prospective study of the clinicopathologic features and response to therapy in 25 patients. Am J Med 71:517, 1981.

30. Tsairis P, Dyck PJ, Mulder DW: Natural history of brachial plexus neuropathy. Arch Neurol 27:109, 1972.

31. Raff MC, Asbury AK: Ischemic mononeuropathy and mononeuropathy multiplex in diabetes mellitus. N Engl J Med 279:17, 1968.

32. Peet RM, Hendricksen JD, Gunderson TP, et al.: Thoracic outlet syndrome: evaluation of a therapeutic exercise program. Mayo Clin Proc 31:281, 1956.

33. Pecina MM, Krmpotic-Nemanic J, Markiewitz AD: Tunnel Syndromes. Boca Raton, Florida: CRC Press, 1991, pp 1–84.

34. Brannon EW: Cervical rib syndrome: an analysis of nineteen cases and twenty-four operations. J Bone Joint Surg 45A:977, 1963.

35. Adson AW: Surgical treatment for symptoms produced by cervical ribs and scalenus anticus muscle. Clin Orthop 207:3, 1986.

36. Liu JE, Tahmoush AJ, Roos DB, et al.: Shoulder-arm pain from cervical bands and scalene muscle anomalies. J Neurol Sci 128:175, 1995.

37. Wilbourn AJ: Thoracic outlet syndrome surgery causing severe brachial plexopathy. Muscle Nerve 11:66, 1988.

38. Frankel SA, Hirata I Jr: The scalenus anticus syndrome and competitive swimming: report of two cases. JAMA 215:1796, 1971.

39. Mackinnon SE, Novak CB: Clinical commentary: pathogenesis of cumulative trauma disorder. J Hand Surg 19A:873, 1994.

40. Novak CB, MacKinnon SE, Patterson GA: Evaluation of patients with thoracic outlet syndrome. J Hand Surg 18A:292, 1993.

41. Dawson DM: Entrapment neuropathies of the upper extremities. N Engl J Med 329:2013, 1993.

42. Kenny RA, Traynor GB, Withington D, et al.: Thoracic outlet syndrome: a useful exercise treatment option. Am J Surg 165:282, 1993.

43. Cherington M, Happer I, Machanic B, et al.: Surgery for thoracic outlet syndrome may be hazardous to your health. Muscle Nerve 9:632, 1986.

44. Lindgren K, Oksala I: Long-term outcome of surgery for thoracic outlet syndrome. Am J Surg 169:358, 1995.

45. Winsor T, Brow R: Costoclavicular syndrome: its diagnosis and treatment. JAMA 196:109, 1966.

46. Gergouldis R, Barnes RW: Thoracic outlet arterial compression: prevalence in normal persons. Angiology 31:538, 1980.

47. Sadler TR Jr, Rainer WG, Twombley G: Thoracic outlet compression: application of positional arteriographic and nerve conduction studies. Am J Surg 130:704, 1975.

48. Toby EB, Koman LA: Thoracic outlet compression syndrome. In: Szabo RM: Nerve Compression Syndromes: Diagnosis and Treatment. Thorofare, New Jersey: Slack Inc, 1989, pp 209–226.

49. Fields WS, Lemak NA, Ben-Menachem Y: Thoracic outlet syndrome: review and reference to stroke in a major league pitcher. AJR 146:809, 1986.

50. Beyer JA, Wright IS: The hyperabduction syndrome: with special reference to its relationship to Raynaud's syndrome. Circulation 4:161, 1951.

51. Ross MA, Kimura J: AAEM case report #2: the carpal tunnel syndrome. Muscle Nerve 18:567, 1995.

52. Szabo RM, Chidgey LK: Stress carpal tunnel pressures in patients with carpal tunnel syndrome and normal patients. J Hand Surg 14A:624, 1989.

53. Barrett DS, Donnell ST: Entrapment neuropathies: 1: upper limb. Br J Hosp Med 46:94, 1991.

54. Tanaka S, Wild DK, Seligman PJ, et al.: The US prevalence of self-reported carpal tunnel syndrome: 1988 national health interview survey data. Am J Public Health 84:1846, 1994.

55. Stevens JC, Sun S, Beard CM, et al.: Carpal tunnel syndrome in Rochester, Minnesota, 1961 to 1980. Neurology 38:134, 1988.

56. Franklin GM, Haug J, Heyer N, et al.: Occupational carpal tunnel syndrome in Washington State, 1984–1988. Am J Public Health 81:741, 1991.

57. Hoppmann RA, Patrone NA: A review of musculoskeletal problems in instrumental musicians. Semin Arthritis Rheum 19:117, 1989.

58. Masear VR, Hayes JM, Hyde AG: An industrial cause of carpal tunnel syndrome. J Hand Surg 11A:222, 1986.

59. Rempel DM, Harrison RJ, Barnhart S: Work-related cumulative trauma disorders of the upper extremity. JAMA 267:838, 1992.
60. Katz JN, Larson MG, Fossel AH, et al.: Validation of a surveillance case definition of carpal tunnel syndrome. Am J Public Health 81:189, 1991.
61. Nathan PA, Meadows KD, Doyle LS: Relationship of age and sex to sensory conduction of the median nerve at the carpal tunnel and association of slowed conduction with symptoms. Muscle Nerve 11:1149, 1988.
62. Stevens JC, Beard CM, O'Fallon WM, et al.: Conditions associated with carpal tunnel syndrome. Mayo Clin Proc 67:541, 1992.
63. Jablecki CK, Andary MT, So YT, et al.: Usefulness of nerve conduction studies and electromyography for the evaluation of patients with carpal tunnel syndrome. Muscle Nerve 16:1392, 1993.
64. Nathan PA, Keniston RC, Meadows KD, et al.: Predictive value of nerve conduction measurements at the carpal tunnel. Muscle Nerve 16:1377, 1993.
65. Uncini A, DiMuzio A, Awad J, et al.: Sensitivity of three median-to-ulnar comparative tests in the diagnosis of mild carpal tunnel syndrome. Muscle Nerve 16:1366, 1993.
66. Seror P: Sensitivity of various electrophysiologic studies for the diagnosis of carpal tunnel syndrome. Muscle Nerve 16:1418, 1993.
67. Werner RA, Albers JW: Relation between needle electromyography and nerve conduction studies in patients with carpal tunnel syndrome. Arch Phys Med Rehabil 76:246, 1995.
68. Biundo JJ Jr, Mipro RC Jr, Djuric V: Peripheral nerve entrapment, occupation-related syndromes, sports injuries, bursitis, and soft tissue problems of the shoulder. Curr Opin Rheumatol 7:151, 1995.
69. Osterman AL: The double crush syndrome. Orthop Clin North Am 19:147, 1988.
70. Seyfert S, Boegner F, Hamm B, et al.: The value of magnetic resonance imaging in carpal tunnel syndrome. J Neurol 242:41, 1994.
71. Harter BT Jr, McKiernan JE Jr, Kirzinger SS, et al.: Carpal tunnel syndrome: surgical and nonsurgical treatment. J Hand Surg 18A:471, 1993.
72. Kaplan SJ, Glickel SZ, Eaton RG: Predictive factors in the non-surgical treatment of carpal tunnel syndrome. J Hand Surg 15B:106, 1990.
73. Cseuz KA, Thomas JE, Lambert EH, et al.: Long-term results of operation for carpal tunnel syndrome. Mayo Clin Proc 41:232, 1966.
74. Haupt WF, Wintzer G, Schop A, et al.: Tunnel decompression. J Hand Surg 18B:471, 1993.
75. O'Malley MJ, Evanoff M, Terrono AL, et al.: Factors that determine reexploration treatment of carpal tunnel syndrome. J Hand Surg 17A:638, 1992.
76. Chang B, Dellon AL: Surgical management of recurrent carpal tunnel syndrome. J Hand Surg 18B:467, 1993.
77. Bracker MD, Ralph LP: The numb arm and hand. Am Fam Physician 51:103, 1995.
78. Stern MB: The anterior interosseous nerve syndrome (The Kiloh-Nevin syndrome): report and followup study of three cases. Clin Orthop 187:223, 1984.
79. Miller RG, Camp PE: Postoperative ulnar neuropathy. JAMA 242:1636, 1979.
80. Heithoff SJ, Millender LH, Nalebuff EA, et al.: Medial epicondylectomy for the treatment of ulnar nerve compression at the elbow. J Hand Surg 15A:22, 1990.
81. Adelaar RS, Foster WC, McDowell C: The treatment of the cubital tunnel syndrome. J Hand Surg 9A:90, 1984.
82. Spinner MJ: The arcade of Frohse and its relationship to posterior interosseous nerve paralysis. J Bone Joint Surg 50B:809, 1968.
83. Lister GD, Belsole RB, Kleinert HE: The radial tunnel syndrome. J Hand Surg 4A:52, 1979.
84. Werner CO: Lateral elbow pain and posterior interosseous nerve entrapment. Acta Orthop Scand 174(Suppl):1, 1979.
85. Paice E: Reflex sympathetic dystrophy. BMJ 310:1645, 1995.
86. Kozin F: Reflex sympathetic dystrophy syndrome: a review. Clin Exp Rheumatol 10:401, 1992.
87. Amadio PC, Mackinnon SE, Merritt WH, et al.: RSDS: consensus report of an ad hoc committee of the American Association for Hand Surgery on the definition of RSDS. Plast Reconstr Surg 87:371, 1991.
88. Drummond PD, Finch PM, Smythe GA: Reflex sympathetic dystrophy: the significance of differing plasma catecholamine concentrations in affected and unaffected limbs. Brain 114:2025, 1991.
89. Hannington-Kiff JG: Does failed natural opioid modulation in regional sympathetic ganglia cause reflex sympathetic dystrophy? Lancet 338:1125, 1991.
90. Van Houdenhove B, Vasquez G, Onghena P, et al.: Etiopathogenesis of RSD: a review and biopsychosocial hypothesis. Clin J Pain 8:300, 1992.
91. Ochoa JL, Verdugo RJ: Reflex sympathetic dystrophy: a common clinical avenue for somatoform expression. Neurol Clin 13:351, 1995.
92. Bonica JJ: Causalgia and other reflex sympathetic dystrophies. Advances in Pain Research and Therapy 3:141, 1979.
93. Veldman PHJM, Reynen HM, Arntz IE, et al.: Signs and symptoms of reflex sympathetic dystrophy: prospective study of 829 patients. Lancet 342:1012, 1993.
94. Teasell RW, Potter P, Moulin D: Reflex sympathetic dystrophy involving three limbs: a case study. Arch Phys Med Rehabil 75:1008, 1994.
95. Laukaitis JP, Varma VM, Borenstein DG: Reflex sympathetic dystrophy localized to a single digit. J Rheumatol 16:402, 1989.
96. Genant HK, Kozin F, Bekerman C, McCarty DJ, et al.: The reflex sympathetic dystrophy syndrome: a comprehensive analysis using fine-detail radiography, photon absorptiometry and bone and joint scintigraphy. Radiology 117:21, 1975.
97. O'Donoghue JP, Powe JE, Mattar AG, et al.: Three-phase bone scintigraphy: asymmetric patterns in the upper extremities of asymptomatic normals and reflex sympathetic dystrophy patients. Clin Nucl Med 18:829, 1993.
98. Hord AH, Rooks MD, Stephens BO, et al.: Intravenous regional bretylium and lidocaine for treatment of reflex sympathetic dystrophy: randomized, double-blind study. Anesth Analg 74:818, 1992.
99. Kleinert HE, Cole NM, Wayne L, et al.: Post-traumatic sympathetic dystrophy. Orthop Clin North Am 4:917, 1983.
100. Prough DS, McLeshey CH, Poehling GG, et al.: Efficacy of oral nifedipine in the treatment of reflex sympathetic dystrophy. Anesthesiology 62:796, 1985.
101. Becker WJ, Ablett DP, Harris CJ, et al.: Long-term treatment of intractable reflex sympathetic dystrophy with intrathecal morphine. Can J Neurol Sci 22:153, 1995.
102. Smith DL, Campbell SM: Painful shoulder syndromes: diagnosis and management. J Gen Intern Med 7:328, 1992.
103. Glockner SM: Shoulder pain: a diagnostic dilemma. Am Fam Physician 51:1677, 1995.

PSYCHIATRIC DISORDERS

Capsule Summary

P—psychiatric disorders
CP—chronic pain
M—malingering
Frequency of neck pain
    P—rare
    CP—common
    M—common
Location of neck pain
    P—neck
    CP—neck
    M—neck
Quality of neck pain
    P—unremitting, persistent, requires descriptive language ("burning through my neck")
    CP—continuous with irregular fluctuations
    M—unremitting, unresponsive to all therapies, disabling
Symptoms and signs
    P—neurotic
    CP—traumatic injury, loss of control over life
    M—incapacitating pain, attempt to impress with severity of lesion, nonanatomic examination: entire neck, entire limb affected
Laboratory and x-ray tests
    P—normal
    CP—normal
    M—normal
Treatment
    P—antipsychotic drugs
    CP—antidepressants, pain clinic
    M—none

PSYCHIATRIC DISORDERS

Patients with psychiatric disorders may develop pain as part of their symptoms associated with their illness. The prevalence of pain as a symptom in psychiatric patients ranges from 22% to 66%, depending on the population studied (inpatient versus outpatient, Veterans Administration system versus private clinic).[1–3] In many of these patients, pain is recognized as a result of their mental illness but is not a major complaint. However, in at least 25% of psychiatric patients, pain is severe.[3]

Patients with psychiatric disorders use medical services frequently. Katon and colleagues reported on frequent medical care users at a clinic.[4] About 33% of all services were used by 10% of patients. Of this 10%, about 50% were psychologically distressed. In this group, psychiatric diagnoses were prevalent, including major depression, panic disorder, and somatization disorder. Somatoform disorders are defined as those in which the presentation of psychological conflicts and issues has taken the form of physical illness.[5]

Somatization accompanies genuine physical disease as excessive worry, elaboration of symptoms, or disproportionate disability.[6] Components of the somatoform disorders include hypochondriasis, conversion disorder, somatization disorder, pain disorder, and body dysmorphic disorder.[7]

The pain that these patients with psychiatric illness experience is as "real" to them as to those with a fractured femur. Pain is defined by the International Association for the Study of Pain as "an unpleasant sensory and emotional experience which we primarily associate with tissue damage or describe in terms of such damage, or both."[8] The definition of pain has two parts. One part deals with tissue damage or the threat of damage. It is necessary to experience an emotional response to that injury in order to experience pain. Therefore, those psychiatric patients who experience an emotional response to an event that they believe to be damaging have felt pain.

Walters was one of the first to report on pain in psychiatric patients.[9] In a study of 430 patients referred for evaluation of pain, the head and neck were areas of discomfort mentioned by patients. The low back was most frequently affected in 112 patients (26%). Pain was usually described dramatically. The most common diagnoses in these 430 patients was "other neuroses and situational states" in 336, conversion hysteria in 26, and psychoses in 68. Psychiatric patients with minor physical trauma had greater levels of pain than would have been expected given the extent of tissue damage.

Merskey reported his experience with 76 patients with mental illness and pain. The occurrence of neurosis and pain was more common than the occurrence of pain associated with schizophrenia or endogenous depression.[10] Merskey discovered a relatively high association of neurosis, hysteria, and conversion symptoms with pain. Spear also found an increased number of neurotic patients with pain.[2] He found a similar proportion of neurotic patients with pain, compared with the psychotic individuals in Merskey's study.

Psychological test studies have used the Minnesota Multiphasic Personality Inventory

(MMPI) scores for hypochondrosis and conversion reaction. Those scores were elevated compared with those for depression in psychiatric patients. Sternbach has demonstrated that the conversion pattern on the MMPI was found in patients who had pain that was chronic in duration. An unexpected finding was the relative absence of depression as a psychiatric diagnosis.[11] In a comparison between chronic pain–clinic patients and psychiatric patients with pain, depression was identified more commonly in the psychiatric population, but even then represented only 10% of the psychiatric patients with pain.[12, 13]

Merskey has suggested four reasons why psychological illness causes the appearance or exacerbation of pain.[14] The first relates to a state of anxiety. Increased anxiety or worry about a lesion or experience heightens the intensity of pain. The mechanism of anxiety-associated pain remains speculative, but from a clinical standpoint, alleviation of anxiety has a beneficial effect in the reduction of pain.

A second mechanism is associated with psychiatric hallucination. This mechanism is a rare cause of pain and is most closely associated with schizophrenic patients. Schizophrenic patients may experience hallucinatory damage to their person but infrequently associate that with pain.[15]

The third mechanism is a hypothesis concerning increased tension in muscles, which is associated with inadequate circulation and the accumulation of metabolic byproducts (lactic acid).[16] Individuals in ordinary life who use muscles in a new way may develop aching and discomfort in a body part, whereas those with chronic anxiety and stress have generalized muscle tension and pain. This hypothesis has not been proved. In a number of studies of pain, particularly headache, increased muscle tension accounted for only a small percentage of pain in chronic pain patients. The pain was more closely related to a patient's personality disorder than to the level of muscle contraction.[17, 18]

The fourth mechanism of pain production in psychiatric patients is hysteria with conversion reactions. Conversion reaction or hysterical conversion is a mechanism, supplied by the voluntary portion of the nervous system, for transforming anxiety or other emotions into a dysfunction of bodily structures or organs. The symptoms lessen anxiety and symbolize the underlying mental conflict. The patient may gain benefits from the situation and may not be overly concerned about the dysfunction. The mental anguish associated with the condition is difficult to recognize by the people around the patient, but a somatic complaint, such as neck pain, is one that is readily accepted and understood. Some traditional associated phenomena such as symbolism, la belle indifférence, and histrionic personality do not occur with adequate frequency to be useful in differentiating conversion from physical disease.[19]

Psychogenic rheumatism is a term that may be used in patients who have musculoskeletal symptoms, such as neck pain, associated with a psychiatric disorder.[20] The criteria for this diagnosis include the absence of an organic disease or insufficient disease present to account for the complaints, "functional" character of the complaints, and a positive diagnosis for a psychiatric illness. In one large population of rheumatology patients, approximately 7% had a diagnosis of psychogenic rheumatism. However, the separation of psychogenic rheumatism and organic disease was seldom distinct.

Rotes Querol has suggested a list of symptoms and signs for patients with psychogenic rheumatism.[20] The presence of these symptoms does not have diagnostic importance until the possibility of organic disease has been ruled out. The symptoms and signs include the following:

1. Dramatic urgency for an appointment not justified by the severity of disease.
2. A written list of complaints so that no fact is left out.
3. Multiple test results, including electrocardiogram, electromyogram, electroencephalogram, barium enema, upper gastrointestinal scan, computerized tomography scan, myelograms, and MR imaging.
4. The need to review the laboratory data first to determine the cause of the patient's symptoms. Any minor abnormalities are highlighted by the patient.
5. Preoccupation with future disability from minor physical changes.
6. Those who accompany the patient may be entirely separated from the patient's condition or intensively supportive, highlighting every abnormality and frequently using the pronoun "we" during the description of test or medication taken.
7. Inability to relax during the examination.
8. Marked theatrical responses to questions concerning pain.
9. Patient frequently holds on to the physician during the course of the examination as a gesture of seeking support.

Specific psychogenic syndromes involving

the cervical spine and areas of referred pain are listed in Table 15–3. Benign dorsalgia is associated with pain in the interscapular area. The pain is variable in quality, consisting of components of fatigue, aching, and burning. Diffuse pain over the corresponding spinous processes is common. In contrast, pain in a band-like pattern may be of nerve root origin. Plain roentgenograms are unremarkable for alterations that are commensurate with the level of pain expressed by the patient. The syndrome is seen most frequently in light-duty workers who require a slight flexion of the spine, such as typists and computer operators. Cervicocranial psychogenic rheumatism affects older patients and involves the nuchal area, with radiation of pain to the vertex of the skull. These individuals experience persistent headaches and an unsteady gait. These episodes may be differentiated from vertebrobasilar insufficiency by the lack of reproducibility of symptoms and signs with specific rotatory and extension movements of the neck.[20]

The evaluation of the psychiatric patient must be complete. A thorough history evaluation is essential to remove the possibility of an organic cause of a patient's pain. This type of evaluation also gains the patient's confidence that the physician has been thorough and concerned about the problem. At a second session, the possibility of stress as a cause of the patient's pain should be raised. Additional portions of the patient's history concerning job or family stresses or conflicts are asked. The patient may be willing to talk about the faults of others in the workplace but remains reticent about sexual conflicts with the spouse or conflicts with parents or children unless specifically asked.

The patient must be told that the pain is of psychogenic origin. Statements by the physician denying the presence of an illness are inappropriate ("It is all in your own imagination"). The explanation of the fact that people who are anxious, threatened, or stressed experience real pain is reassuring to the patient. Such a patient is referred to a mental health professional for care of the psychiatric disorder. While the patient is undergoing psychiatric therapy, the referring physician should encourage the patient to be as physically active as possible. Interaction with other people in an exercise class may be useful.

TABLE 15–3. PSYCHOGENIC RHEUMATISM SYNDROMES OF THE CERVICAL SPINE

Benign dorsalgia
Cervicocranial syndromes
  Pain in the cervical and nuchal areas
  Fronto-occipital headaches
  Paresthesias over the vertex
  Sensations of giddiness and instability on walking;
    agoraphobia
  Feelings of weight and pain in the eyes or in the
    periorbital region
  Functional disturbances of eyesight including
    transitory blindness and central scotomata
  Dryness and irritation of the mouth and larynx and
    intermittent loss of voice
  Feelings of unreality
Nocturnal acroparesthesias
  Sensory abnormalities similar to carpal tunnel
    syndrome
  Occur always at night
  Relieved by moving arms in morning
  Absence of motor abnormalities
  Frequent proximal radiation of pain to the shoulder
  Symptoms increased with anxiety and tension, not
    position
  Difficult to differentiate from median nerve
    compression

Modified from Rotes Querol J: The syndrome of psychogenic rheumatism. Clin Rheum Dis 5:797, 1979.

CHRONIC PAIN

Patients with acute injuries recognize the linkage between pain (nociception) and tissue injury. The stimulation of nociceptors results in communication of injury to the spinal cord and cerebral cortex. Acute pain is localized, measured, qualified, and experienced as an emotional response. Reflex response results in muscle contraction surrounding the injured site, moving the body away from the painful stimulus and protecting the injured area. The pain that remains after the immediate injury results in decreased use of that body part during the healing process. That portion of the body is protected. Once the lesion heals, the pain disappears.

From a psychological perspective, neck pain is particularly disturbing to the host because the location of discomfort is close to the spinal cord and central nervous system. Referred pain from neck injury may radiate up to become a headache or down the spine to cause low back pain. Pain may also radiate into the arms, hands, or thighs. Although the pain may be severe, gradual resolution of the pain is the rule. In the usual circumstance, the process resolves with increasing improvement over 8 weeks.

The patient with chronic pain does not follow this scenario. Chronic pain is defined as pain that has been present for 6 months or longer.[21] The most significant factor differentiating chronic from acute pain is that the pain is no longer serving a useful biologic or survival function and has become a disease itself. The emotional state of patients, involving affective, vegetative, cognitive, and behavioral components of their personality, is affected. This was noted during the Civil War by Mitchell and colleagues, who described the development of dejection and anger in soldiers who developed chronic causalgia.[22] The patient undergoes a progressive physical and emotional deterioration caused by loss of appetite, insomnia, depression, anxiety, decreased physical activity, demoralization, and depressive symptoms of worthlessness, helplessness, and hopelessness. The patient has the clinical signs and symptoms of chronic pain syndrome.[23]

The effects of chronic pain syndrome vary, depending on the patient's ethnic background, coping skills, self-image, and support system contributed by family and coworkers. Understanding the patient's psychosocial dynamics has a profound effect on the prognosis of the patient and the choice of therapy. A psychosocial assessment can identify the strengths and weaknesses of the patient's personality structure, which influences the manifestations of the patient's pain syndrome and identifies those factors that may hinder compliance with the treatment regimen.

The psychological assessment of the patient with chronic pain may include evaluation of the patient's personality, conceptualization of the pain, and a rating scale for the severity of pain. The MMPI is the most widely used personality test.[24] The purpose of the test is to categorize psychiatric patients and to discriminate between psychiatric and normal patients through answers to 566 true-or-false questions. The questions are divided into 10 clinical scales, consisting of hypochondriasis, depression, hysteria, psychopathic deviance, masculinity and femininity, paranoia, psychasthenia, schizophrenia, hypomania, and social introversion.

Patients with chronic pain indicate an elevation in neuroticism manifested by increases on the hypochondriasis, depression, and hysteria scales. The basic interpretation of this profile is that it reflects a preoccupation with physical symptoms, bodily functions, depression, negativism, and hostility and use of denial to cope with psychological conflicts. Data for patients who have less depression form a V on the data record, which is referred to as a "conversion V" pattern. These patients somatize their

problems when under stress. Physical symptoms are easier for these patients to understand than psychological conflicts.

The results of the MMPI taken by chronic pain patients have been reported by a number of investigations. Sternbach reported neurotic scale elevation in patients with chronic back pain compared with those with acute low back pain.[25] Neurosis was not a permanent part of the patient's personality, as shown by a reduction in neurotic scales in patients who had pain relief after back surgery.[26] Fordyce has noted that the degree of neuroticism in MMPI studies is related more to the chronicity of the pain than to the physical lesion.[27]

The McGill Pain Questionnaire assesses how patients conceptualize their pain by using words to qualify and quantify it. There are 78 pain descriptors in the questionnaire. In one study, psychiatric disturbance was associated with a greater total number of pain descriptors.[28] Patients may also use visual pain analog scales to quantify their pain. A daily log of a patient's pain level, along with extent of physical activity and medication usage, can be used to assess the patient's functional status and monitor progress. Whether estimations of pain intensity are correlated with the clinical status and health care use by a patient has been challenged by Fordyce.[29] Patient's self-reports of pain may not accurately describe their level of functioning. However, the ratings of pain by the patient do help in monitoring progress in treatment.

In addition to those tests already mentioned, a mental status examination along with a social and work history is essential. These evaluations focus on the patient's thought processes and self-image. The work history is important for listing a patient's work experiences and testing those job skills the patient retains, which may be used in vocational rehabilitation.

The classification of psychiatric diagnoses of pain patients is difficult. *The Diagnostic and Statistical Manual of Mental Disorders,* 4th edition (DSM-IV), is the standard for the nomenclature of psychiatric diagnoses. In a study of 1801 patients seen by a psychiatric consultation service, 167 pain patients were compared with the remainder in regard to their DSM-III diagnosis. The pain patients had more serious medical problems, lacked improvement in medical condition, and had decreased mobility. Non-pain patients had more serious psychiatric disorders. The psychiatric diagnoses of the pain patients were nonspecific for the problem of pain, including dysthymic disorder, and depressed mood. DSM does not provide specificity of the clinical state of pain, including the separation of chronic and acute syndromes.[30]

A variety of DSM diagnoses, including depression, somatosensory conversion disorder, anxiety, and personality disorders, were used for the characterization of 283 chronic pain patients at a pain center.[31] Diagnosis of schizophrenia and psychogenic disorders was rare. The authors of this study agreed that difficulties exist in characterizing patients with chronic pain with the current DSM classification.

All the patients with chronic neck pain have received medical therapy consisting of NSAIDs, muscle relaxants, and physical therapy, including temperature modalities and exercises, but have not had a satisfactory response. Many of these patients seek multiple medical consultations and undergo a variety of unconventional therapies including acupuncture and spinal manipulation. Other chronic pain patients may have undergone multiple surgical procedures or suffered substance abuse in the form of alcohol or narcotics.

Treatment of patients with chronic pain must be directed at physical-structural abnormalities if they persist and, equally importantly, at pain behavior of the patient. The four most important factors determining successful outcome in rehabilitation of chronic pain patients are the following in order of importance: (1) motivation, (2) social support system, (3) chronicity, and (4) degree of tissue pathology.[32] Correction of tissue pathology is important but may not be adequate to alter pain behavior. If the condition has been chronic, patients may have altered their behavior because of the pain to the point where they have lost control over their lives.[33] These individuals, in response to the loss of control, develop reduced motivation to initiate responses to the environment, inability to learn new responses, depression, and anxiety disorders. Depression was noted in over 50% of patients with chronic low back pain who were resistant to medical and surgical therapy.[34] The reality of being in pain and out of work can also contribute to psychological dysfunction. Dependency becomes all-encompassing in a patient who is unemployed, financially insecure, experiencing deteriorating interpersonal relationships with family members, and socially isolated. Therapy for these individuals must be directed at returning control of their lives to them.

A patient with chronic, resistant neck pain benefits from an evaluation by a pain center. Pain centers have the resources to deal with a patient's situation in a multidisciplinary fashion. Psychiatrists, psychologists, neurosurgeons, anesthesiologists, physical therapists, vocational rehabilitation counselors, and social workers are part of the treatment team. Through the concerted effort of all these health professionals and the motivation of the patient, improvement in the patient's condition can occur. A study of 38 patients with disabling chronic pain at a 3-week inpatient/outpatient pain center demonstrated an improvement in patient function. Patients at the pain center had significant reduction in addictive medications, subjective pain ratings, the number of functional activities that caused pain, and the number of health professional visits.[35]

MALINGERING

Malingering, which may be defined as conscious misrepresentation of thoughts, feelings, and facts, is a condition in which symptoms and signs associated with pain are entirely feigned for secondary gain.[36] Most commonly, malingering occurs in the workplace for workers' compensation. However, the secondary gain may not be just financial. Individuals may feign neck symptoms to continue in a less strenuous job at work. They may receive a parking space closer to their place of employment. These individuals may feign symptoms to gain control over family members or co-workers. The injured person may allow others to do the work that person would ordinarily do.

The actual percentage of chronic neck pain patients who are malingering is undetermined. Obviously, judging the inaccuracy of a patient's report of pain and disability is a difficult process. It is difficult to prove conscious misrepresentation of thoughts, feelings, and facts by the patient. Also, each health care provider has an individual standard of symptoms and signs by which to judge those with chronic neck pain. However, most physicians who see a large population of neck pain patients believe that the number of individuals who are true malingerers—those who feign injury and pain in willful manner to collect workers' compensation or disability payments—is quite low.

The possibility of malingering should be

raised in the mind of the treating physician when major discrepancies or inconsistences appear in a patient's medical situation. These inconsistencies may involve the patient's history or physical examination. The inconsistencies are useful in documenting one's suspicions. Research suggests that patients are able to fool clinicians into diagnosing disorders that are functional.[37] These difficulties have been documented for a variety of physicians.[38] A patient may describe excruciating pain that is incapacitating for any activities of daily living. The pain is continuous and has not been affected by any therapy. The patient is unable to sleep but seems rested. The patient may describe a history of multiple visits to physicians without any benefit. The patient may also try to flatter the physician by complimenting his or her reputation.

Two separate sets of criteria have been developed to document the likelihood of malingering.[39, 40] Although the Emory Pain Control Center "inconsistency profile" and Ellard's profile of inconsistency were developed independently, they are remarkably similar. The Emory profile is an amalgam of factors that can lead the examining physician to a suspicion of malingering. The profile includes the following:

1. Discrepancy between a patient's complaint of "terrible pain" and an attitude of calmness and well-being.

2. Completely normal workup for organic disease by two or more physicians.

3. "Dramatized" complaints that are vague or that have global implications ("It just hurts." or "I hurt bad.").

4. Exaggeration of trivial problems, embellished with medical terms learned from previous contacts with physicians ("My back spasms paralyze my legs.").

5. Overemphasized gait or posture abnormalities that develop suddenly, persist, and cannot be substantiated objectively (such as the presence of a limp that is not confirmed by a specific pattern of wear of old shoes, the use of a cane, the daily use of a back brace that shows little wear).

6. Resistance to evaluation or rehabilitation when the goal of therapy is return to gainful employment.

7. Lack of motivation to learn new coping skills, despite verbal reports of compliance with treatment (such as no increase in back motion despite claims of completing range of motion exercises on a daily basis).

8. Missed appointments for studies that measure function, motion, or vocational capabilities.

9. Unconventional response to treatment (such as no discrimination between saline and analgesic injection into affected areas), with reports of increased symptoms with therapy that follow no anatomic or physiologic pattern (such as tranquilizers being stimulants and vice versa).

10. Resistance to treatment especially in the presence of intense complaints of pain.

11. Absence of psychological or emotional disturbances.

12. Psychological test profile inconsistent with clinical presentation (such as MMPI profile indicative of a psychotic disorder with no clinical signs of psychosis).

13. Discrepancies between reports of patient and those of spouse or other close relatives.

14. Unstable personal and occupational history.

15. A personal history that reflects a character disorder such as drug or alcohol abuse, criminal behavior, erratic personal relationships, and violence.

As suggested by the inconsistency profile, physical examination of the malingerer is often helpful and revealing. The patient may refuse to cooperate with components of the examination.[41] A normal cervical curvature without paraspinous muscle spasm is unusual in the patient with persistent neck pain in whom straightening would be expected. Gently touching the skin over the neck results in intense pain with reflex spasm. The area of tenderness may vary during the examination. It is worthwhile to retest the area of tenderness during the course of the physical examination. The physician may mark the location of maximum pain. Frequently, the patient does not remember the exact location of the tenderness and an inconsistency is noted. Later in the examination, the patient designates a different location. A patients will be unable to bend the neck forward more than 5° despite the absence of muscle spasm. Simultaneous hand strength should be checked after each hand is tested independently. The strong arm becomes weak in the simultaneous test. Sensory abnormalities may include extreme pain with pinprick, a midline loss of sensation, stocking-glove anesthesia, whole arm numbness, differences in loss in supination and pronation, and inconsistent response to vibratory stimuli with a tuning fork. Deep tendon reflexes are hyperactive and out of proportion to the stimulus. Cogwheel rigidity is noted in the affected arm with sudden giving way. Patients should also complete a pain drawing documenting all areas of involvement. Many malingerers believe that more is better. Patients tend to fill out areas of involvement far from the cervical spine.

Once all the data have been collected, the physician should make a determination of malingering. This is a difficult process that requires the diagnostic and detective skill of the physician. Very few malingerers are totally without pain or the fear of being placed back in a job situation that may be perceived as harmful.

Some physicians prefer to remove themselves from the determination of malingering, leaving it to others, including lawyers, to determine impairment and disability. If the process is allowed to function without medical input, those who do not deserve compensation or consideration will diminish the resources that rightfully belong to those individuals who have organic difficulties who are attempting to function at their maximum capacity. If the physician believes the patient is a malingerer, the physician should terminate further treatment of the patient. The patient should be told there is no anatomic abnormality that can explain the pain. If the patient has been evaluated only once, the patient should be referred to another physician for a second opinion. If the first physician was in error, the second physician can initiate appropriate therapy. If the first physician was correct, no additional investigations are ordered, and therapy is discontinued.

References

PSYCHIATRIC DISORDERS

1. Klee GD, Ozelis S, Greenberg I, Gallant LJ: Pain and other somatic complaints in a psychiatric clinic. Maryland St Med J 8:188, 1959.
2. Spear FG: Pain in psychiatric patients. J Psychosom Res 11:187, 1967.
3. Delaplaine R, Ifabumuyi OI, Mersky H, Zarfas J: Significance of pain in psychiatric hospital patients. Pain 4:361, 1978.
4. Katon W, Von Korff M, Lin E, et al.: Distressed high utilizers of medical care. DSMIII-R diagnoses and treatment needs. Gen Hosp Psychiatry 12:355, 1990.
5. American Psychiatric Association: Diagnostic and Statistical Manual of Mental Disorders, 3rd ed. Washington, D.C.: American Psychiatric Press, 1987.
6. Mabe PA, Hobson DP, Jones LR, et al.: Hypochondriacal traits in medical inpatients. Gen Hosp Psychiatry 10:236, 1988.
7. Ford CV: Dimensions of somatization and hypochondriasis. Neurol Clin 13:241, 1955.
8. International Association for the Study of Pain (Subcommittee on Taxonomy): Pain terms: a list with definitions and notes on usage. Pain 6:249, 1979.
9. Walters A: Psychogenic regional pain alias hysterical pain. Brain 84:1, 1961.
10. Merskey H: The characteristics of persistent pain in psychological illness. J Psychosom Res 9:291, 1965.
11. Sternbach RA: Pain Patients: Traits and Treatment. New York: Academic Press, 1974.
12. Pilowsky I, Chapman CR, Bonica JJ: Pain, depression, and illness behavior in a pain clinic population. Pain 4:183, 1977.
13. Pelz M, Merskey H: A description of the psychological effects of chronic painful lesions. Pain 14:293, 1982.
14. Merskey H: Pain and psychological medicine. In: Wall PD, Melzack R (eds): Textbook of Pain, 2nd ed. Edinburgh: Churchill Livingstone, 1989, pp 656–666.
15. Watson GD, Chandarana PC, Merskey H: Relationships between pain and schizophrenia. Br J Psychiatry 138:33, 1981.
16. Lewis T, Pickering GW, Rothschild P: Observations upon muscular pain in intermittent claudication. Heart 15:359, 1931.
17. Sainsbury P, Gibson JG: Symptoms of anxiety and tension and the accompanying physiological changes in the muscular system. Psychosom Med 17:216, 1954.
18. Harper RC, Steger JC: Psychological correlates of frontalis EMG and pain in tension headache. Headache 18:215, 1978.
19. Ford CV, Folks DG: Conversion disorders: an overview. Psychosomatics 26:371, 1985.
20. Rotes Querol J: The syndrome of psychogenic rheumatism. Clin Rheum Dis 5:797, 1979.
21. Sternbach RA: Pain: A Psychophysiological Analysis. New York: Academic Press, 1968.
22. Mitchell SW, Moorehouse GR, Keen WW: Gunshot Wounds and Other Injuries of Nerves. Philadelphia: JB Lippincott, 1864.
23. Black RG: The chronic pain syndrome. Surg Clin North Am 4:999, 1975.
24. Dahlstrom WG, Welsh GS, Dahlstrom LE: An MMPI Handbook, vols 1, 2. Minneapolis: University of Minnesota Press, 1972.
25. Sternbach RA, Wolf SR, Murphy RW, et al.: Traits of pain patients: the low-back "loser." Psychosom 14:226, 1973.
26. Sternbach RA, Timmermans G: Personality changes associated with reduction of pain. Pain 1:177, 1975.
27. Fordyce WE: Behavioral methods in chronic pain and illness. St Louis, CV Mosby, 1976.
28. Kremer EF, Atkinson JH, Kremer AM: The language of pain: affective descriptors of pain are a better predictor of psychological disturbance than sensory and effective descriptors. Pain 16:185, 1983.
29. Fordyce WE, Lansky D, Calsyn DA, et al.: Pain measurement and pain behavior. Pain 18:53, 1984.
30. King SA, Strain JJ: The problem of psychiatric diagnosis for the pain patient in the general hospital. Clin J Pain 5:329, 1989.
31. Fishbain DA, Goldberg M, Meagher BR, et al.: Male and female chronic pain patients categorized by DSM-III psychiatric diagnostic criteria. Pain 26:181, 1986.
32. Ng LKY (ed): New Approaches to Treatment of Chronic Pain: A Review of Multidisciplinary Pain Clinics and Pain Centers. HEW, NIDA, Monograph Series 36, 1981.
33. Woodforde JM, Merskey H: Personality traits of patients with chronic pain. J Psychosom Res 16:167, 1972.

34. Maruta T, Swanson DW, Swenson WM: Low back pain in a psychiatric population. Mayo Clin Proc 51:57, 1976.

35. Smith GT, Hughes LB, Duvall RD, Rothman S: Treatment outcome of a multidisciplinary center for management of chronic pain: a long-term follow-up. Clin J Pain 4:47, 1988.

36. Finneson BE: Low Back Pain, 2nd ed. Philadelphia: JB Lippincott Co., 1981, pp 179–197.

37. Faust D: The detection of deception. Neurol Clin 13:255, 1995.

38. Rosenhan D: On being sane in insane places. Science 179:250, 1973.

39. Ellard J: Psychological reactions to compensable injury. Med J Aust 8:349, 1970.

40. Brena SF, Chapman SL: Pain and litigation. In: Wall PD, Melzack R (eds): Textbook of Pain. Edinburgh: Churchill Livingstone, 1984, pp 832–839.

41. Cunnien AJ: Psychiatric and medical syndromes associated with deception. In: Rogers R (ed): Clinical Assessment of Malingering and Deception. New York: The Guilford Press, 1988, pp 13–33.

16

Referred Pain

Neck pain occurs not only with diseases that affect the bones, joints, ligaments, tendons, and other components of the cervical spine but also may be a significant symptom of disorders of the vascular, pulmonary, and gastrointestinal systems. Some of the visceral organs of the throat lie in proximity to the cervical spine. Inflammation, infection, and thrombosis that originate in the carotid artery, thyroid, or lymph glands may spread beyond the confines of these organs, stimulating sensory nerves within the cervical spine. This direct stimulation of sensory nerves not only results in pain that is localized to the damaged area but also may be experienced in a location other than the one being stimulated. The pain occurs in superficial tissues supplied by the same segment of the spinal cord that sends afferent sensory fibers to the diseased area. This is called "referred pain."

Referred pain occurs as a result of the organization of the nervous system and the embryologic location of the visceral organs. Sensory impulses of somatic origin (skin) travel by somatic afferent neurons to the dorsal root ganglia and then into the posterior horn of the spinal cord. They synapse either with a second neuron, which crosses to the opposite side of the cord and ascends to the cerebral cortex through the lateral spinothalamic tract, or with motor neurons in the anterior horn of the spinal cord at the same level. Sensory impulses from visceral structures, such as the myocardium, travel in visceral afferent nerve fibers, which accompany fibers of the sympathetic nervous system, through the rami communicates and the posterior horn to join somatic sensory neurons in the posterior horn of the spinal cord. The visceral afferent fibers may travel cranially or caudally in the gray matter of the dorsal horn before synapsing with neurons of the spinothalamic tract.

Sensory impulses of visceral origin travel the same path to the brain as somatic afferent nerves. The radiation of visceral afferents to a number of spinal cord segments may explain the diffuse, poorly localized character of visceral and somatic pain. Sensory stimulation that is of a visceral origin may spill over in the dorsal horn to affect somatic sensory nerves and result in pain that is felt only in the corresponding segmental somatic distribution (a dermatome of skin). Sensory input may also stimulate motor fibers in the anterior horn; their stimulation results in muscle contraction and spasm.

The segment of the spinal cord that supplies a visceral structure is not dependent on its anatomic location in the fully developed adult but on its original location in the developing human embryo. Visceral organs migrate to their final location, taking along their nerve and vascular supplies, and referred pain from these organs is sensed in the somatic distribution of their embryologic origin. For example, because the third, fourth, and fifth cervical nerves supply the visceral sensory input of the central part of the diaphragm, referred somatic pain originating in the diaphragm is felt in the neck and shoulder, which receive their somatic sensory input from the same cervical segments.

Patients with visceral disease in the thorax may experience three types of pain. True visceral pain is felt at the site of primary stimulation and is dull and aching in character. It has a diffuse and deep location. This is particularly true of visceral structures that originate in the midline (esophagus) and have visceral sensory input from both sides of the spinal cord.

Deep somatic pain in the thorax is related to stimulation of the parietal pleura. These impulses are transmitted by somatic pathways.

The pain is localized, sharp, and intense in character. The pain is frequently associated with reflex chest wall muscle splinting.

Referred pain to the neck from lesions in the myocardium is characteristically sharp and relatively well localized to the skin. Hyperalgesia may be noted in the area of referred pain, and reflex muscle contraction may also be present. Although referred pain usually occurs in combination with visceral and somatic pain, it may occasionally exist in the absence of visceral pain or symptoms of an underlying disease.

In the setting of neck pain and no associated visceral symptoms, a complete history, physical examination, and laboratory evaluation are essential to discovering the source of the visceral referred pain. Characteristically, neck pain that is referred from visceral structures is not aggravated by activity or relieved by recumbency. Cardiac examination may uncover abnormal heart sounds or cardiomegaly indicative of a silent myocardial infarction. Laboratory evaluation with electrocardiogram or abdominal roentgenogram may show evidence of myocardial infarction or cholecystitis. Referred pain from a visceral structure must be considered as the cause of neck pain when mechanical, rheumatologic, infectious, metabolic, and neoplastic origins of the pain have been eliminated as possibilities.

CARDIOVASCULAR

MYOCARDIAL PAIN

Capsule Summary

Frequency of neck pain—rare
Location of neck pain—anterior, left arm: C8 distribution
Quality of neck pain—crushing
Symptoms and signs—chest pain: not affected by position; increased with activity, hypertension, smoking history
Laboratory and x-ray tests—electrocardiogram with ischemic changes, angiographic evidence of coronary artery stenosis
Treatment—medical therapy, angioplasty, bypass procedure

Angina and Myocardial Infarction

The sensory fibers of the heart, parietal pleura, and diaphragmatic surface of the pari-etal pericardium are supplied by nerves in the thoracic and cervical spinal cord levels. The sensory fibers of the heart are supplied by the superior, middle, and inferior cardiac nerves that are conducted through the cervical and upper thoracic sympathetic ganglia to the posterior sensory roots at levels T1 to T5, with expansion to C8. Cardiac pain may radiate into the left arm in a C8 (ulnar nerve) distribution.

The central diaphragmatic pleura has innervation from the phrenic nerve, with contribution from nerve roots C3, C4, and C5. Disorders that affect the central portion of the diaphragm may refer pain to the superior ridge of the trapezius muscle.[1] Inflammation of the diaphragm may occur secondary to bacterial pneumonia, pulmonary infarction, or pleurisy secondary to systemic lupus erythematosus. Right shoulder pain may occur secondary to diaphragmatic inflammation secondary to cholecystitis. Left shoulder pain may occur secondary to splenic inflammation. In instances of inflammation of the diaphragm, respirations tend to exacerbate the symptoms.

The epidemiology and pathophysiology of coronary artery disease are beyond the scope of this book. A wide range of articles is available that reviews individuals at risk for developing this disorder and the factors that predispose to coronary artery disease.[2-4]

Angina occurs with increased activity or stress due to, for example, cold weather, a large meal, and emotional upset. Resting or relieving the stress results in a decrease of the pain or pressure. The pressure or pain may be perceived as a pressure sensation or chest pain. With increasing severity, the pain may remain localized to the chest or may radiate to the anterolateral neck, left shoulder, left arm to hand, or lower jaw. Anginal pain may last up to 30 minutes. Relief is obtained within 3 minutes with sublingual nitroglycerin. Myocardial infarction causes pain in a similar distribution but of greater severity and duration. In addition, sympathetic stimulation characterized by marked sweating, nausea, and vomiting is frequent. Physical examination demonstrates amounts of cardiac dysfunction in proportion to the location and severity of cardiac muscle damage. Angina may result in a transient S_4 gallop that occurs with episodes of pain. Myocardial infarction may result in alterations of blood pressure, faint heart sounds, an S_3 gallop indicative of ventricular dysfunction, and arrhythmias. Electrocardiography is the most readily available diagnostic method for detecting cardiac ischemia associated with angina or myocardial infarction. A number of other diagnostic tests—exercise electrocardiography, radioisotope imaging, and angiography—are available to document the extent of coronary artery stenosis with associated increased risks.[5, 6]

The differential diagnosis of arm pain is the clinical symptom shared by patients with coronary artery insufficiency and patients with cervical radiculopathy. The determination of the cause of chest and arm pain may be quite difficult. Mechanical factors that are unassociated with significant physical exertion (such as rolling over in bed and coughing) may identify patients with arm pain secondary to nerve impingement.[7, 8] Patients who have a herniated cervical disc with radiculopathy may present with all the symptoms associated with myocardial ischemia (diaphoresis, nausea, vomiting, and dyspnea).[9] Patients with cervical disease may complain of radiation to the posterolateral neck and scapula. The diagnosis of herniated cervical disc may be considered only after the possibility of myocardial ischemia has been eliminated as a diagnosis.

Brodsky reported on a group of 438 patients with chest pain unassociated with myocardial ischemia.[10] Of this group, 88 patients underwent cervical spine surgery to improve chest and arm pain. These patients had arm pain with or without numbness, tender chest wall, and absence of neurologic signs. Neck pain and interscapular pain were uncommon symptoms. These patients underwent normal coronary angiography prior to spine surgery. Cervical laminectomy was associated with an excellent or fair outcome, with decreased arm pain in 84% of patients with cervical angina.

Acute pericarditis may develop secondary to myocardial infarction or from a wide variety of disorders that inflame serosal surfaces, including viruses, uremia, systemic lupus erythematosus, rheumatoid arthritis, tuberculosis, and drugs. Patients have chest pain that may radiate to the shoulder or lateral neck that is exacerbated by the supine position and relieved by sitting forward. Physical examination may reveal a triphasic pericardial rub. Electrocardiography demonstrates characteristic diffuse ST segment elevation. Therapy is usually symptomatic.[11]

Carotid Artery Dissection

Dissection of the internal carotid artery is an unusual cause of anterolateral neck pain. In a study of 147 patients with this entity, 9% (13) had neck pain as an associated symptom.[12] In another study of 36 patients with carotid dissection, neck pain was noted in 19% (7).[13] The disorder occurs in hypertensive individuals who have no evidence of atherosclerotic vessel disease. Other risk factors include smoking and fibromuscular dysplasia. Dissection may occur with hyperextension and lateral flexion of the neck as the artery is stretched over the transverse processes of the upper cervical vertebrae.[14] Dissection may also occur with trauma involved with chiropractic manipulation.[15] Focal unilateral headache is the most common symptom in association with dissection. The headache is steady, nonthrobbing, of variable intensity, and is located in the frontal, auricular, or periorbital area. Neurologic manifestations may include stroke (resulting in contralateral hemiparesis, paresthesias, aphasia, ipsilateral blindness, or abducens paralysis) or oculosympathetic palsy with ptosis and miosis without anhidrosis. Focal neurologic deficits may follow the onset of headache or neck pain within minutes or hours. In rare circumstances, major strokes may be associated with severe deficits or death.[16] Bruits may be heard over the carotid. The diagnosis may be identified by arteriography or magnetic resonance (MR) imaging.[12, 17] Heparinization is the most commonly used form of therapy for symptomatic dissection.[18] Surgery may be required for recurrent or progressive dissections resistant to medical therapy. Traumatic dissections require surgical therapy more often than spontaneous internal carotid dissections.[19]

Vertebral Artery Dissection

Vertebral artery dissection occurs most commonly in middle-aged women.[20] People with hypertension or fibromuscular dysplasia are at greater risk of dissection. Cervical manipulation has also been reported as a cause of vertebral artery damage.[21] Pain in the occiput or posterior neck is the presenting symptom in 80% of patients, preceding ischemic symptoms by minutes to 30 days. Most patients present with a completed stroke, with a minority presenting with transient ischemic attacks. The lateral medullary syndrome (pain, numbness, ipsilateral face [trigeminal], ataxia, vertigo, nystagmus, Horner's syndrome [descending sympathetic tract], dysphagia, numbness of ipsilateral appendages) is the most common neurologic manifestation. Severe cases may have basilar artery involvement with associated quadriparesis, dysphagia, diplopia, with preserved sensation. The diagnosis is documented by angiography. Treatment with heparin followed by warfarin has been helpful in decreasing risk of thrombosis. The majority of patients improve without the need for surgical intervention.

Thoracic Aortic Dissection

Neck pain associated with disease of the thoracic aorta occurs secondary to aneurysmal dilatation or dissection of the vessel. An arterial aneurysm is a localized or diffuse enlargement of an artery. One or all three layers (intima, media, and adventitia) of the aorta make up the wall of the aneurysm. A dissecting aneurysm is caused by the formation of a false channel in the wall of the aorta that splits apart the layers of the vessel. Saccular aneurysms are bulbous protrusions of all three layers on one side of the vessel. A fusiform aneurysm is a diffuse, circumferential expansion of a segment of the vessel.

Thoracic aneurysms and dissections occur most commonly in elderly patients with hypertension and atherosclerosis. Hypertension is noted in up to 90% of aneurysm patients, particularly those with distal dissections.[22] Dissections in the ascending aorta occur in middle-aged patients without hypertension who have cystic medionecrosis of the aorta.[23] Aneurysms in the ascending aorta are relatively uncommon. Dissections predominate in males in a ratio of 3:1. Pregnant women younger than 40 years who are in the third trimester have half the dissections in that age group.[24]

The pathogenesis of the aneurysm is related to atherosclerotic degeneration with structural weakening of the connective tissue (collagen) of the vessel wall. Patients with aneurysms are usually hypertensive and may demonstrate manifestations of generalized atherosclerosis including angina, previous myocardial infarction, stroke, or peripheral vascular disease.[25]

Two theories have been proposed as to the cause of aneurysmal enlargement. The first theory is that a genetic-linked deficit in the quantity and quality of collagen and elastin in the arterial wall cause generalized arteriomegaly. This explains the fact that a number of vessels may be affected in an individual patient. The second theory is that plaque from atherosclerosis interferes with the blood supply of the arterial wall, resulting in weakening.[26] Inflammatory mediators, such as interleukin-8 and monocyte chemoattractant protein-1, have been identified in aortic aneurysms. These factors are chemoattractant to leukocytes and recruit inflammatory cells to the arterial wall, causing weakening.[27] Atherosclerosis may represent a secondary, nonspecific response to vessel-wall injury.

Pain associated with thoracic aortic dissection occurs secondary to expansion of the aneurysm. Extension of the aneurysm is associated with severe chest pain, with maximal intensity at the initiation of the dissection. A distinguishing feature of pain associated with aortic dissection is its tendency to migrate from its initial site to other areas as the dissection advances through the aorta. Patients complain of a tearing pain in the chest that radiates to the lateral and posterior neck, and to the interscapular, low back, and abdominal regions. Syncope, in the absence of a stroke, is frequently associated with proximal dissection and the development of cardiac tamponade.[28] Neurologic complications include stroke, ischemic peripheral neuropathy, and paralysis related to impaired flow to the spinal cord.

The physical findings in patients with thoracic aortic dissection demonstrate diaphoresis, vasoconstriction, and normal blood pressure in a majority with distal lesions.[24] Hypotension is common in proximal dissections. Loss of one or more peripheral pulses may be found with proximal or distal lesions.

Laboratory tests may be normal. Patients with ruptured aneurysms may have mild to profound anemia at time of evaluation, depending on the amount of extravascular blood loss and moderate leukocytosis.

There is controversy about the most appropriate noninvasive method for detecting the presence of thoracic aneurysms and dissections. Recent studies have reported the superior sensitivity of MR for detecting aneurysms in patients who are hemodynamically stable.[29] In patients who are unable to be moved, transesophageal echocardiography has sufficient sensitivity to identify the presence of aortic defects.[30]

Aortography is done in patients with thoracic dissection to delineate vascular anatomy. Aortography determines the site of the intimal tear and the extent of the dissection and assesses aortic insufficiency and the involvement of branch arteries.[24]

Therapy for thoracic dissection in the early phase is lowering of blood pressure while protecting cerebral, cardiac, and renal blood flow. Therapy for acute proximal dissection is surgical. Therapy for distal dissections may be medical or surgical, depending on the extent of the aneurysm. The overall 10-year survival of dissection patients is 40%.[31]

References

CARDIOVASCULAR

1. Bauwens DB, Paine R: Thoracic pain. In: Blacklow RS (ed): MacBryde's Signs and Symptoms: Applied Pathologic Physiology and Clinical Interpretation, 6th ed. Philadelphia: JB Lippincott Co, 1983, pp 139–164.
2. Sempose C, Cooper R, Kovar MG, et al.: Divergence of the recent trends in coronary mortality for the four major race-sex groups in the United States. Am J Public Health 78:1422, 1988.
3. Sytkowski PA, Kannel WB, D'Agostino RB: Changes in risk factors and the decline in mortality from cardiovascular disease: the Framingham study. N Engl J Med 322:1635, 1990.
4. Ross R: The pathogenesis of atherosclerosis: a perspective for the 1990s. Nature 362:801, 1993.
5. Zaret BL, Wackers FJ: Nuclear cardiology. N Engl J Med 329:775, 1993.
6. Guidelines for coronary angiography: a report of the American College of Cardiology/American Heart Association Task Force on Assessment of Diagnostic and Therapeutic Cardiovascular Procedures (Subcommittee on Coronary Angiography). J Am Coll Cardiol 10:935, 1987.
7. Allison DR: Pain in the chest wall simulating heart disease. Br Med J 332, 1950.
8. Davis D, Rivito M: Osteoarthritis of the cervicodorsal spine (radiculitis) simulating coronary artery disease. N Engl J Med 238:857, 1948.
9. Mitchell LC, Schafermeyer RW: Herniated cervical disc presenting as ischemic chest pain. Am J Emerg Med 9:343, 1991.
10. Brodsky AE: Cervical angina: a correlative study with emphasis on the use of coronary arteriography. Spine 10:699, 1985.
11. Permanyer-Miralda G, Sagrista-Sauleda J, Soler-Soler J: Primary acute pericardial disease: a prospective series of 231 consecutive patients. Am J Cardiol 56:623, 1985.
12. Anson J, Crowell RM: Cervicocranial arterial dissection. Neurosurgery 29:89, 1991.
13. Mokri B, Sundt TM Jr, Houser OW, et al.: Spontaneous dissection of the cervical internal carotid artery. Ann Neurol 19:126, 1986.
14. Stringer WL, Kelly DL: Traumatic dissection of the extracranial internal carotid artery. Neurosurgery 6:123, 1980.
15. Sherman DG, Hart RG, Easton JD: Abrupt change in head position and cerebral infarction. Stroke 12:2, 1981.
16. Hart RG, Easton JD: Dissections of cervical and cerebral arteries. Neurol Clin North Am 1:255, 1983.
17. Waespe W, Niesper J, Imhof H, et al.: Lower cranial nerve palsies due to internal carotid dissection. Stroke 19:1561, 1988.
18. McNeil DH, Dreisbach J, Marsden RJ: Spontaneous dissecting aneurysm of the internal carotid artery: its conservative management with heparin sodium. Arch Neurol 37:54, 1980.
19. Mokri B, Piepgras DG, Houser OW: Traumatic dissections of the extracranial internal carotid artery. J Neurosurg 68:189, 1988.
20. Mas J, Bousser M, Hasboun D, et al.: Extracranial vertebral artery dissections: a review of 13 cases. Stroke 18:1037, 1987.
21. Mas JL, Henin D, Bousser MG, et al.: Dissecting aneurysm of the vertebral artery and cervical manipulation: a case report with autopsy. Neurology 39:512, 1989.
22. Leonard JC, Hasleton PS: Dissecting aortic aneurysms: a clinicopathological study. Q J Med 48:55, 1979.
23. Hirst AE, Gore I: Is cystic medionecrosis the cause of dissecting aortic aneurysm? Circulation 53:915, 1976.
24. DeSanctis RW, Doroghazi RM, Austen WG, et al.: Aortic dissection. N Engl J Med 317:1060, 1987.
25. Spittell JA: Hypertension and arterial aneurysm. J Am Coll Cardiol 1:533, 1983.
26. Giordano JM: Vascular versus spinal disease as a cause of back and lower extremity pain. Semin Spine Surg 2:136, 1990.
27. Koch AE, Kunkel SL, Pearce WH, et al.: Enhanced production of the chemotactic cytokines interleukin-8 and monocyte chemoattractant protein-1 in human abdominal aortic aneurysms. J Pathol 142:1423, 1993.
28. Slater EE, DeSanctis RW: The clinical recognition of dissecting aortic aneurysm. Am J Med 60:625, 1976.
29. Nienaber CA, von Kodolitsch Y, Nicolas V, et al.: The diagnosis of thoracic aortic dissection by noninvasive imaging procedures. N Engl J Med 328:1, 1993.
30. Wiet SP, Pearce WH, McCarthy WJ, et al.: Utility of transesophageal echocardiography in the diagnosis of disease of the thoracic aorta. J Vasc Surg 20:613, 1994.
31. DeBakey ME, McCollum CH, Crawford ES, et al.: Dissection and dissecting aneurysms of the aorta: twenty-year follow-up of five hundred twenty-seven patients treated surgically. Surgery 92:1118, 1982.

GASTROINTESTINAL TRACT

Capsule Summary

Frequency of neck pain—rare

Location of neck pain—lateral neck, shoulder, interscapular

Quality of neck pain—dull ache, colicky

Symptoms and signs—dysphagia, fatty food intolerance, neck mass

Laboratory and x-ray tests—abnormal alkaline phosphatase level, bilirubin, white blood cell count; contrast radiograph: abnormal filling defects; scintiscan: decreased function

Treatment—surgical removal of mass or stones, antibiotics

The organs of the gastrointestinal tract associated with neck pain are those with referred pain distribution to the neck and shoulder. Diseases of the esophagus and gallbladder may be associated with neck pain of visceral, somatic, or referred origin. A common finding in the history of patients with neck pain secondary to a gastrointestinal disorder is the relationship between pain and eating or bowel function.[1]

GALLBLADDER

The gallbladder receives its innervation from both greater splanchnic nerves (T5–T9). The brain interprets biliary pain to be in the midline in relation to the bilateral innervation of the gallbladder. When biliary pain is severe, the discomfort may radiate to the back in a T5–T9 distribution, corresponding to an interscapular location. Occasionally patients may experience pain that radiates to the right shoulder.

Acute Cholecystitis

In certain patients, the bile that is stored in the gallbladder crystallizes to form gallstones (cholelithiasis). The presence of these stones may cause inflammation of the gallbladder, which results in chronic cholecystitis. Gallstones are a common medical problem, with 5 million men and 15 million women affected in the United States.[2] Women younger than 30 years of age who have had more than three pregnancies are at greatest risk of developing gallstones.[3] A majority of gallstones are asymptomatic. When the cystic duct is obstructed by a gallstone, acute cholecystitis occurs. Cholelithiasis is present in 95% of patients with acute cholecystitis. Acalculous cholecystitis is usually associated with previous surgery, trauma, or sepsis.[4] Bacterial infection and ischemia may play a role in the pathogenesis of acute cholecystitis. Lodging of a gallstone in the cystic duct, or common bile duct, causes severe, steady pain lasting 15 minutes to 1 hour. The pain typically occurs in the midepigastrium and moves to the right upper quadrant. Pain may radiate around the sides to the back or directly through to an area below the tip of the right scapula or occasionally to the right shoulder.[5] The pain is intense, begins abruptly, and subsides gradually. The quality of the pain varies from excruciating or lancinating to aching or cramping. Patients may develop nausea, vomiting, and dyspepsia.

Physical examination demonstrates an abnormal Murphy's sign (inspiratory arrest on palpation in the right subcostal area), abdominal guarding, rebound tenderness, fever, and jaundice. The gallbladder is palpable in 30% of patients. Generalized rebound tenderness suggests the possibility of rupture. In a study of patients referred for gallstones, the most characteristic signs and symptoms were pain in the upper abdomen, radiation to the back, a steady quality, duration for 1 to 24 hours,

and onset more than an hour after meals. These clinical findings required confirmation by radiographic imaging.[6]

Laboratory tests demonstrate an elevated white blood cell count to 15,000 cells/mm³. Increased alkaline phosphatase level suggests a common bile duct stone. Elevated amylase level also suggests pancreatic inflammation and a common bile duct stone.

The primary imaging modality for diagnosis of cholelithiasis is ultrasonography. Ultrasonography has 93% sensitivity and 96% specificity for the diagnosis of cholelithiasis and acute cholecystitis[7] (Fig. 16–1). Ultrasonography is able to detect biliary duct obstruction as well as the presence of an abscess or tumor. However, the technique is unable to determine the extent of inflammation in the gallbladder.[8–10] Cholescintigraphy is a reasonably specific test to confirm the diagnosis of acute cholecystitis.[8] Under normal circumstances, technetium-labeled iminodiacetic acid (IDA) is preferentially concentrated in the biliary tree and enters the gallbladder. In acute cholecystitis, radio-labeled material enters the common bile duct but does not enter the gallbladder. The scan may not be helpful in patients with severe hyperbilirubinemia. These tests have taken the place of the oral cholecystogram.

Frequently, treatment for acute cholecystitis is surgical removal of the gallbladder, once the patient's condition has been optimized with the use of antibiotics, fluid replacement, and nasogastric suction. Patients who do not elect cholecystectomy may be at risk of perfo-

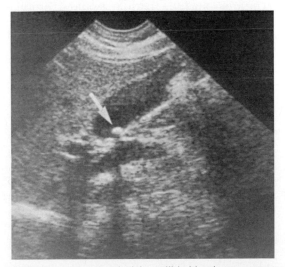

Figure 16–1. Ultrasound of the gallbladder demonstrates a large gallstone (arrow). (Courtesy of Michael Hill, M.D.)

ration. Laparoscopic cholecystectomy has become the surgical method of choice for removal of the gallbladder.[11] Compared to laparotomy, postoperative pain is reduced, hospitalization is shortened, and a quicker return to normal function is common.[12]

For those who choose to forego surgery, symptoms may resolve in as little time as 48 hours or continue for weeks despite antibiotics. The interscapular pain associated with cholecystitis follows a similar course. Those who have had one attack of cholecystitis are at risk of developing another. Those patients with recurrent attacks should consider surgical removal of the gallbladder.

ESOPHAGUS

The esophagus is a midline structure that is innervated with a distribution from C7 to T12. Most esophageal pain is substernal in location. Acid-reflux disorders are associated with substernal, burning pain that may radiate to the anterior neck and between the shoulder blades.[13] Other esophageal disorders that may cause chest, posterior thoracic, and anterior neck pain include esophageal spasm, dysmotility disorders, and carcinoma.[14] Hiatal hernia, resulting from slippage of the lower esophageal sphincter through the diaphragm, may also be associated with left arm, anterior neck, and posterior thorax pain. In general, esophageal pain is altered by eating and recumbent position. Esophageal pain is relieved by antacid therapy or by nitroglycerin therapy in the setting of esophageal spasm. Diagnostic techniques include barium swallow, esophagoscopy, and manometry to evaluate the cause of esophageal dysfunction. Therapy is directed both at decreasing damage caused by acid secretion and at normalization of peristalsis.

Esophageal Diverticulum

Zenker's diverticulum occurs in the upper esophagus at the level of the cricopharyngeal muscle. Symptoms are insidious in onset, with dysphagia and regurgitation being most common. As the diverticulum expands, food lodges in the sac and is regurgitated hours after eating. Increasing size may result in a neck mass and local neck pain. Patients are at risk of aspiration pneumonia. A barium esophagram is useful in identifying the location and size of the diverticulum. Esophagoscopy is not recommended because of the risk of perforation, unless a malignancy is suspected.[14] Surgical removal of the diverticulum in a one-step procedure is indicated if the size of the lesion is large enough to cause obstruction.[15]

Esophageal Cancer

Esophageal cancer is one of the more common malignant tumors, but it affects the upper portion of the esophagus in a minority of patients.[16] The middle and lower esophagus are involved more frequently. The tumors arise from the squamous epithelium of the lumen and cause squamous cell carcinomas. Adenocarcinomas occur in the columnar epithelium near the end of the esophagus (Barrett's esophagus) and comprise the remainder of the tumors.[17] Dysphagia and weight loss are frequent early symptoms. The esophagus does not have a serosal layer allowing neoplasms to grow to significant size and extent before evaluation is undertaken. The rich lymphatic supply to the esophagus allows for early metastatic spread before diagnosis is considered. Upper esophageal cancer may present with upper neck discomfort along with dysphagia and weight loss. Difficulty with solids progresses to dysphagia with liquids. Advanced tumors may cause local mass lesions, infections, and fistulas. The prognosis is poor for most individuals with esophageal cancer whose presentation is neck pain.[14]

MISCELLANEOUS

Anterior Neck Lesions

Lesions of the oropharynx, thyroid, cervical lymph glands, salivary glands (parotid and submandibular), and vascular structures (carotid) may cause anterior and lateral neck pain. These lesions may refer pain to the throat, anterior chest wall, and occasionally to the posterior neck. Many of these disorders are mass lesions. Among patients 60 years of age or older, a mass in the lateral neck has an 80% chance of being malignant. Lesions found in the upper portion of the anterior neck have sources in lesions of the tongue, larynx, mouth floor, or salivary glands. Lesions in the lower portion of the neck have an origin in the thyroid gland. Enlarged lymph glands are the most frequent cause of masses in the anterior cervical triangle.

History and physical examination are essential in determining potential etiologies of neck lesions. Duration and amount of smoking is an essential part of the history. A change in voice quality, dysphagia, onset of cough, fever, chills, and night sweats have implications of tumor or infection as a cause of anterior neck pain. History of migraine headaches may be associated with vascular pain. Physical examination, including bimanual palpation of the oropharynx, may identify small masses in the parotid and submandibular regions and in the base of the tongue and tonsillar areas. Careful examination of the thyroid identifies any nodules and the free movement of the gland anterior to the trachea.

Technological advances, including fiberoptic laryngoscopy, computerized tomography (CT) and MR imaging, and fine-needle biopsies, have improved the opportunity to identify the location and pathologic condition of lesions with less invasive procedures. Laryngoscopy allows for direct visualization of lesions in the nasal cavity, base of the tongue, epiglottis, larynx, and vocal cords. CT and MR scans visualize the extent of soft tissue lesions and the number of masses present. Fine-needle aspiration is able to obtain specimen samples for cytopathology, Gram's stain, and cultures.

Benign masses in the neck are most frequently lymph glands (cervical lymphadenitis). Primary infections in the mouth, pharynx, tonsils, dental structures, and skin over face or head cause lymph gland enlargement.[18] Midline masses are of thyroid origin or from thyroglossal cysts. The thyroid gland may be involved with acute infection (suppurative thyroiditis), subacute thyroiditis (de Quervain's thyroiditis), Hashimoto's thyroiditis, Riedel's struma, or thyroid malignancy.[19–22] Branchial cleft cysts are lateral masses with a fistulous opening found near the anterior border of the sternocleidomastoid muscle. These congenital cysts may be asymptomatic masses or acutely inflamed and associated with suppurative infections.[23] Infections unassociated with congenital cysts or lymph glands may occur from superficial structures (skin), or deep structures such as the parotid gland, mastoid process, mandible, or muscles in fascial compartments. Superficial infections cause a tender mass at the anterior border of the sternocleidomastoid muscle. Deep fascial infections require radiographic evaluation to identify the location of the abscess in the lateral pharyngeal, pretracheal, submandibular, or deep fascial planes (retropharyngeal and prevertebral).[24, 25] Deep fascial infections are rare but potentially catastrophic if swelling in soft tissue planes results in airway compromise. Ludwig's angina is the term associated with submandibular space infection. Most of these infections are associated with dental abscesses or postextraction infections.[26] Carotidynia may be caused by vascular and soft tissue structures near the carotid sheath. Carotid body tumors are found close to the bifurcation of the carotid artery. Migraine headaches may cause carotid tenderness. Calcification or inflammation of tendons (stylohyoid), bone (hyoid), and muscles (digastric and stylohyoid) may cause pain in the lateral aspect of the neck.[27, 28]

Lymphomas may present as cervical lymphadenopathy or as mass lesions in Waldeyer's ring, involving the tonsils. Metastatic lesions may also cause lymph gland swelling. The presence of metastatic lesions in the upper portion of the neck suggests that the primary lesion (squamous cell carcinoma, melanoma, or adenocarcinoma) is localized to the head or neck. Unknown primary neck metastases are the most common cause of node swelling in the lower third of the neck. Surgical intervention in the form of neck dissection depends on the location of the mass and the likely primary source of the tumor.[29]

References

GASTROINTESTINAL TRACT

1. Roberts I: Gastrointestinal disorders presenting with back pain. Semin Spine Surg 2:141, 1990.
2. Friedman GD, Kannel WB, Dawber TR: The epidemiology of gallbladder disease: observations in the Framingham study. J Chronic Dis 19:273, 1966.
3. Maringhini A, Ciambra M, Baccelleria P, et al.: Sludge, stones, and pregnancy. Gastroenterology 95:1160, 1988.
4. Frazee RC, Nagorney DM, Mucha P Jr: Acute acalculous cholecystitis. Mayo Clin Proc 64:163, 1989.
5. French EG, Robb WAT: Biliary and renal colic. Br Med J 2:135, 1963.
6. Diehl AK, Sugarek NJ, Todd KH: Clinical evaluation for gallstone disease: Usefulness of symptoms and signs in diagnosis. Am J Med 69:29, 1990.
7. Marton KI, Doubilet P: How to image the gallbladder in suspected cholecystitis. Ann Intern Med 109:722, 1988.
8. Boucher IAD: Imaging procedures to diagnose gallbladder disease. Br Med J 288:1632, 1984.
9. Laing FC, Federle MP, Jeffrey RB, et al.: Ultrasonic evaluation of patients with acute right upper quadrant pain. Radiology 140:449, 1981.
10. Fink-Bennett D, Freitas JE, Ripley SD, et al.: The sensitivity of hepatobiliary imaging and real time ultrasonography in the detection of acute cholecystitis. Arch Surg 120:904, 1985.
11. The Southern Surgeons Club: A prospective analysis

of 1518 laparoscopic cholecystectomies. N Engl J Med 324:1073, 1991.

12. McMahon AJ, Russell IT, Baxter JN, et al.: Laparoscopic versus minilaparotomy cholecystectomy: a randomized trial. Lancet 343:135, 1994.

13. Pope CE: Acid-reflux disorders. N Engl J Med 331:656, 1994.

14. Castell DO: The Esophagus, 2nd ed. Boston: Little, Brown, 1995, p 795.

15. Payne WS, King RM: Pharyngoesophageal (Zenker's) diverticulum. Surg Clin North Am 63:815, 1983.

16. Puhakka HJ, Aitsalo K: Oesophageal carcinoma: endoscopic and clinical findings in 258 patients. J Laryngol Otol 102:1137, 1988.

17. Cameron AJ, Ott BJ, Payne WS: The incidence of adenocarcinoma in columnar-lined (Barrett's) esophagus. N Engl J Med 313:857, 1985.

18. Brook I: The swollen neck: cervical lymphadenitis, parotitis, thyroiditis, and infected cysts. Infect Dis Clin North Am 21:221, 1988.

19. Szabo S, Allen DB: Thyroiditis: differentiation of acute suppurative and subacute—case report and review of the literature. Clin Pediatr 28:171, 1989.

20. Hamburger JI: The various presentations of thyroiditis: diagnostic considerations. Ann Intern Med 104:219, 1986.

21. Shervo J, Gal R, Avidor I, et al.: Anaplastic thyroid carcinoma: a clinical, histologic, and immunohistochemical study. Cancer 62:319, 1988.

22. Tupchong L, Phil D, Hughes F, et al.: Primary lymphoma of the thyroid: clinical features, prognostic factors, and results of treatment. Int J Radiat Oncol Biol Phys 12:1813, 1986.

23. McManus K, Holt R, Aufdemorte TM, et al.: Bronchogenic cyst presenting as deep neck abscess. Otolaryngol Head Neck Surg 92:109, 1984.

24. Blomquist IK, Bayer AS: Life-threatening deep fascial space infections of the head and neck. Infect Dis Clin North Am 2:237, 1988.

25. Hall MB, Arteaga DM, Mancuso A: Use of computerized tomography in the localization of head-and-neck-space infections. J Oral Maxillofac Surg 43:978, 1985.

26. Moreland LW, Corey J, McKenzie R: Ludwig's angina: report of a case and review of the literature. Arch Intern Med 148:461, 1988.

27. Sarkozi J, Fam AG: Acute calcific retropharyngeal tendinitis: an unusual cause of neck pain. Arthritis Rheum 27:708, 1984.

28. Lim RY: Carotodynia exposed: hyoid bone syndrome. South Med J 80:444, 1987.

29. Vokes EE, Weichselbaum RR, Lippman SM, et al.: Head and neck cancer. N Engl J Med 328:184, 1993.

17

Miscellaneous Diseases

PAGET'S DISEASE OF BONE

Capsule Summary

Frequency of neck pain—rare
Location of neck pain—cervical spine
Quality of neck pain—deep, boring ache
Symptoms and signs—decreased spine motion
Laboratory and x-ray tests—increased alkaline phosphatase level; lytic and sclerotic enlarged vertebrae on plain roentgenogram
Treatment—bisphosphonates, calcitonin, nonsteroidal anti-inflammatory drugs

Prevalence and Pathogenesis

Paget's disease of bone is a localized disorder of bone characterized by a remarkable amount of bone resorption and subsequent formation of disorganized and irregular new bone. The disease was first described by Sir James Paget in 1877.[1]

Paget's disease is common in certain areas of the world, including Western Europe, Australia, and New Zealand. Most Americans with Paget's disease are of Western European or Mediterranean descent. Paget's disease is rare in blacks in Africa, but it has been reported in blacks in the United States.[2] It affects up to 3% of people older than 40 years of age.[3] The prevalence of Paget's disease increases to 10% in people 80 years of age and older.[4] This prevalence increases to 20% in people with a positive family history.[5] Men are slightly more often affected than women, with a rate of 1.3:1.[6] In New York State from 1980 to 1983, the incidence of Paget's disease for hospitalized patients was 26 per 100,000 for people 65 to 74 years of age and 34 per 100,000 for 75 years of age and older. The average length of hospitalization for these two groups was 9 and 11 days, respectively.[7]

The pathogenesis of Paget's disease is unknown. There is little evidence to support abnormalities in hormone secretion, vascular supply, or connective tissue metabolism as the cause of this disease. The primary abnormality is in the osteoclasts, cells that resorb bone. Histologic examination of pagetic bone reveals increased numbers of osteoclasts with marked increase in size and number of nuclei. Pagetic osteoclasts in long-term marrow cultures have a 10-fold to 20-fold increase in number compared to normal marrow cultures, are larger in size, have more nuclei per cell, have increased levels of tartrate-resistant acid phosphatase activity, and are hyperresponsive to $1,25(OH)_2$ vitamin D.[8] Levels of interleukin-6 (IL-6) are also increased. IL-6 is an important regulator of bone function, acting as a stimulator of osteoclast cell formation.[9] The change in number of osteoclasts results in increased bone resorption and inadequate new bone formation. New pagetic bone is less compact, more vascular, and weaker than normal bone.[10]

Other investigators have suggested that the osteoblast is the source of the primary abnormality of Paget's disease.[11, 12] The evidence for this hypothesis is the focal nature of Paget's disease and the presence of viral genome in cells other than osteoclasts in bone, including the osteoblast. Osteoblasts are not distributed by the blood stream. The osteoclasts are derived from progenitor cells in bone marrow and are distributed through the peripheral circulation. If osteoclasts were the putative cause of Paget's disease, the illness should be systemic, following the bodywide distribution of the osteoclasts. In addition, osteoblasts produce large amounts of IL-6. Additional evidence

425

has been reported suggesting the importance of deregulation of c-*fos* proto-oncogene expression in bone cells by the insertion of a paramyxovirus may be the primary lesion of Paget's disease.

Ultrastructural studies of pagetic bone have demonstrated the presence of nuclear and cytoplasmic inclusions that resemble portions of paramyxoviruses.[13] The characteristics of a slow virus infection, long latent period, single organ disease, and lack of inflammatory response, closely match those of Paget's disease. However, the infectious agent has not been isolated from cultured pagetic cells, and the specific virus has not been identified. Polymerase chain reaction techniques have been used to screen for paramyxovirus sequences in ribonucleic acid (RNA) extracted from bone from Paget's patients. No evidence of viral products was identified in RNA extracts from 10 Paget's disease patients.[14] Therefore, any conclusion concerning the role of viruses as the etiologic agent of Paget's disease cannot be made at this time.

Clinical History

Most patients with Paget's disease are asymptomatic.[15] Frequently the possibility that a patient may have the disease is raised by the presence of an elevated serum alkaline phosphatase level on screening chemistry tests or by the discovery of an area of bony change on radiographs. Skeletal involvement of Paget's disease is concentrated in the femur, skull, tibia, humerus, and axial skeleton. A recent study has documented spine involvement in 35% of 248 Paget's disease patients.[16] Axial skeletal disease occurs in the sacrum, lumbar spine, thoracic spine, and cervical spine in decreasing order. Cervical spine disease occurs in only 3% to 8% of patients with axial skeleton disease.[16, 17] The problem arises that Paget's patients may have osteoarthritis of the spine, which may be the actual cause of bone pain. A recent study investigating this point reported only 12% of patients (3 of 25) with Paget's disease having back pain directly related to their underlying illness. The remaining patients had back pain that could be related to Paget's disease or coexistent osteoarthritis or both.[18] A similar frequency (13%) of back or neck pain related to Paget's disease alone was reported in the study of 248 patients, and mechanical causes of back and neck pain were present in 27%.[16]

Pain of Paget's disease is of a deep boring quality and does not increase at night. Pain secondary to Paget's disease uncomplicated by mechanical disorders is unrelated to activity, not relieved by rest, and is not significantly relieved with nonsteroidal anti-inflammatory drugs (NSAIDs).[16] The pain may radiate with a radicular pattern in the shoulders, arms, or hands. Paget's disease may affect the upper portion of the cervical spine, resulting in symptoms of radiculopathy, myelopathy, or quadraparesis.[17-26]

The pain of Paget's disease involving the axial skeleton may be of bone, joint, or nerve origin. Vertebral bodies may fracture, facet joints may develop secondary osteoarthritis owing to deformity, and neural elements may become compressed by new bone growth, including extradural structures such as the ligamentum flavum.[27] Monostotic Paget's disease affecting a vertebral body may be associated with pain unassociated with fracture or compression of neural elements.[20, 28] Pain may also be generated by compression of neural elements by intraspinal soft tissue, neural ischemia produced by arterial steal phenomenon, interference with blood supply to the cord by compression by expanding bone, or platybasia with compression of the medulla.[16] The increased vascularity associated with Paget's disease has been implicated as the cause of spontaneous spinal epidural hematomas associated with neurologic dysfunction. Neurologic complications are relatively uncommon but may cause significant disability such as myelopathy, radiculopathy, and cranial nerve signs, including optic atrophy, deafness, and cerebellar dysfunction.[29] Spinal cord compression occurs most commonly in the thoracic spine where vertebral width is narrowed.[30] Cervical spinal stenosis secondary to Paget's disease may occur with or without neck pain.[16] Occasionally, cord compression develops suddenly as a result of a collapse of a vertebra.[31]

Other frequently affected sites are the skull, pelvis, femora, and tibias. Patients may experience pain on walking in weight-bearing bones. Paget's disease may also cause deformities in bones and result in increased size of the skull, hip joint disease (osteoarthritis), and bowing of the legs. Bone softening may give rise to invagination of the base of the skull, which may result in obstructive hydrocephalus.[2]

Other complications of Paget's disease include hyperuricemia with gout, hypercalcemia in the immobilized patient, and high-output cardiac failure owing to the increased blood flow to bones.[32] Malignant degeneration develops in patients with polyostotic Paget's disease but is a rare occurrence. Less than 1% of Paget's disease patients develop osteosarcoma or fibrosarcoma.[33] Metastases may also involve pagetic bone and may be differentiated from sarcomas only by tissue biopsy.[34]

Physical Examination

Physical examination may be entirely normal in the patient with asymptomatic Paget's disease. Increasing disease activity, manifested by rapid bone growth, may correspond to physical findings consistent with rapid bone metabolism, and the temperature over bones may be elevated from increased blood flow. Bone growth of the skull is manifested by increased skull circumference and dilated scalp veins. Angioid streaks are an occasional finding on funduscopic examination. Resting tachycardia is seen in patients with high cardiac output.

Musculoskeletal abnormalities may include a pagetic stature (dorsal kyphosis) and abnormal gait. In the weight-bearing bones, new bone formation leads to lateral bowing in the femur and anterior bowing in the tibia. Decreased motion may be demonstrated in the cervical spine, and point tenderness may be elicited over vertebral bodies that have sustained fractures. The cervical spine may be straightened, fixed, or reversed on examination. Patients with upper cervical involvement have decreased rotation.[19] Neurologic examination may be remarkable for cranial nerve, sensory, motor, or cerebellar dysfunction if bone growth has resulted in nerve compression in the cervical area.

Laboratory Data

The most characteristic laboratory abnormality is an elevation of the serum alkaline phosphatase level because this mirrors the extent of new bone, osteoblastic activity. A measure of bone resorption is 24-hour total urinary hydroxyproline. This amino acid is formed from the collagen matrix during bone breakdown. Together the tests can provide an indication of bone disease, its progression, and its response to therapy. From a practical standpoint, serum alkaline phosphatase level is used routinely as 24 urine collections are difficult to obtain on a regular basis.

Serum levels of calcium and phosphorus are normal because bone resorption and formation are closely linked. Elevations of calcium

level occur in pagetic patients who are immobilized, who have coexistent primary hyperparathyroidism, or who have metastatic disease to bone. In rare circumstances, hypercalcemia has been reported in monostotic Paget's disease unassociated with immobilization.[35] Serum uric acid concentrations may be increased in men with extensive disease. Serum osteocalcin is a vitamin K–dependent protein that has a high affinity for hydroxyapatite, binds calcium, and is produced by osteoblasts. Osteocalcin levels have lower sensitivity and specificity than other biochemical markers for activity of Paget's disease.[36] Histocompatibility testing of a small group of patients has demonstrated a greater frequency of human leukocyte antigen HLA-DR2 compared with controls.[37] This test has no diagnostic significance at this time.

Abnormalities of early disease are characterized by an increased number of osteoclasts. Subsequently new bone is produced in a chaotic, mosaic pattern, and woven bone, as opposed to normal lamellar bone, is produced. The amount of minerals in pagetic new bone appears normal. Histologically, the bone contains irregular, broad trabeculae, with numerous osteoclasts and fibrous vascular tissue replacement of the bone marrow space (Fig. 17–1A). Malignant tumors may arise in pagetoid lesions. The most common is osteosarcoma. Other neoplasms include fibrosarcoma and malignant giant cell tumor.[38]

Radiographic Evaluation

Radiographic abnormalities vary with the stage of disease. The osteolytic phase corresponds to localized lytic lesions of bone. There is a well-demarcated area of lucency without associated bony reaction. These lesions are most commonly discovered in the skull and are called osteoporosis circumscripta. Lytic lesions may be seen in long bones but are rarely seen in the spine.[39] Paget's disease is monostotic in 35% of cases[40] (Fig. 17–1).

The mixed phase consists of bone sclerosis combined with osseous demineralization. The bone increases in size with greatly thickened and widely spaced trabeculae, cortical thickening, and irregularly distributed zones of increased and reduced density. A "cotton wool" appearance is a term used to describe the patchy involvement.

The sclerotic phase of disease appears as areas of homogeneous increase in bone density. This form of disease may be too difficult to

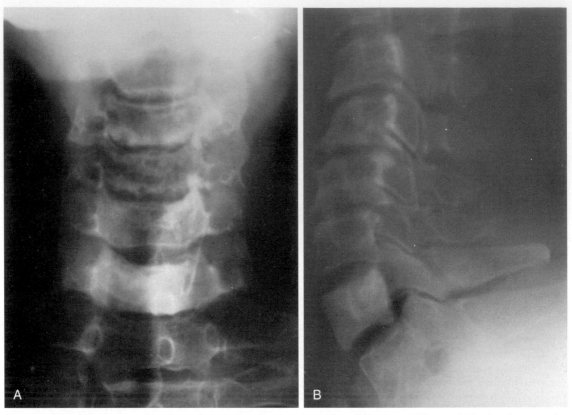

Figure 17–1. Paget's disease: "ivory" vertebra. Posteroanterior, *A,* and lateral, *B,* views of the cervical spine demonstrating "ivory" vertebra at the C7 level. (Courtesy of Anne Brower, M.D.)

clearly distinguish from the mixed form of disease.

In the spine, mixed or sclerotic radiographic changes are usually demonstrated.[41] Vertebral bodies may develop coarse, parallel, vertical striations that may simulate the appearance of a hemangioma. Increased cortical thickening at the inferior and superior vertebral borders may result in a "picture frame" appearance. Marked osteoblastic changes may result in a homogenously sclerotic "ivory" vertebra. The ivory vertebra is usually enlarged in Paget's disease; this helps differentiate it from metastatic disease.[20] Compression fractures and large osteophytes may also be seen. Paget's disease may invade soft tissue and cartilage structures such as intervertebral discs. This process, causing disc space narrowing, may be entirely asymptomatic.[42]

Bone scintiscans are sensitive in detecting increased bone activity even in locations where plain radiographs are normal. In a patient with localized disease and normal biochemical parameters, a bone scan may give the only objective indication of the presence and activity of disease.[43] In a patient with Paget's disease, an abnormal scan in a "normal" area of skeleton suggests involvement at that location.[44] Multiple areas of increased activity may also be associated with diffuse skeletal metastases. Roentgenographic evaluation of areas of increased scintiscan activity may be able to differentiate those with Paget's disease from those with a malignancy.[45] Response to treatment is characterized by radiographic changes in an area of normal activity on scan. Paget's disease may be noted on indium-111 white blood cell scintigraphy as "cold" areas. The cold bone defects are related to the loss of the bone marrow component in pagetic bone.[46]

Computerized tomography (CT) is generally not required for the evaluation of uncomplicated Paget's disease.[47] CT demonstrates the coarsened trabeculae of Paget's disease. CT is most useful at identifying complications of Paget's disease including articular disease, neoplastic degeneration, and neurologic impingement secondary to vertebral involvement.[48]

Magnetic resonance (MR) imaging is also not required for the diagnosis of Paget's disease. However, the frequent use of MR in a variety of skeletal conditions often results in the identification of Paget's disease. Complications of spinal stenosis secondary to Paget's disease are readily identified by MR.[49]

Differential Diagnosis

In the majority of patients, the history, physical examination, and chemical, radiographic, and bone scan abnormalities are adequate to confirm the diagnosis of Paget's disease. In an occasional patient with unusual clinical or radiologic presentation, bone biopsy may be necessary to confirm the diagnosis.

The problem for the clinician may not be discovering the presence of Paget's disease in the spine but rather the association of the patient's neck symptoms with the cervical spine pagetoid lesion. Altman and colleagues have suggested guidelines for differentiating Paget's disease from osteoarthritis of the lumbar spine.[18] These same criteria may be applied to lesions of the cervical spine. For a patient's symptoms to be directly related to Paget's disease and not to another disorder (osteoarthritis), they should have the following characteristics: (1) nonspecific neck pain without radiculopathy, (2) normal or minimal findings on examination, (3) roentgenograph revealing vertebral sclerosis (ivory vertebra) with facet sclerosis and normal disc space and facet joint, (4) bone scan revealing isolated vertebral Paget's disease, and (5) CT revealing an enlarged vertebra and neural arch, but the facet joint not being arthritic and no bony impingement being present.[18]

The differential diagnosis of Paget's disease is broad because all lesions that may cause sclerosis of bone must be included. Diseases associated with sclerotic vertebral bodies, including metastatic tumor, lymphoma, myelofibrosis, fluorosis, mastocytosis, renal osteodystrophy, tuberous sclerosis, axial osteomalacia, and fibrogenesis imperfecta ossium, may be confused with Paget's disease. Abnormalities on physical and radiologic examination, such as hepatosplenomegaly (myelofibrosis) and anemia (metastatic tumor), help differentiate these disorders from Paget's disease. A history of renal disease along with laboratory evidence of renal failure helps with the diagnosis of renal osteodystrophy. A history of urticaria pigmentosa is common in patients with mastocytosis. Fibrous dysplasia may also cause sclerosis of vertebral bodies in the cervical spine (see Chapter 13).

Treatment

Most patients with Paget's disease are asymptomatic and do not require therapy. Indications for treatment include disabling bone pain that is not relieved by NSAIDs, progressive skeletal deformity with frequent fractures, vertebral compression, acetabular protrusion, neurologic complications, deafness, high-output congestive heart failure, or immobilization. Siris has proposed a more aggressive approach to therapy, based on her extensive experience with the illness.[50] She recommends treating asymptomatic disease at a site where progression will lead to future complications. For example, acetabular disease may lead to secondary osteoarthritis.[50]

A number of agents have been developed for treating Paget's disease (Table 17–1). Many of these agents are available in Europe and will be released in the United States.[51] Some of the agents that will be available include alendronate, risedronate, and tiludronate disodium.[50]

None of the three classes of agents used for Paget's disease to produce symptomatic improvement and better control of bone metabolism cure the illness. Calcitonin, a polypeptide hormone from the parafollicular cells of the thyroid gland, slows osteoclastic bone resorption. Injection of 50 to 100 units of calcitonin three or more times per week results in a gradual decrease in serum alkaline phosphatase level to about half of the initial elevated concentration and resolution of bone pain; however, patients may develop antibodies to calcitonin, which abrogates its beneficial effects.[52] Salmon calcitonin is the most commonly used form of calcitonin and the type most commonly associated with antibody production. Human calcitonin differs from salmon calcitonin at 16 of the 32 amino acid sites.[53] Anti–salmon calcitonin antibodies do not bind human calcitonin. Patients resistant to salmon calcitonin have responded to human calcitonin.[54] Intranasal salmon calcitonin is available in Europe for the treatment of Paget's disease.[55] Intranasal calcitonin is more convenient than parenteral calcitonin, but its efficacy relative to parenteral calcitonin remains to be determined. The absence of side effects is probably related to the 60% reduction in plasma levels obtained from intranasal installation compared with the same dose given by subcutaneous injection. Intranasal calcitonin produces a maximum reduction in bone turnover of 30% to 40% after 6 months

TABLE 17–1. RECOMMENDED THERAPY FOR PAGET'S DISEASE

	DRUG	DOSE	DURATION	EFFECT
Initial	Etidronate	5 mg/kg/day; 200–400 mg; middle of 4-hour fast	6 months on; 6 months off	50% decrease in alkaline phosphatase level; not appropriate because of increased pain in patients with long lytic fronts; increased fracture risk
Secondary	Calcitonin (salmon)	50 units (U) subcutaneously (SQ) daily first week; 100 U SQ daily 6 months; 100 U SQ three times a week	Indefinite	50% decrease in alkaline phosphatase level; escape of efficacy related to neutralizing antibodies
	Calcitonin (human)	50 U SQ daily first week; 100 U SQ daily 6 months; 100 U SQ three times a week	Indefinite	50% decrease in alkaline phosphatase; nausea, flushing more common than for salmon calcitonin
	Pamidronate	60 mg 500 mL 5% dextrose 3 hours; once weekly for 2 weeks; multiple infusions 30–60 mg biweekly up to 480 mg total for severe disease	Yearly	Alkaline phosphatase level below 400 U/L; low-grade fever with flu-like symptoms with first dose; mineralization defect at higher doses

Modified from Siris ES: Paget's disease of bone. J Clin Endocrinol Metab 80(2):335–338, 1995. © The Endocrine Society.

of therapy. Intranasal calcitonin has been released in the United States.

Bisphosphonates, including etidronate, are structural analogues of pyrophosphate, which, when ingested by osteoclasts, decrease the osteoclast's ability to resorb bone. In addition, they interfere to a variable extent with the mineralization of normal bone, and this limits the dose and duration of a course of bisphosphonate therapy. Bisphosphonates are given at a dose of 5 mg/kg/day for 6 months of the year. The dose is given with water during the middle of a 4-hour fast. Some physicians give a course for 6 months and then discontinue therapy for 6 months; others give therapy every other month for 6 months and then reevaluate the response. Bisphosphonates may increase the tendency of Paget's disease patients to develop pathologic fractures if given at too large a dose for too long a time.[56] Etidronate has been the most commonly used bisphosphonate. Many physicians initiate therapy with etidronate.

Pamidronate, an aminohydroxypropilidene bisphosphonate, has been used in the United States for intravenous treatment of hypercalcemia associated with malignancy.[57] In Europe, pamidronate is used regularly for the control of Paget's disease. The drug may be used orally or intravenously. As opposed to other bisphosphonates, pamidronate is able to inhibit bone resorption without any significant detrimental effect on bone growth and mineralization.[58]

Pamidronate is able to decrease serum alkaline phosphatase level to near normal values, almost completely relieve bone pain, and maintain the response for 6 months or longer after the cessation of therapy.[59] The dose range of pamidronate has been from 300 mg to 1,200 mg per day. An oral dose of 600 mg per day has been associated with low back pain relief in 56% (87) of 156 Paget's disease patients.[60]

Bisphosphonate therapy has been shown to cause improvement of symptoms in 60% or more of patients, even in the presence of secondary osteoarthritis.[61] Bisphosphonates may be helpful in patients with skeletal pain secondary to Paget's disease alone or to Paget's disease and associated osteoarthritis.[18]

Plicamycin, previously known as mithramycin, is an antibiotic that binds to deoxyribonucleic acid and inhibits RNA synthesis. It has a cytotoxic effect on osteoclasts and is used as a treatment for hypercalcemia related to cancer. The drug is potent and rapidly effective but, because it is associated with toxicity, it cannot be used as a first-line agent.[62] It is administered intravenously in patients with progressive neurologic compression syndromes secondary to Paget's disease. Pamidronate is able to control hypercalcemia secondary to malignancy with less toxicity than plicamycin.[63]

Other therapies used for Paget's disease have included gallium nitrate and oral tiludronate disodium. These agents have been associated with a beneficial effect on the clinical symptoms and biochemical parameters of Paget's disease.[64, 65] Gallium nitrate, administered subcutaneously, is able to decrease elevated enzyme activity by 50% or more in patients with advanced Paget's disease who have not benefited from other therapies.[66]

Physicians usually use one agent at a time, following the patient's symptoms, serum alkaline phosphatase level, and bone activity on bone scan. Many patients have remission of their disease after a course of therapy and may not need to resume the drug for an extended period. More complete biochemical suppression is associated with more prolonged clinical remission not requiring a resumption of therapy.[67] Patients with persistent neurologic syndromes may require a combination of agents for adequate control.[68]

Prognosis

Most patients with Paget's disease have an asymptomatic illness. Others with more active disease are controlled with NSAIDs and agents that modify bone metabolism. Patients with Paget's disease uncomplicated by osteoarthritis may respond to a combination of calcitonin and bisphosphonates or to bisphosphonates alone.[28, 69] Improvement may be manifested by a decrease in bone scintiscan activity. However, complete resolution of increased activity is unusual.[70]

The complications of Paget's disease that cause disability and death are rare. Occasionally patients develop neurologic symptoms from spinal cord compression. Patients with Paget's disease of the skull and cervical spine may develop obstruction of cerebrospinal fluid flow. These patients are at risk of developing a syringomyelia.[71] Increased drug therapy or laminectomy can be effective in controlling these complications. Many of the patients with cervical spine disease in association with spinal cord compression require decompression for improvement of neurologic dysfunction.[19, 21, 23]

Malignant transformation of Paget's disease is associated with a poor prognosis but is fortunately a rare occurrence. In a series of 22 cases of sarcoma complicating Paget's disease, one patient had involvement of the sacrum, another patient, the thoracic spine. None of the cases involved the cervical spine.[72] Sarcoma occurred in areas of advanced disease and presented as a destructive lesion without periosteal reaction. The 5-year survival rate is 15% of Paget's disease patients with sarcoma.[73]

References

PAGET'S DISEASE OF BONE

1. Paget J: On a form of chronic inflammation of bones (osteitis deformans). Trans R Chir Soc London 60:37, 1877.
2. Siris ES, Jacobs TP, Canfield RE: Paget's disease of bone. Bull NY Acad Med 56:285, 1980.
3. Schmorl G: Ueber osteitis deformans Paget. Virchows Arch A Pathol Anat Histopathol 283:694, 1932.
4. Barker DJ: The epidemiology of Paget's disease of bone. Metab Bone Dis 3:231, 1981.
5. Rosenthal MJ, Hartnell JM, Kaiser FE, et al.: Paget's disease of bone in older patients. J Am Geriatr Soc 37:639, 1989.
6. Altman RD: Musculoskeletal manifestations of Paget's disease of bone. Arthritis Rheum 23:1121, 1980.
7. Polednak AP: Rates of Paget's disease of bone among hospital discharges, by age and sex. J Am Geriatr Soc 35:550, 1987.
8. Kukita A, Chenu C, McManus LM, et al.: Atypical multinucleated cells form in long-term marrow cultures from patients with Paget's disease. J Clin Invest 85:1280, 1990.
9. Roodman GD, Kukihara N, Ohsaki Y, et al.: Interleukin-6: a potential autocrine/paracrine factor in Paget's disease of bone. J Clin Invest 89:46, 1992.
10. de Deuxchaisnes CN, Krane SM: Paget's disease of bone: clinical and metabolic observations. Medicine 43:233, 1964.
11. Kahn AJ: The viral etiology of Paget's disease of bone: a new perspective (editorial). Calcif Tissue Int 47:127, 1990.
12. Bataille R: Etiology of Paget's disease of bone: a new perspective (letter). Calcif Tissue Int 50:293, 1992.
13. Singer FR, Mills BG: Evidence for a viral etiology of Paget's disease of bone. Clin Orthop 178:245, 1983.
14. Ralston SH, Digiovine FS, Gallacher SJ, et al.: Failure to detect paramyxovirus sequences in Paget's disease of bone using the polymerase chain reaction. J Bone Miner Res 6:1243, 1991.
15. Collins DH: Paget's disease of bone: incidence and subclinical forms. Lancet 2:51, 1956.
16. Hadjipavlou A, Lander P: Paget disease of the spine. J Bone Joint Surg 73A:1376, 1991.
17. Freeman DA: Southwestern internal medicine conference: Paget's disease of bone. Am J Med Sci 295:144, 1988.
18. Altman RD, Brown M, Gargano GA: Low back pain in Paget's disease of bone. Clin Orthop 217:152, 1987.
19. Rosen MA, Wesolowski DP, Herkowitz HN: Osteolytic monostotic Paget's disease of the axis: a case report. Spine 13:125, 1988.
20. Lewis RJ, Jacobs B, Marchisello PJ, Bullough PG: Monostatic Paget's disease of the spine. Clin Orthop 127:208, 1977.
21. Mawhinney R, Jones R, Worthington BS: Spinal cord compression secondary to Paget's disease of the axis. Br J Radiol 58:1203, 1985.
22. Brown HP, LaRocca H, Wickstrom JK: Paget's disease of the atlas and axis. J Bone Joint Surg 53A:1441, 1971.
23. Feldman F, Seaman WB: The neurologic complications of Paget's disease in the cervical spine. AJR 105:375, 1969.
24. Janetos GP: Paget's disease in the cervical spine. AJR 97:655, 1966.
25. Ramamurthi B, Visvanathan GS: Paget's disease of the axis causing quadraplegia. J Neurosurg 14:580, 1957.

26. Whalley N: Paget's disease of atlas and axis. J Neurol Neurosurg Psychiatry 9:84, 1946.
27. Frank WA, Bress NM, Singer FR, Krane SM: Rheumatic manifestations of Paget's disease of bone. Am J Med 56:592, 1974.
28. Chines A, Villareal D, Pacifici R: Paget's disease of bone affecting a single vertebra: clinical, radiologic, and histopathologic correlations. Calcif Tissue Int 50:115, 1992.
29. Chen JR, Rhee RS, Wallach S, et al.: Neurologic disturbances in Paget disease of bone: response to calcitonin. Neurology 29:448, 1979.
30. Schmidek HH: Neurologic and neurosurgical sequelae of Paget's disease of bone. Clin Orthop 127:70, 1977.
31. Schreiber MH, Richardson GA: Paget's disease confined to one lumbar vertebra. AJR 90:1271, 1963.
32. Lluberas-Acosta G, Hansell JR, Schumacher HR Jr: Paget's disease of bone in patients with gout. Arch Intern Med 146:2389, 1986.
33. Wick MR, Siegal GP, Unni KK, et al.: Sarcomas of bone complicating osteitis deformans (Paget's disease): fifty years' experience. Am J Surg Pathol 5:47, 1981.
34. Schajowicz F, Velan O, Santini Araujo E, et al.: Metastases of carcinoma in the pagetic bone. Clin Orthop 228:290, 1988.
35. Bannister P, Roberts M, Sheridan P: Recurrent hypercalcaemia in a young man with mono-ostotic Paget's disease. Postgrad Med J 62:481, 1986.
36. Coulton LA, Preston CJ, Couch M, Kanis JA: An evaluation of serum osteocalcin in Paget's disease of bone and its response to diphosphonate treatment. Arthritis Rheum 31:1142, 1988.
37. Foldes J, Shamir S, Brautbar C, et al.: HLA-D antigens and Paget's disease of bone. Clin Orthop 266:301, 1991.
38. Dahlin DC, Unni KK: Bone Tumors: General Aspects and Data on 8,542 Cases, 4th ed. Springfield, Illinois: Charles C Thomas, Publisher, 1986, pp 458–459.
39. Rosen MA, Matasar KW, Irwin RB, et al.: Osteolytic monostotic Paget's disease of the fifth lumbar vertebra: a case report. Clin Orthop 262:119, 1991.
40. Resnick D: Paget disease of bone: current status and a look back to 1943 and earlier. AJR 150:249, 1988.
41. Steinbach HL: Some roentgen features of Paget's disease. AJR 86:950, 1961.
42. Lander P, Hadjipavlou A: Intradiscal invasion of Paget's disease of the spine. Spine 16:26, 1991.
43. Waxman AD, Ducker S, McKee D, et al.: Evaluation of 99m Tc diphosphonate kinetics and bone scans in patients with Paget's disease before and after calcitonin treatment. Radiology 125:761, 1977.
44. Khairi MRA, Wellman HN, Robb JA, Johnston CC Jr: Paget's disease of bone (osteitis deformans): symptomatic lesions and bone scan. Ann Intern Med 79:348, 1973.
45. Shih W, Riley C, Maggoun S, Ryo Y: Paget's disease mimicking skeletal metastases in a patient with coexistent prostatic carcinoma. Eur J Nucl Med 14:422, 1988.
46. Dunn EK, Vaquer RA, Strashun AM: Paget's disease: a cause of photopenic skeletal defect in indium-111 WBC scintigraphy. J Nucl Med 29:561, 1988.
47. Resnick D, Niwayama G: Paget's disease. In: Resnick D (ed): Diagnosis of Bone and Joint Disorders, 3rd ed. Philadelphia: WB Saunders Co, 1995, pp 1923–1968.
48. Zlatkin MB, Lander PH, Hadjipavlou AG, Levine JS: Paget's disease of the spine: CT with clinical correlation. Radiology 160:155, 1986.
49. Roberts MC, Kressel HY, Fallon MD, et al.: Paget disease: MR imaging findings. Radiology 173:341, 1989.
50. Siris ES: Paget's disease of bone. J Clin Endocrinol Metab 80:335, 1995.
51. Hosking DJ: Advances in the management of Paget's disease of bone. Drugs 40:829, 1990.
52. De Rose J, Singer FR, Avramides A, et al.: Response of Paget's disease to porcine and salmon calcitonins: effects of long-term treatment. Am J Med 56:858, 1974.
53. Human calcitonin for Paget's disease. Med Lett Drugs Ther 29:47, 1987.
54. Altman RD, Collins-Yudiskas B: Synthetic human calcitonin in refractory Paget's disease of bone. Arch Intern Med 147:1305, 1987.
55. D'Agostino HR, Barnett CA, Zielinski XJ, Gordan GS: Intranasal salmon calcitonin treatment of Paget's disease of bone: results in nine patients. Clin Orthop 230:223, 1988.
56. Canfield R, Rosner W, Skinner J, et al.: Diphosphonate therapy of Paget's disease of bone. J Clin Endocrinol Metab 44:96, 1977.
57. Pamidronate. Med Lett Drugs Ther 34:1, 1992.
58. Fitton A, McTavish D: Pamidronate: a review of its pharmacological properties and therapeutic efficacy in resorptive bone disease. Drugs 41:289, 1991.
59. Mallette LE: Successful treatment of resistant Paget's disease of bone with pamidronate. Arch Intern Med 149:2765, 1989.
60. Harinck HI, Bijvoet OL, Blanksma HJ, Dahlinghaus-Nienhuys PJ: Efficacious management with aminobisphosphonate (APD) in Paget's disease of bone. Clin Orthop 217:79, 1987.
61. Altman RD: Long-term follow-up of therapy with intermittent etidronate disodium in Paget's disease of bone. Am J Med 79:583, 1985.
62. Ryan W, Schwartz TB, Perlia CP: Effects of mithramycin on Paget's disease of bone. Ann Intern Med 70:549, 1969.
63. Siris ES: Paget's disease of bone. In: Favus MJ (ed): Primer on the Metabolic Bone Disease and Disorders of Mineral Metabolism, 2nd ed. New York: Raven Press, 1993, pp 375–384.
64. Warrell RP Jr, Bosco B, Weinerman S, et al.: Gallium nitrate for advanced Paget disease of bone: effectiveness and dose-response analysis. Ann Intern Med 113:847, 1990.
65. Reginster JY, Colson F, Morlock G, et al.: Evaluation of the efficacy and safety of oral tiludronate in Paget's disease of bone: a double-blind, multiple-dosage, placebo-controlled study. Arthritis Rheum 35:967, 1992.
66. Bockman RS, Wilhelm F, Siris E, et al.: A multicenter trial of low-dose gallium nitrate in patients with advanced Paget's disease of bone. J Clin Endocrinol Metab 80:595, 1995.
67. Gray RES, Yates AJP, Preston CJ, et al.: Duration of effect of oral diphosphonate therapy in Paget's disease of bone. Q J Med 64:755, 1987.
68. Hosking DJ, Bijvoet OLM, van Aken J, Will EJ: Paget's bone diseases treated with diphosphonate and calcitonin. Lancet 1:615, 1976.
69. Jawad ASM, Berry H: Spinal cord compression in Paget's disease of bone treated medically. J R Soc Med 80:319, 1987.
70. Ryan PJ, Gibson T, Fogelman I: Bone scintigraphy following intravenous pamidronate for Paget's disease of bone. J Nucl Med 33:1589, 1992.
71. Pryce AP, Wiener SN: Syringomyelia associated with Paget disease of the skull. AJR 155:881, 1990.
72. Moore TE, King AR, Kathol MH, et al.: Sarcoma in

Paget disease of bone: clinical, radiologic, and pathologic features in 22 cases. AJR 156:1199, 1991.
73. Healey JH, Buss D: Radiation and pagetic osteogenic sarcomas. Clin Orthop 270:128, 1991.

SARCOIDOSIS

Capsule Summary

Frequency of neck pain—rare
Location of neck pain—cervical spine
Quality of neck pain—intermittent, dull, or stabbing pain
Symptoms and signs—cough, dyspnea, vertebral percussion tenderness
Laboratory and x-ray tests—increased calcium and gamma globulin levels, mixed lytic-sclerotic lesions on plain roentgenogram
Treatment—corticosteroids, surgical decompression

Prevalence and Pathogenesis

Sarcoidosis is a disease whose causes are unknown. Sarcoidosis causes the formation of granulomas, a form of inflammation consisting of epithelioid cells surrounded by a border of mononuclear cells, in any organ in the body. It is most closely associated with granuloma formation in the lung and thoracic lymph nodes. Less commonly, patients develop bony involvement, including vertebral bodies. The disease was first described by Hutchinson in 1877.[1]

The exact prevalence of sarcoidosis is unknown but may be as high as one case per 10,000 population. Autopsy studies suggest that the prevalence of sarcoidosis may be as high as 641 cases per 100,000 population in Scandinavian countries.[2] In the United States sarcoidosis is 14 times more common in blacks than whites.[3] The age of onset for sarcoidosis is from 20 to 40 years. The male-to-female ratio is 1:1. Vertebral sarcoidosis is rare, with 20 reported cases.[4] Most patients with vertebral sarcoidosis are black males with a mean age of 26 years.

The pathogenesis of sarcoidosis is unknown. The presence of granulomas in the lung and other tissues suggests an abnormality in immune function. Bronchoalveolar lavage has been used to sample immune cells from the lungs of sarcoid patients. Lavage fluid has a high proportion and absolute number of lymphocytes.[5] Normally, macrophages comprise 90% and lymphocytes 10% of lavage fluid. In sarcoidosis, the number of cells is increased several times the number of normal individuals, and the number of lymphocytes may be increased to 60% of total recovered cells.[6] T lymphocytes from patients with active sarcoidosis release substances that promote the formation of granulomas. Helper T cells, as opposed to suppressor T cells, are found in increased numbers in the lung, whereas the ratio of helper to suppressor cells in the peripheral blood is decreased. In addition to their increased numbers, T lymphocytes are in an activated state, manifested by active proliferation and release of migration inhibiting factor, interleukin-2, and gamma interferon.[5] Macrophages are also activated to produce interleukin-1. In addition, T lymphocytes from sarcoid patients cause B lymphocytes to produce immunoglobulin. These abnormalities in the number and function of immune cells correlate with the clinical findings of granuloma formation, anergy to delayed hypersensitivity reaction, and hypergammaglobulinemia.[7–9] The granuloma in an organ causes disorganization of normal tissue, and the process of healing results in the production of fibrosis in areas of granulomatous inflammation. Granuloma-associated fibrosis in the lungs, heart, kidney, eyes, musculoskeletal system, and nervous system may be associated with dysfunction in all these organ systems and correlates with the wide range of clinical findings associated with this illness.

Osseous involvement in sarcoidosis has been estimated to be 15% to 20%. A proportion of sarcoid patients as high as 34% has been reported if consistent radiologic evaluation of patients is performed.[2] This proportion of patients with osseous involvement may still be an underestimate because granulomata may be present in bone and not detected by radiographic techniques. Bone lesions are more common in patients with more persistent disease with chronic skin involvement.[10] The areas of involvement include the bones of the hands and feet, skull, pelvis, femurs, humerus, and ribs. The spine is rarely involved.

Clinical History

Osseous sarcoidosis almost invariably occurs when there is clinical or radiographic pulmonary involvement. Pulmonary symptoms include cough and shortness of breath. Osseous lesions may be asymptomatic or discovered by chance on radiographs, but this is rarely the case in vertebral sarcoidosis because it is usually painful. Patients complain of a dull or stabbing pain localized at the involved vertebrae. It may radiate from the neck to the shoulders; it is relieved by rest and increased with activity. Patients with spinal cord compression and spinal cord infiltration complain of neurologic symptoms, including lower extremity weakness, loss of sensation, and abnormalities of bladder and bowel function.[11–15] Symptoms related to a single nerve root infiltrated with sarcoid have also been reported.[16] Patients with generalized sarcoidosis may also give a history of anorexia, weight loss, and fever.

Physical Examination

Physical examination of patients with vertebral sarcoidosis demonstrates percussion tenderness over the involved area of the axial skeleton. Limitation of motion of the spine may be an accompanying finding. Those with neurologic involvement may demonstrate impaired sensation, weakness, and depressed or absent lower extremity reflexes.[17] General physical examination may demonstrate other organ system involvement with sarcoidosis, including skin rash (erythema nodosum and macules or papules containing granulomas), abnormal breath sounds, splenomegaly, generalized lymphadenopathy, and eye inflammation (iridocyclitis, choroidoretinitis, conjunctivitis, and enlarged lacrimal glands).[18]

Laboratory Data

Several biochemical abnormalities have been described in sarcoidosis. These include hypercalcemia, increased serum alkaline phosphatase levels, and hypergammaglobulinemia. The level of serum angiotensin-converting enzyme (ACE) is elevated in patients with sarcoidosis.[19] ACE is most active in lung lining cells. Granulomatous inflammation of the lung and lymph nodes may be the source of increased concentrations of ACE. ACE level is elevated in 43% to 88% of patients with sarcoidosis.[20] This variability is in part due to differences in sensitivity of the test in different laboratories. The test also lacks specificity: miliary tuberculosis, histoplasmosis, Gaucher's disease, and biliary cirrhosis are associated with increased ACE levels. Therefore, an elevated ACE level is supportive but not diagnostic of sarcoidosis. Cutaneous anergy (loss of

delayed hypersensitivity) when tested with exposure to three antigens (purified protein derivative, Candida, and Trichophyton) occurs in a minority of patients.[21] Bronchoalveolar lavage has been used for determination of elevated proportions of helper T lymphocytes in sarcoidosis patients.[22] The results are nonspecific for sarcoidosis, and difficulty in obtaining fluid has limited its usefulness as a diagnostic test.

Pathologic specimens from patients with sarcoidosis demonstrate multiple noncaseating granulomas consisting of multinucleated giant cells. They are present in any organ involved with sarcoid, including the lung, skin, bone, and muscle. Nonsarcoid causes of granulomas (such as tuberculosis and berylliosis) must be considered before a diagnosis of sarcoidosis is entertained.

Radiographic Evaluation

Radiographic abnormalities associated with vertebral sarcoidosis include bone lysis with marginal sclerosis that involves the vertebral body.[23] Occasionally the posterior elements of vertebra may also be affected.[24] Contiguous vertebrae may be involved, some with narrowing of the intervertebral disc.[25] Other patients have noncontiguous vertebral body disease[26] (Fig. 17–2). The inflammatory process may progress to cause vertebral body collapse.[27] The lower thoracic and upper lumbar vertebrae are the ones most frequently involved in vertebral sarcoidosis. Paravertebral ossification with anterior bony bridges simulating ankylosing spondylitis has been reported.[11] A report suggests that patients with sarcoidosis may develop sacroiliitis in addition to nonmarginal syndesmophytes and paravertebral ossification.[28] Occasionally, sarcoidosis may produce sclerotic lesions of bone that may be confused with metastatic disease of bone.[29] Sarcoidosis may cause severe disc destruction that may mimic radiographic changes of discitis.[4] Cervical spine involvement has included pathologic fracture of the odontoid process.

Myelography may demonstrate defects compatible with soft tissue compression of spinal cord elements.[23] Rarely, the spinal cord and cauda equina may be affected directly. Myelography may reveal intramedullary or intradural masses, arachnoiditis, or meningeal thickening.[30] CT and MR scans are particularly well suited to the evaluation of neurosarcoidosis. CT and MR scans are sensitive to detecting space-occupying lesions in the spinal cord and other parts of the central nervous system.[17, 31]

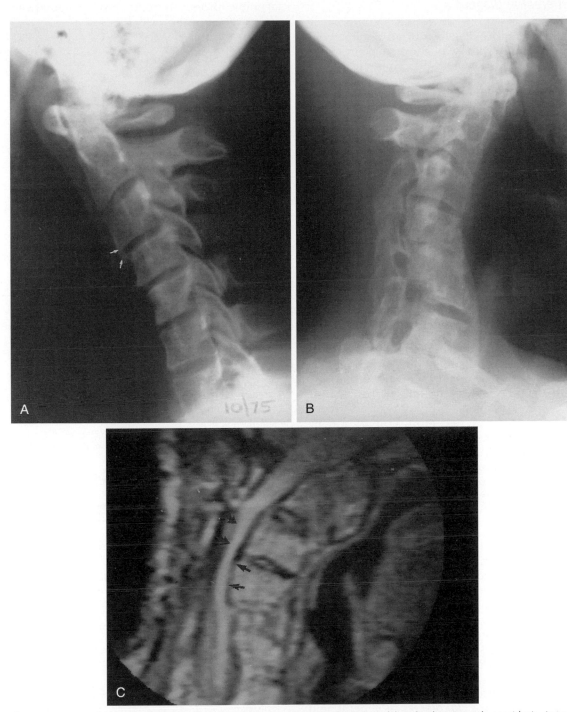

Figure 17–2. Vertebral sarcoidosis. A black male 27 years of age with neck and low back pain and sarcoidosis. Lateral view, *A,* of the cervical spine (10/75) reveals early bridging of the C3–C4 interspace *(arrows)*. In 11/76 he developed the abrupt onset of quadriparesis secondary to a fall. A lateral roentgenogram and myelogram (not shown) revealed collapse of C5 as well as C3–C7 extradural blockage. An anterior C4–C6 spinal fusion was completed. Lateral view, *B,* of the cervical spine in 1980 demonstrates continued paravertebral calcification. In 1986 he developed increasing neck pain and angulation. Magnetic resonance scan, *C,* reveals reversal of normal spinal curvature, with most marked angulation at C3–C5, close adherence of the spinal cord to the posterior margin of the vertebral bodies *(straight arrows),* and atrophy of the spinal cord *(curved arrows).* The patient developed hemoptysis secondary to an aspergilloma and died in 1989. (Courtesy of Werner Barth, M.D.)

Differential Diagnosis

The definitive diagnosis of vertebral sarcoidosis requires a biopsy of the lesion in patients with posterior element involvement or disc space narrowing. Diseases that may mimic sarcoid involvement of the spine include tuberculosis, pyogenic osteomyelitis, Hodgkin's disease, and metastatic carcinoma. These diseases may also cause posterior element destruction and disc space narrowing. Biopsy of the bone lesion may not be necessary in the patient with biopsy-proven pulmonary and skin disease secondary to sarcoidosis. However, if an anterior lytic lesion of a vertebral body does not respond to therapy, further diagnostic tests, including biopsy, are indicated.

Treatment

Most patients with vertebral sarcoidosis require corticosteroids in the range of 15 to 80 mg/day to control the symptoms and the granulomatous inflammation.[11, 25, 27] Bone lysis and sclerosis may remain the same or improve with therapy. In patients with persistent neck pain with neurologic symptoms of cord compression, surgical decompression of the involved vertebrae is required.[11, 32] Surgical decompression may also be necessary to relieve radicular pain for nerve roots infiltrated with sarcoid granulomas.[33]

Prognosis

The prognosis of patients with vertebral sarcoidosis has been generally good.[34] Surgical intervention for biopsies of lesions is important in eliminating other causes of vertebral lysis and sclerosis and confirming the presence of noncaseating granuloma. Decompression and fusion of severely affected areas of the axial skeleton have helped prevent the progression of potentially life-threatening neurologic complications. In most circumstances, corticosteroids for sarcoidosis in general, and vertebral sarcoidosis in particular, have been effective in controlling the systemic inflammatory component of this disease. MR scan may be used in a serial manner to document the response to corticosteroids of neurosarcoidosis, including spinal cord and nerve roots.[35] Patients with vertebral sarcoidosis have extrathoracic disease, and patients with extensive systemic manifestations of sarcoidosis have a less favorable prognosis than those patients with exclusively intrathoracic disease.[36]

References

SARCOIDOSIS

1. Hutchinson J: Illustrations of Clinical Surgery, vol. 1. London: Churchill, 1877, p 42.
2. Sharma OP: Sarcoidosis: Clinical Management. London: Butterworth, 1984.
3. Johns CJ, Scott PP, Schonfeld SA: Sarcoidosis. Annu Rev Med 40:353, 1989.
4. Kenney CM III, Goldstein SJ: MRI of sarcoid spondylodiskitis. J Comput Assist Tomogr 16:660, 1992.
5. Thomas PD, Hunninghake GW: Current concepts of the pathogenesis of sarcoidosis. Am Rev Respir Dis 135:747, 1987.
6. Soskel NT, Fox R: Sarcoidosis or something like it. South Med J 83:1190, 1990.
7. Hunninghake GW, Crystal RG: Mechanisms of hypergammaglobulinemia in pulmonary sarcoidosis: site of increased antibody production and role of T-lymphocytes. J Clin Invest 67:86, 1981.
8. Hunninghake GW, Crystal RG: Pulmonary sarcoidosis: a disorder mediated by excess helper T-lymphocytes activity at sites of disease activity. N Engl J Med 305:429, 1981.
9. Daniele RP, Dauber JH, Rossman MD: Immunologic abnormalities in sarcoidosis. Ann Intern Med 92:406, 1980.
10. Neville E, Carstairs LS, James DG: Sarcoidosis of bone. Q J Med 46:215, 1977.
11. Perlman SG, Damergis J, Witrosch P, et al.: Vertebral sarcoidosis with paravertebral ossification. Arthritis Rheum 21:271, 1978.
12. Moldover A: Sarcoidosis of the spinal cord: report of a case with remission associated with cortisone therapy. Arch Intern Med 102:414, 1958.
13. Delaney P: Neurologic manifestations in sarcoidosis: review of literature and report of 23 cases. Ann Intern Med 87:336, 1977.
14. Clifton AG, Stevens JM, Kapoor R, Rudge P: Spinal cord sarcoidosis with intramedullary cyst formation. Br J Radiol 63:805, 1990.
15. Tuel SM, Meythaler JM, Cross LL: Rehabilitation of quadriparesis secondary to spinal cord sarcoidosis. Am J Phys Med Rehabil 70:63, 1991.
16. Atkinson R, Ghelman B, Tsairis P, et al.: Sarcoidosis presenting as cervical radiculopathy: a case report and literature review. Spine 7:412, 1982.
17. Chapelon C, Ziza JM, Piette JC, et al.: Neurosarcoidosis: signs, course and treatment in 35 confirmed cases. Medicine 69:261, 1990.
18. James DG, Williams WJ: Sarcoidosis and Other Granulomatous Disorders. Philadelphia: WB Saunders Co, 1985.
19. Lieberman S: The specificity and nature of serum angiotensin-converting enzyme in sarcoidosis. Ann NY Acad Sci 278:488, 1976.
20. Fanburg BL: Angiotensin-1-converting enzyme. In: Fanbourg BL (ed): Sarcoidosis and Other Granulomatous Disease of the Lung. New York, Marcel Dekker, 1983, pp 263–272.
21. Tannenbaum H, Rocklin RE, Schur PH, Sheffer AL: Immune function in sarcoidosis. Clin Exp Immunol 26:511, 1976.
22. Yeager J Jr, Williams MC, Beekman JF: Sarcoidosis:

analysis of cells obtained by bronchoalveolar lavage. Am Rev Respir Dis 116:951, 1977.

23. Brodey PA, Pripstein S, Strange G, Kohout ND: Vertebral sarcoidosis: a case report and review of the literature. AJR 126:900, 1976.

24. Berk RN, Brower TD: Vertebral sarcoidosis. Radiology 82:660, 1964.

25. Baldwin DM, Roberts JG, Croff HE: Vertebral sarcoidosis: a case report. J Bone Joint Surg 56A:629, 1974.

26. Zener JC, Alpert M, Klainer LM: Vertebral sarcoidosis. Arch Intern Med 11:696, 1963.

27. Goobar JE, Gilmer S Jr, Carrol DS, Clark GM: Vertebral sarcoidosis. JAMA 178:162, 1961.

28. Curran JJ, Dennis GJ, Boling EP: Sarcoidosis and spondyloarthropathy. Arthritis Rheum 30:S42, 1986.

29. Abdelwahab IF, Norman A: Osteosclerotic sarcoidosis. AJR 150:161, 1988.

30. Bernstein J, Rival J: Sarcoidosis of the spinal cord as the presenting manifestation of the disease. South Med J 71:1571, 1978.

31. Sharma OP, Sharma AM: Sarcoidosis of the nervous system: a clinical approach. Arch Intern Med 151:1317, 1991.

32. Rodman R, Funderburk EE Jr, Myerson RM: Sarcoidosis with vertebral involvement. Ann Intern Med 50:213, 1959.

33. Baron B, Goldberg AL, Rothfus WE, Sherman RL: CT features of sarcoid infiltration of a lumbosacral nerve root. J Comput Assist Tomogr 13:364, 1989.

34. James DG, Neville E, Carstairs LS: Bone and joint sarcoidosis. Semin Arthritis Rheum 6:53, 1976.

35. Lexa FJ, Grossman RI: MR of sarcoidosis in the head and spine: spectrum of manifestations and radiographic response to steroid therapy. AJNR 15:973, 1994.

36. Wurm K, Rosner R: Prognosis of chronic sarcoidosis. Ann NY Acad Sci 278:732, 1976.

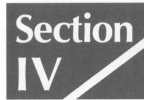

Section IV

THERAPY

There is no single form of therapy that is effective for all forms of neck pain. The various therapies that are effective treatment for specific diseases have been listed in Section III. Section IV concentrates on a more detailed review of the component parts of therapy. The indications for the use of the specific therapies and the toxicities and complications associated with each are discussed. Whenever possible, recommendations are based on published clinical trials. Recommendations based on personal clinical experience are also given and are stated as such. Medical treatment in general and a specific therapeutic regimen that has been used successfully in the care of patients with uncomplicated neck strain is presented in Chapter 18. Chapter 19 describes the indications and expected results from neck surgery. The success of surgery is based on careful selection of patients; the patient's physician can help the surgeon decide whether the individual is an appropriate candidate from a general medical and musculoskeletal standpoint. The epidemiologic factors, impact, and cost of occupational neck pain are presented in Chapter 20.

Therapy for patients with neck pain is arduous and taxing. Physicians should keep the following axioms of therapy in mind in order to provide appropriate care to their neck pain patients.

AXIOMS OF THERAPY

1. Most neck pain is mechanical in origin.
2. Most mechanical neck pain resolves by the end of 2 months.
3. Common sense is the most important part of therapy. Both the patient and physician should use it as much as possible during the course of treatment.
4. The goals of therapy must be the same for the patient and physician.

5. The physician must clearly state the goals at the start of therapy. Inform the patient.

6. Do the patient no harm. Limit the patient's exposure to addictive medications and operative procedures of questionable benefit.

7. Accept the placebo response (an endogenous opiate effect) as an effective part of therapy.

8. Improving the patient's general physical condition is an important component of neck therapy.

9. Consider improved physical function, increased self-reliance, and improved self-esteem as good outcomes of patient therapy.

10. Modify the therapeutic regimen according to changes (improvement or deterioration) in the patient's condition.

In general, therapy for neck pain is directed at decreasing pain in the acute situation. In patients with mechanical causes of neck pain, restoration of normal physiology (muscle length and strength) should begin as soon as pain is decreased. Patients who are at risk of continuous "injuries" that result in neck dysfunction (such as muscle strain in computer programmers) should be instructed in appropriate body mechanics (good posture and appropriate sitting position) to help prevent recurrent episodes of neck strain.[1] Patients who do not follow these recommendations may improve in any case or may develop chronic pain that persists despite healing of the injury that initiated the pain in the acute situation.

Another important component of medical therapy for neck pain is the prevention of injury to the cervical spine. For example, diving accidents are a common cause of cervical spine injury in young adults.[2] Approximately 50% of individuals were intoxicated with alcohol at the time of their accidents. Many of these individuals were injured at their homes in backyard pools.

In a study similar to a report concerning lumbar spine disease, the Quebec Task Force published a review concerning the diagnosis and treatment of whiplash-associated disorders.[3] Few scientific studies are available to demonstrate the efficacy of therapeutic interventions in the course of this cervical injury. Of a review of 1,204 studies, only 62 were found to be scientifically valid. Recommendations of rest and the use of a cervical collar may be counterproductive and may slow improvement in some individuals with whiplash injuries. Some of the recommendations for increasing movement in cases of whiplash may be applicable to therapy for other neck disorders. However, an approval of all the recommendations for other forms of cervical spine disorders should not be assumed. Additional research is required to determine the efficacy of a wide range of therapeutic interventions for neck pain. The clinician should use "scientifically unproven" therapies that improve functional capacity of the patient, in the absence of scientific data demonstrating an unacceptable amount of harm associated with a specific intervention.

Controversy exists in regard to the appropriate use of surgery in the therapy of cervical spine disorders. The rates of cervical spine surgery have been increasing from 1979 to 1990. The rate of cervical spine fusion operations increased more than 70% during this period.[4] There are wide variations in the rate of cervical spine surgery within different geographic areas.[5] Reasons for the rate of increase of neck procedures include an increase in the incidence of cervical spine disease, increasing numbers of physicians available to perform surgery, a lower threshold for surgical treatment, and altered patient expectations for treatment. Additional data are needed to determine the efficacy of these invasive procedures and whether the rate of surgery is appropriate.

References

1. Grandjean E: Fitting the Task to the Man: A Textbook of Occupational Ergonomics, 4th ed. London: Taylor & Francis, 1988.
2. Kluger Y, Jarosz D, Paul DB, et al.: Diving injuries: a preventable catastrophe. J Trauma 36:349, 1994.
3. Spitzer WO, Skovron ML, Salmi LR, et al.: Scientific monograph of the Quebec Task Force on whiplash-associated disorders: Redefining ''whiplash'' and its management. Spine 20:21, 1995.
4. Davis H: Increasing rates of cervical and lumbar spine surgery in the United States, 1979–1990. Spine 19:1117, 1994.
5. Einstadter D, Kent DL, Fihn SD, et al.: Variation in the rate of cervical spine surgery in Washington State. Med Care 31:711, 1993.

Medical Therapy

CONTROLLED PHYSICAL ACTIVITY (BED REST)

Patients with acute neck pain have difficulty walking. Decreased physical activity, frequently in the form of bed rest, is recommended for the therapy for a variety of neck pain patients. Upright positions exacerbate their pain, with an increase in their neck, arm, and head discomfort. These patients spontaneously take to bed to relieve their symptoms. Patients with a herniated cervical intervertebral disc with radiculopathy may find that bed rest with a supporting, appropriately fitted cervical pillow relieves their neck and arm pain (Fig. 18–1). An alternative to a cervical pillow is the arrangement of two pillows in a V with the apex located cranially, with a third pillow placed across the apex of the V. This allows mild traction on the neck and internal rotation of the shoulder, resulting in decreased traction on the cervical nerve roots.[1] Patients should avoid lying prone.

The amount of scientific evidence to prove these clinical observations is relatively small. No studies have been reported that evaluate the independent effect of rest on mechanical neck pain.[2] Data determining the appropriate duration of bed rest are also limited. In general, cumulative evidence suggests that *prolonged* periods of bed rest are detrimental to recovery of patients. Prolonged immobilization promotes decreased neck motion.[3–5]

In fact, patients who are busy rarely stay at bed rest for even a day unless their neck pain is severe. Most patients, however, strictly limit their recreational activities and try to minimize

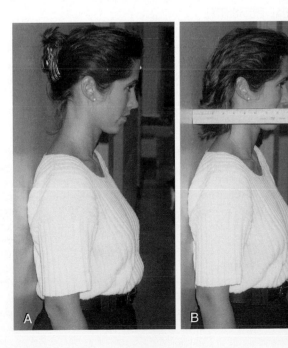

Figure 18–1. Correctly measuring height of cervical pillow: *A*, Patient stands against the wall with head in a comfortable position. *B*, The recommended height of a cervical pillow is the distance from the wall to the base of the skull. (Courtesy of Tom Welsh, R.P.T.)

their time at work. An explanation of the appropriate role of controlled physical activity is important at the outset of therapy. Informing patients of the benefits of rest and gradual mobilization results in their understanding the basic components of the treatment program. Bed rest may be poorly tolerated by older patients including those with trauma to the cervical spine.[6] Prolonged bed rest may result in a number of detrimental alterations in physiologic function, including decreased pulmonary and cardiac function.[7]

References

CONTROLLED PHYSICAL ACTIVITY (BED REST)

1. Murphy MJ, Lieponis JV: Nonoperative treatment of cervical spine pain. In: The Cervical Spine Research Society Editorial Committee: The Cervical Spine, 2nd ed. Philadelphia: JB Lippincott Co, 1989, pp 670–677.
2. Spitzer WO, Skovron ML, Salmi LR, et al.: Scientific monograph of the Quebec Task Force on whiplash-associated disorders: redefining "whiplash" and its management. Spine 20:21, 1995.
3. McKinney LA: Early mobilization and outcome in acute sprains of the neck. Br Med J 299:1006, 1989.
4. McKinney LA, Dornan JO, Ryan M: The role of physiotherapy in the management of acute neck sprains following road-traffic events. Arch Emerg Med 6:27, 1989.
5. Mealy K, Brennan H, Fenelon GC: Early mobilization of acute whiplash injuries. Br Med J 292:656, 1986.
6. Lieberman IH, Webb JK: Cervical spine injuries in the elderly. J Bone Joint Surg 76B:877, 1994.
7. Harper CM, Lyles YM: Physiology and complications of bed rest. J Am Geriatr Soc 36:1047, 1988.

PHYSICAL MODALITIES

In addition to exercises, physical therapists may use temperature modalities to relieve patient symptoms. Treatment programs may include ice massage, hot packs, whirlpool, diathermy, ultrasonography, transcutaneous electrical nerve stimulation, and high-voltage electrical stimulation. All of these counterirritant modalities offer transient relief of symptoms. These modalities do not alter the underlying physical abnormality. Modalities may be used with other therapies (such as exercises) that allow for greater motion and fewer postactivity symptoms.

Cold (Cryotherapy)

Patients with neck pain may experience analgesia with ice massage and cold packs. Therapeutic cold reduces pain, swelling, and muscle spasm during an acute phase of an injury within the first 48 hours. Cold also reduces local metabolic activity, decreases muscle spindle activity, and slows nerve conduction.[1, 2] Cold vasoconstricts peripheral vessels of the skin, resulting in increased blood flow to deeper vessels and tissues, increased muscle tone, reduced swelling, increased patient tolerance to deep massage, and enhanced voluntary motion.[3]

Initially, the patient experiences a burning sensation that dissipates as the application is continued. The ice is applied in a stroking direction following the course of the muscle fibers. A cold pack is used first if a patient cannot tolerate ice massage. The cold pack may be placed in a wet towel to limit contact with the skin. Cold packs with silica gel can be refrozen and used again for patients who experience continued pain. Vapor-coolant spray, flouromethane or ethyl chloride, is another form of cryotherapy. Flouromethane is nonvolatile and does not irritate the skin as much as ethyl chloride. For neck muscles, a cold pack or chipped ice wrapped in a terry cloth towel, applied for 15 minutes, may be the best choice.[4] A comparison of ice massage and cold packs reveals that ice massage cools the skin more so than the underlying muscle and may facilitate alpha motor neuron discharge.[5] Clinically, this correlates with the occasional patient who experiences increased muscle spasm with ice massage.

The anesthetic effect of cold increases patients' tolerance of stretching of contracted neck muscles by the physical therapist. The "spray and stretch" technique may be particularly helpful for patients with contracted paracervical muscles. The skin is sprayed with repeated parallel sweeps over the length of the muscle in the radiation of the neck pain.[6] The neck should be positioned to allow maximal stretching of the injured muscle, with the onset of analgesia associated with application of the spray. A spray period of 3 seconds is sufficient to allow for deep massage and active assisted stretching. If the skin reddens after deep massage, the patient's circulatory status is normal. Persistence of blanching suggests decreased circulatory capacity and potential toxicity from cold application. The duration of relief from pain and spasm is longer with cold than with superficial heat. Cryotherapy should not be used in patients with Raynaud's phenomenon, impaired circulation, peripheral vascular disease, loss of thermal sensitivity, or extreme sensitivity of the skin to temperatures. Cryotherapy is also not indicated for patients with longstanding contracted muscles. For these patients, cryotherapy facilitates the return of shortened muscles to their contracted length after lengthening with stretching exercises. Cold should not be used as the sole treatment for neck pain. Cold is used as an adjunct to facilitate the benefit of other therapies, such as exercises.

Heat (Thermotherapy)

Heat is useful in easing pain and reducing muscle spasm. Heat has a relaxing effect on pathologic tonic activity of skeletal muscle. Moist heat is used prior to cervical traction, mobilization, massage, and therapeutic exercise. Heat cannot be used for patients with impaired mental status, diminished circulation, or impaired sensation. These patients can develop thermal damage of the skin if heat is applied for an excessive time. Heat is also not indicated for patients with neck pain secondary to trauma when swelling and inflammation may increase with heating. Heat causes vasodilatation with increased blood flow, increases the elastic properties of connective tissue, and decreases gamma fiber activity, thereby decreasing muscle spindle excitability and resting muscle tension. Heat to skin and deeper structures has the beneficial effects of decreasing pain through counterirritant mechanisms and decreasing muscle ischemia associated with increased muscle spasm. Hot packs have been reported to reduce muscle spasms.[7]

Superficial Heat. Superficial heat provides mild heating of less than 40°C and penetrates to the level of the subcutaneous tissues. Hydrocollator packs, moist heating pads, infrared heat, and microwavable gel packs generate superficial heat. Hydrocollator packs (heated to 65°C) are wrapped in two or more towels and placed on the prone patient's neck (not underneath to prevent skin burn) for 15 to 20 minutes. Whirlpool baths provide massaging effects as well as heat. A warm shower may also offer temporary heating to the neck and shoulder region, allowing for greater compliance with range of motion exercises.

Infrared Heating. Infrared heating allows the therapist to observe the area as it is treated. The amount of heat applied to the skin is determined by the size of the bulb generating the infrared radiation and the distance of the bulb from the skin. The duration of therapy is 30 minutes.

Another form of superficial heating is generated through the application of topical agents. Capsaicin excites nociceptive fibers to release substance P. Prolonged application of this agent depletes substance P from nociceptive fibers, resulting in inhibition of pain sensation. Application of capsaicin to the neck four times a day may result in pain relief in those individuals unable to tolerate other forms of medical therapy.[8]

Deep Heat. Deep heat penetrates to structures below the subcutaneous tissues. Diathermy and ultrasound are some of the heat modalities that generate deep heat.

Shortwave Diathermy. Shortwave diathermy penetrates the soft tissues and delivers heat to deeper structures. Although diathermy has been shown to be effective at decreasing pain in trigger points, other heat modalities have been used in its place for deep-heat therapy.[9] Microwave diathermy uses electromagnetic waves to transfer heat.

Ultrasonography. Ultrasonography delivers heat to deeper tissues, like muscle, bone, and ligaments. It is not used in the acute situation, because heat causes additional swelling to the area that has been traumatized. Ultrasound reaches structures that are deeper than those reached by diathermy. Ultrasound is used for 20-minute sessions three times a week for 2 to 3 weeks. Ultrasound is used on paraspinous structures, not over the spinal cord itself, gas-containing organs, or on patients with bleeding disorders.

A patient with neck pain may participate in a home program that may include a hydrocollator, hot showers with a thick towel around the neck, or an electric moist heating pad. Hydrocollators are cheaper than electric pads but are less convenient. Heat should not be applied to the neck for longer than 30 minutes because of the risk of increased blood flow with resultant swelling and stiffness.

References

PHYSICAL MODALITIES

1. Lehman JF, Delateur BJ: Diathermy and superficial heat and cold therapy. In: Kottke FJ, Lehmann JF (eds): Krusen's Handbook of Physical Medicine and Rehabilitation, 4th ed. Philadelphia, WB Saunders Co, 1990, pp 283–367.
2. Ottoson D: The effects of temperature on the isolated muscle spindle. J Physiol 180:636, 1965.
3. Welsh TM: Physical therapy, ergonomics, and rehabilitation. In: Wiesel SW, Boden SD, Borenstein DG, Feffer HL (eds): Neck Pain, 2nd ed. Charlottesville: The Michie Co, 1992, pp 377–453.
4. Belitsky RB, Odam SJ, Hubley-Kozey C: Evaluation of the effectiveness of wet ice, dry ice, and cryogen packs in reducing skin temperature. Phys Ther 67:1080, 1987.

5. Hartviksen K: Ice therapy in spasticity. Acta Neurol Scand 38(Suppl 3):79, 1962.
6. Travell JG, Simons DG: Myofascial Pain and Dysfunction, The Trigger Point Manual: The Upper Extremities. Baltimore: Williams & Wilkins, 1983, p 66.
7. Fountain FP, Gersten JW, Sengu O: Decrease in muscle spasm produced by ultrasound, hot packs and infrared radiation. Arch Phys Med Rehabil 41:293, 1960.
8. Mathias BJ, Dillingham TR, Zeigler DN, et al.: Topical capsaicin for chronic neck pain. Am J Phys Med Rehabil 74:39, 1995.
9. McCray RE, Patton NJ: Pain relief at trigger points: a comparison of moist heat and shortwave diathermy. J Orthop Sports Phys Ther 5:175, 1984.

PHYSICAL THERAPY AND EXERCISES

Physical therapy together with personal exercise regimens are recommended to many patients with neck pain. In the past, it was common practice to tear off a sheet of exercises that would be given to all patients with neck pain. The course of events and therapeutic results of these exercises, given to patients without physicians' instructions, were the following: some had improvement; some had exacerbation of symptoms; some would follow the instructions incorrectly; and some would not do the exercises at all. The results of this haphazard attempt at physical therapy exercises left some physicians skeptical of the benefit of this aspect of treatment.

Exercise Programs

Therapeutic exercise may be defined as structural and controlled body movement to correct an impairment, improve musculoskeletal function, or maintain a state of well-being. Exercises can increase muscle strength, elasticity, range of motion, and endurance. A prescription for physical therapy must have a specified objective. The program of exercises may be modified as a patient's condition is altered. Therapeutic programs may include passive, active-assisted, active, or active-resistive exercises. Passive exercise is produced entirely by an external force without any voluntary contraction of muscles by the patient. These exercises maintain range of motion and elasticity of soft tissue. Active-assisted exercises require muscular contraction to move a part of the body without an external force. These exercises maintain flexibility and decrease potential for muscle atrophy. Isometric, isotonic, and isokinetic exercises are classified as active-resistive. Isometric contraction is associated with increased muscle tension without change in muscle length. Strength is increased only at the length of muscle contraction. Different lengths of contraction are needed to increase generalized muscle strength. Isotonic exercise decreases fiber length without a change in muscle tension. Strengthening occurs through maximal effort of motion. Isokinetic exercises move body parts through ranges of motion at a constant speed. This kind of therapy is given through the use of a Cybex machine.

The purpose of physical therapy and exercises is to relieve pain and to regain normal movement of the cervical spine.[1] The choice of therapy must correspond to the phase of the neck injury. During the initial stage, pain may be too severe to allow for increased movement. Patients may wear a soft collar to decrease pain. As the initial pain decreases, the collar is removed and range of motion exercises are completed while the patient is supine, with the neck supported by a pillow (Fig. 18–2). Range of motion exercises performed by the patient are encouraged to decrease the possibility of cervical contractures. Stretching exercises are performed by a therapist on a patient. As the patient improves with more tolerable neck pain, the cervical spine is exercised to the limits of mobility and pain. The spine is then returned to the neutral position. With improvement, additional pressure may be applied to the occiput to increase neck movement. Isometric exercises are accomplished by applying external force that prevents movement of the neck, thereby limiting pain (Fig. 18–3). These exercises maintain the strength of agonist-antagonist muscles; they are essential to counteract the atrophy associated with the use of cervical collars. These exercises may be used while patients remain in cervical orthoses.[2] Isokinetic and isotonic exercises are not as helpful for the cevical spine as for other portions of the axial skeleton. In the final stages of improvement, the seated patient starts postural exercises with maximum range of motion (Fig. 18–4).

Exercises are continued as pain decreases and motion improves. Exercises should be discontinued if severity or radiation of pain increases in a manner other than the expected discomfort or stiffness associated with normal exercise. One new exercise should be added per day to better assess the effect of the intervention on the damaged structures. In the early stages of an exercise program, the sessions should be limited to 5 minutes. Patients who are overly aggressive with exercise should be cautioned to limit duration of exercise ses-

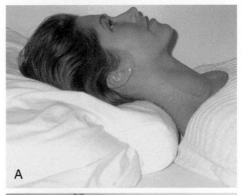

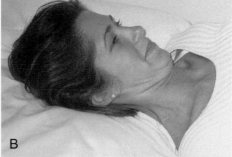

Figure 18–2. Therapeutic exercises, stage 1. *A,* Begin in a supine position with a pillow. *B,* Tuck the chin downward toward the collar bone and at same time force the back of the head into contact with the pillow. Perform slowly and do not hold the contraction. Perform 10 times, three times per day. *C,* Lie on back with small flat pillow under the head. Tuck chin downward and gently rotate head and neck to the left and return to original position. Perform five times. Perform same procedure to opposite side five times. To prevent added pain, do not overturn. Perform three times per day. *D,* Lie on back with or without a pillow. Take a deep breath with upper chest and keep shoulders back. Slowly inhale through the nose and exhale through the mouth. Perform 10 times, three times per day. (Courtesy of Tom Welsh, R.P.T.)

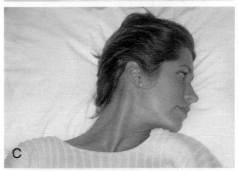

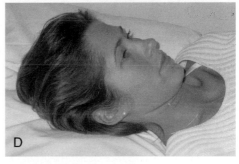

sions so that pain is not increased. Postural exercises should be performed five to six times per day for 1 month or until posture is improved. Subsequently, postural and prevention exercises should be done twice per day to maintain improvement (Fig. 18–5).

General aerobic exercises, such as cycling, walking, and swimming, should be encouraged to limit general deconditioning. However, limits should be placed on activities involving con-

tinuous extension or persistent rotation of the neck. A snorkel may decrease neck movement associated with swimming. Exercises should begin as soon as severe pain decreases.

Just as there is no single therapy for all causes of neck pain, there is no one physical therapy program for all patients with cervical spine disease. Some patients benefit from range of motion exercises, some from stretching, some from isometrics, and some do not

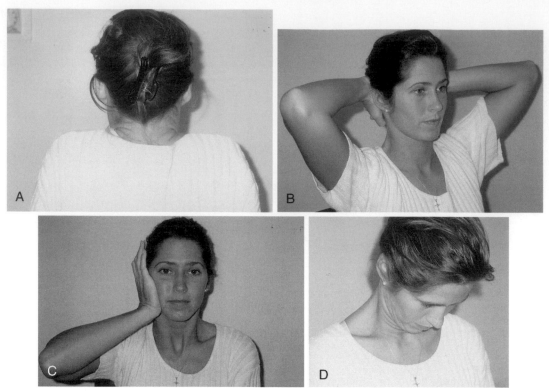

Figure 18–3. Therapeutic exercises, stage 2. *A,* In a seated position with the head in good posture, perform shoulder shrugs by raising shoulders up toward ears. Hold for a count of 3 and rest. Perform 10 times. Repeat hourly. Isometric exercises for sitting or standing position for anterior, posterior, and lateral neck muscles (do not be overaggressive). Perform three times per day: *B,* Place both hands behind the head on occiput and apply equal force to backward motion of the head and neck. Hold for a count of 5 and relax for a count of 3. Perform five times. *C,* Place the right hand against right side of face and apply equal forces of pressure from hands against lateral bending with rotation of the head and neck. Hold for a count of 5 and relax for a count of 3. Perform five times. Perform same procedure on the left side and on the forehead (not shown). *D,* In a seated position, bend the head and neck toward chest without forcing the movement if there is pain. If no pain or stiffness, apply overpressure with hands at end of movement. Perform 10 times hourly. (Courtesy of Tom Welsh, R.P.T.)

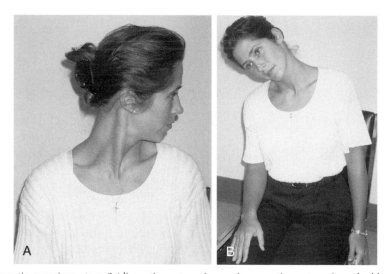

Figure 18–4. Therapeutic exercises, stage 3 (discontinue stage 1 exercises, continue stage 2, and add one exercise daily as tolerated). Lie on back with flat pillow under the neck, raise head off pillow, and bring chin to chest (not shown). Try one time and assess pain. Perform five times if tolerable. If no pain the next day, add one repetition until 10 raises can be performed comfortably. Perform three times per day. *A,* In a seated position, keep chin in and rotate head to look over the left shoulder within pain tolerance, hold for a count of 3, and return to center. Perform same procedure to right side. Perform 10 times hourly. *B,* In seated position, keep chin in and bend head and neck laterally so that right ear moves toward right shoulder. Do not raise shoulder. If there is stiffness and no pain, gentle overpressure may be applied with right hand. Perform same procedure to left side. Perform 10 times hourly. (Courtesy of Tom Welsh, R.P.T.)

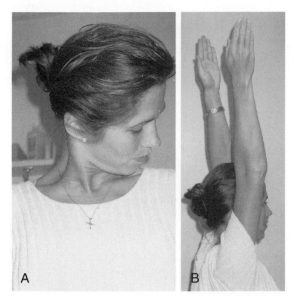

Figure 18–5. Therapeutic exercises, stage 4. *A,* In a seated position, tuck chin in and rotate head and neck toward the right shoulder. Bend neck laterally so that right ear moves toward chest. Apply overpressure with right hand if comfortable. Hold for a count of 3 and relax for a count of 3. Perform five times. Perform same procedure for left side. *B,* In a standing or seated position, raise arms straight toward ceiling. Do not look up. Hold arms up for a count of 3. Perform 10 times. In a standing or seated position, tuck chin in and hold head and neck in good alignment. Bend elbows and raise both arms out to the side so that they are parallel to the ground. Rapidly, move arms backward with elbows moving toward each other behind back. Perform these movements for 10 seconds (not shown). In a standing position with back to wall, tuck chin in and try to flatten the back of the neck against the wall. Hold for a count of 3 (not shown). (Courtesy of Tom Welsh, R.P.T.)

improve at all from exercises. Listening carefully to the patient's symptoms and observing the movements that cause pain help the physician decide which physical therapy program has the greatest chance for success in an individual patient. To increase patient compliance, neck exercises should be simple and easily accomplished. Patients should be supervised to ensure achievement of maximum improvement. Exercise programs should be explained with visual aids, including the number of repetitions, duration, time of exercise, and sequence of progression.[3] No therapy program is unchanging. Communication between the patient, therapist, and physician is essential in optimizing an exercise program. As patients improve, increasingly stressful tasks may be added to the program in an attempt to increase endurance and strength in preparation for return to work. If symptoms increase, exercises may be discontinued or reduced and reinitiated once the patient's symptoms return

to baseline. Conforming exercise programs to patient symptoms results in greater patient compliance and possibilities of improved outcome.

Patients with nonmechanical neck pain may also benefit from physical therapy and exercises. Patients with a spondyloarthropathy need a regular exercise program they can do at home. Therapy may include chest expansion, range of motion, and strengthening exercises for the lumbosacral and cervical spine. The program must be individualized for each patient. This is best achieved under the direction of a physical therapist who communicates with the patient and the physician.

Ergonomics

Ergonomics is a discipline that integrates psychology, physiology, physics, medicine, and engineering to address problems regarding the preservation of health and efficiency at work, in daily living, and in recreation.[4] Ergonomics is concerned with the match between machine, task operations, and work environment and human capacities and limitations. Individuals who are interested in ergonomics include industrial engineers, occupational safety officers, and physical therapists.

Workers may experience fatigue, muscle tension, and postural discomfort even with effective workstation design. An ergonomics team may be able to design modifications of the task to match physical capabilities in order to limit fatigue and strain.

Occupations that require coordination of visual and hand tasks along with a great amount of concentration or stress often result in postural pain problems involving the neck, shoulders, and upper and lower back. Fatigue may continue, resulting in a stressful work environment. Improvement of the work environment may avoid worker injury.

The worker needs to be observed in both dynamic and static tasks. During the dynamic muscular activity, the muscles contract and relax rhythmically. Walking, climbing stairs, and loading boxes are examples of dynamic activity. Static muscle activity supports a weight without movement but with a steady consumption of energy. Examples of static activities include neck posture in front of a computer screen, lateral neck flexion to hold a telephone, or neck posture in painting a ceiling. Some tasks have components of both activities.

Of the two activities, static activity results in overfatigue and muscle strain. Decreased

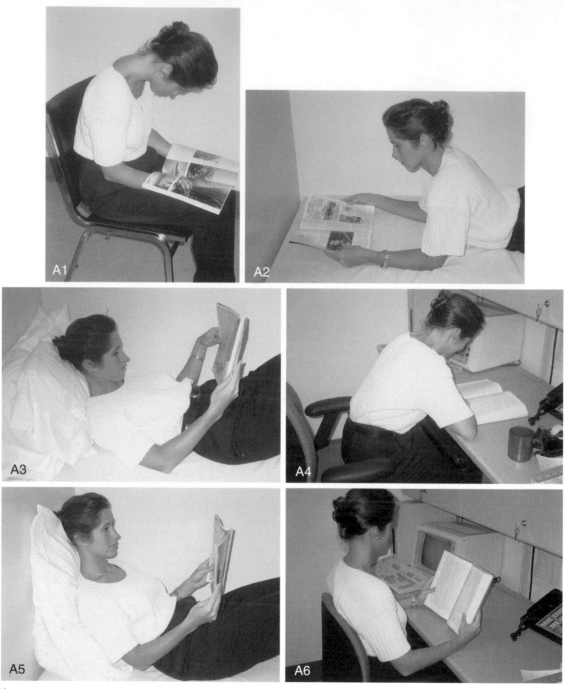

Figure 18–6. Postures for preventing neck pain. **Reading positions.** Incorrect: *A(1),* Avoid reading position that encourages prolonged forward head posture. *A(2),* Avoid prolonged extension of the neck. *A(3),* Avoid pillows under head only. This position promotes stretch in the posterior neck structures. *A(4),* Avoid excessive flexion of the neck. Correct: *A(5),* Reading in bed, pillows should support the back, shoulders, and neck. *A(6),* Reading material should be at appropriate level to maintain normal cervical lordosis. (Courtesy of Tom Welsh, R.P.T.)

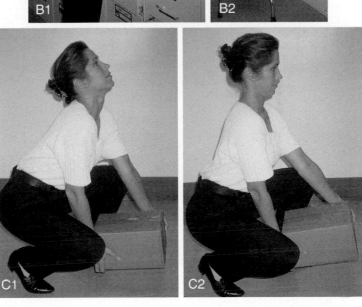

Figure 18–6 *Continued* **Overhead work.** Incorrect: *B(1)*, Avoid continuously reaching overhead and extending neck to look up. *B(2)*, Use a stool to keep objects to be reached at chest level. **Stooping and lifting.** Incorrect: *C(1)*, Avoid extending neck and lifting quickly. Correct: *C(2)*, Keep chin down and neck muscles fixed. Lift with legs and shoulders. (Courtesy of Tom Welsh, R.P.T.)

Illustration continued on following page

blood flow to muscle and soft tissue during tonic contractions may result in relative anoxia and pain. Dynamic tasks are fatiguing only after duration of many hours. Dynamic tasks allow for persistent blood flow to exercising tissues. A brief set of dynamic exercises at the workstation may help the individual with static tasks to increase muscular blood flow and decrease neck pain. These exercises may include deep breathing, shrugging shoulders, moving lower extremities, flattening the lumbar spine, flexion of the lumbar spine, and straightening the cervical spine.[2, 5]

Improvement of posture, workstation (through engineering), and body mechanics may decrease the risk for worker injury (Fig. 18–6).

Good posture is achieved by balancing the head and spine over the center of gravity. Poor posture is fatiguing and may result in instability, falls, and related accidents. The proper position of the head and neck is an angle of 20° to 30° of flexion. Tilting the head backward should be avoided. A range of eye movement within 15° above and below the normal line of sight is most comfortable.[4] The visibility distance between the eye and object should be 1 ft. Continuous deviations from this range may result in neck muscle fatigue and pain. Sitting posture is also important in maintaining static positions that are painless. Knees should be slightly higher than the hips, arm rests and chair back should support arms and spine, and reclined postures are acceptable

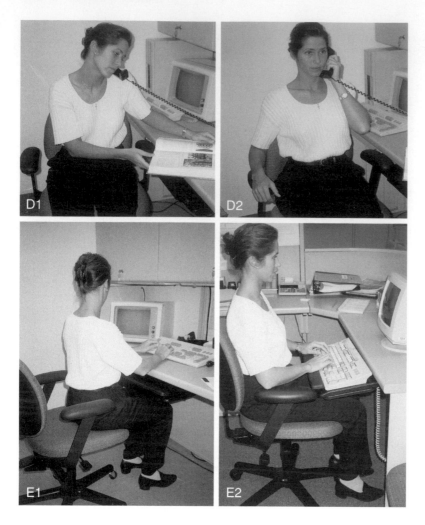

Figure 18–6 *Continued* **Telephone use.** Incorrect: *D(1)*, Avoid cradling the phone between shoulder and ear. Use a receiver cradle to maintain appropriate neck position. Correct: *D(2)*, Head should be maintained in midline position. Use headset if both hands are required for desk tasks. **Computer use.** Incorrect: *E(1)*, Avoid unsupported back and rotation of the neck. Correct: *E(2)*, Low back is supported with head erect with elbows resting comfortably at sides. (Courtesy of Tom Welsh, R.P.T.)

with adequate support of the head (Table 18–1). Work should be at the same height as the elbows.[6]

Engineering of workstations is important in limiting worker fatigue and pain. Placement of machines in awkward places may increase stress on the worker's musculoskeletal system. Evaluation of the components and order of a task may suggest more appropriate placement of machines. Neck stress and upper back pain may develop if the head is held too far forward or backward with sedentary activities. The appropriate placement of visual display terminals may limit the stress on the cervical spine by taking into account the capabilities and limitations of the worker. The head should also not be rotated or bent for any extended period. The work surface should be easily accessible.

A functional capacity evaluation measures the physical capacities of individuals. The evaluation measures strength, maximum effort, ranges of motion, walking pace, squatting ability, and posture.[7] The requirements of job tasks should be assessed. Abilities and preferences of the worker are compared with job demands and modifications made to diminish the risk of reinjury to the worker.

Patient education in a variety of forms may be helpful in informing individuals of their physical capabilities and limitations. Neck school is patterned after the back school concept.[2] Patients receive information on the anatomy and biomechanics of the cervical spine. A group discussion allows presentation of practical techniques for relaxation, exercises, and activities of daily living. Neck school may inform patients but may be too general to help individuals prevent neck pain in the workplace.[2] Cervicothoracic stabilization training is another method of strengthening the cervical spine to improve stability and flexibility and to decrease neck pain.[8]

TABLE 18–1. SELECTION OF ERGONOMICALLY APPROPRIATE CHAIR

1. Back and seat components should be contoured for maximum comfortable support.
2. The chair should have a flexible tilt for better support and variety of movement.
3. Seat and back components should be independently adjustable. The angle between the seat and back should be greater than 90°. The height of support for the thighs should also be greater than 90°.
4. Upholstery of the chair should consist of a porous, rough-textured material to dissipate heat, facilitate circulation, and reduce static pressure.
5. A high back rest is preferable for office work to support the trunk and should be concave to support the head.
6. The back rest should be angled at 10–15° from vertical.
7. An adjustable seat height allows the appropriate placement of the feet on the floor and elbows on the arm rests to allow for correct tension in the cervical musculature. Adequate support of the feet and arms allows for the correct position of the cervical spine to decrease fatigue.
8. Adjustable seat depth allows for correct thigh support and avoidance of pressure on the lower leg.
9. Seat width should allow for movement.
10. A five-spur, swivel pedestal chair with casters allows for stability and mobility.

Modified from Abdel-Moty E, Khalil TM, Rosomoff RS, et al.: Ergonomic considerations and interventions. In: Tollison CD, Satterthwaite JR (eds): Painful Cervical Trauma: Diagnosis and Rehabilitative Treatment of Neuromusculoskeletal Injuries. Baltimore: Williams & Wilkins, 1992, pp 214–229.

References

PHYSICAL THERAPY AND EXERCISES

1. Welsh TM: Physical therapy, ergonomics, and rehabilitation. In: Wiesel SW, Boden SD, Borenstein DG, Feffer HL (eds): Neck Pain, 2nd ed. Charlottesville: The Michie Co, 1992, pp 377–453.
2. Tan JC, Nordin M: Role of physical therapy in the treatment of cervical disk disease. Orthop Clin North Am 23:435, 1992.
3. Glossop ES, Goldenberg E, Smith DS, et al: Patient compliance in back and neck pain. Physiotherapy 68:225, 1982.
4. Abdel-Moty E, Khalil TM, Rosomoff RS, et al.: Ergonomic considerations and interventions. In: Tollison CD, Satterthwaite JR (eds): Painful Cervical Trauma: Diagnosis and Rehabilitative Treatment of Neuromusculoskeletal Injuries. Baltimore: Williams & Wilkins, 1992, pp 214–229.
5. Sundelin G, Hagberg M: The effects of different pause types on neck and shoulder EMG activity during VDU work. Ergonomics 32:527, 1989.
6. Grandjean E: Fitting the Task to the Man: A Textbook of Occupational Ergonomics, 4th ed. London: Taylor & Francis, 1988.
7. Khalil TM, Goldberg ML, Asfour SS, et al.: Acceptable maximum effort (AME): a psychophysical measure of strength in back pain patients. Spine 12:372, 1987.
8. Sweeney T: Neck school: cervicothoracic stabilization training. Occup Med 7:43, 1992.

CERVICAL ORTHOSES

Prescriptions for cervical orthoses must consider the biomechanics and pathophysiology of the disease being treated.[1] Spinal bracing affects the movement and stability of the cervical spine. The major reasons for the need to decrease motion are to decrease or control pain, protect the unstable spine, and limit damage to the traumatized cervical spine.[2] Cervical orthoses also have additional biomechanical effects of transferring partial weight of the head to the trunk when an individual is upright. While decreasing pain, cervical bracing has detrimental effects on the cervical spine structures. Muscle atrophy and weakness occur secondary to reducing the muscular activity necessary to support the skull. Decreased motion associated with the use of cervical braces promotes contracture of soft tissue structures. Psychological dependence and increased energy expenditures are also potential complications.[1] Cervical orthoses (collars and braces) have been used to decrease the motion of the cervical spine and head since the 5th Egyptian dynasty (from about 2750 BC).[3]

The planes of motion of the cervical spine are flexion-extension and rotation and lateral bending and are the greatest of all portions of the entire spinal column. Flexion and extension are coupled with rotation in the cervical spine. Most axial rotation occurs between C1 and C2, with the remainder occurring between segments C4 to C7. Considerable flexion and extension occur between the occiput and C1, with the remainder from the lower segments of the cervical spine. Most lateral bending occurs in the middle portion of the cervical spine at C2 to C6.[4]

Cervical orthoses come in four categories: (1) cervical (CO) (soft, rigid); (2) head-cervical (HCO) (molded, poster); (3) head-cervical-thoracic (HCTO) (molded, poster); and (4) halo. These categories range from least restrictive to most restrictive. In general, cervical orthoses are most effective in limiting flexion and extension and limiting lateral bending by 50% and rotation by 20%.[1] As opposed to lumbar supports that have contact over the entire lumbar spine, cervical orthoses must control motion by contact between the mandible and the thorax. Cervical orthoses should fit snugly but not so tight as to cause discomfort. If fitted too tightly, pressure on soft tissue structures causes pain.[5]

For mild neck pain, the soft cervical collar is the most commonly prescribed orthosis (Fig. 18–7). The collar is made of firm foam cov-

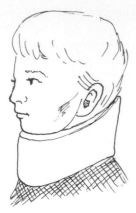

Figure 18–7. Soft cervical collar is the most comfortable orthosis. The soft collar is ineffective at limiting neck motion.

ered with cotton that is held together with a Velcro closure. The foam may vary in thickness or firmness. The soft collar is the least effective orthosis for reducing motion, but it provides comfort and warmth surrounding the neck.[6] The soft collar reduces motion in the sagittal plane by 26% but does not limit rotation or lateral bending.[7] The restriction of motion is mediated through sensory feedback and a reminder to limit head and neck motion more than an actual restriction of motion (Fig. 18–8). Sleep may be the ideal time for the use of a soft collar. The collar may limit awkward positions of the head. The hard collars (polyethylene) may have occipital and mandibular projections for added support. The Thomas collar has adjustments in height with foam edges. The Thomas collar decreases 75% of sagittal motion but does not restrict other planes of motion.[8] A higher anterior part of the collar results in decreased flexion, and a higher posterior part results in decreased extension. Scientific evidence demonstrating the efficacy of soft cervical collars is generally lacking.[9, 10] However, significant decrease in neck pain associated with the use of a cervical collar has been reported on occasion.[11, 12] Variability of results may be related to patient compliance.

HCO collars support the occipital and chin regions.[13] The most common HCO collar is the Philadelphia collar (Fig. 18–9). The collar consists of two pieces of Plastazote foam, with sides reinforced by rigid thermoplastic with Velcro closures. The orthosis may be less irritating to the skin by placing cloth padding under the chin support. The Philadelphia collar limits sagittal movement to 30% of normal.[14] The collar may also be extended along

the thorax and thoracic spine, with a strap around the thorax at the xiphoid level for increased support (Fig. 18–10).

HCTO collars are rigid poster-type supports with two or four upright supports. The four-post collar limits sagittal motion to 5% to 21% of normal, rotation to 27% of normal, and lateral bending to 46% of normal.[7] The Guilford brace has an anterior and posterior support but may be less effective at limiting lateral bending (Fig. 18–11). These orthoses offer less warmth to the neck than closed orthoses.

Another form of HCTO is the sternal-occi-

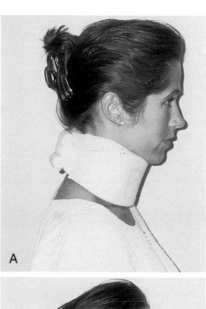

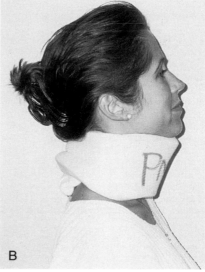

Figure 18–8. Fitting of soft cervical collar. *A,* The width of the collar should allow the neck to be in a slightly forward position. *B,* A collar that is too wide can cause pain secondary to excessive extension. In this circumstance, the collar should be reversed and fastened in front. A smaller collar should be obtained if extension of the spine cannot be corrected. (Courtesy of Tom Welsh, R.P.T.)

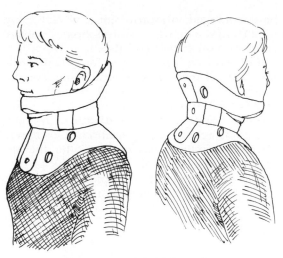

Figure 18–9. Philadelphia collar.

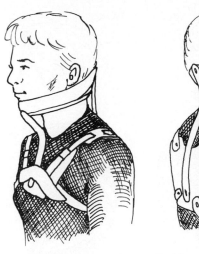

Figure 18–11. Guilford brace.

pital-mandibular immobilizer (SOMI) brace (Figs. 18–12 and 18–13). This brace consists of a broad chest piece that extends down the xiphoid and is hung on shoulder straps that attach behind to an encircling chest strap. The support may attach under the chin or solely to the occiput. The main advantage of this brace is the fitting of supine patients and the ease of adjustment. This brace is effective in immobilizing the upper cervical spine (C1–C5) in flexion. The SOMI brace allows 28% of normal sagittal motion, 34% of rotation, and 66% of lateral bending.[2] The SOMI brace is used after surgical fusions, to immobilize stable fractures of the neck, and to wean patients from bony-contact orthoses like the halo vest.

The halo vest consists of a steel band encir-

cling the head and secured to the skull with metal pins with attachments to a plastic thoracic vest with upright supports (Fig. 18–14). The halo vest requires expert fitting but offers the greatest restriction of cervical motion while the patient remains ambulatory. The vest reduces motion to 4% of sagittal motion, 1% of rotation, and 4% of lateral bending.[7] However, individual cervical segments may move in the lower cervical spine (snaking phenomenon).[15] A Minerva jacket consists of a body jacket with a chin, occipital, and forehead support. Movement of individual segments is decreased with the Minerva jacket compared with the halo vest. The Minerva jacket is also more comfortable than the halo vest.[16]

The most effective orthoses for control of

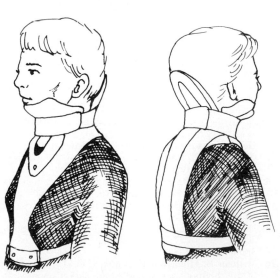

Figure 18–10. Molded cervicothoracic orthosis.

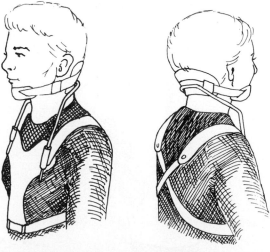

Figure 18–12. Sternal-occipital-mandibular immobilizer orthosis with mandibular support.

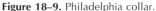

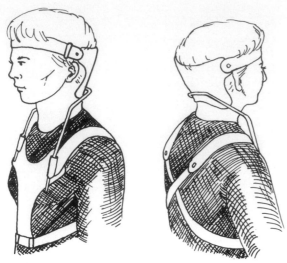

Figure 18–13. Sternal-occipital-mandibular immobilizer orthosis with occipital support.

sagittal motion are the halo vest and Minerva jacket. Rotation is also controlled with these orthoses. No orthosis offers total control of lateral bending. The halo vest limits lateral bending to 4% or less.

In conclusion, the selection of an orthosis must balance the comfort of the patient with the need for restriction of cervical motion. The CO collar is tolerated better than more restrictive braces. The soft collars should be used for a limited time. The patient should

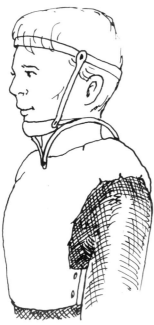

Figure 18–14. Halo vest.

be encouraged to remove the collar at every opportunity. The only orthosis that effectively controls motion between the occiput and C1 is the halo vest; it is required for patients with instability of the upper cervical spine. For patients with lower cervical spine instability, the HCO or SOMI braces are adequate. The more serious conditions associated with neurologic symptoms require more restrictive orthoses. Orthoses should be selected to offer the appropriate restriction of motion at the proper intervertebral level. In complicated patients, an orthotist can be helpful in selecting the correct brace.

References

CERVICAL ORTHOSES

1. Fisher SV: Spinal orthoses. In: Kottke FJ, Lehmann JF (eds): Krusen's Handbook of Physical Medicine and Rehabilitation, 4th ed. Philadelphia: WB Saunders Co, 1990, pp 593–601.
2. Redford JB, Patel AT: Orthotic devices in the management of spinal disorders. Phys Med Rehabil 9:709, 1995.
3. Smith GE: The most ancient splints. Br Med J 1:732, 1908.
4. Punjabi MM, Vasavada A, White AA: Cervical spine biomechanics. Semin Spine Surg 5:10, 1993.
5. Fisher SV: Proper fitting of the cervical orthoses. Arch Phys Med Rehabil 59:505, 1978.
6. Wolf JW Jr, Johnson RM: Cervical orthoses. In: The Cervical Spine Research Society Editorial Committee: The Cervical Spine, 2nd ed. Philadelphia: JB Lippincott Co, 1989.
7. Johnson RM, Hart DL, Simmons EF, et al.: Cervical orthoses. J Bone Joint Surg 59A:332, 1977.
8. Hartman JT, Palumbo F, Hill BJ: Cineradiography of the braced normal cervical spine: a comparative study of five commonly used orthoses. Clin Orthop 109:97, 1975.
9. British Association of Physical Medicine: Pain in the neck and arm: a multicentre trial of the effects of physiotherapy. Br Med J 1:253, 1966.
10. Huston GJ: Collars and corsets. Br Med J 296:276, 1988.
11. Naylor JR, Mulley GP: Surgical collars: a survey of their prescription and use. Br J Rheumatol 30:282, 1991.
12. Barnes MP, Saunders M: The effect of cervical mobility on the natural history of cervical spondylitic myelopathy. J Neurol Neurosurg Psychiatry 47:17, 1984.
13. Harris JD: Cervical orthoses. In: Redford JB (ed): Orthotics, etc, 3rd ed. Baltimore: Williams & Wilkins, 1986, pp 100–121.
14. Fisher SV, Bowar JF, Awad EA, et al.: Cervical orthoses effect on cervical spine motion: roentgenographic and goniometric method of study. Arch Phys Med Rehabil 58:109, 1977.
15. Lind B, Sihlbolm H, Nordwall A: Forces and motions across the neck in patients treated with halo-vest. Spine 13:162, 1988.
16. Maiman D, Millington P, Novak S, et al.: The effect of the thermoplastic Minerva body jacket on cervical spine motion. Neurosurgery 25:363, 1989.

TRACTION

Cervical traction is a nonstandardized conservative treatment modality for neck pain and radiculopathy. Traction has been suggested as a therapeutic intervention to relieve symptoms associated with nerve root compression, osteoarthritis of the zygapophyseal joints, and contracted cervical muscles. Patients with radiculopathy seem to benefit most from traction. Local muscle spasm is less responsive to traction.[1] The basic premise of traction is unloading the components of the spine by stretching muscles, ligaments, and functional spinal units. This stretching results in distraction of articular surfaces, prevention and lysis of adhesions within the dural sleeves, relief of nerve root compression within the neural foramen, decreased pressure within the intervertebral discs, relief of tonic muscle contraction, and improved vascular status within the epidural space and perineural structures.[2]

There are many forms of cervical spinal traction. Traction may be applied manually or mechanically. The tension may be intermittent or continuous. The patient may be upright or supine when tension is applied. Intermittent traction is best applied to the supine patient. The most effective intermittent traction consists of the greatest force and longest duration that causes the least discomfort to the patient's jaw and chin. The force may vary from 5 to 50 pounds for 15 seconds' duration, with 7 seconds' rest, for a 5- to 20-minute period. The weight and duration are increased corresponding to patient tolerance.[3] Intermittent traction may be most helpful for osteoarthritis or muscular strain associated with spondylosis.[4] This form of traction should not be continued if the patient experiences an exacerbation of neck pain.

Continuous traction is less well tolerated than other forms of traction secondary to the constant pressure on the chin and jaw. During an acute phase, maximum traction is limited to five pounds for a brief duration of 5 minutes. The maximum tolerated weight is 50 pounds for 15 minutes. If applied correctly, this form of therapy straightens the cervical spine and enlarges the intervertebral foramina. This therapy may be applied at home by the patient (Fig. 18–15).

The force and duration of traction vary with patient and condition. If posterior vertebral separation is desired, a weight of 25 to 45 pounds is required.[4] An increased degree of neck flexion (20° to 30°) is associated with greater elongation of the cervical spine. Angles

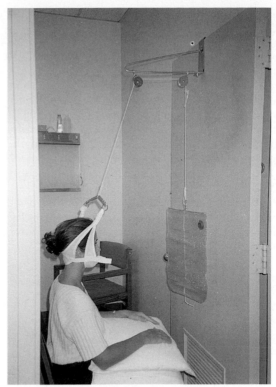

Figure 18–15. Overdoor traction. The patient sits facing the door with arms resting on two pillows. Head harness is adjusted to apply pressure to the back of the head and only slightly under the chin. A resting mandibular splint in a form of gauze or moldable wax may increase comfort on the chin. A 30° angle of tension is desired with a weight of 8 to 12 lbs for 15 minutes. Traction is applied twice daily for pain relief and three times weekly for maintenance. (Courtesy of Tom Welsh, R.P.T.)

of 24° are associated with the most effective widening of the intervertebral foramina.[5] Greater angles of traction increase muscle tension.[6]

Manual traction allows the therapist to control the amount of force applied to the neck at varying angles of cervical flexion, extension, and rotation. The application of the hands to the neck allows the therapist a continuous assessment of the extent of muscle spasm and joint movement associated with stretching. Traction is applied to the supine patient after moist heat is applied to the cervical musculature to promote relaxation.

Contraindications for cervical traction include a variety of disorders. A partial list of examples includes rheumatoid arthritis, spondyloarthropathies, osteomyelitis, malignancies, myelopathy, hypermobility, torticollis, and structural scoliosis.

Special concern is also given to patients with temporomandibular joint (TMJ) dysfunction.

Patients with TMJ may develop pain in the jaw that radiates to anterior and posterior locations in the cervical spine, including the sternocleidomastoid and trapezius muscles. Individuals involved in rear-end automobile accidents may develop injury to discs and ligaments of these joints as the head is thrown posteriorly and the jaw moves anteriorly. The masseter and temporalis muscles are tender and firm to palpation. Attempts to open the jaw result in ear and jaw pain.[7] Patients with TMJ are not candidates for cervical traction. They also may not tolerate cervical orthoses.

A study by Zylbergold and Piper reported on a comparison of three types of cervical traction.[8] Groups given static traction, intermittent traction, and manual traction were compared with a control group given no traction. All groups received education, heat treatments, and exercises. Patients receiving traction (25 pounds at 25° for 15 minutes) had greater range of motion and less need for medication. The authors advocate the use of intermittent traction.[8]

Patients receiving traction must continue with exercises to maintain the benefit of traction. Mechanical traction may be used if active modalities and manual traction have failed.[3] The patient should be supine when therapy is applied by a therapist.[9] This position improves patient comfort and relaxation. Therapy should be given three times a week for 10 to 15 sessions.[3] For home use, a simple pulley system attached over the door is useful. This home system is limited by patient compliance.

References

TRACTION

1. Klaber-Moffett JA, Hughes GI, Griffiths P: An investigation of the effects of cervical traction, part 2: the effects on the neck musculature. Clin Rehabil 4:287, 1990.
2. Rath W: Cervical traction: a clinical perspective. Orthop Rev 13:29, 1984.
3. Tan JC, Nordin M: Role of physical therapy in the treatment of cervical disk disease. Orthop Clin North Am 23:435, 1992.
4. Welsh TM: Physical therapy, ergonomics, and rehabilitation. In: Wiesel SW, Boden SD, Borenstein DG, Feffer HL (eds): Neck Pain. Charlottesville: The Michie Co, 1992, pp 377–453.
5. Colachis SC Jr, Strohm BR: A study of tractive forces and angle of pull on vertebral interspaces in the cervical spine. Arch Phys Med 46:820, 1965.
6. DeLacerda FG: Effect of angle of traction pull on upper trapezius muscle activity. J Orthop Sports Phys Ther 1:205, 1980.
7. Hodges J: Managing temporomandibular joint syndrome. Laryngoscope 100:60, 1990.
8. Zylbergold RS, Piper MC: Cervical spine disorders: a comparison of three types of traction. Spine 10:867, 1985.
9. Deets D, Hands KL, Hopp SS: Cervical traction: a comparison of sitting and supine positions. Phys Ther 57:255, 1977.

MANIPULATION

Spinal manipulation—movement of parts of the axial skeleton through the use of external force—is controversial because, in the United States, this therapy is associated with chiropractic. Manipulation has been used for deformities of the spine since Greek medicine as described by Hippocrates II.[1] The principle behind its use is based on the assumption that subluxation of the vertebra precipitates neck complaints and that these symptoms can be reduced with correction of the subluxation. In conflict with this premise of pain associated with malposition are studies of large groups of patients that have shown no relationship between vertebral malalignment and neck pain.[2] Manipulation may also use massage or stretching techniques to relax muscles that are shortened and in spasm. Other explanations for benefits of manipulation have included reduction of posterior disc herniations by tightening the posterior longitudinal ligament. Manipulation may free adhesions around a prolapsed disc, mechanically stimulating large A-alpha fibers, blocking nociceptive input.[2, 3] Although Mathews and Yates demonstrated a reduction of small lumbar disc protrusions, another study of 39 patients examined by myelography failed to demonstrate any persistent disc reduction after manipulation.[3, 4]

The terminology used by chiropractors must be defined. Mobilization is a less aggressive maneuver than manipulation. Mobilization, or nonthrust manipulation, starts where the active range of motion ends at the physiologic extreme of normal motion of the anatomic structure. Between the physiologic barrier (muscle tension) and an anatomic barrier (joint compression) is the movement associated with manipulation. Chiropractors use the term adjustment for both maneuvers. Mobilization goes past the active range of a joint and stretches the elastic tissues in the joint capsule, resulting in increased range of motion. With manipulation, a high-velocity, short-amplitude force is applied to stretch structures such as the capsule and ligaments. The cracking sound is caused by the negative pressure (vacuum) produced, resulting in the sudden production of joint nitrogen. Adjustments are directed at one specific joint, with force applied in a specific direction.

Evaluation of a patient considered for manipulation therapy involves measurement of active joint motion, passive joint motion, and accessory movements.[5] This is necessary to determine which type of manipulative treatment to use. Movements may be classified as distraction, nonthrust, and thrust. The manipulation may be given with varying force from different positions but is always given in the direction that causes no pain for the patient.[5] Manipulation does not require a forceful action to be effective. The patient is told to relax and is taken to a maximum range of passive motion. A gentle thrust at this point takes the joint or muscle to its maximum range of motion. The specific conditions amenable to cervical manipulation are those with aberrant components of flexion, extension, lateral bending, and rotation.[6]

Patients with decreased range of cervical motion are considered for spinal manipulation. Short-levered, high-velocity thrust therapy is used most often. A course of therapy is given for 4 to 12 weeks. Treatment is given daily for 2 weeks; then, manipulation is administered three times per week for the remainder of the course. To prevent recurrence, one treatment per month is recommended.

Absolute contraindications for mobilization include malignancy, osteomyelitis, osteoporosis, fracture, ruptured ligaments, acute arthritis, herniated nucleus pulposus, neurologic dysfunction, hypermobility, anticoagulant therapy, and acquired bleeding disorders.[6]

In general, spinal manipulation is associated with transient benefit, lasting hours. Evaluations at 3 months or longer do not find any significant difference among patients who have received manipulation and a variety of other therapeutic modalities. Patients who seem to benefit most are those who have a shorter history of pain. Patients who had pain for a longer period do not respond as well. Many of the studies of manipulation are flawed with inappropriate control groups, indefinite entry criteria, and variable outcome measures.[2, 7] Only six studies of manipulation therapy for neck pain have been reported.[2] Some studies used passive mobilization only. Two trials demonstrated significant improvement 1 week after mobilization was initiated but did not analyze the benefit after this period. Another study found no significant difference in treated patients compared with control subjects after 3 and 12 weeks.[8–10]

Spinal manipulation is not a benign procedure. Significant mechanical damage can result from physical force applied to the vertebral column.[2] Complications of cervical manipulation have been reported at a frequency of two to three cases per million treatments.[7, 11] There have been 138 cases of extracranial vascular injury associated with cervical manipulation.[12] Many complications are severe, associated with arterial injuries, stroke, and death.[13] Of the complications associated with spinal manipulation, 81.2% were associated with cervical manipulation.[2] Quadriplegia has been reported in misdiagnosed individuals with cervical vertebral osteomyelitis.[14]

The risk-benefit ratio for cervical manipulation for patients with neck pain remains significantly high. Most patients with neck pain improve spontaneously. Any severe complication is unacceptable for a benign condition. Other conservative modalities have the opportunity to improve neck pain with less serious toxicities. Mobilization, not manipulation, by a physiotherapist has been recommended for the treatment of whiplash patients by the Quebec Task Force.[15]

References

MANIPULATION

1. Adams F (trans): The Genuine Works of Hippocrates. Huntington, New York: Robert E. Krieger Publishing Co, 1972, pp 238–239.
2. Powell FC, Hanigan WC, Olivero WC: A risk/benefit analysis of spinal manipulation therapy for relief of lumbar or cervical pain. Neurosurgery 33:73, 1993.
3. Mathews JA, Yates DAH: Reduction of lumbar disc prolapse by manipulation. Br Med J 3:692, 1969.
4. Jayson MIV, Sims-Williams H, Young S, et al.: Mobilization and manipulation for low back pain. Spine 6:409, 1981.
5. Chrisman OD, Mittnacht A, Snook GA: A study of the results of following rotary manipulation in the lumbar intervertebral disc syndrome. J Bone Joint Surg 46A:517, 1964.
6. Paris SV: Spinal manipulative therapy. Clin Orthop 179:55, 1983.
7. Fitzgerald PB: Manipulation and mobilization. In: Tollison CD, Satterthwaite JR (eds): Painful Cervical Trauma: Diagnosis and Rehabilitative Treatment of Neuromusculoskeletal Injuries. Baltimore: Williams & Wilkins, 1992, pp 120–133.
8. Brodin H: Cervical pain and mobilization. Med Phys 6:67, 1983.
9. Howe DH, Newcombe RG, Wade MT: Manipulation of the cervical spine: a pilot study. J R Coll Gen Pract 33:574, 1983.
10. Sloop PR, Smith DS, Goldenberg E, et al.: Manipulation for chronic neck pain: a double-blind controlled study. Spine 7:532, 1982.
11. Dvorak J, Orelli P: How dangerous is manipulation to the cervical spine? Manual Med 2:1, 1985.

12. Robertson JT: Neck manipulation as a cause of stroke. Stroke 12:260, 1987.
13. Ford RF, Clark D: Thrombosis of the basilar artery with softening of the cerebellum and brain stem due to manipulation in the neck. Johns Hopkins Hosp Bull 98:37, 1956.
14. Lewis M, Grundy D: Vertebral osteomyelitis following manipulation of spondylitic necks: a possible risk. Paraplegia 30:788, 1992.
15. Spitzer WO, Skovron ML, Salmi LR, et al.: Scientific monograph of the Quebec Task Force on whiplash-associated disorders: redefining "whiplash" and its management. Spine 20:1, 1995.

INJECTION THERAPY

Local and regional analgesia, either applied topically or injected locally or regionally, is part of the therapeutic regimen of patients with neck pain. The basic premise on which this therapy is based is that nociceptive input can be interrupted at its source by blocking the function of nociceptive sensory fibers in the peripheral nerve supplying the "injured" area as well as interrupting the afferent limb of abnormal reflexes that increase muscle tension, which also contributes to pain. Depending on the type of agent used (topical cooling spray, short-acting analgesic, or corticosteroid), the concentration of the medicine, and location of the application, the peripheral and central nervous systems can be affected in a number of ways. For example, low concentrations of local anesthetics can block the unmyelinated C and B fibers and small myelinated A-delta fibers without affecting A-alpha or motor fibers. If motor function needs to be blocked to decrease muscle spasm, this effect can be obtained through the use of an appropriate anesthetic at an increased concentration.

Bonica has suggested that blocks are not only therapeutic but also have diagnostic and prognostic indications (Table 18–2).[1] Too much diagnostic importance should not be ascribed to a response to an injection. The clinician should not confuse a response to an anesthetic with a definite diagnosis of the cause of neck pain. Certainly, a response to an injection with relief of pain suggests that the area treated has been the source of nociceptive input, but referred pain may improve from an injection as well. The physician must continue to observe the patient who receives a therapeutic injection. An initial beneficial response may wane if a more sinister problem other than local muscle strain is the cause of pain.

TABLE 18–2. INDICATIONS FOR NERVE BLOCKS WITH LOCAL ANESTHETICS

DIAGNOSTIC BLOCKS

1. Aid in the identification of the site and cause of pain.
2. Identify nociceptive pathways (specific peripheral nerves).
3. Determine mechanism of chronic pain syndromes.
4. Determine patients' reaction to pain relief.

PROGNOSTIC BLOCKS

1. Determine potential response to permanent blocks or neurosurgery.
2. Allow patients to experience the sensations and side effects from permanent procedures on a temporary basis (decision concerning surgery).

THERAPEUTIC BLOCKS

1. Relieve acute postoperative pain and pain from self-limiting diseases.
2. Prolong pain relief by breaking reflex mechanisms.
3. Provide temporary relief to allow the onset of action of other therapies with delayed effects.

Modified from Bonica JJ: Local anesthesia and regional block. In: Wall PD, Melzack R (eds): Textbook of Pain. Edinburgh: Churchill Livingstone, 1984, p 541.

Soft Tissue Injections

A variety of topical and injectable anesthetics are available for use in patients with acute and chronic pain. All have advantages and disadvantages in specific circumstances. A brief review of their characteristics will help the clinician decide which agent is most appropriate for specific patients.

The local anesthetics produce their affects by blocking the depolarization of nerves inhibiting the flux of sodium ions across membranes. The local anesthetic blocks the mouth of the sodium channel and does this to a greater extent in nerves that are actively conducting impulses than in nerves that are inactive.[2] The sensitivity of nerves to local anesthetics relates to fiber size and myelination. Fibers that are thicker and myelinated transmit nerve impulses at a faster velocity and are more resistant to local blockade than thin, unmyelinated fibers. The minimum amount of anesthetic that blocks impulse transmission (Cm) varies for each nerve and each agent. The Cm of A-alpha fibers (motor—fastest velocity) is approximately twice that of A-delta fibers (pain and temperature). B fibers (preganglionic autonomic nervous system) are the most sensitive of all fibers despite thin myelination and have a Cm about one third that of unmyelinated C fibers (pain).[2] Agents also have different onsets of action correlated with diffusion capacity. Agents with greater lipophilic action (increased binding to tissue) have a slower onset of action. The characteristics of the common local anesthetics are listed in Table 18–3.

Toxicities of local anesthetic agents are unusual but potentially serious. Systemic reactions occur when these agents are injected directly into the blood stream. Locally injected anesthetics slowly diffuse into the blood stream. Patients with hypersensitivity to these agents may develop systemic allergic reactions to locally injected medications. The neurologic toxicities range from slight dizziness to grand mal seizures. Seizures occur when high concentrations of anesthetic reach the central nervous system. This complication can be prevented by using low doses of anesthetic, aspirating the area before injection, and injecting at a slow rate. Other toxicities include hypersensitivity reactions and cardiac toxicity in the form of conduction delays.[3, 4] Repeated injections of anesthetic into the same location may cause local irritation and muscle spasm.

Techniques of Injection

Identification of those patients who would benefit from injection is essential for a successful outcome. Patients who describe localized areas of muscle or ligamentous tenderness are candidates. These patients must be reliable; that is, they must be able to limit their activities to avoid increased tissue damage in areas with blocked reflex action. If there is any doubt, do not inject the patient.

The area of tenderness may be secondary to localized trauma or strain or may be a myofascial trigger point. Travell and Simons popularized the notion of localized areas of muscle damage, which undergo increased metabolism and decreased circulation, which accumulate products that result in contracted muscles that are painful.[5] Active myofascial trigger points are those that are painful at rest, prevent full lengthening of muscles, weaken the muscle, refer pain on direct palpation, and cause a local twitch response in the muscle band containing the trigger point. Latent trigger points are those that are tender only with compression.[6]

In the cervical spine, trigger points are located in the trapezius and splenius muscles. Pain from these points may radiate to the neck, head, and shoulder. The locations for injection that correlate with trigger areas, which parenthetically correspond with acupuncture points, include the upper border of the trapezius and the medial portion of the neck near its base.[5]

Whether undertaken to relieve pain associated with trigger points or, as some prefer to consider, local areas of muscle trauma, the use of local anesthetics is helpful in the treatment of neck pain. The procedure is started by identifying the area to be treated. Two cutaneous coolants are available: ethyl chloride, which is flammable and cold when applied, and fluorimethane, which is nonflammable and is the preferred coolant. The spray is applied in sweeps in one direction only that matches the referred pattern of pain. This procedure is used to stretch muscles that are foreshortened due to trigger points. The muscle is gradually stretched after the spray is applied.[5]

In many patients, local cooling with stretching is inadequate, and injection of medication is needed to control local areas of pain. The skin must be cleansed with a suitable antiseptic and a sterile technique must be used. Patients are questioned about any prior sensitivity to injected anesthetics. The possibility of vasovagal reaction is also raised. If a patient has had vagal reactions, the patient should be premedicated with atropine or placed in a supine position to limit potential hemodynamic effects. The choice of anesthetic to be used depends on the desired effect (Table 18–3). Travell and Simons advocate the use of procaine for trigger-point injections because this agent has less systemic and local toxicity in addition to its vasodilator effect.[5] Swezey and Clements have proposed the use of 2 to 5 mL of 1% lidocaine in combination with a depository form of corticosteroid.[7] Raj has used a mixture of 0.5% etidocaine and 0.375% bupivacaine for prolonged analgesia (the former for motor blockade, the latter for sensory blockade).[8] Bonica advocated using lower concentrations of anesthetics (0.25% lidocaine, 0.05% bupivacaine) because they are effective as anesthetics for local injections.[1]

The use of corticosteroids, in addition to anesthetics, is advised for patients with soft tissue inflammation or with postinjection soreness, according to Travell and Simons.[5] Swezey and Clements advocated the use of triamcinolone in conjunction with anesthetics.[7] Raj prefers 4 mg (1 mL) of soluble dexamethasone in 9 mL of local anesthetic.[8] He reports no painful effects other than a burning sensation in the area of the injection that lasts 24 to 48 hours. The authors have used betamethasone sodium phosphate suspension (6 mg/mL) 1 mL/3 mL of anesthetic solution with success.

After allowing the antiseptic to dry, the area

TABLE 18–3. CLINICAL CHARACTERISTICS AND DOSAGE OF LOCAL ANESTHETICS

	PROCAINE (NOVOCAINE)	2-CHLORPROCAINE (NESACAINE)	LIDOCAINE (XYLOCAINE)	MEPIVACINE (CARBOCAINE)	PRILOCAINE (CITANEST)	TETRACAINE (PONTOCAINE)	BUPIVACAINE (MARCAINE)	ETIDOCAINE (DURANEST)
Onset of action	Moderate	Fast	Fast	Moderate	Moderate	Very slow	Fast	Very fast
Dispersion	Moderate	Marked	Marked	Moderate	Moderate	Poor	Moderate	Moderate
Duration of action	Short	Very short	Moderate	Moderate	Moderate	Long	Long	Long
Optimal concentration (%)								
Local	0.5	0.5	0.25	0.25	0.25	0.05	0.05	0.1
Spinal nerve	1.5–2.0	1.0–2.0	0.5–1.0	0.5–1.0	0.5–1.0	0.1–0.2	0.25–0.5	0.5–1.0
Maximum safe dose (mg/kg)	12	15	6	6	6	2	2	2

Modified from Bonica JJ: Local anesthesia and regional block. In: Wall PD, Melzack R (eds): Textbook of Pain. Edinburgh: Churchill Livingstone, 1984, p 541.

to be injected is wiped clean with a sterile alcohol swab and anesthetized with coolant spray. The skin is entered and injection is started only after the area has been aspirated to ensure that the tip of the needle is not in a blood vessel. Fingers are placed on the skin surface to try and localize the maximum point of tenderness. A small amount of solution is injected. If the appropriate area has been entered, the patient experiences an increase in pain before the analgesic effects of the injected solution commence. The tip of the needle is moved in a fanlike pattern to cover the entire area of pain. During the injection, test for tenderness over the injected area to ensure the medication has been placed in the appropriate location. After removal of the needle, the patient is reminded of the potential burning and redness over the area injected. The patient is told to call if symptoms persist or increase during the next 24 to 48 hours. Dry needling, or the injection of saline without anesthetic into trigger points, has also been associated with decreased pain.[9] However, patients who undergo dry needling experience prolonged postinjection soreness compared with those who receive injections with an anesthetic.[9] After injection, patients may begin stretching exercises to maximize the length of muscles that have been contracted. Additional modalities including heat, massage, transcutaneous electrical nerve stimulation, and acupuncture may be used to maximize normal activity in the muscle. This allows adequate blood flow and return of muscle strength. If pain continues, repeated injections may be necessary. These may be done on a weekly basis for three to four additional sessions. If the pain still continues, other therapies are indicated because repeated injections cause irritation and local muscle spasm.

Epidural Corticosteroid Injection

The injection of epidural corticosteroids has been used in patients who have failed conservative therapy for lumbar nerve root compression. The theory supporting the use of corticosteroids in the epidural space is the increased benefit of the direct local effect of the medicine on an inflamed nerve root and its surrounding connective tissue in comparison with oral corticosteroids. Dilke and colleagues performed a double-blind, controlled study in 100 patients.[10] Their study demonstrated a significant difference in pain relief and resumption of usual occupation at 3 months in patients

receiving an extradural injection of 80 mg of methylprednisolone in 10 mL of saline, compared with an injection of 10 mL of saline into the interspinous ligaments in a control group. The procedure has also been used for cervical spine disorders. A number of studies have reported success rates of 55% to 75% with epidural injections for cervical pain secondary to several causes.[11–14]

The procedure is safe when the cervical spine anatomy is considered. The cervical spinous processes form an angle of 45° with the axis of the cervical spine. The C7–T1 interspace is the largest, making access relatively easy.[15] The cervical cord is narrowest at the C7 level. The negative pressure in the cervical epidural space is most pronounced at the C7–T1 level, corresponding to its proximity to the thorax. The C7–T1 and C6–C7 interspaces are the usual locations for epidural injections. A total of 10 to 12 mL of fluid (anesthetic and Depo-Medrol) injected into the C7–T1 interspace spreads cephalad to C2 and caudad to T4. The injection should avoid the subdural space. The maximum effects of the injection may require 7 to 10 days to appear. The ideal frequency of injections for sustained relief of pain is not established. Single injections may be adequate to diminish cervical pain.[16] In a study of 58 patients, good or excellent results were reported in 35 (60.7%) as long as 6 months after a single injection.[16] Complications are associated with cervical epidural injections (Table 18–4). These complications are not frequent but must be considered in reference to the specific patient to evaluate

TABLE 18–4. COMPLICATIONS OF CERVICAL EPIDURAL INJECTIONS

Initial
  Intravascular injection (seizures, cardiac arrest)
  Vasovagal syncope
  Subdural injection
    Total spinal block
    Postinjection headache
  Cervical spinal cord damage
  High cervical block with hypotension, bradycardia
  Transient neurologic deficits

Late
  Epidural hematoma
  Anterior spinal artery thrombosis
  Superficial infection
  Epidural abscess
  Neck stiffness
  Abdominal distention

Modified from Parris WCV: Nerve blocks and invasive therapies. In: Tollison CD, Satterthwaite JR (eds): Painful Cervical Trauma: Diagnosis and Rehabilitative Treatment of Neuromusculoskeletal Injuries. Baltimore: Williams & Wilkins, 1992, pp 134–143.

the relative benefit of the injection. Until larger studies are conducted, epidurally administered steroid injections are an unproven therapy for cervical radiculopathy. In patients who have continued pain and who are poor candidates for surgical intervention, epidural corticosteroid injections may be considered. The course of therapy includes up to three injections at varying intervals (days to weeks) between injections. After the course of injections is completed, patients usually do not receive a second course of injections.

In rare circumstances, patients who are resistent to epidural injection may be considered for a short course of oral corticosteroid therapy. The course is limited to 7 days or less. The highest dose of steroid administered is 40 to 60 mg for 1 or 2 days at most. The drug is rapidly tapered over the next 5 to 6 days. The potential toxicity of the drug (hyperglycemia, fluid retention, hypertension, and infection) must be balanced against the potential benefit. If there is any doubt, the corticosteroid should not be given to the patient. There are no scientific studies to document the efficacy of oral corticosteroid for cervical radiculopathy.

Facet Joint Injection

Patients with facet joint arthritis may develop pain that simulates radicular pain. If these patients do not respond to conservative therapy, they may benefit from facet joint anesthesia. Each facet joint receives sensory innervation from two spinal segment levels. Therefore, facets at and above the level of the involved joint must be blocked or denervated to obtain adequate analgesia.

The procedure requires radiographic surveillance for placement of the spinal needle. Diagnostic block at the initial step uses 2 mL of 1% lidocaine at each level to confirm responsiveness to therapy. Patients then receive a solution of methylprednisolone in 1 mL of bupivacaine at each level to be blocked. Repeated injections may be given every 2 to 4 weeks for three sessions.

The mechanism by which injections cause improvement is not apparent. Patients are told that symptoms may be aggravated by the swelling associated with the injection before they improve.

Uncontrolled studies of facet joint blocks with corticosteroid have reported improvement in neck pain.[17–21] Barnsley and colleagues reported on a double-blind injection study comparing bupivacaine with betamethasone

for chronic pain associated with cervical zygapophyseal joints.[22] The corticosteroid therapy was no better than anesthetic at 1 week and 1 month with regard to relief of pain. Less than 50% of patients reported pain relief of more than 1 week's duration. Facet joint blocks in the cervical spine can be considered to offer only short-term improvement for neck pain.

Peripheral Nerve Blocks

A patient with radicular pain secondary to nerve root irritation of any cause and the patient with neurogenic pain of peripheral nerve origin may develop, in addition, a component of sympathetic nerve pain. Causalgia is the term used to describe this pain, which has a burning, agonizing quality. The pain is constant and is not relieved through mechanical means by changing positions. The area affected with pain also shows alteration in sweating and temperature function along with loss of motor power. The patient with sympathetic dystrophy also develops dyesthesias in the affected area so that the slightest touch causes unpleasant sensations. Reflex sympathetic dystrophies occur in patients with postherpetic neuralgia; carcinomatous invasion of nerves; trauma, including nerve root damage, associated with subsequent scarring; and phantom limb pain.

If patients do not respond to physical therapy and a course of oral medications, including nonsteroidal anti-inflammatory drugs and corticosteroids, stellate ganglion blockade with local anesthesia or other medications is indicated. The procedure can be performed on an outpatient basis. The location for the injection is the C6 transverse process (cricoid cartilage) to minimize the risk of pneumothorax.[15] The needle is inserted to contact with the transverse process and then withdrawn 2 mm. Aspiration for blood is essential to prevent the injection of anesthetic directly into the vertebral arteries. An injection of up to 10 mL of bupivacaine has sufficient volume to anesthetize the sympathetic ganglion. Three injections are usually given to obtain continued blockade. The efficacy of the blockade can be assessed by the development of Horner's syndrome (ptosis, miosis, and enophthalmos). Complications associated with stellate blocks include vertebral artery injection with convulsions, neuralgias, pneumothorax, intradural injections, phrenic nerve blockade, and hematoma. Bilateral injections are not done to prevent the possibility of airway compromise. Patients who have pain secondary to sympathetic nerve irritation notice a change in their pain within 12 to 24 hours of the injection. Increased physical activity is encouraged once pain relief starts. By increasing "normal activity" in the peripheral and central nervous system, the opportunity for "abnormal activity" to predominate in sensory pathways is diminished.

Nerve blocks may also be given to relieve symptoms associated with compression of peripheral nerves. Areas around the suprascapular, greater occipital, and median nerves are injected with a combination of anesthetic and corticosteroid. The reduction of swelling and inflammation results in relief of pain in the distribution of the compressed nerve.[15]

References

INJECTION THERAPY

1. Bonica JJ: Local anaesthesia and regional blocks. In: Wall PD, Melzack R (eds): Textbook of Pain. Edinburgh: Churchill Livingstone, 1984, p 541.
2. de Jong RH: Local anesthetics. In: RAJ PP (ed): Practical Management of Pain. Chicago: Year Book Medical Publishers, Inc., 1986, pp 539–556.
3. Incaudo G, Schatz M, Patterson R, et al.: Administration of local anesthetics to patients with a history of prior adverse reaction. J Allergy Clin Immunol 61:339, 1978.
4. de Jong RH, Ronfeld RA, DeRosa RA: Cardiovascular effects of amide local anesthetics. Anesth Analg 61:3, 1982.
5. Travell JG, Simons DG: Myofascial Pain and Dysfunction, The Trigger Point Manual: The Upper Extremities. Baltimore: Williams & Wilkins, 1983.
6. Simons DG, Travell JG: Myofascial pain syndromes. In: Wall PD, Melzack R (eds): Textbook of Pain, 2nd ed. Edinburgh: Churchill Livingstone, 1989, pp 368–385.
7. Swezey RL, Clements PJ: Conservative treatment of back pain. In: Jayson MIV (ed): The Lumbar Spine and Back Pain, 3rd ed. Edinburgh: Churchill Livingstone, 1987, pp 299–314.
8. RAJ PP: Myofascial trigger point injection. In: RAJ PP (ed): Practical Management of Pain. Chicago: Year Book Medical Publishers, Inc., 1986, pp 569–577.
9. Hong CZ: Lidocaine injection versus dry needling to myofascial trigger point: the importance of the local twitch response. Am J Phys Med Rehabil 73:256, 1994.
10. Dilke TFW, Burry HC, Grahame R: Extradural corticosteroid injection management of lumbar nerve root compression. Br Med J 2:635, 1973.
11. Shulman M. Treatment of neck pain with cervical epidural steroid injection. Reg Anesth 11:92, 1986.
12. Rowlingson JC, Kirschenbaum LP: Epidural analgesic techniques in the management of cervical pain. Anesth Analg 65:938, 1986.
13. Catchelove RF, Braha R: The use of cervical epidural nerve block in the management of chronic head and neck pain. Can Anaesth Soc J 31:188, 1984.
14. Shulman M, Nimmagada U, Valenta A: Cervical epidural steroid injection for pain of cervical spine origin. Anesthesiology 61:A223, 1984.
15. Parris WCV: Nerve blocks and invasive therapies. In: Tollison CD, Satterthwaite JR (eds): Painful Cervical Trauma: Diagnosis and Rehabilitative Treatment of Neuromusculoskeletal Injuries. Baltimore: Williams & Wilkins, 1992, pp 134–143.
16. Cicala RS, Thoni K, Angel JJ: Long-term results of cervical epidural steroid injections. Clin J Pain 5:143, 1989.
17. Roy DF, Fleury J, Fontaine SB, et al: Clinical evaluation of cervical facet joint infiltration. Can Assoc Radiol J 39:118, 1988.
18. Wedel DJ, Wilson PR: Cervical facet arthrography. Reg Anesth 10:7, 1985.
19. Dory MA: Arthrography of the cervical facet joints. Radiology 148:379, 1983.
20. Hove B, Gyldensted C: Cervical analgesic facet joint arthrography. Neuroradiology 32:456, 1990.
21. Dussault RG, Nicolet VM: Cervical facet joint arthrography. J Can Assoc Radiol 36:79, 1985.
22. Barnsley L, Lord SM, Wallis BJ, et al.: Lack of effect of intraarticular corticosteroids for chronic pain in the cervical zygapophyseal joints. N Engl J Med 330:1047, 1994.

MEDICATION

Nonsteroidal Anti-inflammatory Drugs

A number of drugs have been advocated for the treatment of neck pain on a short-term or long-term basis. The nonsteroidal anti-inflammatory drugs (NSAIDs) and analgesics, non-narcotic and narcotic, have been used as part of the therapy for neck pain patients. In general, the scientific evidence demonstrating efficacy of NSAIDs in neck pain is small compared with the frequency of their use. Nevertheless, NSAIDs play a useful role in the control of symptoms of pain.

Several factors need to be considered when deciding on the use of NSAIDs or analgesics. The natural history of acute neck pain is one of resolution throughout a short period in 80% to 90% of patients. Patients may go through this period using only physical measures of cold and heat and physical therapy. On the other hand, the pain some patients experience may be diminished by the use of NSAIDs or analgesics. In making the decision to use these drugs, the physician must remember not to exacerbate the condition or cause serious toxicities while the patient's neck pain resolves. The clinical correlate of this prohibition is that NSAIDs and nonnarcotic analgesics are appropriate agents in some patients with neck pain, but narcotic analgesics are reserved only for a small group of patients with documented anatomic abnormalities and for specified brief periods.

NSAIDs have analgesic properties when

given in single doses and are anti-inflammatory and analgesic when given chronically in larger doses. Pure analgesics have no anti-inflammatory effect, whereas corticosteroids are anti-inflammatory without analgesic effects except for those mediated through reduction of inflammation.

Whereas narcotic analgesics act on the endorphin system in the central nervous system, NSAIDs act at the site of peripheral injury where peripheral nerves send nociceptive impulses to the cortex. Prostaglandins do not cause pain by themselves; they sensitize nociceptive nerve fibers to environmental chemical factors (bradykinin and histamine). In the presence of prostaglandins, small amounts of these chemical factors initiate nociceptive impulses. Cyclo-oxygenase inhibition by NSAIDs with decreased production of prostaglandins seems to play a role in the analgesic action of these agents. Other mechanisms must also play a role in the production of analgesia associated with these drugs; the potency of NSAIDs as prostaglandin inhibitor does not necessarily correlate with their efficacy as analgesics. NSAIDs also have significant effects on other components of the inflammatory response, including oxidative phosphorylation, superoxide production, and cellular activation.[1]

The pharmacokinetics and clinical pharmacology of these agents have little direct bearing on their time course of action. That is, the onset of analgesia does not parallel the peak plasma level. Agents that are rapidly absorbed do not necessarily have more rapid onset of analgesic effect. Determinations of peak plasma levels are not obtained clinically because they have little bearing in predicting qualitative or quantitative responses to a medication. Patient response to medication seems to be individualized and cannot be predicted by the pharmacokinetics of a drug.[2] The anti-inflammatory effect of a medication may have a different duration of action than the analgesic effect. An example given by Huskisson is that of piroxicam with a plasma half-life of 38 hours.[3] The anti-inflammatory effects of this drug are effective for 24 hours with a once-a-day dose, whereas the analgesic effect is only 6 hours in duration similar to the time course of aspirin.

Although the NSAIDs are all weak organic acids, except nabumetone, a pro-drug that is administered as a base, they belong to different chemical groups (Table 18–5). The drugs may be divided by their chemical grouping in a variety of ways depending on the complexity of the classification.[4, 5] For example, aspirin may be considered a salicylate or a heterocarboxylic acid. These groups include the salicylates (heterocarboxylic acids), propionic acid derivative (phenylacetic acid, naphthalene-acetic acid, oxazolepropionic acid, benzene-acetic acid), acetic acid derivatives (indoleacetic acid and pyrrole acetic acid), fenamates (anthranilic acids and heterocarboxylic acids), oxicams, naphthylalkanone derivatives, pyrrolo-pyrrole derivative, and pyrazolones (pyrazolidinediones). Within these groups are agents with short half-lives and rapid onset of action and others with longer half-lives and slower onset of action. In general, the half-life of the drug plays a greater role in selection of a specific NSAID than the chemical grouping. However, when an NSAID is ineffective, the choice of the subsequent NSAID is usually one from a different chemical group with a similar half-life.

NSAIDs that are used as analgesics include aspirin, diflunisal, fenoprofen, ibuprofen, mefenamic acid, naproxen, naproxen sodium, piroxicam, ketoprofen, ketorolac tromethamine, etodolac, and diclofenac potassium. In general, the dosage needed for the production of the analgesic effect of these agents is lower than that required for anti-inflammatory effects. The doses required for analgesic effects might be 2,600 mg aspirin, 1,000 mg diflunisal, 1,600 mg ibuprofen, 500 mg naproxen, 30 mg ketorolac tromethamine, 900 mg etodolac, or 100 mg diclofenac potassium.

Most of the NSAIDs, when given as analgesics, must be given every 4 to 6 hours. The exceptions are diflunisal and piroxicam. The analgesic effect of diflunisal lasts up to 12 hours; therefore, the drug may be given only twice a day. Although the analgesic effect of piroxicam lasts 6 hours, the drug has a long half-life that prevents its use more than once a day because it creates gastrointestinal intolerance. Therefore, piroxicam is not a first-line agent for analgesia.

When NSAIDs are used as anti-inflammatory agents, higher doses are necessary to obtain adequate anti-inflammatory effects. In addition, when NSAIDs are used for diseases that are chronic, the rapid onset of action is not as important a factor in deciding on a drug as eventual efficacy of that agent for that individual patient. Examples of daily dosages of drugs that may be required for the therapy of the spondyloarthropathies or rheumatoid arthritis are 5,300 mg aspirin, 400 mg sulindac, 1,500 mg naproxen, and 3,600 mg ibuprofen. NSAIDs are effective in controlling pain associated with cervical spine disorders.[6]

The toxicities of the NSAIDs are predominantly gastrointestinal and renal.[7] Aspirin ingestion has been associated with acute gastrointestinal bleeding.[7] Other NSAIDs have also been associated with bleeding.[8, 9] The enteric-coated salicylates and sulindac have less risk of causing acute gastric damage, according to endoscopic studies in normal volunteers.[10] Nabumetone may also have less gastrointestinal toxicities. Approximately 10% of patients develop gastrointestinal toxicity, usually dyspepsia.[11]

Another major toxicity associated with NSAIDs is related to renal dysfunction.[12] A small group of patients develops an idiosyncratic reaction with interstitial nephritis. A larger group develops reversible renal failure secondary to diminished renal prostaglandins that are directly associated with diminished renal blood flow. Sulindac, a drug with fewer active metabolites in the renal circulation, has less effect on renal blood flow and is rarely the cause of this form of renal toxicity.[12] Other forms of NSAID toxicity include neurologic, hematologic, and hepatic complications.[1]

A combination of drug and patient characteristics will help the clinician decide which is the best agent for a particular individual (Table 18–6). The most important drug characteristic is efficacy. When choosing an agent for acute neck pain, a drug with rapid onset of action is preferred once efficacy of the agent has been established. Most of the NSAIDs have similar safety profiles. Most individuals tolerate NSAIDs. Geriatric patients may require smaller doses because of their slower metabolism and distribution. If patients find an effective agent but develop gastric toxicity, alternative means of taking the medication may be tried (for example, with meals). Alterations in other habits (alcohol and coffee consumption and smoking) or adding cytoprotective agents may be useful in increasing tolerability of an effective drug. A study of more than 8,000 rheumatoid arthritis patients taking NSAIDs reported the efficacy of misoprostol in preventing severe gastrointestinal complications, including perforation, obstruction, and severe bleeding.[13] Two hundred micrograms of misoprostol twice a day is sufficient to decrease the risk of gastrointestinal ulcers.[14] Misoprostol should be given initially in a dose of 100 μg twice a day with meals. The drug must be given with meals to minimize diarrhea, the major complication of the drug. Food in the stomach slows gastric emptying. Prostaglandin in the small intestine may cause cramps and diarrhea. As the patient tolerates the drug, the frequency of administration is increased to three to four times a day with meals. The dose of the drug should be increased to 200 μg as tolerated. In general, agents that require ingestion of fewer tablets are associated with greater patient compliance. Flexibility in amount of drug per tablet and in the total dose needed to attain and maintain efficacy is useful. Some patients obtain adequate analgesia at low doses, whereas others require greater amounts to obtain pain relief. Some patients prefer aspirin because of its lower cost.

As for patient characteristics, it is impossible to predict which chemical class will be effective in an individual patient. Patients with mechanical problems improve with the analgesic effects of NSAIDs; those with spondyloarthropathies require the anti-inflammatory action of these drugs. Drug interactions may limit choices. Drugs with a shorter half-life may be safer in older patients with diminished capacity to metabolize drugs. The combination of all these factors should be considered before the physician chooses an NSAID for a particular patient. New NSAIDs with greater effects on the inflammatory process are being developed. Tenidap sodium, a drug not chemically related to any other NSAID, causes significant inhibition of the production of a variety of acute phase reactants and eicosanoids.[15] These properties may prove to be effective in decreasing pain and inflammation in patients with cervical spine disease.

Most patients obtain significant relief of pain with an NSAID and are able to stop the drug when resolution of their neck pain occurs. Occasionally after an initial recovery, a patient experiences intermittent recurrent attacks or complains of a chronic neckache. Such a patient benefits from a maintenance dose of an NSAID. Medication should be taken on a regular schedule. Delaying medication until pain is present is not an appropriate way to take an NSAID. NSAIDs work better before pain is maximum. Patients should take the NSAID until pain resolves and then discontinue the drug a few days later.

Analgesics

The analgesic medications are divided into non-narcotic (acetaminophen and tramadol HCl) and narcotic (codeine, oxycodone, and meperidine HCl) groups. Patients who are unable to tolerate NSAIDs may benefit from a non-narcotic analgesic like acetaminophen. Acetaminophen, a paraphenol derivative, is a

TABLE 18–5.   NONSTEROIDAL ANTI-INFLAMMATORY DRUGS

DRUG (CHEMICAL CLASS)	TRADE NAME	TABLET/CAPSULE SIZE (MG)	DOSE (MG/DAY)	FREQUENCY (TIMES/DAY)	ONSET (HOURS)	HALF-LIFE (HOURS)	METABOLISM
(Salicylates)							
Aspirin	Bayer	325	Up to 5200	4–6	1–2	4	Liver
Enteric coated	Ecotrin	325	5200	4–6	1–2	4	Liver
	Easprin	975	3900	4	1–2		Liver
Time release	Zorprin	800	3200	2	2	4	Liver
(Substituted Salicylates)							
Diflunisal	Dolobid	250, 500	500–1500	2–3	1 (with loading dose)	11	Liver
Salsalate	Disalcid	500, 750	3000	2	2	4	Liver
Choline magnesium trisalicylate	Trilisate	500, 750, 1000, liquid (500 mg/5 mL)	3000	2	2	4	Liver
Choline salicylate	Arthropan	650 mg/mL	1950	4–6	1	4	Liver
Magnesium salicylate	Magan	545	3270	3–4	2	4	Liver
Sodium salicylate	Uracel	325	3900	3–6	1	4	Liver
Aspirin/antacids	Ascriptin	325	5200	4–6	2	4	Liver
(Propionic Acid Derivatives)							
Ibuprofen	Motrin	200	1200–3600	4–6	1–2	1–3	Liver
	Rufen	400					
	Advil	600					
	Medipren	800					
	Nuprin	200					
Naproxen	Naprosyn	250, 375, 500	500–1500	2–3	3	13	Liver
Sodium naproxen	Anaprox	275, 550	550–100	2	1–2	13	Liver
Fenoprofen calcium	Nalfon	200, 300, 600	600–3000	3–4	3	2–3	Liver
Ketoprofen	Orudis	25, 50, 75	150–300	3–4	2	3–4	Liver
	Oruvail	200					
Flurbiprofen	Ansaid	50, 100	300	2–3	1–2	6	Liver
Oxaprozin	Daypro	600	1800	1–2	3–5	25	Liver
(Pyrrole Acetic Acid Derivatives)							
Sulindac	Clinoril	150, 200	300–450	2–3	2	18	Liver
Indomethacin	Indocin	25, 50, 75 SR, 50 suppositories	75–225	1–3	2	1–4	Liver
Tolmetin sodium	Tolectin	200, 400	600–1600	4	1	1–4	Liver
(Benzeneacetic Acid Derivatives)							
Diclofenac sodium	Voltaren	25, 50, 75 100 XR	75–225	1–3	2–3	2	Liver
Diclofenac potassium	Cataflam	25, 50	100–150	2–3	1	2	Liver
Oxicam							
Piroxicam	Feldene	10, 20	30	1	5	38–45	Liver
Pyranocarboxylic Acid							
Etodolac	Lodine	200, 300, 400	800–1600	2–4	2	6	Liver
Fenemate							
Meclofenamate sodium	Meclomen	50, 100	200–400	4	1	4	Liver
Mefenamic acid	Ponstel	250	1000	4	3	4	Liver
Pyrrolo-pyrrole							
Ketorolac tromethamine	Toradol	10	10–40	4	1	4–6	Liver
Naphthylalkanone							
Nabumetone	Relafen	500, 750	1000–2000	1–2	4	26	Liver
Pyrazolones							
Phenylbutazone	Butazolidin, Azolid	100	400	4	2 (with loading)	72	Liver

Modified from The Medical Letter 29:24, 1987.
*G = gastrointestinal; R = renal; CNS = central nervous system; BM = bone marrow; SR = slow-release
**Cost as of 1995

TABLE 18–5. NONSTEROIDAL ANTI-INFLAMMATORY DRUGS *Continued*

DRUG (CHEMICAL CLASS)	EXCRETION	MAJOR TOXICITY*	COST ($/MONTH)**	COMMENTS
(Salicylates)				
Aspirin	Kidney	G, R	16.00 (5200 mg)	Less expensive than other NSAIDs
Enteric coated	Kidney	G, R	16.39 (4000 mg)	Less G upset than aspirin
	Kidney	G, R	15.39 (3900 mg)	Less G upset than aspirin
Time release	Kidney	G, R	20.36 (3200 mg)	Less G upset than aspirin
(Substituted Salicylates)				
Diflunisal	Kidney	G, R	51.84 (1000 mg)	Loading dose for rapid onset of action; long half-life twice daily dosing
Salsalate	Kidney	G, R	43.24 (4000 mg)	Less G upset than aspirin
Choline magnesium trisalicylate	Kidney	G, R	43.72 (3000 mg)	Less G upset than aspirin
Choline salicylate	Kidney	G, R	27.30 (1950 mg)	Ease of swallowing
Magnesium salicylate	Kidney	G, R	34.31 (3270 mg)	Magnesium toxicity with impaired renal function
Sodium salicylate	Kidney	G, R	2.43–10.79 (5400 mg)	Simple analgesic, less effective than aspirin; increased sodium intake
Aspirin/antacids	Kidney	G, R	21.58	Antacids do not buffer gastric acid adequately
(Propionic Acid Derivatives)				
Ibuprofen	Kidney	G, R	12.94–23.78 (generic–Motrin)	Need larger doses for anti-inflammatory effect (rheumatoid arthritis)
Naproxen	Kidney, stool	G, R	40.53 (1000 mg)	Effective in a number of musculoskeletal disorders
Sodium naproxen	Kidney, stool	G, R	40.40 (825 mg)	Onset of action more rapid than naproxen
Fenoprofen calcium	Kidney	G, R	28.69 (2400 mg) (generic)	Associated with renal toxicity more often than other NSAIDs
Ketoprofen	Kidney, stool	G, R	65.36 (300 mg)	Newer NSAID (extended release)
Flurbiprofen	Kidney	G, R	56.01 (200 mg)	More powerful form of ibuprofen
Oxaprozin	Kidney, stool	G, R	55.19 (1200 mg)	Convenient daily dosing
(Pyrrole Acetic Acid Derivatives)				
Sulindac	Kidney, stool	G	44.83 (400 mg) (generic)	Effective in a number of musculoskeletal disorders; less renal toxicity
Indomethacin	Kidney, stool	G, R, CNS, BM	15.80 (150 mg) (generic) 38.90 (150 mg SR)	Drug of choice for spondylitis; greatest CNS toxicity of all NSAIDs
Tolmetin sodium	Kidney	G, R	49.60 (1200 mg) (generic)	Cross-reactivity with zomepirac sodium (Zomax)
(Benzeneacetic Acid Derivatives)				
Diclofenac sodium	Kidney, stool	G, R	60.65 (150 mg)	Effective in a number of musculoskeletal conditions
Diclofenac potassium	Kidney, stool	G, R	72.27 (100 mg)	Potassium salt associated with more rapid onset of analgesia
Oxicam				
Piroxicam	Kidney	G, R	59.38 (20 mg) (generic)	Substantial G toxicity; long duration of action, which extends toxicity
Pyranocarboxylic Acid				
Etodolac	Kidney	G, R	57.75 (1200 mg)	Multiple dosage form allows for specific amounts for different disorders
Fenemate				
Meclofenamate sodium	Kidney, stool	G, R	43.34 (400 mg) (generic)	Diarrhea in one third of patients
Mefenamic acid	Kidney, stool	G, R	42.34 (100 mg) (generic)	Dysmenorrhea
Pyrrolo-pyrrole				
Ketorolac tromethamine	Kidney	G, R	77.96 (30 mg)	Effective, rapid onset analgesic
Naphthylalkanone				
Nabumetone	Kidney, stool	G, R	54.00 (1000 mg)	Only basic NSAID, less toxic to G tract
Pyrazolones				
Phenylbutazone	Kidney, stool	G, R, BM	32.72 (300 mg) (generic)	Bone marrow toxicity limits utility in most back pain patients, limited availability

TABLE 18–6. CHOICE OF NONSTEROIDAL ANTI-INFLAMMATORY DRUG

DRUG CHARACTERISTICS	PATIENT CHARACTERISTICS
Efficacy	Individual variations
Safety	Nature of the disease
Tolerance	Other drugs
Compliance potential	Age
Dose	Severity of disease
Formulation	Time factors
Cost	Pregnancy

pure analgesic with antipyretic but without anti-inflammatory effects. Acetaminophen inhibits central nervous system prostaglandin production but not peripheral production; this corresponds to its activity as an analgesic and antipyretic and its lack of effect as an anti-inflammatory agent.[16] The drug is given in doses of 500 to 650 mg every 4 hours. Acetaminophen is packaged in an extended release form. The drug is slowly released for 8 hours, allowing for a more sustained analgesic effect. The drug is probably a little less effective as an analgesic than aspirin, but it is unassociated with gastrointestinal bleeding caused by acetylsalicylic acid. In addition, no cross tolerance exists between NSAIDs and acetaminophen. Added analgesic effects can be demonstrated in patients who take both agents simultaneously. The use of both agents occurs in the occasional patient who is on an NSAID and is prescribed chlorzoxazone (Parafon Forte), a drug containing a muscle relaxant and acetaminophen. Tramadol HCl is a non-NSAID drug with analgesic properties that is equipotent to acetaminophen and codeine preparations. The drug has no prostaglandin inhibition and does not cause gastrointestinal bleeding. Toxicities include constipation, nausea, and dizziness. The drug is formulated in 50 mg tablets. The dosage schedule is up to 100 mg every 6 hours. This drug may be given in combination with NSAIDs. Tramadol should be considered for patients with chronic neck pain who have NSAID-associated toxicities and have had no response to maximum doses of acetaminophen.

A patient who experiences an acute herniated nucleus pulposus may develop severe neck and arm pain that is not relieved by NSAIDs alone. This patient may obtain analgesia with the use of codeine 30 to 60 mg every 4 to 6 hours in combination with acetaminophen or aspirin. These medications are given in conjunction with a therapeutic program of rest and temperature modalities. If stronger analgesia is required, the patient should be admitted to the hospital for parenteral narcotics (meperidine and morphine). These drugs are given on a regular basis, in adequate doses to relieve pain while the patient receives other therapies. The chances of a patient developing addiction to narcotics during a short course of therapy is small. Therefore, physicians should prescribe sufficient doses of narcotics to provide adequate analgesia.[17] Ketorolac is an effective parenteral or oral analgesic with potency similar to that of some narcotics.[18] As pain decreases, non-narcotic analgesics are substituted for the more potent narcotic analgesics.

Narcotic analgesics, such as meperidine and oxycodone, should not be given on an outpatient basis. The potential for abuse of these drugs is great. Patients become tolerant of the analgesic effects of the drugs, require higher and more frequent doses and, if continued on a chronic basis, become addicted.[19] Patients may use narcotics to shortcut the period of gradual mobilization that is an essential part of therapy. The drugs are not a substitute for a gradual exercise program. Patients who use the drugs as a substitute for exercise discover a return of pain once the narcotics are discontinued.

There is no role for the narcotic analgesic in the therapy of chronic neck pain. Chronic pain patients who take narcotics experience the toxicities of the medications and none of the benefits. Many times, these patients need to be detoxified before other therapies can be instituted to control their pain.

References

NSAIDs AND ANALGESICS

1. Abramson SB, Weissmann G: The mechanisms of action of nonsteroidal anti-inflammatory drugs. Arthritis Rheum 32:1, 1989.
2. Dahl SL: Nonsteroidal antiinflammatory agents: Clinical pharmacology/adverse effects/usage guidelines. In: Wilkens RF, Dahl SL (eds): Therapeutic Controversies in the Rheumatic Diseases. Orlando: Grune & Stratton, 1987, pp 27–68.
3. Huskisson EC: Non-narcotic analgesics. In: Wall PD, Melzack R (eds): Textbook of Pain. Edinburgh: Churchill Livingstone, 1984, pp 505–513.
4. Paulus HE, Bulpitt KJ: Nonsteroidal anti-inflammatory agents and corticosteroids. In: Schumacker HR Jr (ed): Primer of the Rheumatic Diseases, 10th ed. Atlanta: Arthritis Foundation, 1993, pp 298–303.
5. Shaw J, Brooks PM, McNeil JJ, et al.: Therapeutic usage of the nonsteroidal anti-inflammatory drugs. Med J Aust 149:203, 1988.
6. Dillin W, Uppal GS: Analysis of medications used in

the treatment of cervical disk degeneration. Orthop Clin North Am 23:421, 1992.

7. Levy M: Aspirin use in patients with major upper gastrointestinal bleeding and peptic ulcer disease. N Engl J Med 290:1158, 197.

8. Hart FD: Naproxen and gastrointestinal hemorrhage. Br Med J 2:51, 1974.

9. Holdstock DJ: Gastrointestinal bleeding: a possible association with ibuprofen. Lancet 1:541, 1972.

10. Lanza FL: Endoscopic studies of gastric and duodenal injury after the use of ibuprofen, aspirin, and other nonsteroidal anti-inflammatory agents. Am J Med 77:19, 1984.

11. Simon LS, Mills JS: Drug therapy: nonsteroidal anti-inflammatory drugs. N Engl J Med 302:1179, 1980.

12. Clive DM, Stoff JS: Renal syndrome associated with nonsteroidal antiinflammatory drugs. N Engl J Med 310:563, 1964.

13. Silverstein FE, Graham DY, Senior JR, et al.: Misoprostol reduces serious gastrointestinal complications in patients with rheumatoid arthritis receiving nonsteroidal anti-inflammatory drugs: a randomized, double-blind, placebo-controlled trial. Ann Intern Med 123:241, 1995.

14. Raskin JB, White RH, Jackson JE, et al.: Misoprostol dosage in the prevention of nonsteroidal anti-inflammatory drug-induced gastric and duodenal ulcers: a comparison of three regimens. Ann Intern Med 123:344, 1995.

15. Loose LD, Sipe JD, Kirby DS, et al.: Reduction of acute-phase proteins with tenidap sodium: a cytokine-modulating anti-rheumatic drug. Br J Rheumatol 32(Suppl 3):19, 1993.

16. Beaver WT: Mild analgesics: a review of their clinical pharmacology. Am J Med Sci 250:577, 1966.

17. Stimmel B: Pain, analgesia, and addition: an approach to the pharmacologic management of pain. Clin J Pain 1:14, 1985.

18. O'Hara DA, Fragen RJ, Kinzer M, et al.: Ketorolac tromethamine as compared with morphine sulfate for treatment of postoperative pain. Clin Pharmacol Ther 41:556, 1987.

19. Inturrisi CE: Narcotic drugs. Med Clin North Am 66:1061, 1982.

Muscle Relaxants

Although muscle relaxants have been used in the treatment of neck pain for a number of years, their use has remained controversial. Not all physicians believe that these agents have a therapeutic role in the care of patients with neck pain. There are several reasons why this may be the case. Muscle spasm in the neck may be caused by a variety of mechanisms, including local conditions and referred mechanisms. No one therapy is effective in all forms of muscle spasm. Muscle relaxants do not relieve spasm in all patients with tonic muscle contraction. Some physicians believe muscle spasm to be a "natural, protective mechanism" by which the body heals itself. The dissipation of spasm should occur naturally as the underlying lesion heals and should not be sped up with medications. Other physicians believe

that patients with neck pain do not experience muscle spasm because muscles are not damaged in this disorder.[1] The anatomic abnormality is in the annular fibers of the intervertebral disc. Therefore, muscle relaxants are not useful in improving the condition because the medications have no effect on healing the disc disorder.

Other reasons for resistance to using this group of drugs involve their site of action. Many of these drugs do not work on the muscles themselves; instead they act on the central nervous system to modify muscle tone. Differences of opinion exist in regard to the concentration of medication needed in the blood stream to achieve muscle relaxation. Some physicians believe that the concentration obtained in the blood is adequate to affect muscle spindle function. Others believe the blood concentration to reach only the level to cause sedation by effects on the central nervous system. Therefore, these physicians consider muscle relaxants to work as sedatives, not as relaxants. They consider these drugs to be ineffective in the therapy of this muscle disorder. In addition, some of these agents have serious potential toxicities, including addiction (diazepam). The use of benzodiazepines causes depression, which compounds the difficulties of the chronic neck pain patients who are depressed from the long duration of their disease. Finally, the number of scientific studies that investigate the role of these agents in the care of patients with neck pain, acute or chronic, is even smaller than the number of studies reporting on low back pain.[2, 3] The number of studies that actually prove efficacy is even smaller.[4] Therefore, anecdotal evidence and clinical experience are offered as proof of efficacy, but to some physicians, that evidence is inadequate to justify the use of muscle relaxants.[5]

Some of these criticisms of muscle relaxants are valid. These agents are not indicated for all patients with neck pain. However, these agents do seem to relieve symptoms in carefully selected patients and should not be condemned outright. In the experience of the authors of this book, the combination of a muscle relaxant and an NSAID has been effective in decreasing symptoms and improving function, including return to work.[6]

PATHOPHYSIOLOGY OF MUSCLE SPASM

The interrelationship of the sensory and motor systems is clearly recognized at the level of the spinal cord. This interrelationship involves the classic reflex arc in which stretching of a tendon (afferent-sensory input) results in a reflex contraction of the corresponding muscle (efferent-motor output). Adding to this simple arc are inputs from other levels of the spinal cord, the brain stem, and the cerebral cortex that alter the threshold of the reflex arc. Increased muscle tension may occur as a consequence of intramuscular (trauma and fatigue), perimuscular (arthritis and bone fracture), and referred pain (carotid dissection) processes.

Local trauma to muscles may cause reflex spasm. Tissue damage activates nociceptive (unmyelinated) nerve fibers that are distributed through tendons, fascial sheaths, and the adventitial sheaths of intramuscular blood vessels. Increased muscle tension decreases muscle movement and allows for the damaged area to heal, usually in a contracted position. In addition to the nociceptive input derived from tissue damage, pain sensations may be generated through muscle fatigue associated with tonic contraction. Muscles that are chronically fatigued become locally painful and tender. This process may occur secondary to chronic contraction associated with trauma or to hyperactivity of muscles associated with poor posture or with occupational or sports activities.[7] Muscle spasm may continue while the patient sleeps, as measured by nocturnal electromyogram recordings.[8] The pain associated with chronic fatigue may be related to inadequate blood flow that occurs during hyperactivity of a muscle.[9] That component of muscle pain related to overuse may be relieved with rest and increased blood flow promoted by heat or massage.

Muscle spasm may also occur in response to disease processes in structures to which muscles and tendons attach. Inflammatory processes affecting joints in the axial skeleton can result in reflex muscle spasm, which limits mobility. Patients with spondyloarthropathies are prime examples of this mechanism of spasm. Patients with spondylitis of the neck may experience associated paracervical muscle spasm. Therapy directed at decreasing joint inflammation, and thereby muscle spasm, decreases the neck stiffness.

Spasm that is secondary to sensory input from organs with common innervation results from the common connections of these nerve fibers in the spinal cord.[10] Abnormalities in the gastrointestinal and vascular systems may cause reflex spasm in the cervical spine. Therapy must be given to alleviate the primary disorder for muscle spasm to be relieved.

ACTION OF MUSCLE RELAXANTS

The exact mechanism of action of the muscle relaxants is not known. Depression of polysynaptic, to a greater extent than monosynaptic, reflexes has been reported in animal studies.[11, 12] These effects are mediated through the central nervous system. The area of the central nervous system affected is the lateral reticular area of the brain stem that monitors the facilitative and inhibitory nerve pathways that affect the activity of the muscle stretch reflexes.[13] The effects of these agents may be mediated through enhanced stimulation of gamma aminobutyric acid (GABA) neurons that play a significant role in the inhibition of tonic facilitory input from supraspinal sources on motor neurons, both alpha and gamma. This action of GABA receptors has been associated with the action of benzodiazepines (diazepam).[14] The oral doses of the muscle relaxants are below the levels needed in animal studies to achieve muscle relaxation. This fact has been used by some investigators to conclude that the beneficial effect of muscle relaxants is, in fact, sedation. Clinically, sedation is noted by most patients who ingest any of the members of this group of agents. Some patients obtain muscle relaxation without associated sedation.

The oral muscle relaxants have been shown to be better than a placebo in acute muscle spasm. Their efficacy in chronic muscle spasm has been more difficult to prove. Combinations of muscle relaxants and analgesics are more effective than their individual components in the control of muscle spasm.[15] The Drug Efficacy and Safety Implementation Program of the Food and Drug Administration has categorized all such combination products as possibly effective. The muscle relaxants alone do not provide analgesia.

The drugs included in the oral muscle relaxant group are cyclobenzaprine (Flexeril), chlorphenesin (Maolate), orphenadrine citrate (Norflex), chlorzoxazone (Paraflex, Parafon Forte DSC), methocarbamol (Robaxin), metaxalone (Skelaxin), carisoprodol (Soma), and diazepam (Valium). Combinations of these agents with analgesics include the drugs Norgesic, Parafon Forte, Robaxisal, Soma Compound, and Soma Compound with Codeine (Table 18–7).

Muscle relaxants have been studied and

TABLE 18–7. ORAL MUSCLE RELAXANTS

DRUG	BRAND NAME	TABLET/CAPSULE SIZE (MG)	DOSE (MG/DAY)	FREQUENCY (TIMES/DAY)	ONSET (HOURS)	DURATION (HOURS)	HALF-LIFE	MAJOR TOXICITY	EXCRETION	COMMENTS
Cyclobenzaprine hydrochloride	Flexeril	10	20–60	3	1–2	12–24	1–3 days	Drowsiness, dry mouth, dizziness	Kidney, stool	10 mg 2 hours before sleep may be adequate dose with half-life (Caution: angle closure glaucoma, prostatic hypertrophy, myocardial infarction)
Chlorphenesin carbamate	Maolate	400	1600–2400	3–4	3	4–6	5 hours	Drowsiness, dizziness	Kidney	
Orphenadrine citrate	Norflex	100	200	2	2	4–6	14 hours	Blurred vision, dry mouth, urinary retention	Kidney, stool	Intravenous form for therapy of acute spasm (Norgesic includes aspirin and caffeine)
	Norgesic	30 mg/dL								
Chlorzoxazone	Paraflex	250	1500–3000	3–4	1	3–4	1 hour	Drowsiness, dizziness	Kidney	Parafon Forte includes acetaminophen
	Parafon Forte DSC	500								Contraindicated—history of liver disease
Methocarbamol	Robaxin	500, 750	6000	4–6	1	3	2 hours	Dizziness, blurred vision	Kidney, stool	Intravenous form for acute spasm, tetanus (Robaxisal includes aspirin)
	Robaxisal	100 mg/dL								
Metaxalone	Skelaxin	400	2400–3200	3–4	1	4–6	2–3 hours	Drowsiness	Kidney	Extreme weakness Temporary loss of vision (rare)
Carisoprodol	Soma	350	1400	4	1	4–6	8 hours	Drowsiness	Kidney	Mild withdrawal symptoms with abrupt cessation Contraindicated—acute intermittent porphyria (Soma compound includes aspirin)
Diazepam	Valium	2, 5, 10 (5 mg/mL, 15 slow release)	4–40	4	1	8–12	24 hours	Drowsiness	Kidney	Withdrawal symptoms with abrupt cessation Depression with prolonged use

been found to be better than placebos in acute and chronic muscle spasm. Both carisoprodol and chlorphenesin were effective in acute but not chronic disorders.[16-19] In studies of acute pain, chlorzoxazone, metaxalone, and methocarbamol were also effective.[20-22] Cyclobenzaprine was compared with a placebo in chronic disorders and was found to be superior.[2, 3, 23] Diazepam was not better than a placebo in acute and chronic pain in hospitalized patients.[23] In a 4-day study of acute cervical muscle spasm, diazepam was significantly better than phenobarbital and a placebo in decreasing symptoms.[24] In unspecified musculoskeletal disorders, chlorphenesin, chlorzoxazone, and methocarbamol were found better than a placebo, whereas diazepam was not.[25-28]

Studies comparing one muscle relaxant with another have been completed but the results are not sufficiently different to identify one agent that is clearly superior to the others.[15] In regard to combination tablets, these medications appear to be better than single agents alone. However, no difference among the products was noted.[15]

The major side effect of these agents is drowsiness. Other central nervous system effects include headache, dizziness, and blurred vision. Cyclobenzaprine causes dry mouth. Nausea and vomiting occur with all these agents, although on a rare basis. Orphenadrine may have a direct depressant and anticholinergic effect on the heart. This may cause arrhythmias and cardiac arrest at lethal doses of 2 to 3 gm. Chronic use of carisoprodol may be associated with tolerance for the drug. Patients may ask for increasing doses of the medicine for the same muscle-relaxing effect.

The authors of this book have found muscle relaxants to be useful in patients who, on examination, have palpable evidence of muscle spasm or who have difficulty sleeping because of muscle pain. These patients may be experiencing spasm although their primary symptom is pain.[1] Although no superiority of efficacy has been demonstrated for any one muscle relaxant, the chemical properties of cyclobenzaprine are useful in the clinical setting. The drug is not combined with any analgesic and therefore can be used with any of the NSAIDs or analgesics. Its long half-life equates with a once-daily dosage for many patients. The medication is given 2 hours before sleep; this time interval allows the medicine to build up in the blood stream so that the patient is sleepy at the appropriate time. The patient awakens the next day feeling rested and not drowsy. If 10 mg causes drowsiness, the tablet may be cut in half; 5 mg is an adequate dose for many patients.

The sedation that occurs in some patients may serve a useful purpose. Many patients stay in bed during the first few days of taking the medicine. The sedation associated with the drug is not a toxicity but is a part of therapy. The sedative effect of the medication diminishes with continued use of the drug. The drug is continued for up to 2 weeks in patients with acute spasm. Patients are easily tapered off the medicine without any withdrawal symptoms. If the patient does not have a response to cyclobenzaprine, then chlorzoxazone, orphenadrine, methocarbamol, or carisoprodol may be substituted (Table 18–7). A greater number of tablets and more frequent dosing are necessary to achieve adequate levels of these other medications. These agents belong to different chemical groups. Just as with the NSAIDs, a lack of response to one agent does not indicate inefficacy of the whole group of drugs. A series of agents may be tried before an efficacious and well-tolerated agent is found. The total dose of medication and frequency of administration must be individualized. Occasionally, combination tablets (Parafon Forte and Robaxisal) are used. The convenience of these preparations is the presence of the muscle relaxant and analgesic in the same tablet. However, the amount of medicine is fixed, limiting the alteration of dose that some patients require.

Diazepam is a muscle relaxant that is not used by the authors of this book. The evidence for efficacy of this agent in neck spasm is meager, whereas its toxicities are real and troublesome. One cannot predict which patient with acute neck pain will go on to develop chronic neck pain and depression. Diazepam only worsens the depression and drug dependence of such a patient. The drug is not indicated in this disorder.

The use of muscle relaxants is not limited to traumatic muscle strain. Patients with arthritic conditions, particularly the spondyloarthropathies, may benefit from long-term use of a muscle relaxant. The following case is presented as an example of a patient with a spondyloarthropathy who had greater mobility because of the use of a muscle relaxant:

Case Study 18–1: J.A. is a 46-year-old white man admitted to the hospital because of the acute onset of neck, right buttock, left index finger, left great toe, and right heel pain that developed during a 3-week period after a fall from a 2-ft garden wall. The patient had marked limitation of cervical motion in all directions, associated with marked paravertebral muscle spasm. Swollen joints included the right knee, ankle, heel, left great toe, and index finger. The diagnosis of incomplete Reiter's syndrome was made, and the patient was started on indomethacin 50 mg three times a day, which was increased to 75 mg slow release 3 times a day. The patient's lower and upper extremity arthritis improved, but severe muscle spasm of the cervical spine continued. Cyclobenzaprine 10 mg two times a day was added, and the patient had a gradual improvement in his neck motion. The patient had an exacerbation of symptoms after discharge from the hospital. Cyclobenzaprine was increased to 30 mg/day, and prednisone 10 mg/day was added. During the next 2 months, the patient's symptoms gradually resolved. One year after discharge, the patient was able to discontinue prednisone therapy. Attempts at reducing cyclobenzaprine were associated with decreased neck motion. The patient remains on indomethacin 75 mg two times a day and cyclobenzaprine 10 mg at night. The patient is active and is able to complete a full day's work without difficulty. He spontaneously volunteers the fact that he believes that the muscle relaxant played a substantial role in his recovery. He has remained on the combination of indomethacin and cyclobenzaprine for 10 years. A recent exacerbation of his arthritis with associated neck stiffness required an increase in his cyclobenzaprine to 20 mg/day.

An anecdotal case report does not prove efficacy scientifically. However, clinical observation is a reasonable means for studying the effects of therapeutic interventions. Muscle relaxants are not indicated for all patients with neck pain. In the carefully chosen patient, however, the use of muscle relaxants can relieve symptoms while the natural course of healing unfolds.

References

MUSCLE RELAXANTS

1. Fischer AA, Chang CH: Electromyographic evidence of paraspinal muscle spasm during sleep in patients with low back pain. Clin J Pain 1:147, 1985.
2. Bercel NA: Cyclobenzaprine in the treatment of skeletal muscle spasm in osteoarthritis of the cervical and lumbar spine. Curr Ther Res 22:462, 1977.
3. Brown BR, Womble J: Cyclobenzaprine in intractable pain syndromes with muscle spasm. JAMA 240:1151, 1978.
4. Deyo RA: Conservative therapy for low back pain: distinguishing useful from useless therapy. JAMA 250:1057, 1983.
5. Hadler NM: Diagnosis and treatment of backache. In: Hadler NM (ed): Medical Management of the Regional Musculoskeletal Diseases. Orlando: Grune & Stratton, 1984, pp 3–52.
6. Borenstein DG, Lacks S, Wiesel SW: Cyclobenzaprine and naproxen versus naproxen alone in the treatment of acute low back pain and muscle spasm. Clin Ther 12:125, 1990.
7. Simons DG: Muscle pain syndrome part II. Am J Phys Med 55:15, 1976.
8. Fischer AA, Chang CH: Electromyographic evidence of paraspinal muscle spasm during sleep in patients with low back pain. Clin J Pain 1:147, 1985.
9. Kuroda E, Klissouras V, Mulsum JH: Electrical and metabolic activities and fatigue in human isometric contraction. J Appl Physiol 29:358, 1970.
10. Kerr FWL: Neuroanatomical substrates of nociception in the spinal cord. Pain 1:325, 1975.
11. Smith CM: Relaxants of skeletal muscle. In: Root WS, Hoffman FG (eds): Physiological Pharmacology vol II. New York: Academic Press, 1965, pp 1–96.
12. Roszkowski AP: A pharmacological comparison of therapeutically useful centrally-acting skeletal muscle relaxants. J Pharmacol Exp Ther 129:75, 1970.
13. Ginzel KH: The blockade of reticular and spinal facilitation of motor function by orphenadrine. J Pharmacol Exp Ther 154:128, 1966.
14. Study RE, Barker JL: Cellular mechanisms of benzodiazepine action. JAMA 247:2147, 1982.
15. Elenbaas JK: Centrally acting oral skeletal muscle relaxants. Am J Hosp Pharm 37:1313, 1980.
16. Cullen AP: Carisoprodol (Soma) in acute back conditions: a double-blind randomized, placebo-controlled study. Curr Ther Res Clin Exp 20:557, 1976.
17. Turner R, Rockwood CA: Chlorphenesin carbamate (Maolate) in the relief of muscle pain. Mil Med 132:371, 1967.
18. Jones AC: Role of carisoprodol in physical medicine. Ann NY Acad Sci 86:226, 1960.
19. Waltham-Weeks CD: The analgesic properties of chlorphenesin carbamate in the treatment of osteoarthrosis. Ann Phys Med 9:197, 1968.
20. Ogden HD, Shackett L: Controlled studies of chlorzoxazone and chlorzoxazone-acetaminophen in treatment of myalgia associated with headache. South Med M 53:1415, 1960.
21. Dent RW, Ervin DK: A study of metaxalone (Skelaxin) vs placebo in acute musculoskeletal disorders: a cooperative study. Curr Ther Res Clin Exp 18:433, 1975.
22. Tisdale SA, Ervin DK: A controlled study of methocarbamol (Robaxin) in acute painful musculoskeletal conditions. Curr Ther Res Clin Exp 17:525, 1975.
23. Basmajian JV: Cyclobenzaprine hydrochloride effect on skeletal muscle in the lumbar region and neck: two double-blind controlled clinical and laboratory studies. Arch Phys Med Rehabil 59:58, 1978.
24. Basmajian JV: Reflex cervical muscle spasm: treatment by diazepam, phenobarbital or placebo. Arch Phys Med Rehabil 64:121, 1983.
25. Valtonene EJ: A double-blind trial of methocarbamol versus placebo in painful muscle spasm. Curr Med Res Opin 3:382, 1975.
26. Kolodny AL: Controlled clinical evaluation of a new muscle relaxant: chlorphenesin carbamate. Psychosomatics 4:161, 1963.
27. Schiener JJ: Evaluation of combined muscle relaxant-analgesic as an effective therapy for painful skeletal muscle spasm. Curr Ther Res Clin Exp 14:168, 1972.
28. Payne RW, Xorenson EJ, Smalley TK, Brandt EN Jr: Diazepam, meprobamate, and placebo in musculoskeletal disorders. JAMA 188:229, 1964.

Antidepressants

During the past 30 years, tricyclic antidepressants (TCAs) have been widely used for the treatment of chronic pain in patients with or without depression.[1, 2] The mechanism of action that results in pain relief remains unknown, although a number of theories have been proposed. In addition, the factors that might better predict a beneficial response to these drugs by chronic pain patients remain to be determined.[3]

MECHANISM OF ACTION

The basis for a response of pain to TCAs seems to be related to alterations in the central nervous system associated with chronic pain. Sternbach postulated that chronic pain results in depression, which is associated with depletion of serotonin in the brain.[4] TCAs that increase serotonin levels might therefore be associated with pain relief. This hypothesis was tested in a study using fenfluramine, a drug that causes a relatively selective release of serotonin, at a dose of 40 mg/day. This drug transiently reduced both chronic pain and depression in some patients, supporting this hypothesis.[5]

Another popular hypothesis involves the activation of the endogenous opiate system in the central nervous system by TCAs. TCAs can exert analgesic effects either directly or indirectly on the endogenous opiate system.[6] TCAs can increase the low levels of endogenous opiates in patients with organic pain.[7]

As a neurotransmitter, serotonin may also play an important role as an inhibitor of pain. The pain inhibitory pathway descends from the raphe nuclei in the brain stem via the lateral columns of the dorsal spinal cord to the superficial laminae (substantia gelatinosa) of the dorsal horn.[8] Antinociceptive effects are generated by the application of serotonin and norepinephrine to the substantia gelatinosa in animal models.[9] From anatomic and neurophysiologic data, serotonergic pathways significantly modify transmission of nociceptive impulses.

Reduction of anxiety and relief of muscle tension may also decrease neck pain. Amitriptyline, a sedating antidepressant, has been associated with pain relief in individuals with chronic muscle tension.[10]

Pain relief by antidepressants may also be ascribed to therapy of masked depression. Pain may be a part of the symptom complex of the depressed patient. Although this may play a part in the resolution of symptoms, studies have demonstrated improvement of pain but not of depression in patients treated with TCAs.[11]

TCAs work by inhibiting the uptake of serotonin and norepinephrine by the nerve terminal that released them, thereby increasing the concentration of the neurotransmitter in the synapse. Increased neurotransmitter concentrations amplify the tone in corresponding neural pathways where these substances are neurotransmitters. TCAs that have been associated with potentiation of serotonin and related pain relief have included imipramine, amitriptyline, doxepin, and desipramine.

The role of TCAs and low back pain has been evaluated to a greater extent than that in chronic neck pain. A few clinical studies have investigated the use of TCAs in patients with chronic low back pain. Two double-blind studies comparing imipramine and placebo generated conflicting results. In a study using low-dose imipramine for 4 weeks, no difference was noted between imipramine and the placebo.[12] In contrast, a study using higher doses for 8 weeks found statistically significant improvement with imipramine compared with the placebo.[2] Doxepin has been found to be effective in reducing pain compared with placebo in clinical studies. Hameroff and colleagues showed antidepressant doses of doxepin to be superior to placebo.[1]

Ward demonstrated that 60% of patients experienced pain reduction in response to doxepin and desipramine.[3] The study's findings supported the hypothesis of low serotonin concentrations being associated with chronic pain. Those patients who responded to fenfluramine were the same patients who were more likely to have pain relief with either antidepressant. Levels of endorphins, pain tolerance, and electromyogram findings were unaltered by the medications. Sedation was not a key factor in that the nonsedating drug (desipramine) was as effective as the sedating agent (doxepin). Patients with or without depression and with or without physical trauma responded equally well. Doxepin has also been shown to be effective in patients with back pain who have failed other therapies.[13]

Amitriptyline, the agent with the greatest serotonergic activity, is also associated with pain relief in patients with chronic back pain. In a double-blind study, amitriptyline was associated with a significant decrease in the use of analgesics but no measurable change in activity level in patients with low back pain.[14]

The use of TCAs in the treatment of chronic pain is not totally benign. In one study, 100% of patients taking TCAs developed side effects, however minor in severity.[15] The toxicities of these agents are nicely summarized by Hart.[16]

[The TCA] should be used with extreme caution in cardiovascular disease, liver disorders, epilepsy, patients with known suicidal tendencies, conditions where an anticholinergic agent would be undesirable, for example, glaucoma, urinary retention and pyloric stenosis, prostatic hypertrophy, pregnancy. Barbiturates alter the pharmacological effects of tricyclic antidepressants, which can in turn alter the action of other drugs administered concurrently including other antidepressants (especially MAOIs); alcohol; some antihypertensives, for example methyldopa and guanethidine; anticholinergics and local anaesthetics with noradrenaline.

These toxicities are particularly troublesome in the elderly, who are more prone to the diseases and drug-related complications.[17]

As opposed to the use of TCAs in depression, the dose of medication should be kept low and raised slowly in light of the patient's clinical response.[18] Reaching antidepressant levels of 150 mg of amitriptyline has not been necessary in chronic pain patients. The drug is taken as a single dose 2 hours before bed time. Ten milligrams of amitriptyline is the initial dose, which may be increased to 25 mg within 2 to 3 weeks. During the following 8 weeks, the patient's dose may be increased to 75 to 100 mg. It is rare to use larger doses unless the patient is clinically depressed. The therapeutic ranges of the TCAs are listed in Table 18–8.

New antidepressants—fluoxetine, sertraline, paroxetine, and bupropion—are effective for treating depression, but their efficacy for pain relief similar to the TCAs has not been estab-

lished.[19] The TCAs are relatively safe drugs at the doses that are effective in patients with chronic pain. In patients with neck pain who have failed other therapies, a trial of TCAs is indicated. The choice of agent is related to the physician's familiarity with the individual TCAs and the need for sedation (amitriptyline). The trial should be continued for a number of weeks unless toxicity intervenes.

References

ANTIDEPRESSANTS

1. Hameroff SR, Crago BR, Cork RC, et al.: Doxepin effects on chronic pain, depression, and serum opioids. Anesth Analg 61:187, 1982.
2. Alcoff J, Jones E, Rust P, Newman R: Controlled trial of imipramine for chronic low back pain. J Fam Pract 14:841, 1982.
3. Ward NG: Tricyclic antidepressants for chronic low back pain: mechanisms of action and predictors of response. Spine 11:661, 1986.
4. Sternbach RA: The need for an animal model of chronic pain. Pain 2:2, 1976.
5. Clineschmidt BV, Zacchei AG, Totaro JA, et al.: Fenfluramine and brain serotonin. Ann NY Acad Sci 305:222, 1978.
6. Spiegel K, Kalb R, Pasternak GW: Analgesic activity of tricyclic antidepressants. Ann Neurol 13:462, 1983.
7. Ward NG, Bloom VL, Dworkin S, et al.: Psychobiological markers in coexisting pain and depression: toward a unified theory. J Clin Psychiatry 43:32, 1982.
8. Oliveras JL, Bourgoin S, Hery F, et al.: The topographical distribution of serotonergic terminals in the spinal cord of the cat: biochemical mapping by the combined use of microdissection and microassay procedures. Brain Res 138:393, 1977.
9. Headley PM, Duggan AW, Griersmith BT: Selective reduction by noradrenaline and 5-hydroxytryptamine of nociceptive responses of cat dorsal horn neurons. Brain Res 145:185, 1978.
10. Lance JW, Curran DA: Treatment of chronic tension headache. Lancet 1:1236, 1964.
11. Watson CP, Evans RJ, Reed K, et al.: Amitriptyline versus placebo in postherpetic neuralgia. Neurology 32:671, 1982.
12. Jenkins DG, Ebbutt AF, Evans CD: Tofranil in the treatment of low back pain. J Int Med Res 4(Suppl 2):28, 1976.
13. Hameroff SR, Cork RC, Weiss JL, et al.: Doxepin effects on chronic pain and depression: a controlled study. Clin J Pain 1:171, 1985.
14. Pheasant H, Bursk A, Goldfarb J, et al.: Amitriptyline and chronic low-back pain: a randomized double-blind crossover study. Spine 8:552, 1983.
15. Pilowsky I, Hallett EC, Basset DL, et al.: A controlled study of amitriptyline in the treatment of chronic pain. Pain 14:169, 1982.
16. Hart FD: The use of psychotropic drugs in rheumatology. J Int Med Res 4(Suppl 2):15, 1976.
17. Shillcutt SD, Easterday JL, Anderson RJ: Geriatric pharmacology part I: antidepressant medications. Hosp Formul 19:941, 1984.
18. Hollister LE: Treatment of depression with drugs. Ann Intern Med 88:78, 1978.
19. Backonja M, Fitzthum J: Pharmacologic management

TABLE 18–8. SELECTED ANTIDEPRESSANTS

CLASS	PAIN DOSE (MG)	DEPRESSION DOSE (MG)	SEDATION
Tricyclic Tertiary Amines			
Imipramine (Tofranil)	10–75	200	3 +
Amitriptyline (Elavil)	10–100	300	4 +
Doxepin (Sinequan)	10–100	300	4 +
Nortriptyline (Pamelor)	10–100	300	3 +
Tricyclic Secondary Amines			
Desipramine (Norpramin)	10–100	300	1 +

of noncancer spinal pain syndromes. Phys Med Rehabil 9:765, 1995.

ELECTROTHERAPY

Transcutaneous Electrical Nerve Stimulation

During the past decade, evidence has been reported suggesting that transcutaneous electrical nerve stimulation (TENS) therapy may alleviate chronic pain. The exact mechanism by which electrical current decreases pain is unknown, although there are a number of hypotheses. Most reports have assumed that TENS activates large-diameter afferent A-alpha nerve fibers. The input through these nerves presumably activates an intraneural network that presynaptically or postsynaptically inhibits ongoing transmission of nociceptive impulses supplied through the small C unmyelinated and A-delta fibers or inhibits the C fibers directly.[1, 2] TENS preferentially stimulates the low-threshold A-alpha fibers.[3] The effect of TENS on pain modulation does not seem to be directly related to endogenous opiates. Naloxone, an inhibitor of endogenous and exogenous opiates, failed to reverse the effect of high-frequency TENS in patients with acute and chronic pain.[4]

Electrical stimulation of the nerves may be accomplished by TENS using surface electrodes applied to the skin, subcutaneously implanted electrodes, or electrodes implanted directly on the nerve or dorsal column with stimulation applied directly to the spinal cord or through the dura. The transcutaneous stimulator is used most frequently.

The basic equipment for TENS therapy is an electrical pulse generator and transcutaneous electrodes. The pulses produced by the generator may be high-frequency, low-frequency, or variable-frequency. The pulse generator feeds its output to an amplifier that increases the signal to a level that delivers current to the electrodes. The waveforms most commonly used are rectangular and spike. The rectangular waveform can be adjusted for amplitude and pulse width, and the spike form can be modified by amplitude alone. TENS therapy uses alternating current to limit the flow of material on the surface of the skin (electrode gel) into subdermal structures, resulting in irritation.

The electrodes receive the current and produce an electric field that excites the afferent fibers in the neighboring peripheral nerve. The current must be delivered without damaging the skin. The most widely used electrodes are silicone rubber impregnated with carbon particles. The electrodes are flexible and follow the contours of the body. An aquaphilic gel is needed to reduce skin resistance to facilitate current transmission, and the electrodes must be taped appropriately to maintain a tight fit with the underlying skin. Poor contact may result in sparking and damaging of the skin. Disposable and reusable electrodes that have pre-applied gel and adhesive are available, but they are more expensive and detach from the skin more easily, particularly when the patient perspires.

The choice of electrode placement is dependent on the location of the pain. The electrodes may be placed directly over the area, within the dermatome or myotome, or over a superficial peripheral nerve. The optimal site of stimulation is proximal to the painful area. The closer the electrodes are to the nerve, the lower the current required to stimulate the appropriate nerve fibers. It is not possible to predict the most effective site for electrode placement. Different locations may need to be tested before optimal placement is identified. Some patients need bilateral stimulation even in the circumstance of unilateral pain.[5] For bilateral neck pain, crisscrossed electrode placement is preferred.[6]

Once the electrodes are placed, waveform parameters are altered to maximize pain relief. The parameters that can be modified are pulse rate, width, and amplitude. The rate regulates the number of electrical impulses delivered per second (pps). The range is from 2 to 200 pps, with 2 to 150 pps the most commonly used rates. The pulse width determines the duration of each impulse. A range of 50 to 250 μsec is commonly used. The amplitude of the signal is measured in milliamperes (mA).

Various combinations of rate, width, and amplitude have a marked effect on the signal that reaches the stimulated area. The conventional mode of TENS therapy was a high rate (80 to 100 pps) and low pulse width (less than 100 μsec). The amplitude is increased until a tingling sensation is felt in the stimulated area. The aim of this setting is to activate large sensory myelinated fibers without producing muscle contraction or dysesthesias.

Other signal forms may be uncomfortable and are used only for short periods. High pulse width at low rates (2 to 4 pps) stimulates nerves at superficial to deep levels and may cause muscle contraction. Like acupuncture, this form of TENS may stimulate endogenous opiate (endorphin) production.[7] Burst mode uses a low rate (4 pps) of a series of impulses (seven in number). The pulse width is wide and the amplitude high. The burst mode is useful for chronic, deep pain.[8] In this mode, rhythmic muscle contraction occurs. The subcutaneous and cutaneous nerves are stimulated with high-rate, wide-width, and high-amplitude settings. Newer units allow for alternating modes between those that stimulate deep and those that stimulate superficial structures. Switching between modes may help prevent adaptation to TENS therapy. Once the effective mode is determined, that single mode is used, instead of multiple modes, to produce more lasting effects.[9]

The induction time for TENS to produce analgesia ranges from immediately to several hours, the average time being 20 minutes. The effect of TENS therapy may be cumulative in patients with chronic pain. Patients may not experience pain relief if stimulation is limited to a duration of 30 minutes or less.[10] Therefore, TENS therapy should be used for a minimum of 30 minutes at a time. TENS should be given at 2-hour intervals, with a maximum of 8 hours per day. This regimen should be given for 3 weeks, with a reduction of the time of application of TENS during the next 12 weeks.[9] The pain relief from TENS may be present only during the stimulation or may last for a considerable period during poststimulation.[11]

TENS therapy may be indicated for patients with acute or chronic pain. In treating patients with acute cervical pain, caution must be used so that electrodes are not placed over the carotid sinus or epiglottis.[12]

Although TENS therapy has been shown to be helpful in pain conditions, a controlled trial of TENS therapy has not been reported.[13] TENS, like other forms of pain therapy, has a significant placebo component.[14] In the early stages of therapy, TENS produces a 60% to 80% relief of chronic pain. The placebo effect portion of the response falls off quickly while the therapeutic efficacy of TENS decreases more slowly so that from 20% to 30% of patients continue with pain relief at 1 year.[15] TENS may cause a more rapid restoration of cervical mobility when used with other modalities in patients with acute cervical pain.[16]

The authors offer TENS therapy applied by our physical therapists to patients with localized, chronic neck pain of traumatic origin. This therapy is most useful in patients who are limited at work because of pain. The use of TENS therapy allows these patients to complete a usual day's work with much less discomfort. They also use the TENS units during recreational activities or activities of daily living. These patients use the units on an intermittent basis and have found the units a way to sustain the beneficial effect of the therapy. Patients are always advised to rent, not buy, units initially. Only after a period of months of sustained pain relief do these patients buy their units. Whether it is placebo effect or direct effect on the nervous system, TENS therapy does help patients with neck pain become more functional.

Iontophoresis

Iontophoresis, also called common ion transfer, uses direct current, as opposed to TENS's alternating current, to induce the transfer of an ion across a body surface. A variety of medications, including corticosteroids, epinephrine, and local anesthetics, may enter an area of soft tissue without an injection. A study by Russo and colleagues demonstrated an equal amount of analgesia derived by injection of lidocaine and lidocaine iontophoresis.[17] Harris reported on 50 patients with inflammatory musculoskeletal conditions.[18] About 76% of those patients had marked relief of pain with iontophoresis of a solution composed of lidocaine and dexamethasone. This technique may be of benefit to a patient with localized areas of pain that are irritated from injection. Pain may be diminished by iontophoresis with the instillation of a local anesthetic (lidocaine 4% solution) alone or in combination with a soluble corticosteroid.

High-Voltage Stimulation

High-voltage stimulation is a form of TENS that uses high-voltage, monophasic pulses of short duration to stimulate soft tissue structures in the cervical spine. High-voltage stimulation may be particularly helpful in eliminating persistent muscle spasm. Repeated electrical stimulation relaxes protective muscle spasm, decreasing muscle fatigue. Patients may be able to exercise or stretch the muscle in spasm once electrical stimulation has been applied to the superficial area over the muscle.

References

ELECTROTHERAPY

1. Woolf CJ: Transcutaneous and implanted nerve stimulation. In: Wall PD, Melzack R (eds): Textbook of

Pain. Edinburgh: Churchill Livingstone, 1984, pp 679–690.

2. Campbell JN, Taub A: Local analgesia from percutaneous electrical stimulation. Arch Neurol 28:347, 1973.

3. Bloedel J, McCreery D: Organization of peripheral and central pain pathways. Surg Neurol 4:65, 1975.

4. Abrams SE, Reynolds AC, Cusick JF: Failure of naloxone to reverse analgesia from transcutaneous electrical stimulation in patients with chronic pain. Anesth Anal 60:81, 1981.

5. Picaza J, Cannon BW, Hunter SE, et al.: Pain suppression by peripheral nerve stimulation part 1: observation with transcutaneous stimuli. Surg Neurol 4:105, 1975.

6. Mannheimer JS: Transcutaneous electrical nerve stimulation: Its uses and effectiveness with patients in pain. In: Echternach JL (ed): Pain. New York: Churchill Livingstone, 1987, pp 213–254.

7. Sjolund B, Eriksson M: Endorphins and analgesia produced by peripheral conditioning stimulation. In: Bonica JJ, Liebeskind JC, Albe-Fessard DG: Advances in Pain Research and Therapy, vol 3. New York: Raven Press, 1979, pp 587–591.

8. Eriksson MBE, Sjolund BH, Nielzen S: Long-term results of peripheral conditioning stimulation as an analgesia measure in chronic pain. Pain 6:335, 1979.

9. Tan JC, Nordin M: Role of physical therapy in the treatment of cervical disk disease. Orthop Clin North Am 23:435, 1992.

10. Wolf SL, Gersh MR, Rao VK: Examination of electrode placement and stimulating parameters in treating chronic pain with conventional transcutaneous electrical nerve stimulation (TENS). Pain 11:37, 1981.

11. Meyer GA, Fields HL: Causalgia treated by selective large fiber stimulation of peripheral nerves. Brain 95:163, 1972.

12. Soric R, Devlin M: Role of physical medicine. In: Tollison CD (ed): Handbook of Chronic Pain Management. Baltimore: Williams & Wilkins, 1988, pp 147–162.

13. Deyo RA: Conservative therapy for low back pain: distinguishing useful from useless therapy. JAMA 250:1057, 1983.

14. Thorsteinsson G, Stonnington HH, Stillwell GK, et al.: The placebo effect of transcutaneous electrical stimulation. Pain 5:31, 1978.

15. Bates JAV, Nathan PW: Transcutaneous electrical nerve stimulation for chronic pain. Anaesthesia 35:817, 1980.

16. Nordemar R, Thorner C: Treatment of acute cervical pain: a comparative group study. Pain 10:93, 1981.

17. Russo J Jr, Lipman AG, Comstock TJ, et al.: Lidocaine anesthesia: comparison of iontophoresis, injection, and swabbing. Am J Hosp Pharm 37:843, 1980.

18. Harris PR: Iontophoresis: clinical research in musculoskeletal inflammatory conditions. J Orthop Sports Phys Ther 4:109, 1982.

MISCELLANEOUS THERAPY

Acupuncture

The basic principle of acupuncture follows the theory that the production of brief, moderate pain in specific locations abolishes severe, chronic pain. The same principle has long been used in many forms, including cupping, scarification, and cauterization. These counterirritant therapies have been referred to by Melzack as "hyperstimulation analgesia."[1] Acupuncture points can be stimulated by heat, cold, pressure, electricity, ultrasonography, and lasers. The most common method of stimulation is insertion of tiny needles into acupuncture points.[2]

The efficacy of acupuncture in diminishing pain is related to endorphin release and to stimulation of large myelinated fibers blocking nociceptive transmission from small unmyelinated C fibers. Stimulation of large-fiber mechanoreceptors in a dermatome inhibits the small-fiber pain input in the ipsilateral or contralateral dermatome by "closing the gate" in the spinal cord that allows nociceptive impulses to reach the cerebral cortex.[3, 4] This mechanism explains the lack of effect of acupuncture in patients with large-fiber destruction, such as postherpetic neuralgia.[5] The importance of afferent transmission to achieve analgesia is also demonstrated by observations that the analgesic effect is blocked by procaine infiltration of acupuncture points. Acupuncture may also produce analgesia by stimulating a location distant to the site of pain. Acupuncture causes the release of endorphins, the endogenous opiates.[6] The effect of analgesia with acupuncture can be partially abolished with injection of naloxone, an opiate antagonist.[7, 8] The long-term relief of pain associated with acupuncture may occur by two mechanisms: (1) a stimulated area may resume normal physical activity and normal large-fiber proprioceptive input is reestablished, which blocks nociceptive input[9]; and (2) pain that may be a learned response, or part of memory, is "forgotten" with brief intense stimulation.[1]

Acupuncture analgesia is obtained by stimulation of particular areas of the skin with fine needles (30-gauge steel, silver, or gold) that are twisted slowly after insertion. The specific areas to be stimulated follow specific meridians (14 in all) that have been plotted on charts.[10] The most effective acupuncture points are often located where nerves enter muscle.[11] The location of acupuncture points and the location for injection for nerve blocks are similar.[12] Acupuncture points may have greater concentrations of pain fibers and vascular structures, which explains the enhanced sensitivity of these points. Most points are at or near the site of pain and a few are distant from it. The needles are left in place for 20 to 40 minutes. The needle insertion feels like a small prick, followed by an ache, numbness, and warmth in the area.[2] Electrical stimulation that directs current with a square or spike wave with variable frequency, pulse width, and voltage may be applied to the needles in situ. Low-frequency electrical stimulation increases the efficacy of the acupuncture procedure.[13] Patients who are overanxious or who have visceral pain should not receive acupuncture.[14] Potential complications of acupuncture include hemorrhage, pneumothorax, hepatitis, and endocarditis.[14–16]

Acupuncture has been studied in the treatment of neck pain. In a placebo-controlled, double-blind, crossover study of neck pain, acupuncture demonstrated an 80% remission rate of neck pain compared with a placebo rate of 33%.[17] Teng and colleagues reported the efficacy of acupuncture in combination with physical therapy in the treatment of cervical spondylosis.[18] Tan reported long-term beneficial effects of electroacupuncture on 64.9% of patients with chronic neck and shoulder pain.[19]

Auriculotherapy is acupuncture of the auricle. Nogier proposed that an inverted homunculus is represented on the auricle.[20] In a double-blind study, Oleson and colleagues were able to find abnormalities in other parts of the body by detecting areas of increased skin conductivity and tenderness over the ear.[21] Areas of the body that have been injured have altered conductivity of electrical current. Electrical current follows the path of least resistance and bypasses injured areas. Diseased areas of the body may be located by measuring the electrical conductivity of the skin over suspicious areas, including the auricle, with an ohmmeter.[2] A hypothesis has been proposed that visceral disorders may also be discovered by identification of abnormal electroconductivity in specific meridians corresponding to individual organs.[22] The explanation for this phenomenon is the viscero-skin-sympathetic nerve reflex. Abnormalities in the viscera are transmitted to the spinal cord and are reflected onto the skin via the efferent sympathetic nerves as longitudinal areas of electrical resistance. Electrostimulation of areas of the auricle has been demonstrated to increase cerebrospinal fluid endorphin levels.[23] Others have not been able to reproduce these results.[1] The efficacy of this therapy may be related to anatomic organization of the nervous system. Inputs from the ear project to central nervous system structures that play a role in referred sensation. Low-frequency versus high-frequency electroacupuncture may have a dif-

ferential effect on the type of neurotransmitters (low-frequency endogenous opioids, high-frequency nonopioid neurotransmitters) resulting in analgesia.[24] Whether specific auricular stimulation or placebo stimulation alone accounts for analgesia with auriculotherapy remains to be determined. A study by Katz and Melzack was unable to demonstrate any increased benefit of stimulating "Nogier" points compared with placebo points in the auricle.[25] However, about one third of patients reported warmth and other sensations in distant parts of the body with ear stimulation. This suggests that referred sensations are generated by ear stimulation. Acupuncture of the ear is associated with toxicities including auricular chondritis that is resistant to therapy.[26]

The same mechanism that results in analgesia with acupuncture may also be the same for pain relief associated with TENS, ice massage, and needle effect (dry needling of trigger points). The counterirritation of superficial structures may have analgesic effects of short, intermediate, or prolonged duration.[27, 28]

Acupuncture should be considered adjunctive therapy for patients with chronic neck pain. Patients should be considered candidates for this therapy even if they have not responded to TENS therapy. Acupuncture of the body and ear may be tried. Success of acupuncture as a therapy relies on the practitioner having thorough knowledge of the anatomy of the acupuncture points. Placement must be exact and the stimulation given correctly.[29] Obviously, the availability of this therapy depends on the accessibility of an experienced acupuncturist.

References

ACUPUNCTURE

1. Melzack R. Folk medicine and the sensory modulation of pain. In: Wall PD, Melzack R (eds): Textbook of Pain, 2nd ed. Edinburgh: Churchill Livingstone, 1989, pp 897–905.
2. McLean B, Fives HE: Stimulation-induced analgesia. In: Warfield CA (ed): Principles and Practice of Pain Management. New York: McGraw-Hill, Inc, 1993, pp 413–425.
3. Fitzgerald M: The contralateral input to the dorsal horn of the spinal cord in the decerebrate spinal rat. Brain Res 236:275, 1982.
4. Melzack R, Wall PD: Pain mechanisms: a new theory. Science 150:971, 1965.
5. Levine JD, Gormley J, Fields HL: Observations on the analgesic effects of needle puncture (acupuncture). Pain 2:149, 1976.
6. Pomerantz B, Chiu D: Naloxone blockade of acupuncture analgesia: endorphin implicated. Life Sci 19:1757, 1976.

7. Mayer DJ, Price DD, Raffi A: Antagonism of acupuncture analgesia in man by the narcotic antagonist naloxone. Brain Res 121:368, 1977.

8. Chapman CR, Colpitts YM, Beneditti C, et al.: Evoked potential assessment of acupunctural analgesia: attempted reversal with naloxone. Pain 9:183, 1980.

9. Melzack R: Prolonged relief of pain by brief, intense transcutaneous somatic stimulation. Pain 1:357, 1975.

10. Duke M: Acupuncture: The Meridians of Ch'i. New York: Pyramid House, 1972.

11. Gunn CC: Motor points and motor lines. J Acupunc 6:55, 1978.

12. Omura Y: Electro-acupuncture: its electrophysiologic basis and criteria for effectiveness and safety, part 1. Acupunct Electrother Res 1:157, 1975.

13. Matsumoto T, Lyu BS: Anatomical comparison between acupuncture and nerve block. Am Surg 41:11, 1975.

14. Macdonald AJR: Acupuncture analgesia and therapy. In: Wall PD, Melzack R (eds): Textbook of Pain, 2nd ed. Edinburgh: Churchill Livingstone, 1989, pp 906–919.

15. Scheel O, Sundsfjord A, Lunde P, et al.: Endocarditis after acupuncture and injection: treatment by a natural healer. JAMA 267:56, 1992.

16. Kent GP, Brondum J, Keenlyside RA, et al.: A large outbreak of acupuncture-associated hepatitis B. Am J Epidemiol 127:591, 1988.

17. Coan RM, Wong G, Coan PL: The acupuncture treatment of neck pain: a randomized controlled study. Am J Chin Med 9:326, 1982.

18. Teng C, Liu T, Chang W: Effect of acupuncture and physical therapy in the management of cervical spondylosis. Arch Phys Med Rehabil 54:601, 1973.

19. Tan JC, Nordin M: Role of physical therapy in the treatment of cervical disk disease. Orthop Clin North Am 23:435, 1992.

20. Nogier PFM: Treatise of auriculotherapy. Maisonneuve, France: Moulin-les-Metz, 1972.

21. Oleson TD, Kroening RJ, Bressler DE: An experimental evaluation of auricular diagnosis: the somatotopic mapping of musculo-skeletal pain at ear puncture points. Pain 8:217, 1980.

22. Pert A, Dionne R, Ng L, et al.: Alterations in rat central nervous system endorphins following transauricular electroacupuncture. Brain Res 224:83, 1981.

23. Hyodo M: Modern scientific acupuncture as practiced in Japan. In: Lipton S, Miles J (eds): Persistent Pain: Modern Methods of Treatment. London: Grune & Stratton, 1985, pp 129–156.

24. Lee JH, Beitz AJ: Electroacupuncture modifies the expression of c-*fos* in the spinal cord induced by noxious stimulation. Brain Res 577:80, 1992.

25. Katz J, Melzack R: Referred sensations in chronic pain patients. Pain 28:51, 1987.

26. Melzack R, Jeans ME, Stratford JG, et al.: Ice massage and transcutaneous electrical stimulation: comparison of treatment for low-back pain. Pain 9:20, 1980.

27. Lewit K: The needle effect in the relief of myofascial pain. Pain 6:83, 1979.

28. Gilbert JG: Auricular complication of acupuncture. NZ Med J 100:142, 1987.

29. Evans D: Acupuncture. In: Raj PP (ed): Practical Management of Pain, 2nd ed. St Louis: Mosby-Year Book, 1992, pp 934–944.

Biofeedback

Chronic pain is associated with the development of a depressed or vegetative state. Pain, when associated with change in personality and mentation, may persist despite resolution of the physical trauma associated with the initial pain. In these circumstances, therapies directed primarily at analgesia alone without attempting to modify the psychological state of the patient may not be successful.

A number of techniques are available to alter the psychological state of chronic pain patients. Biofeedback is a technique by which alterations in biologic processes are presented to an individual by a proportional change in a sensory signal (visual or auditory). The biologic processes measured include muscle tension measured by electromyogram, skin temperature, pulse volumes, and waveforms on electroencephalograms. Biofeedback techniques are valuable in reducing anxiety and stress, emphasizing self-control, and manifesting the psychological and somatic relationship. Biofeedback treatment is based on the premise that patients with neck pain have elevated levels of muscular tension.[1] Melzack reported decreased pain in patients using biofeedback who felt in greater control of their symptoms.[2]

Biofeedback requires several weeks of training. It is indicated only for patients who have persistent chronic pain. Patient motivation must be high. In many circumstances, biofeedback is used in conjunction with relaxation training for control of pain. Patients who may have the best outcome from biofeedback were studied by Keefe and colleagues.[3] These individuals initially rated their pain as severe, were less likely to be receiving disability payments, had fewer years of continuous pain, and had fewer surgical procedures.[3]

The efficacy of biofeedback in neck pain remains to be determined.[4] The reliance on control of a physiologic function ignores the complex psychological, affective, and behavioral components of the pain experience. Biofeedback may work by allowing the patient to improve focused thinking, thereby resulting in increased relaxation.[5]

Relaxation

The basic premise of relaxation is that elicitation of this response results in an altered stated of consciousness. This state is associated with a sense of well-being and peace of mind, which also results in decreased oxygen consumption, respiratory rate, and heart rate.[6] The proposed mechanisms include increased endorphin levels and presence of electroencephalography.[7] The scientific data to support these proposed mechanisms are inconclusive. The relaxation response leads to generalized decreased sympathetic nervous system activity. This response may be mediated by an area in the hypothalamus.[8] More than one technique is able to elicit the relaxation response.[9]

Relaxation may be induced by a simple technique as proposed by Beary and Benson.[10] The instructions are as follows:

1. Sit quietly with your eyes closed.
2. Relax all your muscles, starting with the feet and progressing to the head. Keep all muscles deeply relaxed.
3. Breathe through the nose. Say the word "one" silently after each breath. Continue for 20 minutes. Eyes are opened to check the time, but no alarm is used. After 20 minutes, rest with the eyes closed, then opened.
4. Do not attempt within 2 hours of any meal.

This technique may be used alone or in conjunction with biofeedback or hypnosis to achieve the desired response.

Other relaxation techniques besides deep breathing may also be effective in achieving an appropriate relaxation response. Progressive muscle relaxation training decreases muscular tension and pain. Mindfulness meditation uses imagery techniques to focus on distinguishing pain from other sensations.[10] Few studies have been completed comparing the efficacy of relaxation techniques with other therapies. Relaxation techniques may not be proven better than a placebo but are relatively cost-effective and lack lasting harmful side effects. Although the specific physiologic mechanisms resulting in pain relief are unproven, relaxation reduces muscle tension, decreases sympathetic nervous system tone, and provides a cognitive distraction from distress.

Hypnosis

Hypnosis is an altered state of awareness in which the patient experiences increased suggestibility. The hypnotic state restricts attention so as to exclude extraneous stimulation while narrowing attention. Chronic pain is not purely a physical trauma but is also associated with emotions and thoughts that alter the patient's perceptions. Hypnosis, through its effects on emotions and thoughts, can alter the perception of pain. Hypnotic suggestions may decrease pain in a number of ways. A patient may attain a level of deep relaxation. The pain may be directly diminished by suggestion or by transfer to another part of the body. The quality of the pain may be altered to tingling or numbness. A patient may be distracted from the pain or told to think of a time prior to the onset of pain.[11] Hypnotic therapy is most useful if the patient can be taught self-hypnosis, eliminating the need for a hypnotherapist on a continuous basis. Hypnosis may also be helpful with the headaches associated with cervical neck pain.[12]

References

BIOFEEDBACK, RELAXATION, HYPNOSIS

1. Evaskus DS, Laskin DM: A biochemical measure of stress in patients with myofascial dysfunction syndrome. J Dent Res 51:1464, 1972.
2. Melzack R, Perry C: Self-regulation of pain: the use of alpha-feedback and hypnotic training for the control of chronic pain. Exp Neurol 46:452, 1975.
3. Keefe FJ, Block AR, Williams RB, et al.: Behavioral treatment of chronic low back pain: clinical outcome and individual differences in pain relief. Pain 11:221, 1981.
4. Reich BA: Biofeedback and relaxation therapies. In: Tollison CD, Satterthwaite JR (eds): Painful Cervical Trauma: Diagnosis and Rehabilitative Treatment of Neuromusculoskeletal Injuries. Baltimore: Williams & Wilkins, 1992, pp 144–167.
5. Blancard EB, Ahles TA: Biofeedback therapy. In: Bonica JJ (ed): The Management of Pain, 2nd ed. Philadelphia: Lea & Febiger, 1990, pp 1722–1732.
6. Domar AD, Friedman R, Benson H: Behavioral therapy. In: Warfield CA (ed): Principles and Practice of Pain Management. New York: McGraw-Hill, Inc, 1993, pp 437–444.
7. Wallace RK: Physiological effects of transcendental meditation. Science 167:1751, 1970.
8. Benson H, Pomeranz B, Kutz I: The relaxation response and pain. In: Wall PD, Melzack R (eds): Textbook of Pain. Edinburgh, Churchill Livingstone, 1984, pp 817–822.
9. Benson H, Arns P, Hoffman J: The relaxation response and hypnosis. Int J Clin Exp Hypn 29:259, 1981.
10. Beary JF, Benson H: A simple psychophysiologic technique which elicits the hypometabolic changes of the relaxation response. Psychosom Med 36:115, 1974.
11. Pawlicki RE, Wester WC II: Hypnosis. In: Raj PP (ed): Practical Management of Pain. Chicago: Year Book Medical Publishers Inc, 1986, pp 829–833.
12. Carasso RL, Klienhautz M, Peded O, et al.: Treatment of cervical headache with hypnosis, suggestive therapy, and relaxation techniques. Am J Clin Hypn 27:216, 1985.

RECOMMENDED THERAPEUTIC REGIMEN

With so many different recommended forms of therapy, it is clear to the treating physician that there is no one therapeutic intervention that is effective for the universe of patients with neck pain (Table 18–9). The physician faced with this myriad of therapeutic options should refer back to the axioms of therapy that introduced this section. These guidelines

TABLE 18–9. RECOMMENDED THERAPEUTIC REGIMEN

ACUTE NECK PAIN

1. Controlled physical activity:
    Limit bed rest, encourage walking
2. Physical modalities:
    Cryotherapy—ice pack or
    Thermotherapy—hot towel in plastic bag;
    hot shower
3. Nonsteroidal anti-inflammatory drugs (NSAIDs):
    Analgesic NSAIDs
        Aspirin 650 mg q.i.d. or ketorolac 10 mg q.i.d. or diflunisal 500 mg b.i.d. (after loading with 1000 mg) or diclofenac potassium 50 mg b.i.d. or naproxen sodium 550 mg b.i.d. or etodolac 300 mg t.i.d. or ketoprofen 75 mg t.i.d. or ibuprofen 800 mg q.i.d.
4. Muscle relaxants (palpable spasm or difficulty sleeping):
    Cyclobenzaprine 10 mg 2 hours before bedtime increased to 10 mg t.i.d. as needed and tolerated
    If ineffective, not tolerated:
    Orphenadrine citrate 100 mg b.i.d. or chlorzoxazone 500 mg q.i.d.
5. Injection therapy: anesthetic with/without corticosteroids
6. Optional therapy—prevent recurrence:
    Home exercise program

CHRONIC NECK PAIN

1. Physical modalities:
    Cryotherapy or thermotherapy
2. Nonsteroidal anti-inflammatory drugs (NSAIDs):
    Aspirin 650 mg q.i.d. or diclofenac sodium 75 mg t.i.d. or oxaprozin 1200 mg q.d. or etodolac 400 mg q.i.d. or sulindac 200 mg b.i.d. or naproxen 500 mg b.i.d. or piroxicam 20 mg q.d. or ketoprofen 200 mg q.d.
    Other choices: ibuprofen, indomethacin, tolmetin (non-acetylated salicylates or coated preparations for patients with GI intolerance to the other NSAIDs)
3. Muscle Relaxants (palpable spasm or difficulty sleeping):
    Cyclobenzaprine 10 mg q.d.; increase to t.i.d. as tolerated
        If ineffective:
        Amitriptyline 10 mg increasing to 100 mg q.h.s. or doxepin 10 mg increasing to 100 mg q.h.s. (less sedating)
4. Physical Therapy:
    a. Exercises
        Flexion, extension, or isometric
    b. Modalities
        Temperature (with exercise)
        Transcutaneous electrical nerve stimulation
        Electric stimulation
5. Other modalities:
    Acupuncture
    Biofeedback

should help the physician decide on the forms of appropriate therapy for each specific patient with neck pain.

Acute neck pain of any cause is usually a self-limited illness in the majority of patients. Educating patients to this fact is worth the effort. The time spent with patients increases the confidence patients place in the physician's recommendations and facilitates the therapeutic process. Patients are told that they will improve. Patients with acute pain of short duration should experience total relief of their pain and should expect to return to their usual activities. The physician will be right 80% to 90% of the time. During the initial period of injury, controlled physical activity is recommended to reduce pain and hasten return to work. Non-narcotic analgesics in the form of aspirin or other rapid-onset NSAIDs (diflunisal, naproxen sodium, ibuprofen, diclofenac potassium, and ketorolac) should be added to decrease pain. Ketorolac may be used by an intramuscular route for emergency room patients. Ketorolac is as effective as narcotics but lacks anti-inflammatory effects. A different analgesic NSAID must be chosen if anti-inflammatory effects are required. If patients experience muscle spasm, which is noted on physical examination, or develop difficulty sleeping, muscle relaxants, which are nonaddictive, are indicated. Therapeutic modalities in the form of heat or cold may be applied to the symptomatic area of the neck while the patient is at home.

With resolution of neck pain, patients may resume their usual activities with or without additional education. A session with a physical therapist is useful for those patients interested in learning how to prevent recurrence of pain.

Patients who do not improve on this regimen are candidates for additional therapy. This may take the form of local injection of painful sites. A change in NSAID and muscle relaxant after a trial of 2 to 3 weeks may be warranted if pain continues. If a patient had a partial response to the NSAID without toxicity, the dose of the drug should be increased to the maximum.

Patients who have improved and who will resume strenuous physical activities are candidates for physical therapy. Exercises improve their general physical condition and prepare them for increased strain on the cervical spine. Patients learn good posture and range of motion exercises.

The therapy for chronic neck pain patients is more difficult. The goal of therapy for these patients is maximum physical function despite continued pain. The general internist or family practitioner may offer therapies that may diminish but not abolish discomfort. Patients must understand from the outset the goal of therapy and the likelihood of only partial pain relief. This understanding is an essential part of therapy. If these patients do not accept the goals and outcomes, they are quickly disappointed and frustrated. These patients do not improve.

Patients are instructed at the initial meeting with the physician that maximum function and return to work is the goal of therapy. Pain may continue and may exacerbate at times but is not necessarily indicative of past or present disease-associated damage. Patients can be functional despite pain. Patients with organic pain readily accept these goals. Malingerers are frequently disappointed with this regimen and miss appointments.

Patients with chronic neck pain are treated with NSAIDs, muscle relaxants, and injection therapy when indicated. The medications are substituted for the initial agents if they prove to be ineffective. Tricyclic antidepressants are used if patients have chronic pain and clinical symptoms of depression. Referral to a physical therapist is given for exercises to improve general conditioning as well as correcting any imbalance in the spine with stretching and strengthening exercises of the flexion, extension, and isometric variety.

Patients who continue to experience pain should try transcutaneous electrical nerve stimulation (TENS) therapy. Patients are fitted with the machine by the therapist. Patients who find the unit useful can rent the units for varying periods. Patients should buy units only if they obtain benefit from the TENS machine for a period of months.

Patients who continue to experience pain after receiving these therapies need to be considered for referral to a pain clinic. Pain clinics offer a multidisciplinary approach to pain. Pain clinics offer the expertise of neurosurgeons, anesthetists, psychiatrists, physical therapists, vocational rehabilitation counselors, and other professionals interested in the therapy of chronic pain. The number of people who require this type of therapy in comparison with those who present with neck pain is extremely small. However, the opportunity for this group of chronic pain patients to improve without this combined therapeutic approach is limited.

The clinician treating patients with chronic neck pain may become frustrated with a lack of response to a variety of therapies. The clinician must remain supportive to maintain the trust and hope of the patient. The physician must remain resourceful, using all treatment modalities in a variety of combinations to improve the patient's condition. Educate the patient about the benefits and potential toxicities of every change in therapy. Remember that increased function, despite the persistence of neck pain, is an improvement.

19

Surgical Therapy

INDICATIONS FOR CERVICAL SPINE SURGERY

Surgical intervention, when indicated, provides predictable results to the patient with cervical spine disease. Despite areas of minor controversies, the indications for surgical procedures have been well established. Unlike surgery on the lumbar spine, surgery on the cervical spine is not as easily mastered, and the complications, when present, can be quite serious. With the establishment of strict criteria for patient selection, results ranging from good to excellent can approach 90% to 95% in most cases. The purpose of this chapter is not to detail the surgical procedures but to provide a general discussion of the role of surgery in the treatment of cervical spine disorders.

Surgery on the cervical spine is performed to relieve pain (usually radicular or arm pain), bony instability, and neural element compression (spinal cord and nerve roots). The procedures performed may be grouped into one of three categories: decompression (with or without disc excision), stabilization (fusion or bony ankylosis), or both. Furthermore, the cervical spine surgeon must decide whether the problem area should be approached from the front or back of the spine and in one or two stages.

INDICATIONS FOR SURGERY: HERNIATED NUCLEUS PULPOSUS

When nonoperative therapeutic measures have proven unsuccessful in managing the patient with symptoms from an acute herniated disc, surgical intervention can and should be considered.[1, 2] This occurs in 10% to 15% of all cases. Patients with a herniated disc can present predominantly with neck pain, arm pain, or a combination of both.

Neck Pain

Failure of nonoperative treatment is not an indication for operative treatment for patients mainly with neck pain associated with a cervical disc. Axial or predominant neck pain responds poorly to disc excision, with good to excellent results attainable only in 65% of patients. Disc surgery for neck pain alone is unpredictable and should be undertaken with great caution.

Profound Spinal Cord Impingement

The most dramatic, but fortunately the most rare, presentation of a cervical herniated nucleus pulposus is sudden and profound neurologic loss produced by a large central disc displacement. This disc displacement produces a profound or progressive acute myelopathy with quadriparesis or quadriplegia below the level of the herniation. If not decompressed urgently, the potential for lasting weakness, spasticity, loss of bowel and bladder function, and sexual dysfunction is increased.[3] In some cases, even prompt treatment does not reverse the spinal cord damage thought to be the result of lack of blood supply. Once this clinical condition is identified, the patient should undergo emergent myelography or magnetic resonance (MR) scan, followed by decompression of the offending disc by anterior discectomy and interbody fusion. Despite the potential lack of total recovery, the surgery often prevents further damage to the spinal cord and loss of neurologic function.

Progressive Neurologic Deficit

If the physician can document a worsening in a patient's neurologic examination, prompt surgical intervention should be considered. Commonly, a patient presents with arm pain radiating into the index and long fingers. A diminished brachioradialis and possibly a diminished biceps reflex are noted on initial examination. Conservative treatment is instituted and the patient is later reevaluated. Subsequent evaluation might reveal a further loss in the arm reflexes associated with demonstrable motor weakness in the biceps muscle. This constellation of findings represents a progressive neurologic deficit. Because this is usually not reversible with medications and rest, and the surgeon wants to prevent further permanent nerve damage, surgical decompression should be done once confirmatory evidence of the location of the lesion is provided by computerized tomography (CT) (with myelography), or MR evaluation.

The more common patient presentation is one of an acute stable neurologic deficit. If the deficit is profound with significant motor weakness, for example complete paralysis of the hand intrinsic muscles (C8 and T1), surgical intervention is a viable option and most spine surgeons consider it mandatory.[4] Although often difficult to quantitate, clinical experience suggests that the more prolonged and severe the pressure on a spinal nerve, the less likely the nerve is to recover function. Unfortunately, there are no good prospectively controlled series to document the recovery of cervical nerve root function. Every spine surgeon remembers cases in which the return was noted within days and those in which it never improved or even worsened. Presently, recommendations for surgery have to be individualized for each patient, based on the clinical picture and the significance of the neurologic findings.

It is an even more difficult clinical judgment when the patient presents with a partial neurologic lesion (weakness) or the clinical situation is subacute. A stable neurologic finding, by itself, is not a good criterion for surgery because it is unpredictably reversed. One must keep in mind the temporal relationship because acute or subacute pain may not correlate with the patient's neurologic findings. Previ-

ous medical records and examination are often helpful in making this decision.

Unrelenting Radicular Arm Pain (Brachialgia)

Occasionally an acute episode of brachialgia without neurologic deficit fails to respond to conservative treatment. The exact timing of surgical treatment varies from patient to patient, depending on individual pain tolerance, socioeconomic factors, and emotional stability. In most instances, if a patient has an abnormal electromyogram, has an abnormal myelogram or MR scan, and has not improved with a minimum of 6 weeks of nonoperative treatment, the patient may be considered for surgery. However, if some improvement is realized, waiting up to an additional 6 weeks may result in continued resolution of symptoms. The results of surgery are not as predictable as with those of neurologic deficits, but they can be dramatic.

Recurrent Episodes of Arm Pain

A small group of patients with arm or radicular pain has recurrent episodes of incapacitating pain. Most often the arm or radicular pain is low-grade or smoldering between the incapacitating episodes, suggesting chronic cervical spondylosis. The time between episodes is tolerable for the patient. If the recurrent acute-pain episodes are within the patient's tolerance and minimally affect activities of daily living, nonoperative therapy should be provided. Less commonly, the frequency and intensity of the pain are severe enough to interfere with the patient's employment and avocational endeavors such that surgery should be considered. As a guideline, if the patient experiences three or more episodes in a year, surgery should be offered if the confirmatory tests of nerve compression are positive.

The relief of the painful condition requires that the surgeon find evidence of a physical or organic cause of the patient's pain. This means that, ideally, mechanical compression of the suspicious nerve root is demonstrable from either a bony spur (also known as a hard disc) or a soft tissue abnormality such as a herniated disc (soft disc). On the contrary, if one undertakes to decompress a nerve root that is not the focus of a mechanical or organic lesion, the results are no better than a placebo (about

50%). The so-called exploratory spinal operation should be avoided for pain relief.

When the patient with brachialgia is considered for surgery, the following three criteria should be met if an excellent result is to be anticipated: (1) clear radicular pain pattern, (2) neurologic deficit, and (3) positive confirmatory test (myelogram or MR).[5] The results of surgery cannot be expected to be excellent unless the patient has at least a neurologic examination and a correlative MR or myelogram showing abnormalities.

Patient Factors

The key to a successful outcome in any surgery, especially spine surgery, is patient selection. Even the most expertly performed surgical procedure, if done in an inappropriate patient, is doomed to an unfavorable outcome. A patient's emotional, psychological, and socioeconomic condition must be considered. A patient's concern or depression about his or her condition should not be misinterpreted; physical and psychological factors interrelate. In a patient with a complicated clinical situation, organic problems may coexist with psychological difficulties.

The emotional factor is difficult to quantitate; it is a subjective measure best ascertained by patient interview. The Minnesota Multiphasic Personality Inventory, a questionnaire that measures relative levels of hysteria, depression, and hypochondriasis, among others, may be of use preoperatively in predicting the surgical outcome. If the patient presents with minor complaints and a paucity of physical findings but has a significant emotional overlay or even overt depression, continued nonoperative treatment is warranted. If, on the other hand, definite physical findings are present (such as a neurologic deficit) and emotional problems preexist, a psychiatric consultation is recommended. The patient may need to have optimal medical and psychiatric management prior to surgery or, as is often the case, once the psychological overlay is treated, the symptoms improve enough that surgery is no longer required. As a rule, emotional and psychological factors should be addressed and treated before surgical intervention.

Socioeconomic factors include litigation and work-related injury. Patients with cervical spine problems who were involved in an automobile accident (usually minor) or injured at work are some of the most difficult patients to treat successfully.[6] These patients, unlike those with psychological overlays, do not exhibit emotional problems. It is often difficult to pinpoint a reason for their less than optimal response to treatment. Unless these patients have a profound or progressive neurologic condition with objective findings that warrants emergency surgery, the wisest course is to continue conservative treatment until the litigation or compensation is settled. Although these problems are not as prominent in cervical spine disease as in lumbar spine disease, their presence should not be overlooked or underemphasized. Finally, a small group of patients, usually women who have domestic problems, warrants special mention. These patients may have been injured at home or may have spouse-related problems but do not have compensation or litigation claims. They have so-called "domestic neuroses." The secondary factors that preclude a good response to surgery are the patient's home environment and marital problems, resulting in varying levels of emotional overlay and depression.

Selection of the Type of Surgery

The goals of surgery for cervical disc herniation are to decompress the spinal nerve by removing the mechanical impingement on the nerve root and to relieve the patient's radicular arm pain. Two surgical options of nearly equal efficacy can be undertaken in patients with a posterolateral disc herniation.[5] The first involves a partial removal of the offending facet through a posterior approach and is called a "keyhole" foraminotomy.

The second surgical procedure is the anterior disc excision with bony fusion. This procedure involves an anterior or frontal approach to the cervical spine and directly addresses the problem.[7, 8] This procedure is clearly superior in a true central disc herniation with acute spinal cord compression. In general, the anterior approach provides about a 90% to 95% chance of good-to-excellent results in relief of the radicular arm pain (Fig. 19–1). The long-term results of this operation have been documented to a greater degree in the literature than results of the posterior approach.

In general, the authors favor an anterior procedure for two reasons: (1) the procedure approaches the offending problem most directly, and (2) the long-term results, excluding bone graft donor site pain, are slightly better. Either procedure is adequate for treating radicular arm pain and may be chosen based on the surgeon's preference and experience.

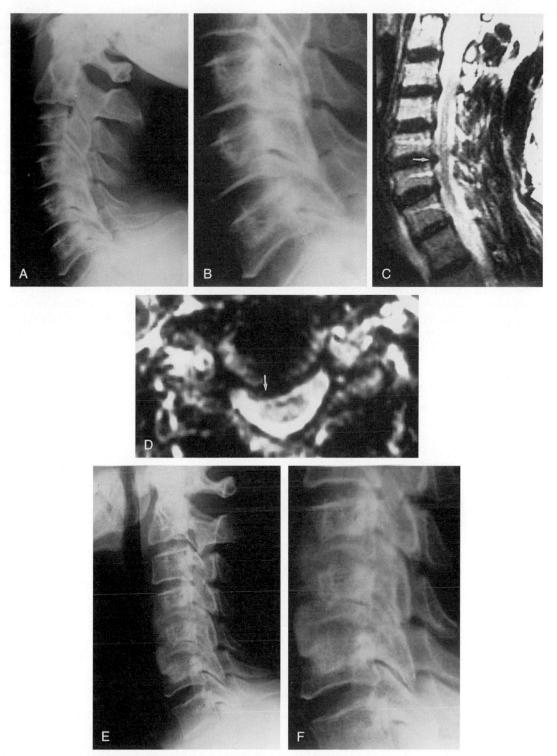

Figure 19–1. Herniated cervical disc. A patient presented with right arm pain in a C6 dermatomal pattern and neck pain suggestive of discogenic pain in a C4–C5 distribution. Lateral views, *A* and *B*, of the cervical spine. Preoperative views on plain roentgenograms do not reveal significant discogenic disease. Preoperative magnetic resonance sagittal, *C*, and axial, *D*, views reveal a herniated nucleus pulposus at the C5–C6 level *(arrows)*. Postoperative roentgenograms, *E* and *F*, after anterior cervical discectomy and fusion with autogenous iliac crest bone graft from C4–C5 to C5–C6. The patient had total postoperative relief of arm and neck pain.

Anterior surgery, however, is clearly the procedure of choice for central disc herniation.

Herkowitz and colleagues designed a prospective study to compare anterior fusion versus laminotomy-foraminotomy in patients with cervical disc herniation.[9] The success rate for anterior fusion was 85% versus 75% for laminotomy. Zeidman and Ducker described their experience with posterior cervical laminoforaminotomy for radiculopathy.[10] A success rate of 97% was reported for 172 patients with cervical radiculopathy, but follow-up was limited.

INDICATIONS FOR SURGERY: CERVICAL SPONDYLOSIS

Cervical spondylosis, or chronic cervical disc degeneration, produces pathologic changes in the diameter of the cervical spinal canal or neural foramina, or both. The reduction in area can compress the spinal cord and either directly or secondarily, owing to spinal cord ischemia, lead to spinal cord damage or myelopathy. Once myelopathy has been diagnosed, surgery should be considered.[11, 12] The goals of surgery are to relieve the pressure on the spinal cord and thereby prevent the progression of the myelopathic symptoms. Improvement of myelopathy is harder to achieve and relates to the duration and severity of the spinal cord compression. Neck pain relief is not a goal of the surgery, but fortunately not a significant part of the clinical symptoms either. Furthermore, the patient must understand that myelopathy, unlike radicular arm pain, is less predictable in its response to decompression.

Routine radiographs of the cervical spine are helpful in cervical spine stenosis because they reveal degenerative disc space narrowing, spur formation, and a diminished spinal canal diameter. Unfortunately, the mere presence of these findings does not explain the patient's clinical picture; further confirmation is required. A CT scan with small amounts of intrathecal water-soluble dye (called CT/myelogram) aids in the diagnosis as an alternative to plain myelography or MR scanning.

Selection of the Type of Surgery

The goal of an operation for cervical spinal stenosis is to remove all pressure from the neural elements completely. The type of problem dictates the nature and extent of the decompression required. If a large, central, soft disc herniation is encroaching on the spinal canal, the herniation must be removed. More commonly, anterior spondylotic or bony spurs (hard discs) compress the neural elements, which are further exacerbated by the posterior changes in the ligamentum flavum and facet joints. Unlike in the lumbar spine, complete removal of all the offending elements is not possible or even necessary to provide an adequate decompression.

When cervical spinal stenosis involves four or more levels, a posterior laminectomy or laminoplasty is favored. If radicular symptoms coexist from foraminal narrowing, foraminal decompression at the appropriate level is also done. If more than two foraminotomies are required, they may best be done anteriorly despite the need for a large bone graft, which incorporates slowly. On the other hand, if the spinal canal stenosis involves three or fewer adjacent vertebral levels, anterior disc fusion without removal of posterior osteophytes is favored. Anterior cervical discectomy without fusion results in decompression but may result in a risk of 50% of patients developing autofusion in kyphosis. The results of the surgery in cervical spinal stenosis are satisfactory in about 80% of cases, with the anterior procedures providing slightly better results.[13]

RESULTS OF OPERATIVE TREATMENT

A general statement regarding the results of cervical spine surgery is not possible. Each category of cervical degenerative disc disease and inflammatory cervical processes has its own peculiar problems that influence the end results. The results of cervical spine surgery for acute herniated disc with radicular arm pain, cervical spondylosis with neck pain only, cervical spondylosis with myelopathy and myeloradiculopathy, and for cervical instability in rheumatoid arthritis will be reviewed.

Surgery for acute cervical herniated disc has been moving slowly from the posterolateral keyhole foraminotomy to the anterior disc excision with fusion. The results of these two procedures are similar in long-term reviews, but the anterior approach with discectomy and fusion is slightly better, despite requiring bone grafting. If proper indications are followed in the appropriate patient population, one can expect a 90% chance of good-to-excellent results. This is the most common type of surgery performed in the cervical spine.[9]

Surgery for cervical spondylosis with neck pain only is much less satisfactory and unpredictable. Good or excellent results were achieved only in 63% of these patients. The quality of the result does not deteriorate with time, and older patients tend to have a higher percentage of satisfactory results.

Results of decompressive laminectomy for cervical spondylosis are variable. The goal is mainly prophylactic—to prevent further neurologic deficit. On occasion, improvement of the clinical state present 6 months prior to surgery can be achieved, and sometimes more dramatic recovery occurs. The procedure has yielded a rate of 70% to 85% satisfactory (good to excellent) results.

Rheumatoid arthritis (RA) commonly involves the neck but infrequently requires surgery. RA patients with atlantoaxial subluxation with posterior atlantodental intervals of 14 mm or less are candidates for posterior arthrodesis from the first to second cervical vertebrae. Patients with atlantoaxial subluxation and 5 mm of basilar invagination are candidates for posterior arthrodesis of the occiput to the second cervical vertebra after halo traction to reduce subluxation.[14] The results of surgery in RA are not as good as for cervical degenerative disc disease. In large part, this is explained by the nature of the systemic progressive rheumatoid process. These patients tend to be quite ill, and the perioperative mortality rate is about 10%. A second problem is the severe bone loss and erosion that are a consequence of RA and disuse osteoporosis. The bones of the neck are weak and do not hold instrumentation well. Fusion fails to occur in 20% to 50% of cases. Patients are also at risk of infection.[15] Other complications of surgery of the rheumatoid cervical spine include wound dehiscence, wire breakage, nonunion, and late subaxial subluxation below a fused segment.[16]

In summary, surgery for acute herniated cervical disc provides satisfactory long-term results in 90% of cases, whereas surgery for myelopathy provides satisfactory long-term results in 70% to 80% of cases. Surgery for patients with cervical disc disease with neck pain only has the worst rate, with long-term satisfactory results of about only 60%. Finally, in RA patients, the results are not always satisfactory, with high rates of perioperative morbidity with persistent neurologic deficits, pseudoarthrosis, and mortality.[17]

COMPLICATIONS

Even with meticulous surgical exposure and the surgeon's intimate knowledge of anatomy, complications occur during cervical spine surgery.[18] Some complications are unique to the anterior or posterior approach; others are common to both. The overall complication rate is estimated at 3% to 4%, and the frequency of neurologic complications is 1% to 2%. Although the anterior approach has a lower rate of neurologic complications (less than 1%) than the posterior approach (1% to 2%), it is associated with a higher rate of complications related to the bone graft used for fusion (1% to 5%). In a study of 384 surgical patients with cervical myelopathy, 21 (5.5%) sustained neurologic deterioration related to spinal cord or nerve root dysfunction.[19] Surgical failure may occur if inadequate decompression is obtained in patients with multiple levels of neurologic compression. Complete decompression with adequate stabilization with fusions is necessary in these patients with multilevel disease.

Intraoperative complications unique to the anterior approach include complications associated with soft-tissue manipulation, including perforation of the pharynx, trachea, and esophagus, which can be devastating if unrecognized during surgery.[20] Vascular injury to the carotid artery, jugular vein, vertebral artery, and thoracic duct must be avoided. The most frequent neurologic complication is injury to the recurrent laryngeal nerve, but injury to the spinal cord, nerve roots, and sympathetic chain may also occur. Complications associated with the autogenous iliac crest bone graft include improper graft positioning with cervical canal compromise, anterior extrusion of the graft, and graft donor site problems such as injury to the cutaneous femoral nerve and hematoma.

Intraoperative complications associated with the posterior approach include injury to the spinal cord or nerve roots, most frequently those of C5. Late instability or kyphosis due to aggressive decompression without fusion may occur. The most common complications of posterior cervical fusion include wire pull-out and pseudarthrosis.

Postoperative complications that are common to both approaches include hematoma, cerebrospinal fluid leakage from dural tears, infection, and failure of fusion with subsequent kyphosis. The anterior approach may also rarely be complicated by discitis. Pulmonary atelectasis, deep venous thrombosis, and intestinal ileus may occur. Positioning of the patient with cervical instability in the appropriate manner and intubation with the patient awake limits the postoperative complications of increased extrinsic cord compression during induction of general anesthesia.[21] The sitting position is beneficial for decreasing bleeding, but it increases the risk for venous air embolism.[22] The preferred prone position is not associated with the complication of air embolism, but it may cause venous engorgement and retinal artery thrombosis secondary to increased intraocular pressure.[20] Most of these complications can be prevented or at least minimized if recognized and treated early.

Some patients do not improve after surgery because their condition is the result of two diseases. Approximately 10% of patients with cervical spondylosis have concomitant lumbar spinal stenosis associated with lower extremity symptoms.[23] Central nervous system diseases (multiple sclerosis and spinal cord tumors) have symptoms and signs similar to those of compressive myelopathy. These primary neurologic disorders need to be considered in the differential diagnosis of the patient with cervical myelopathy.

Patients who undergo decompression and fusion may develop progressive symptoms during the next 12 to 24 months secondary to the breakdown of the fusion mass.[24] Pseudarthrosis rates vary from 0% to 26%.[25, 26] A variety of salvage surgery techniques are available to stabilize the cervical spine in those patients who experience nonunion of their grafts.[27]

References

1. DePalma AF, Rothman RH: The Intervertebral Disc. Philadelphia: WB Saunders Co, 1970, p 225.
2. Brodsky AE: Management of radiculopathy secondary to acute cervical disc degeneration and spondylosis by the posterior approach. In: Sherk HH, Dunn EJ, Eismont FJ, et al. (eds): The Cervical Spine. Philadelphia: JB Lippincott Co, 1989, pp 617–624.
3. Fager CA: Results of adequate posterior decompression in the relief of spondylitic cervical myelopathy. J Neurosurg 38:684, 1973.
4. DePalma AF, Rothman R, Lewinnek G, et al.: Anterior interbody fusion for severe cervical disc degeneration. Surg Gynecol Obstet 134:755, 1972.
5. Herkowitz HN, Simeone FA, Blumberg KD, Dillin WH: Surgical management of cervical disc disease. In: Rothman RH, Simeone FA: The Spine, 3rd ed. Philadelphia: WB Saunders Co, 1992, pp 597–639.
6. MacNab I: The "whiplash" syndrome. Orthop Clin North Am 2:389, 1971.
7. Aronson NI: The management of soft disc protrusions using the Smith-Robinson approach. Clin Neurosurg 20:253, 1973.
8. Clements DH, O'Leary PF: Anterior cervical discectomy and fusion. Spine, 15:1023, 1990.
9. Herkowitz HN, Kurz LT, Overholt DP: Surgical management of cervical soft disc herniation: a comparison between the anterior and posterior approach. Spine 15:1026, 1990.
10. Zeidman SM, Ducker TB: Posterior cervical laminoforaminotomy for radiculopathy: review of 172 cases. Neurosurgery 33:356, 1993.
11. Clark CR: Cervical spondylitic myelopathy: history and physical findings. Spine 13:847, 1988.
12. Nurick S: The natural history and the results of surgical treatment of the spinal cord disaster associated with cervical spondylosis. Brain 95:101, 1972.
13. Herkowitz HN: A comparison of anterior cervical fusion, cervical laminectomy, and cervical laminoplasty for the surgical management of multiple level spondylotic radiculopathy. Spine 13:774, 1988.
14. Boden SD, Dodge LD, Bohlman HH, Rechtine GR: Rheumatoid arthritis of the cervical spine. J Bone Joint Surg 75A:1282, 1993.
15. Conaty JP, Mongan ES: Cervical fusion in rheumatoid arthritis. J Bone Joint Surg 63A:1218, 1981.
16. Boden SD: Rheumatoid arthritis of the cervical spine: surgical decision making based on predictors of paralysis and recovery. Spine 19:2275, 1994.
17. Peppelman WC, Kraus DR, Donaldson WF, Agarwal A: Cervical spine surgery in rheumatoid arthritis: improvement of neurologic deficit after cervical spine fusion. Spine 18:2375, 1993.
18. Graham JJ: Complications of cervical spine surgery. In: Sherk HH, et al.: The Cervical Spine, 2nd ed. Philadelphia, JB Lippincott Co, 1989, pp 831–837.
19. Yonenbu K, Hosono N, Iwasaki M, et al.: Neurologic complications of surgery for cervical compression myelopathy. Spine 16:1277, 1991.
20. Ullman JS, Camins MB, Post KD: Complications of cervical disk surgery. Mt Sinai J Med 61:276, 1994.
21. Blair J, Garfin S: Complications of cervical laminectomy in degenerative disorders of the cervical spine. Semin Spine Surg 7:52, 1995.
22. Ducker T, Zeidman S: The posterior operative approach for cervical radiculopathy. Neurosurg Clin North Am 4:61, 1993.
23. Edwards W, LaRocca SH: The developmental segmental sagittal diameter in combined cervical and lumbar spondylosis. Spine 10:42, 1985.
24. Brodsky AE, Khalil MA, Sassard WR, et al.: Repair of symptomatic pseudoarthrosis of anterior cervical fusion: posterior versus anterior repair. Spine 17:1137, 1992.
25. Whitecloud TS, LaRocca SH: Fibular strut graft in reconstruction surgery of the cervical spine. Spine 1:33, 1976.
26. White A, Southwick W, Deponte R, et al.: Relief of pain by anterior cervical spine fusion for spondylosis. J Bone Joint Surg 55A:525, 1973.
27. Fellrath RF Jr, Hanley EN Jr: The causes and management of pseudoarthrosis following anterior cervical arthrodesis. Semin Spine Surg 7:43, 1995.

20

Occupational Neck Pain

Neck pain is an illness of all people, not just workers. However, neck pain poses special problems in the industrial setting. Despite their magnitude, surprisingly little has been done to provide an organized approach. Thus, the potential for abuse of the Workers' Compensation system persists. This chapter first discusses the epidemiology of occupational neck injuries and then presents a system for impairment rating of neck injuries.

MAGNITUDE OF THE PROBLEM

Of all the injuries that occur in the workplace, it is the musculoskeletal injuries that are responsible for the greatest number of employee disabilities.[1-3] Other conditions, such as contact dermatitis, are often cited as having a higher rate of occurrence, but it is the musculoskeletal injuries that most often result in employees being absent from work, being on modified work programs, or being placed on long-term disability. Occupational musculoskeletal injuries range from simple muscle strains to fractures to amputation of an appendage.

Neck pain that develops as the result of an accident is perceived as a common problem and is a concern that is familiar to most individuals. Post-traumatic neck pain is frequently discussed by physicians, lawyers, and the general public. Even radio and television programs featuring neck pain and associated work issues are not unusual.

With this widespread interest in neck pain, it might be anticipated that significant short-term or long-term medical investigations of neck pain occurring in the workplace would be conducted. Unfortunately, this is not the case. There is a surprising lack of scientific medical information available on occupational neck pain. The limited information that is available is often confusing because of the variety of terms used to describe post-traumatic neck injuries. Terms such as whiplash, acute neck sprain, acute cervical strain, cervical syndrome, hyperextension-hyperflexion neck injury, acceleration-deceleration neck injury, tension neck syndrome, and others are frequently used to describe what appear to be similar conditions. Because these cervical injury syndromes have not been clearly defined, meaningful analysis of recorded neck injuries is difficult. In addition, when looking at occupational injuries, one must also consider other types of neck injuries, such as bruises, lacerations, and fractures of a cervical vertebra, that may result from an occupational accident.

INCIDENCE OF OCCUPATIONAL NECK PAIN

A review of the medical literature available on neck injuries in an occupational setting completed for this book highlights several problems. Head and shoulder injuries are often combined with neck injuries when occupational accidents are reported. Because head and neck injuries may produce shoulder and arm symptoms, it is a common practice in epidemiologic studies to combine head, neck, shoulder, and arm injuries into one category of injury and not specifically isolate those injuries that primarily involve the neck.

Another major difficulty is that other groups of investigations have considered back or neck pain as a whole. Because many different medical conditions, each with specific etiologic characteristics, can result in low back or neck pain, these conditions have been reviewed as a part of a single musculoskeletal system without more specific differentiation into areas of the spine. The exception to this is in motor vehicle accidents, in which whiplash injuries are often specifically designated.

After reviewing the limited available medical literature on occupational neck injuries and comparing this information with data concerning other common occupational musculoskeletal injuries, the incidence of neck injuries in the general working population is low. Information from the National Council on Compensation Insurance shows an incidence rate for neck injuries of 1.1%.[4] The majority of these injuries were the result of vehicle accidents.

A review was also made of the type of occupational accidents that result in neck injuries. This review determined that 43% of the accidents were the result of rear-end automobile accidents and an additional 10% were the result of other types of automobile accidents. Falls, either from an elevation or on the same level, accounted for 10%; 13% were the result of being hit by some type of object; 12% were the result of working in an awkward position, and 10% were the result of lifting, pushing, or pulling heavy objects.

CERVICAL SPINE IMPAIRMENT RATING

Physical disability and physical impairment are not synonymous. The physical impairment rating is the objective assessment of body dysfunction. Physical disability, on the other hand, is complex and difficult to measure. Disability is affected by the culture, socioeconomic background, education, experience, and psychological makeup of the individual. Whereas a physician should be able to rate physical impairment objectively as well as have a valid opinion concerning disability, a full assessment of disability is not strictly a medical matter and is best done by nonmedical individuals.

These nonmedical individuals are rehabilitation specialists who have been trained as vocational experts. They are trained to take a physician's objective physical impairment rating and translate it into a disability assessment. In essence, this assessment reflects an individual's ability to procure employment generally and is called "Residual Occupational Access." It is an evaluation system conceived on the premise that all individuals, based on their age, education, and previous work experience, qualify for a certain percentage of the jobs found in the labor force. Personal injury, when it results in permanent impairment and functional restrictions, reduces that percentage. Therefore, by comparing an individual's preinjury and postinjury access to the labor force, one has a measure of reduced employability or reduced (residual) occupational access and, accordingly, a measure of loss of earning power. Thus, if vocational experts get a consistent impairment rating, they can calculate a consistent disability.

Unfortunately, there are no standardized guidelines to aid the physician in determining a physical impairment rating for the neck. The best available is the American Medical Association's (AMA) *Guide to the Evaluation of Permanent Impairment.*[5] However, many experienced evaluators have given up on this test for guidance on neck injuries because earlier versions of these tables considered range of motion as the major criterion of impairment and did not adequately consider pain in the determination of neck impairment except when associated with peripheral nerve injury or when "substantiated by clinical findings." As happens so often, chronic neck pain is often associated with few or no objective clinical signs, and these are frequently unrelated to the injury or disability in question. In addition, accurate measurement of cervical spine motion, even by the most experienced people, is often just about impossible. One report evaluated a group of asymptomatic people according to AMA criteria and found that all the subjects had some amount of impairment (2% to 18%).[6] Thus, range of motion cannot be used with any accuracy to distinguish between symptomatic and asymptomatic people. In effect, the facts that are frequently used by most physicians, such as patients' motivation, age, education, personality, I.Q., and social environment, strongly suggest that disability is being rated rather than impairment. Other factors used in the determination of impairment in the AMA guidelines include documented neurologic dysfunction (radiculopathy with evidence of muscle atrophy, asymmetric reflexes, long-tract signs, paresis, and incontinence) or evidence of vertebral fracture.[5]

The AMA guidelines do, however, present one useful concept. This is the "whole person" idea. Each part of the body is considered to represent only a part of the whole; the percentage each part contributes is based only on a notion of function. Because the spine (low back and neck) is important to many functions, it contributes a maximum of 60% of the whole person. Thus, once the impairment for the given part is estimated, the whole-person impairment can be easily determined.

The only other reference for rating impairment with any credibility is the *Manual for Orthopaedic Surgeons in Evaluating Permanent Physical Impairment*, published by the American Academy of Orthopaedic Surgeons.[7] However, this manual for the neck relies on subjective symptoms for the most part and is of little practical value to the examining physician. The problem is that information regarding bending and twisting of the neck simply does not furnish the answers. The patient twists as far as desired, and certainly there is a wide discrepancy among individuals with normal necks. To evaluate one extremity, it can be compared with the other, but unfortunately the neck stands alone in this respect. Some attempt must be made to correlate the objective symptoms available with the subjective complaints to achieve a consistent impairment rating system.

Finally, if a patient does warrant a permanent partial impairment secondary to a neck problem, there must also be some permanent modification of activities. It does not make sense for an individual to be awarded a 10% permanent partial impairment and then to be also told to engage in any type of work. Intermittent symptoms that do not stop the individual from engaging in normal activities do not warrant an award. Intermittent symptoms that are sufficiently frequent or severe enough to cause an individual to avoid usual duties, such as overhead work, do warrant an impairment rating.

Neck pain during the acute phase may be totally disabling; however, there are few cases that warrant a significant impairment rating after adequate treatment. Many neck problems can have a functional component; that is, a patient can use the real or imagined condition for some type of personal gain, whether it is to get more attention at home, get an easier job, or make more money from a minor accident. Additionally, a patient can have a preexisting neck problem, such as osteoarthritis, and sustain a superimposed injury that results in the subjective complaints not returning to their baseline (preinjury) level. In all these situations, physicians should try to make their evaluations reflect, as much as possible, the true state of impairment in a way that is organized and replicable.

The manual does present the best guidelines for dealing with patients who complain of neck pain but have no objective findings to substantiate their complaint. Pain is a complex entity that can be defined as a disagreeable sensation to varying degrees of severity. The intensity of pain may be verified by an experienced observer with a thorough history and physical examination. Factitious pain may be detected by inconsistent responses to the standard clinical examination. The manual has an impairment classification for pain and discomfort, but by the nature of the problem the classification is based on some arbitrary guidelines. These guidelines divide pain into four grades, each with associated complaints.

Grade I—Mild. There is a firm conviction established, through thorough observation and clinical tests, that pain actually exists even though there may be no organic manifestations. Pain of this grade does not contribute to physical impairment.

Grade II—Moderate. The examination reveals definite evidence of a pathologic state of the involved structures that would reasonably produce the amount of pain indicated to be present. This grade of pain might require treatment and could be expected to contribute to a minor extent to permanent physical impairment.

Grade III—Severe. The pathologic changes and clinical findings indicate that permanent physical function is limited by pain requiring treatment for relief and contributing extensively to permanent physical impairment.

Grade IV—Very Severe. The pathologic changes and clinical signs indicate limitation of physical function by pain to such an extent that physical impairment is nearly complete.

Additionally, malingering or psychogenic overlay may make it difficult to obtain an accurate estimation of impairment. The patient whose complaints are not justified by objective findings or whose response to testing varies widely from time to time should put the examiner on guard. It may be impossible to identify the malingerer without the help of evidence gathered away from the examining room when the patient thinks he or she is not being observed.

Experience is far more important than any reference guide in making these determinations.[8, 9] Pain is the chief limiting factor in spinal disease, and there is a great deal of variation between individuals in their response to pain. Although there is no foolproof method of assessing pain, one can, through experience, use objective observations that are of assistance in evaluating its effects. In addition to limitation of movement, factors such as muscle spasm, wasting, deformity, tension signs, and irrefutable evidence of neurologic damage must be taken into consideration.

STANDARDIZED NECK EVALUATION GUIDELINES

To try to establish a standardized impairment rating system, a questionnaire was circulated among 53 members of the Cervical Spine Research Society. They were asked to fill out the impairment ratings they used in 33 specific clinical situations. The responses from these experts were anything but consistent. However, the responses could be handled statistically so that in most cases an average range was obvious. The figures ranged from 0% in the completely recovered acute neck sprain to 20% following failed neck surgery. The overall goal was to establish a valid link among a specific diagnosis, impairment rating, and physical exertion requirement.

The physical exertion requirements that were related to each impairment rating have been defined by the Social Security Administration. They are relatively simple and easy to use because the terms have the same meaning as they have in the *Dictionary of Occupational Titles* published by the U.S. Department of Labor.[10] Even though the Social Security Administration does not use the permanent partial physical impairment (PPPI) rating system, it is relatively easy to modify the classification to conform to a compensation and litigation setting in the following way:

Very heavy work involves lifting multiple objects weighing more than 100 lb at a time, with frequent lifting or carrying of objects weighing 50 lb or more.

Heavy work involves lifting no more than 100 lb at a time, with frequent lifting or carrying of objects weighing up to 50 lb.

No one with any neck-related PPPI can be expected to perform safely within either of the preceding two categories. If a patient cannot possibly be qualified to do anything lighter, the patient would have to be approved for social security payments.

Medium work involves lifting no more than 50 lb at a time, with frequent lifting or carrying of objects weighing up to 25 lb. Workers with 5% or less neck-related PPPI can qualify in this category, but those with higher ratings cannot.

Light work involves lifting no more than 20 lb at a time, with frequent lifting or carrying of objects weighing up to 10 lb. Workers with 10% to 15% neck-related PPPI because of a neck problem should be able to do this type of work.

Sedentary work involves no more than the lifting of 10 lb at a time and occasional lifting or carrying of articles like docket files, ledgers, and small tools. Workers with 20% to 25% neck-related PPPI should be capable of this type of work.

People with more than 25% neck-related PPPI rarely qualify for any type of productive occupational activity unless they have special sedentary qualifications that enable the work to be done part-time or at home. These work restriction classifications are summarized in Table 20–1.

Table 20–2 presents neck pain impairment ratings in a standardized set of diagnostic situations. It also matches physical exertion requirements with each diagnostic category. Some of the more common diagnostic entities are discussed in the following paragraphs.

An "acute neck sprain" is a soft tissue injury of an otherwise normal neck. Radiographs are normal and there is no radiating pain. Patients should be able to return to their normal activity within 2 to 3 weeks. If recovery is delayed, some nontraumatic medical or psychosocial problem should be suspected.

Most patients who have a cervical "herniated nucleus pulposus" rarely fully recover without some residual physical impairment. In the majority of cases, it can be assumed that none of them will return to very heavy work. No surgical procedure should be performed with the goal to return a patient to heavy work. An individual with a single-level healed fusion of the cervical spine may be able to return to heavy labor after appropriate rehabilitation. Surgery is indicated to relieve an unacceptable level of pain. As a rule, a patient who has had a discectomy in the cervical spine may be expected to have a 10% to 20% PPPI. A perfect operative result rates at least 10%, whereas a patient with a painful neck and a substantial neurologic deficit rates 20%.

Finally, one of the more difficult situations to evaluate relates to on-the-job injuries incurred by workers with preexisting osteoarthritis. Neck sprain in this circumstance can be slow to respond. The symptoms from the osteoarthritis tend to be perceived as being more disabling than they were before the compensable injury. In spite of this, the spinal experts surveyed were in favor of awarding a 5% PPPI rating to those who were subjectively worse and a 10% rating to those who were both

TABLE 20–1. WORK RESTRICTION CLASSIFICATION OF COMPENSABLE LOW BACK AND NECK INJURIES

WORK CATEGORY	WORK RESTRICTION	PPPI*	RELEVANT LOW BACK DIAGNOSIS	RELEVANT NECK DIAGNOSIS
Very Heavy	Occasional lifting in excess of 100 pounds Frequent lifting of 50 pounds or more	0%	Recovered acute back strain Herniated nucleus pulposus treated conservatively with complete recovery	Neck strain with complete recovery Hyperextension injury with complete recovery
Heavy	Occasional lifting of 100 pounds Frequent lifting of up to 50 pounds	0%	Healed acute traumatic spondylolisthesis Healed transverse process fracture	Herniated nucleus pulposus treated conservatively, with complete recovery Preexisting degenerative disease or cervical canal stenosis with secondary neck strain, with complete recovery
Medium	Occasional lifting of 50 pounds Frequent lifting of 25 pounds	<5%	Chronic back strain Degenerative lumbar intervertebral disc disease under reasonable control Herniated nucleus pulposus treated by surgical discectomy and completely recovered Spondylolysis/spondylolisthesis under reasonable control Healed compression fracture with 10% residual loss of vertebral height	Chronic back strain Degenerative cervical disc disease under reasonable control Herniated nucleus pulposus treated by surgical discectomy with complete recovery Hyperextension injury with residual pain Healed odontoid/hangman's fracture treated nonoperatively Preexisting radiologically evident degenerative disease with secondary hyperextension injury, with moderate pain and restriction
Light	Occasional lifting of no more than 20 pounds Frequent lifting of up to 10 pounds No overhead work	10%–15%	Degenerative lumbar intervertebral disc disease with chronic pain and restriction Herniated nucleus pulposus treated conservatively or operatively, but left with some discomfort, restriction, and neurologic deficit Acute traumatic spondylolysis/spondylolisthesis, treated conservatively or operatively, but with residual discomfort and restriction Lumbar canal stenosis Moderately severe osteoarthritis accompanied by instability Healed compression fracture with 25% to 50% residual loss of vertebral height	Degenerative cervical disc disease with chronic pain and restriction Herniated nucleus pulposus treated conservatively or operatively, with residual discomfort, restriction, and neurologic deficit Hyperextension injury with chronic pain and restriction Cervical canal stenosis Moderately severe osteoarthritis accompanied by instability Hangman's fracture treated with fusion Odontoid fracture treated with fusion Burst/compression fracture of lower cervical spine with no neurologic deficit treated with external fixation or fusion
Sedentary	Occasional lifting of 10 pounds Frequent lifting of no more than lightweight articles and dockets	20%–25%	Multiply operated back (failed back syndrome)	Multiply operated neck (constant pain) Preexisting cervical stenosis with neck injury treated by surgery, with patient subjectively and objectively worse

Adapted from Social Security Administration regulations
*PPPI = permanent partial physical impairment

TABLE 20–2. DISABILITY EVALUATION OF THE CERVICAL SPINE

Note: Compensable injuries are <u>underlined</u>. Please indicate percentage of permanent impairment for each subheading.

WORK PERMITTED		(PPPI) % IMPAIRMENT
	(1) <u>Acute neck sprain</u> ⬦ conservative care ⬥	
Very Heavy Work	(a) complete recovery	0
Medium Work	(b) chronic neck strain (no x-ray findings)	5
	(2) Pre-existing, radiologically evident degenerative disease ⬦ <u>acute neck sprain</u> ⬦ nonoperative care ⬥	
Heavy Work	(a) complete recovery	0
Medium Work	(b) acceptable level of discomfort and restriction	5
Light Work	(c) chronic pain and restriction	10
	(3) <u>Herniated nucleus pulposus</u> ⬦ nonoperative care ⬥	
Heavy Work	(a) complete recovery	0
Light Work	(b) acceptable level of discomfort and restriction, with or without neurologic deficit	10
	(4) <u>Herniated nucleus pulposus</u> ⬦ surgical diskectomy, with or without fusion ⬥	
Medium Work	(a) complete recovery	5
Light Work	(b) acceptable level of discomfort, with or without neurologic deficit	10
Light Work	(c) pain and restriction without neurologic deficit	15
Sedentary Work	(d) pain and restriction with neurologic deficit	20
	(5) <u>Herniated nucleus pulposus</u> ⬦ surgical diskectomy (x times), with or without fusion ⬥	
Medium Work	(a) complete recovery	10
Light Work	(b) moderate pain and restriction (employable)	15
Sedentary to No Work	(c) failed neck (constant pain)	20
	(6) <u>Hyperextension injury</u> (no objective findings) ⬦ nonoperative care ⬥	
Very Heavy Work	(a) complete recovery	0
Medium Work	(b) moderate pain and restriction (employable)	5
Light Work	(c) chronic pain and restriction	10
	(7) Pre-existing, radiologically evident degenerative disease ⬦ <u>hyperextension injury:</u> ⬦ nonoperative care ⬥	
Heavy Work	(a) complete recovery	0
Medium Work	(b) moderate pain and restriction (employable)	5
Light Work	(c) chronic pain and restriction	10
	(8) Pre-existing cervical canal stenosis ⬦ <u>acute neck strain</u> ⬦ nonoperative care ⬥	
Heavy Work	(a) status quo	0
Light Work	(b) subjectively worse	10
Light Work	(c) subjectively and objectively worse	15

TABLE 20–2. DISABILITY EVALUATION OF THE CERVICAL SPINE *Continued*

Note: Compensable injuries are <u>underlined</u>. Please indicate percentage of permanent impairment for each sub-heading.

WORK PERMITTED		(PPPI) % IMPAIRMENT
	(9) Pre-existing cervical canal stenosis ♦ <u>acute neck strain</u> ♦ decompression, with or without fusion ⌾	
Medium Work	(a) status quo	5
Light Work	(b) subjectively worse	15
Sedentary to No Work	(c) subjectively and objectively worse	20
Medium Work	(10) <u>Acute neck strain</u> ♦ nonoperative care ♦ NL no objective residuals ♦ confirmed neurosis	0
Medium Work	(11) <u>Odontoid fracture</u> ♦ external fixation ◊	10
Light Work	(12) <u>Odontoid fracture</u> ♦ fusion ◊	20
Medium Work	(13) <u>Hangman's fracture</u> ♦ external fixation ◊	10
Light Work	(14) <u>Hangman's fracture</u> ♦ fusion ◊	15
Light Work	(15) <u>Burst/compression fracture, lower cervical spine,</u> with no NL neurologic deficit ♦ external fixation ◊	15
Light Work	(16) <u>Burst/compression fracture, lower cervical spine,</u> with no NL neurologic deficit ♦ fusion ◊	15

From Wiesel SW, Boden SD, Borenstein DG, Feffer HL: Neck Pain, 2nd ed. Charlottesville, Virginia: The Michie Co., 1992, pp 466–469. PPPI = permanent partial physical impairment

subjectively and objectively worse. In either situation, light work was the most that could be required of these patients.

References

1. Abenhaim L, Suissa S: Importance and economic burden of occupational back pain: a study of 2,500 cases representative of Quebec. J Occup Med 29:670, 1987.
2. Andersson GBJ: Low back pain in industry: epidemiological aspects. Scand J Rehabil Med 11:163, 1979.
3. Bauer W: Scope of industrial low back pain. In: Wiesel SW, Feffer H, Rothman R (eds): Industrial Low Back Pain. Charlottesville, Virginia: The Michie Co, 1985, pp 1–35.
4. National Safety Council: Accident Facts. Chicago, National Safety Council, 1978, p 26.
5. American Medical Association: Guides to the Evaluation of Permanent Impairment, 4th ed., Chicago, 1993.
6. Lowery WD, Horn TJ, Boden SD, Wiesel SW: Impairment evaluation based on spinal range of motion in normal subjects. J Spinal Disorders 5:398, 1992.
7. American Academy of Orthopaedic Surgeons: Manual for Orthopaedic Surgeons in Evaluating Permanent Physical Impairment, St. Louis, 1962.
8. Brand RA, Lehmann TR: Low-back impairment rating practice of orthopaedic surgeons. Spine 8:75, 1983.
9. Ziporyn T: Disability evaluation—a fledgling science? JAMA 250:873, 1983.
10. Social Security Rulings. Title 20—Employees' Benefits. 404.1567—Physical Exertion Requirements.

Appendix

DISEASE ENTITY	NECK PAIN			ADDITIONAL HISTORY	PHYSICAL EXAMINATION
	Character	*Location*	*Radiation*		
Mechanical					
Muscle strain (deep somatic)					
Mild	Sharp (acute) Ache (chronic)	Neck	Interscapular Top of shoulders	None	Point tenderness
Moderate	Sharp (acute) Ache (chronic)	Neck	Interscapular Top of shoulders	None	Point tenderness Spasm Decreased range of motion of neck
Severe	Sharp	Neck	Interscapular Top of shoulders	Tension headache	Point tenderness Spasm Decreased range of motion of neck
Herniated nucleus pulposus (radicular) C3–C4 (C4 nerve root)	Sharp pain with numbness	Neck	Levator scapulae Anterior chest	Associated headaches	Decreased range of motion Point tenderness Normal neurologic
C4–C5 (C5 nerve root)	Sharp pain with numbness	Neck	Tip of shoulder Anterior chest	Associated headaches	Decreased range of motion Point tenderness Sensory change: deltoid area Motor deficit: deltoid, biceps Reflex change: biceps
C5–C6 (C6 nerve root)	Sharp pain with numbness	Neck	Shoulder Medial border of scapula Lateral arm Dorsal forearm	None	Decreased range of motion Point tenderness Sensory change: thumb, index finger Motor deficit: biceps Reflex change: biceps
C6–C7 (C7 nerve root)	Sharp pain with numbness	Neck	Shoulder Medial border of scapula Lateral arm Dorsal forearm	None	Decreased range of motion Point tenderness Sensory change: middle and ring finger Motor deficit–triceps Reflex change–triceps
Cervical spondylosis (deep somatic)	Ache	Neck	—	Pain increases with activity, especially rotation of the neck	Decreased range of motion

LABORATORY ABNORMALITIES	RADIOGRAPHS	DIAGNOSIS	THERAPY	COMMENTS
Normal	Normal	Clinical history Physical exam	Controlled physical activity NSAIDs Collar (intermittent)	Pain relief in 3–4 days
Normal	Normal	Clinical history Physical exam	Controlled physical activity NSAIDs Collar (intermittent)	Pain relief in 7–10 days
Normal	Normal	Clinical history Physical exam	Controlled physical activity NSAIDs Collar	Pain relief in 2 weeks
Normal	Plain radiographs − Myelogram/CT + MR +	Clinical history Physical exam Radiographs	Initial: rest, NSAIDs After 4–6 weeks with no response: trigger point injection, epidural steroids Continued pain: surgery	Up to 70% of patients with an HNP should respond to noninvasive therapy
Normal	Plain radiographs − Myelogram/CT + MR +	Clinical history Physical exam Radiographs	Initial: rest, NSAIDs After 4–6 weeks with no response: trigger point injection, epidural steroids Continued pain: surgery	Up to 70% of patients with an HNP should respond to noninvasive therapy
Normal	Plain radiographs − Myelogram/CT + MR +	Clinical history Physical exam Radiographs	Initial: rest, NSAIDs After 4–6 weeks with no response: trigger point injection, epidural steroids Continued pain: surgery	Up to 70% of patients with an HNP should respond to noninvasive therapy
Normal	Plain radiographs − Myelogram/CT + MR +	Clinical history Physical exam Radiographs	Initial: rest, NSAIDs After 4–6 weeks with no response: trigger point injection, epidural steroids Continued pain: surgery	Up to 70% of patients with an HNP should respond to noninvasive therapy
Normal	Plain radiographs + MR +	Clinical history Physical exam Radiographs	Controlled physical activity Collar (intermittent) NSAIDs	Majority of patients have resolution of symptoms

Appendix continued on following page

DISEASE ENTITY	NECK PAIN			ADDITIONAL HISTORY	PHYSICAL EXAMINATION
	Character	*Location*	*Radiation*		
Myelopathy (radicular)	Ache	Neck	Interscapular and into one or both arms	Difficulty walking, associated with clumsiness and weakness	Decreased range of motion Long tract signs in lower extremities
Hyperextension injuries: whiplash (deep somatic)	Ache	Neck	Interscapular Shoulders	Headaches Pain with motion	Decreased range of motion Muscle spasm
Rheumatologic Rheumatoid arthritis (deep somatic)	Ache	Neck	Interscapular	Headaches	Generalized involvement of hands and feet Decreased range of motion Positive long tract signs with neural compression
Ankylosing spondylitis (deep somatic)	Sharp (acute) Ache (chronic)	Neck	Interscapular	Male predominance: morning stiffness, back pain	Decreased range of motion Entire spine
Psoriatic spondylitis (deep somatic)	Ache	Neck	Interscapular	Morning stiffness Skin lesions	Psoriatic plaques Decreased motion of cervical spine in all planes
Reiter's syndrome (deep somatic)	Ache	Neck	Interscapular	Conjunctivitis urethritis	Decreased range of motion Cervical spine
Enteropathic arthritis (deep somatic, referred)	Ache	Neck	Interscapular	Morning stiffness Abdominal pain Cramps	Abnormal abdominal examination Joint tenderness Decreased motion of cervical spine in all planes
Diffuse idiopathic skeletal hyperostosis (deep somatic)	Mild ache	Midline	None	Dysphagia	Mild limitation of cervical spine motion
Polymyalgia rheumatica (deep somatic)	Muscle soreness	Shoulders Thighs	Arms Legs	Severe morning stiffness No muscle weakness	Muscle tenderness on palpation
Fibromyalgia (deep somatic)	Ache	Generalized	Tender points	Morning stiffness Fatigue Sleeplessness	Localized pain (tender points)
Infections Vertebral osteomyelitis (deep somatic) Bacterial	Sharp	Area infected	Paraspinous muscles	Extraosseous source of infection Fever	Percussion tenderness over involved bone Decreased motion
Meningitis (deep somatic)	Sharp ache	Neck Occiput	Head Lower spine	Fever	Neck rigidity Brudzinski's sign
Discitis (deep somatic)	Severe, sharp	Disc infected	Shoulder	Male predominance	Localized tenderness Marked limitation of motion
Herpes zoster (superficial somatic, radicular)	Burning	Dermatomal	—	Fever Malaise	Vesicular dermatomal rash

LABORATORY ABNORMALITIES	RADIOGRAPHS	DIAGNOSIS	THERAPY	COMMENTS
Normal	Plain radiographs + MR + for compression of spinal cord	Clinical history Physical exam Radiographs	Surgery: decompress neural elements	Goal of surgery to prevent further neurologic deficit; many patients do recover some neural function
Normal	None	History Physical exam	NSAIDs Muscle relaxants Collar (intermittent) Physical therapy	Majority of patients improve but may take an extended period of therapy to recover
Decreased Hct level Increased ESR Rheumatoid factor 80%	Plain radiographs + C1–C2 subluxation MR + neural compression	History Physical exam Laboratory radiographs	NSAIDs Antirheumatics Corticosteroids Surgery: significant neural compression	Most patients do not require surgery Subluxation: atlantoaxial basilar invagination Subaxial instability
Increased ESR HLA-B27 90%	Marginal syndesmophytes Bilateral sacroiliitis	History Plain radiographs (HLA)	Exercises NSAIDs Muscle relaxants Surgery: instability	Pain improved with motion Iritis HLA confirmatory: not diagnostic
Increased ESR HLA-B27 60%	Nonmarginal syndesmophytes Unilateral or bilateral sacroiliitis +/−	Clinical history Skin rash Plain radiographs (HLA)	Exercises Topical skin care NSAIDs Methotrexate	Spondylitis may precede skin manifestations by many years Spondylitis may occur in absence of sacroiliitis
Increased ESR HLA-B27 75%	Nonmarginal syndesmophytes Unilateral or bilateral sacroiliitis +/−	History Plain radiographs (HLA)	Exercises NSAIDs Muscle relaxants Methotrexate	Cervical spine involvement is uncommon
Increased ESR Blood in stool HLA-B27 50%	Marginal syndesmophytes Bilateral sacroiliitis	Clinical history Gastrointestinal x-ray, biopsy	Exercises NSAIDs	Activity of bowel and axial skeletal disease do not correlate
None	Flowing calcification on anterolateral aspect of four contiguous vertebral bodies	Plain radiographs	NSAIDs Exercises	Surgical removal for severe dysphagia
Increased ESR Isolated increased alkaline phosphatase	None	Clinical history	Corticosteroids	Diagnosis by exclusion
None	None	Clinical history	Rest Graduated exercises NSAIDs Antidepressants	Diagnosis by exclusion
Elevated ESR Blood cultures (50%) Bone cultures (60%)	Subchondral bone loss Endplate loss Narrow disc space Contiguous endplate erosion	Positive culture Radiographs	Antibiotics Immobilization	Severe pain exacerbated by motion Meningeal signs
CSF leukocytosis + Gram's stain	Parameningeal focus	Positive culture	Antibiotics	Rapid diagnosis essential for good prognosis
Increased ESR Increased WBC Blood culture Disc culture	Decreased disc height Reactive sclerosis adjoining vertebral bodies	Positive culture	Antibiotics Immobilization	Pain exacerbated with motion Severe muscle spasm Bone scan positive before plain radiograph MR positive before bone scan
Increased CSF WBC (33%)	Normal	Clinical history Physical exam	Analgesics Corticosteroids	Occult malignancy Often lymphoreticular

Appendix continued on following page

DISEASE ENTITY	NECK PAIN			ADDITIONAL HISTORY	PHYSICAL EXAMINATION
	Character	*Location*	*Radiation*		
Lyme disease (deep somatic, radicular)	Ache	Cervical	Arms	Tick bite Erythema chronica migrans	Skin rash Radicular pain
Tumors and Infiltrative Disease *Benign* Osteoblastoma (deep somatic)	Dull ache	Affected bone	Paravertebral muscles Shoulders	Male predominance Young	Localized tenderness and swelling, scoliosis
Osteochondroma (deep somatic)	Mild ache	Affected bone	Paravertebral muscles	Male predominance Slowly progressive	Restricted spinal motion
Giant cell (deep somatic)	Intermittent ache	Affected bone		Female predominance Neurologic dysfunction	Localized bone tenderness and swelling
Aneurysmal bone cyst (deep somatic)	Acute onset Increasing severity	Affected bone		Female predominance Young	Localized bone tenderness Skin erythema and warmth
Hemangioma (deep somatic)	Throbbing	Affected bone		Midlife onset	Localized bone tenderness Limitation of motion with muscle spasm
Eosinophilic granuloma (deep somatic)	Persistent ache	Affected bone		Male predominance Young	Nontender swelling
Malignant Multiple myeloma (deep somatic, radicular)	Mild ache (onset) Acute pain (fractures)	Affected bone	Radicular	Generalized bone pain Generalized fatigue Nausea, vomiting Mental status alterations Renal dysfunction (40 years of age and older)	Diffuse bone tenderness Fever Pallor
Chondrosarcoma (deep somatic, radicular)	Mild discomfort	Affected bone	Radicular	Male predominance (40–60 years of age)	Painless swelling
Chordoma (deep somatic, radicular)	Dull or sharp Persistent	Cervical	Shoulder	Male predominance (40–70 years of age)	Muscle flaccidity

LABORATORY ABNORMALITIES	RADIOGRAPHS	DIAGNOSIS	THERAPY	COMMENTS
Elevated ESR Borrelia antibodies CSF pleocytosis	None	History Erythema migrans	Antibiotics: early disease—oral; late disease—IV	Lyme antibodies are confirmatory, not diagnostic
Bone biopsy: osteoblasts, osteoid, giant cells	Posterior vertebral body expansile, well delineated, with periosteal new bone	Bone biopsy	Excision	Confused with osteosarcoma, but no cartilage or anaplastic cells in osteoblastoma
Bone biopsy: cartilage cap, woven bone with nests of cartilage	Posterior vertebral body well-demarcated sessile or pedunculated bone with cartilage cap	Radiographs Normal laboratory findings	Excision	Nerve impingement requires decompression Malignant degeneration with multiple osteochondromas
Bone biopsy: osteoclastic giant cells, mononuclear stromal cells, thin-walled vessels	Anterior vetebral body expansile lesion Thin cortical margin No bony reaction	Radiographs Bone biopsy	En bloc excision	Recurrence common with partial excision Malignant transformation rate
Bone biopsy: cystic cavities lined with fibroblasts, osteoid, multinucleated giant cells	Posterior vertebral body osteolytic expansile lesion Thin demarcated periosteal shell of bone	Radiographs	En bloc excision	Local recurrence with partial excision Pathologic fracture
Bone biopsy: increased capillary and venous vessels with sparse trabecular tissue	Anterior vertebral body prominent vertical striations with unchanged body configuration	Radiographs	Radiation therapy for symptomatic lesions	Most lesions asymptomatic Surgical excision for neural compression
Peripheral eosinophilia (10%) Increased ESR Bone biopsy: eosinophils, benign pleomorphic histiocytes	Osteolytic areas without sclerosis Vertebra plana Epidural extension on MR	Bone biopsy	Curettage	Bone biopsy findings confused with Hodgkin's disease
Decreased Hct level Increased WBC Decreased platelets Coombs's test + Increased ESR Increased calcium Increased uric acid Increased creatinine M-protein + Bence-Jones proteinuria	Diffuse vertebral body osteolysis without reactive sclerosis Spares posterior elements CT scan more sensitive	Abnormal plasma cells M-protein Electrophoresis	Chemotherapy Decompressing laminectomy and/or local radiotherapy for cord compression	Most common primary malignant tumor Bone scan does not identify bone lesion
Decreased Hct level Increased ESR (late in course) Bone biopsy: verifying degree of malignant chondrocyte atypia with abnormal matrix production	Expansile, interior fluffy or lobular calcifications Thickened cortex CT scan: soft tissue extension	Bone biopsy	En bloc resection	Grade 1—slowly progressive Grade 3—more malignant, locally invasive
Decreased Hct level Increased ESR (late in course) Bone biopsy: gelatinous tumor, physaliphorous cells interspersed in fibrous tissue	Osteolysis with calcific soft tissue mass Vertebral body without disc involvement initially	Bone biopsy	En bloc resection Radiotherapy for inaccessible tumors	Unpredictable clinical course, slow and indolent or rapid and destructive 10-year survival 10%–40%

Appendix continued on following page

DISEASE ENTITY	NECK PAIN			ADDITIONAL HISTORY	PHYSICAL EXAMINATION
	Character	*Location*	*Radiation*		
Lymphoma (deep somatic, radicular)	Persistent ache	Affected bone	Radicular	Male predominance Pain increases with recumbency or alcohol ingestion	Localized tenderness and swelling
Skeletal metastases (deep somatic, radicular)	Gradual onset with increasing intensity	Affected bone	Radicular	Increased pain with recumbency, cough, motion Prior malignancy (over 50 years of age)	Tenderness with palpation Limited motion Fever
Intraspinal neoplasms Extradural (deep somatic, radicular)	Increasing intensity Unrelenting	Affected bone	Radicular	Increased with recumbency or activity Unresponsive to mild analgesics	Tenderness with palpation Abnormal neurologic signs with compression
Intradural-extramedullary (deep somatic, radicular)	Slowly progressive	Neck and arm	Radicular	Increased with recumbency, not by activity Neurofibromatosis	Sensory changes Muscle atrophy
Intramedullary	Painless			Sensory deficits Weakness	Abnormal pain and temperature sensation Hyperreflexia Spasticity
Endocrinologic and Metabolic *Microcrystalline Disease (deep somatic)* Gout	Acute (sharp) Chronic (ache)	Neck Midline		Chronic peripheral gouty arthritis Male predominance	Straightening cervical spine Tophi
Calcium pyrophosphate dihydrate disease	Acute (sharp) Chronic (ache)	Neck Midline		Male predominance	Straightening cervical spine Loss of motion
Genetic Disorders Mucopolysaccharidoses Morquio's syndrome (deep somatic)	Chronic ache	Diffuse		Onset in childhood Decreased hearing Normal intelligence	Short stature Kyphoscoliosis Clouded corneas Ligamentous laxity Hepatomegaly

LABORATORY ABNORMALITIES	RADIOGRAPHS	DIAGNOSIS	THERAPY	COMMENTS
Decreased Hct level Immunoglobulin abnormalities Disseminated disease	Osteolytic (75%) Sclerotic (15%) Mixed (5%) Periosteal (5%) Vertebral body compression fracture Spares disc space	Bone biopsy	Chemotherapy and/or radiotherapy	Potential for cure if diagnosed before extensive disease
Decreased Hct level Increased ESR Urinalysis: RBC Increased alkaline phosphatase, prostatic acid phosphatase Bone biopsy: may or may not show characteristics of primary tumor	Osteolytic: lung, kidney, breast, thyroid Osteoblastic: prostate, breast, colon, bronchial carcinoid Spares disc Bone scan: 85% symptomatic and asymptomatic areas Myelography: cord compression MR: most sensitive test	Bone biopsy if no primary neoplasm is identified	Palliative Radiotherapy Corticosteroids Decompressive laminectomy for spinal cord compression	Most common malignant lesion of the spine
Decreased Hct level Increased ESR Bone biopsy: metastasis	Rapid bone destruction, body or posterior elements Myelogram: complete block, varying densities, displaces cord MR: contrast agent increases sensitivity	Lesional biopsy	Radiotherapy Corticosteroids Decompressive laminectomy	Metastatic lesions
Increased cerebrospinal fluid protein	Posterior scalloping of vertebral bodies Uniform dilatation of neural foramen Myelogram: sharp, smooth outline of lesion MR: contrast agent increases sensitivity	Radiographs	Surgical removal	Neurofibromas Meningiomas
	Myelogram: fusiform enlargement MR +	Lesional biopsy	Surgical removal	Ependymomas Gliomas
Monosodium urate monohydrate crystals Increased serum uric acid	Vertebral erosions Marginal sclerosis	Monosodium urate monohydrate crystals	Colchicine NSAIDs Corticosteroids (acute) Uricosurics Xanthine oxidase inhibitors (chronic)	
Calcium pyrophosphate dihydrate crystals	Disc calcification and narrowing Osteophytes	Calcium pyrophosphate dihydrate crystals	NSAIDs Colchicine (33%)	Secondary forms: Hyperparathyroidism Hemochromatosis Hypothyroidism Wilson's disease Ochronosis
Increased urinary keratan sulfate	Platyspondyly Central beaking of vertebral bodies Increased kyphosis	Increased keratan sulfate	Bracing	Galactosamine-6-sulfate sulfatase deficiency Mild form of β-galactosidase deficiency

Appendix continued on following page

DISEASE ENTITY	NECK PAIN			ADDITIONAL HISTORY	PHYSICAL EXAMINATION
	Character	Location	Radiation		
Neurologic and Psychiatric Disorders					
Neuropathy (radicular)	Burning	Paraspinous	Arm Hand	Episodes of lancinating pain, increased at night Pain not increased with cough	Arm or hand weakness Absent biceps reflex
Psychogenic rheumatism (psychogenic)	Dull ache	Neck Shoulder		Listlessness Sleepiness Anorexia Constipation	Normal
Malingering (psychogenic)	Severe, constant	Entire neck and back	Nondermatomal	No relief with any therapy Job-related	Inconsistent abnormalities Nondermatomal sensory loss Pain with head compression
Referred Pain *Vascular (visceral referred)* Myocardial infarction	Crushing	Anterior neck	Arm—C8 distribution	Angina, hypertension increased with exertion	Diaphoresis Abnormal cardiac sounds
Carotid artery dissection	Sharp constant	Unilateral neck	Head	Smoking Fibromuscular dysplasia	Focal neurologic deficits Carotid bruits
Thoracic aortic dissection	Tearing	Chest	Lateral posterior neck	Older male Arteriosclerotic cardiovascular disease	Hypotension with proximal dissections
Biliary Tree Gallbladder Acute cholecystitis	Severe Colicky	Right paraspinous Right scapula	From right upper quadrant	Nausea Vomiting Female predominance 40 years of age	Fever Abdominal guarding
Hollow Viscus Esophagus diverticulum	Ache	Throat	Lateral neck	Dysphagia, regurgitation	Local neck mass
Esophageal cancer	Ache	Chest	Upper neck	Dysphagia Weight loss	Local neck mass
Miscellaneous Disorders Paget's disease (deep somatic, radicular)	Deep, boring	Affected bone	Shoulders	40 years of age and older Pain with walking Increasing skull size Deafness	Decreased spine motion Percussion tenderness with bone fracture Scalp veins Angioid streaks
Vertebral sarcoidosis (deep somatic)	Intermittent stabbing Dull	Involved bone	Shoulders	Black males Cough Dyspnea Anorexia Weight loss	Percussion tenderness Limitation of motion Skin rash Lymphadenopathy Abnormal breath sounds

NSAIDs = nonsteroidal anti-inflammatory drugs; MR = magnetic resonance; CT = computerized tomography; HNP = herniated nucleus pulposus; HLA = human leukocyte antigen; ESR = erythrocyte sedimentation rate; CSF = cerebrospinal fluid; WBC = white blood cell; Hct = hematocrit; RBC = red blood cell; CK = creatine kinase.

LABORATORY ABNORMALITIES	RADIOGRAPHS	DIAGNOSIS	THERAPY	COMMENTS
Abnormal nerve conduction electromyogram	Normal	Clinical exam Slowed nerve conduction	Analgesics Mexiletene	Carpal tunnel most common form
Normal	Normal	History	Antidepressants	
Normal	Normal	History Physical exam	Psychiatric	
Electrocardiogram: ischemia	Angiogram Stenosis	Angiogram Elevated CK	Reversal of stenosis	Cervical disc may mimic myocardial infarction
Normal	Arteriogram: dissection	Arteriogram	Heparin	Vertebral artery dissection has similar abnormalities affecting posterior circulation
Normal	Aortograph: dissection	Aortography	Control hypertension Surgical repair	
Increased WBC count Increased bilirubin Increased amylase level	Scintiscan: nonvisualization of gall bladder Sonography: stones	Scintiscan Sonography	Fluids Analgesics Antibiotics Nasogastric suction Surgery: perforation, abscess	Pain begins abruptly, subsides gradually Chronic cholecystitis and choledocholithiasis have similar clinical patterns Episodic pain
Normal	Barium eosphagram	Esophagram	Surgical removal	Esophagoscopy contraindicated: perforation
Decreased Hct level	Barium esophagram	Biopsy	Diversion: bypass procedure	Neck pain poor prognostic sign
Increased alkaline phosphatase, urinary hydroxyproline Bone biopsy: increased osteoclastic activity with mosaic and woven bone osteoblastic response	Lytic and sclerotic areas in vertebrae "Picture frame" appearance Enlarged "ivory" vertebrae Scintiscan: increased bone activity	Laboratory abnormalities Biopsy rarely	NSAIDs Calcitonin Bisphosphonates	Bone involvement Asymptomatic in many Slow virus infection
Increased calcium Increased alkaline phosphatase Increased gamma globulins Increased angiotensin converting enzyme Increased ESR Cutaneous anergy Biopsy: noncaseating granuloma	Bone lysis with marginal sclerosis Vertebral body collapse Paravertebral ossification Disc space narrowing	Bone biopsy	Corticosteroids Surgical decompression	Patients with extrathoracic disease have worse prognosis

DIFFERENTIAL DIAGNOSIS OF NECK PAIN

Evaluation	Neck Strain	Herniated Nucleus Pulposus	Instability	Degenerative Disc Disease	Myelopathy	Tumor	Spondylo-arthropathy	Infection	Visceral
Predominant pain (arm vs. neck)	Neck	Arm	Neck	Neck	Neck	Neck	Neck	Neck	Neck/Throat
Constitutional symptoms						+	+	+	+/−
Compression test		+							
Neurologic exam		+	+/−		+	+/−			+/−
Plain x-rays			+/−	+	+/−	+/−	+	+/−	
Lateral motion x-rays			+						
Bone scan				+/−		+	+	+	
CT scan		+		+/−	+	+		+	+
Myelogram		+			+				
MR scan		+		+	+	+	+	+	+
ESR						+		+	+/−
Serum chemistries						+			

+/− = positive in only some patients with the condition
CT = computerized tomography; MR = magnetic resonance; ESR = erythrocyte sedimentation rate

Note: Page numbers in *italics* indicate figures; those followed by t indicate tables.